New Frontiers in Immunology

New Frontiers in Immunology

Edited by Dallas Ford

STATES
ACADEMIC PRESS
www.statesacademicpress.com

States Academic Press,
109 South 5th Street,
Brooklyn, NY 11249, USA

Visit us on the World Wide Web at:
www.statesacademicpress.com

ISBN: 978-1-63989-375-1

Cataloging-in-Publication Data

New frontiers in immunology / edited by Dallas Ford.
p. cm.
Includes bibliographical references and index.
ISBN 978-1-63989-375-1
1. Immunology. 2. Serology. I. Ford, Dallas.

QR181 .N49 2022
616.079--dc23

Table of Contents

Preface

Immunology is a branch of medical sciences that is concerned with the study of the immune system. It is a system that protects the body from several infections through various lines of defense. Defects in the immune system can cause various diseases such as allergy, autoimmunity and cancer. The immune system is composed of structures and processes that have evolved to protect the body from diseases. There are two types of immunity, namely, innate immunity and adaptive immunity. Innate immunity is non-specific and the responses are same for all potential pathogens. It is the first line of defense. Adaptive immunity builds up memory of encountered infections to generate enhanced response specific to a foreign substance. Most of the topics introduced in this book cover new applications of immunology. It studies, analyses and upholds the pillars of this field and its utmost significance in modern times. The topics covered in this book offer the readers new insights in the field of immunology.

This book is a comprehensive compilation of works of different researchers from varied parts of the world. It includes valuable experiences of the researchers with the sole objective of providing the readers (learners) with a proper knowledge of the concerned field. This book will be beneficial in evoking inspiration and enhancing the knowledge of the interested readers.

In the end, I would like to extend my heartiest thanks to the authors who worked with great determination on their chapters. I also appreciate the publisher's support in the course of the book. I would also like to deeply acknowledge my family who stood by me as a source of inspiration during the project.

Editor

1

Asymmetry of cell division in CFSE-based lymphocyte proliferation analysis

Gennady Bocharov[1]*, Tatyana Luzyanina[2], Jovana Cupovic[3] and Burkhard Ludewig[3]

[1] Institute of Numerical Mathematics, Russian Academy of Sciences, Moscow, Russia
[2] Institute of Mathematical Problems in Biology, Russian Academy of Sciences, Pushchino, Russia
[3] Institute of Immunobiology, Kantonal Hospital St. Gallen, St. Gallen, Switzerland

Edited by:
Rob J. De Boer, Utrecht University, Netherlands

Reviewed by:
Vitaly V. Ganusov, University of Tennessee, USA
Ollivier Hyrien, University of Rochester, USA

***Correspondence:**
Gennady Bocharov, Institute of Numerical Mathematics, Russian Academy of Sciences, Gubkina Street 8, Moscow 119333, Russia
e-mail: bocharov@inm.ras.ru

Flow cytometry-based analysis of lymphocyte division using carboxyfluorescein succinimidyl ester (CFSE) dye dilution permits acquisition of data describing cellular proliferation and differentiation. For example, CFSE histogram data enable quantitative insight into cellular turnover rates by applying mathematical models and parameter estimation techniques. Several mathematical models have been developed using different types of deterministic or stochastic approaches. However, analysis of CFSE proliferation assays is based on the premise that the label is halved in the two daughter cells. Importantly, asymmetry of protein distribution in lymphocyte division is a basic biological feature of cell division with the degree of the asymmetry depending on various factors. Here, we review the recent literature on asymmetric lymphocyte division and CFSE-based lymphocyte proliferation analysis. We suggest that division- and label-structured mathematical models describing CFSE-based cell proliferation should take into account asymmetry and time-lag in cell proliferation. Utilization of improved modeling algorithms will permit straightforward quantification of essential parameters describing the performance of activated lymphocytes.

Keywords: T cells, CFSE assay, asymmetric division, mathematical modeling

INTRODUCTION

The ability of the immune system to protect the host organism against live-threatening infections and tumors directly depends on the reactivity of lymphocytes to antigenic stimulation, with a key role of clonal T cell responses (1). The perception of infections as a race between the invading pathogen and immunity suggests that it is the knowledge of the proliferation and death rates of T cells which provides a quantitative basis for assessing the quality of the host immunity (2). For almost 20 years, flow cytometry-based analysis of intracellular fluorescent dye distribution has been used to assess the proliferative performance and differentiation patterns of lymphocytes (3–5). Since the prototype dye for this analysis is CFSE, the assay is commonly referred to as CFSE dilution assay or – more simply – CFSE assay. A quantitative characterization of T cell turnover which can be elaborated from time series of CFSE histograms ranges from "static" measures such as precursor cell frequency or mean generation number, to "dynamic" parameters characterizing the cell cycle progression and apoptosis rates (6). However, estimation of turnover parameters requires formulation of mathematical models of cell growth which can take various forms and differ in their complexity depending on the parameters of interest and the richness of the available data [comprehensively reviewed by De Boer and Perelson (7)]. Importantly, current approaches to the analysis of CFSE proliferation data are based on the assumption that cell division is symmetric, i.e., the fluorescent label is halved in the two daughter cells (3, 5, 9). However, a random and uneven partition of mass between the sister cells is considered as an axiom in cell biology since many years (10). Although the detailed knowledge of the intracellular reactions which affect the turnover and intracellular heterogeneity of CFSE labeled proteins is currently limited (11), it is broadly accepted that CFSE binds indiscriminately to intracellular proteins and the fluorescence intensity of any single cell is roughly proportional to the total number of CFSE molecules bound to proteins within that cell (12). The latter study proposed a method for the analysis of CFSE-labeling experiments which also considered the possibility of an unequal division of CFSE molecules between the daughter cells.

The inequality of the mass (protein) distribution to the daughter cells directly suggests that CFSE labeled proteins are unequally partitioned between daughter cells. Indeed, recent studies describing T cell activation showed that asymmetric cell division can be an inherent part of T cell growth and differentiation (13–16). However, direct experimental evidence for asymmetric partition of CFSE between daughter cells is still missing. Nevertheless, the existing deterministic mathematical frameworks should be amended to facilitate a quantitative analysis of CFSE-based lymphocyte proliferation when asymmetry of cell division associated with unequal partition of CFSE labeled proteins between the two daughter cell results in a poor resolution of divisional clusters in CFSE histograms. Here, we briefly summarize recent findings describing asymmetric lymphocyte division and progress in the analysis of CFSE-based lymphocyte activation. Moreover, cell proliferation is not an instantaneous process and it takes a finite time for a cell to progress from the G1-phase of the cell cycle to the completion of the M-phase. The duration of the continuous progression is called a time-lag and in general, needs to be explicitly parameterized in the model equations. Finally, we suggest that mathematical models describing CFSE-based lymphocyte proliferation should consider both asymmetry in division and time-lag in proliferation.

ASYMMETRIC LYMPHOCYTE DIVISION

Symmetric or asymmetric cell divisions refer to the mode of cell division which results in two phenotypically identical- or different-daughter cells, respectively. The phenotypic features could be the cell size, cell surface receptors, intracellular components such as proteins (including those labeled with CFSE), transcription factors, or messenger RNA (17). Hence, these phenotypic differences provide the basis for the functional differences in the daughter cells, i.e., their cell fates.

Following encounter with their antigen displayed in the context of major histocompatibility complex molecules, naïve T lymphocytes go through well-orchestrated series of divisions generating different populations of cells that fulfill immediate effector functions or generate long-lived immunological memory. Two basic models explain the generation of such functionally distinct T cell phenotypes. According to the "one naïve cell – one fate" model, naïve lymphocytes are instructed to generate either effector or memory progeny (18). In this model, instruction of T cells, for example, is achieved through interaction with professional APCs (19). Hence, to preserve the instructing signal(s) received during activation and to maintain equality of the cells throughout division, T cells should divide in a symmetric fashion. The alternative model proposes asymmetric cell division as the mechanism that allows naïve T cells to give rise to two different daughter cells. These are referred to as proximal or distal daughter cell depending on their proximity to the APC. Such asymmetric T cell division represents a process that allows single cells to give rise to two, phenotypically and functionally different daughter cells, and thereby permits diversification of cell populations. In other words, one of the daughter cells inherits the potential to differentiate into full effector cell (proximal daughter), while the second daughter maintains the stemness of the mother cell. This principle feature of asymmetric cell division has also been described in developmental studies examining neurogenesis (20). Likewise, adaptation of adult tissues to changing environmental conditions such as the content of the gut requires rapid adaptation of one cell fraction while other cells maintain their high proliferative potential (21).

The processes involved in activation and differentiation of T cells, for example during infection have to swiftly generate cells with direct effector function to efficiently restrict viral replication (1). At the same time, some T cells should retain their ability to proliferate in order to prevent exhaustion of certain T cell subsets (22) and to facilitate generation of long-lived memory T cells (23). Indeed, Chang et al. (13) demonstrated that division of $CD8^+$ T cells specific for a viral peptide leads to the generation of daughter cells with different characteristics. CFSE-based assays revealed that asymmetry is established already during the first round of division and is dependent on the presence of the cognate antigen (13). Assessment of the protein content in the daughter cells generated during the first cell division showed that asymmetry established during mitosis is preserved throughout cytokinesis. Moreover, proximal and distal daughter cells exhibit different protein expression profiles and functional properties with proximal daughter cells exhibiting higher immediate protective capacity (13). The finding that proximal daughter cells exhibit higher CD8 co-receptor and LFA-1 expression facilitating formation of more frequent and longer lasting interactions with antigen presenting APCs (14) further emphasized that asymmetric division critically determines both T cell phenotype and function.

Asymmetric cell division is not only an important feature of $CD8^+$ T cell activation (13, 14), but also occurs during the activation and differentiation of $CD4^+$ T cells (13, 24) and B cells (25, 26). While naïve $CD8^+$ T cells require only one or only few encounters with APCs to proliferate and differentiate into effector cells, naïve $CD4^+$ T cells depend on multiple encounters in order to differentiate and to exhibit specialized effector functions (27). Hence, it is likely that $CD4^+$ T cells acquire their distinct phenotypes, e.g., Th1, Th2, or Th17, through multiple sequential asymmetric cell divisions. However, recent studies suggest that asymmetric cell division cannot be considered as the only mechanism that leads to the profound heterogeneity of T cell lineages (16). Thus, more research is required to resolve the contribution of sequential asymmetric T cell division to the generation of diverse T cell phenotypes. We suggest that a combination of CFSE-based T cell proliferation analysis with mathematical modeling may help – at least in part – to clarify this issue.

CURRENT MATHEMATICAL MODELS FOR CFSE-BASED LYMPHOCYTE PROLIFERATION ANALYSIS

Several mathematical models have been established for the analysis of CFSE-based proliferation assays (7, 9, 12, 28–32). The existing modeling frameworks can be subdivided on the basis of the major requirements for CFSE histogram data processing into two main categories (**Table 1**). The first group requires a decomposition of the CFSE histograms characterizing the distribution of cells with respect to the fluorescent dye into the distinct generations of cells. The procedure is based on fitting the CFSE histogram with a series of log-normal Gaussian distributions differing in their means and standard deviation and is implemented in commercially available standard software packages. Importantly, the assignment of distinct cell generations to CFSE clusters has remained an empiric process which depends heavily on initial labeling homogeneity, label degradation, cellular auto-fluorescence, and other factors including experimental skills of the researcher (33). As long as the division is symmetric (or almost symmetric) (**Figure 1A**), these factors can be tuned in a proper way to enable resolution of successive generations as distinct CFSE clusters (**Figure 1B**). Under these conditions a range of existing mathematical models can be tuned to estimate the turnover parameters of the stimulated lymphocyte population. The key features of the corresponding families of the models are outlined in **Table 1**, rows one to three. These models describe the population dynamics of cells which differ in the number of completed divisions and ignore the heterogeneity of the cells within a generation with respect to the CFSE content. The immunologically relevant issues that were addressed with the models of this group include regulatory effects of IL-2 on the T cell responses (34, 35), regulation of hematopoietic stem cells cycling (36), and kinetics of mouse erythroid progenitor cell differentiation (37).

Table 1 | Major features of mathematical models describing CFSE-based proliferation assays.

Cell proliferation model[1]	Input data	Estimated parameters	Mathematical approach[2]	Primary sources
A–B state model	Generation structure	Division entry-, apoptosis-rates, duration of division	DDE	Nordon et al. (6), Ganusov et al. (28)
G_0 model	Generation structure	Division entry-, apoptosis rates, duration of division	hPDE	Bernard et al. (51)
Random birth-death	Generation structure	Division-, apoptosis rates, progressor fraction	ODE, IE, branching processes	Ganusov et al. (28), Yates et al. (29), Lee et al. (30), Zilman et al. (31), Hyrien et al. (41), Veiga-Fernandes et al. (52), Revy et al. (53), Hawkins et al. (54)
Random birth-death, CFSE-structured	CFSE histograms	Division-, apoptosis-, CFSE decay rates	hPDE	Luzyanina et al. (38)
Random birth-death, generation-, CFSE-structured	CFSE histograms	Division-, apoptosis-, CFSE decay rates, auto-fluorescence	hPDE	Hasenauer et al. (40), Banks et al. (32)
Asymmetric division, G_0-model, generation-, CFSE-structured	CFSE histograms	Asymmetry, division-, apoptosis-, CFSE decay rates, time-lag of proliferation	hPDE	See text for details

[1]The following notations are used: "A–B state model" refers to the model of cell cycle in (55) in which the intermitotic period is composed of an A-state (major part of G1-phase) and a B-phase (conventional S, G2, and M phases); "G0 model" refers to the view of the cell cycle with two states (47), i.e., resting- (G0) and cycling-states (G1, S, G2, M). Conceptually, it is equivalent to the A–B state model. "Random birth-death" model refers to a discrete compartmental (generation structured) model of cycling cells (56). "Generation structured" refers to the mathematical model in which the cell population is decomposed into cohorts of cells which differ with respect to the number of completed division cycles; "CFSE-structured" represents the mathematical description of cell population in which the distribution (heterogeneity) of cells with respect to the fluorescence intensity is followed by considering the cell distribution function.

[2]DDE, delay differential equations; hPDE, hyperbolic partial differential equations; ODE, ordinary differential equations; IE, integral equations.

The second group of models which refer directly to the CFSE histograms seems to be more appropriate when the generational structure of the labeled population cannot be easily resolved (**Table 1**, rows four to five). The initially proposed model describes the evolution of the labeled cells distribution with respect to the CFSE level (38). Although this and similar models proved to be functional in estimating the proliferation- and death rates as functions of the structure variable directly from the histogram data (38, 39), the problem of translating the estimated functions into biologically meaningful parameters still requires the knowledge of the division structure of the lymphocyte population. A major breakthrough in the improvement of the distributed parameter models for the dynamics of heterogeneous CFSE labeled cell populations were recently proposed division- and label-structured mathematical models (32, 40). The major potential of this framework as an analytical tool is based upon the following features: (i) no need for CFSE histogram decomposition, (ii) characterization of cell growth in terms of generation dependent division- and death rates, (iii) an explicit form of the dependence of solution on the turnover parameters.

Another class of recently developed mathematical models which allow a direct fitting of the CFSE histograms is based on branching processes (12, 41). The approach allows for probabilistic characterization of cell activation, proliferation, and death from the CFSE dilution data and does not require the assumption about equality of CFSE division between the two daughter cells.

The first and the second group of models rely on the premise of symmetric cell division. However, tracing proliferation of other cell types such as cancer cells has been reported to be difficult (42) due to poorly resolved peaks of the different cell generations. Since cytokinesis is not perfect, it was suggested that the two daughter cells are unlikely to inherit exactly half of the CFSE fluorescence dye of the mother cell. An increase in the degree of the asymmetry of mass partition between daughter cells and hence disparate distribution of fluorescently labeled proteins should result in a poorer resolution of generational clusters as shown in **Figures 1C,D** for lower asymmetry and in **Figures 1E,F** for higher asymmetry. This in turn will lead to the generations overlap in CFSE histograms thus posing a limit to experimentalists' ability to resolve the individual generations using conventional decomposition methods.

MODELING ASYMMETRIC DIVISION OF CFSE LABELED T CELLS

We have been recently dealing with the analysis of the proliferative performance of monoclonal $CD8^+$ T cells recognizing an H2-Kb-binding epitope derived from the S protein of the mouse hepatitis virus (MHV). Clearance of MHV during acute infection is achieved through the combined action of type I interferons (43) and $CD8^+$ T cells (44). Moreover, $CD8^+$ T cells essentially contribute to control of the virus during persistent infection, for example in the central nervous system (45). We have initiated a project on the generation of avidity-tuned, antigen-specific T cells

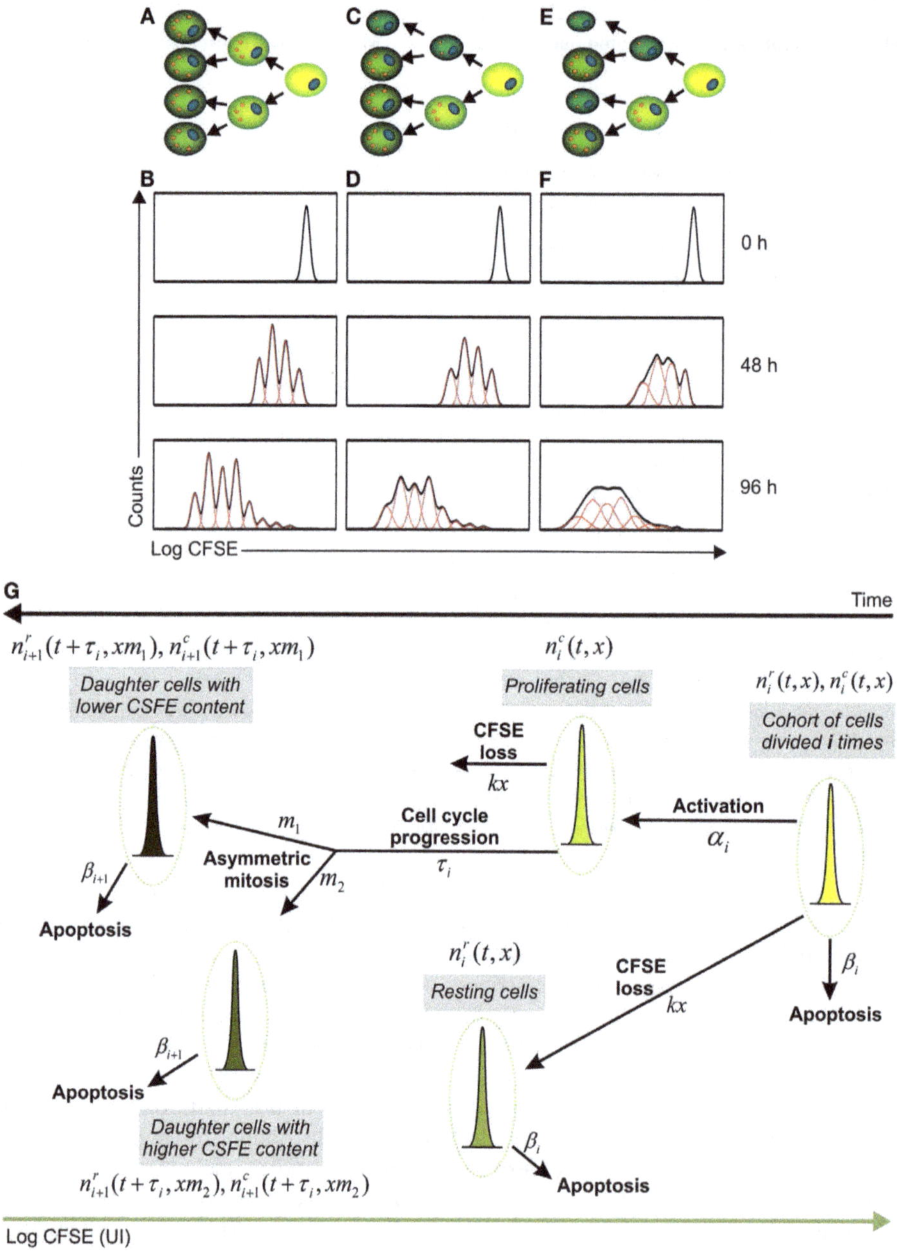

FIGURE 1 | Impact of asymmetry in T cell division impinges on fluorescent protein partition between daughter cells. **(A,B)** Symmetric cell division with equal distribution of the fluorescent dye between daughter cells **(A)** and modeled time course analysis of T cell proliferation as determined by flow cytometry [**(B)**, solid black lines]. Dashed red lines in **(B)** indicate the evolution of CFSE intensity of the cohorts (generations) of cell which differ in the number of completed divisions with the assumption of symmetric division. **(C,D)** Asymmetric cell division with "low" asymmetry **(C)** and modeled flow cytometric time course analysis of CFSE dilution [**(D)**, solid black lines] that corresponds to an asymmetry 46/54% [**(D)**, dashed red lines describe the CFSE distributions for cell cohorts differing in terms of the completed divisions]. **(E,F)** T cells dividing with "high" asymmetry **(E)** and corresponding model-generated flow cytometric CFSE dilution patterns [**(F)**, solid black lines] with asymmetry values of 42/58% describing the behavior of the T cells in this setting [**(F)**, dashed red lines describe the cell cohorts corresponding to different generations]. **(G)** Schematic representation of the structure of a mathematical approach which considers the division- and CFSE label-heterogeneity of proliferating cells as well as asymmetry and time of cell division. Some cells from the cohort of cells which completed "*i*" divisions are activated (α_i characterizes the activation rate) and progress through the cell cycle (τ_i stands for the duration of the progression through S-G_2-M phases), resulting to the generation of daughter cells which differ with respect to their CFSE content. Asymmetric mitosis refers to cell division which results into appearance of two phenotypically different daughter cells with a smaller and larger cell mass, respectively. These cells are characterized by an unequal amount of CFSE labeled proteins (m_1 and $m_2 = 1 - m_1$, describe the fractions of CFSE from the mother cell inherited by the two daughter cells). The natural decay of the CFSE fluorescence intensity is taken into account (*kx* – stands for an exponential decay of CFSE loss).

for adoptive transfer as an option to augment antiviral immune responses during chronic infection. To this end, MHV-specific T cell receptors (TCRs) were cloned and tested in retrogenic systems (46). *In vitro* re-stimulation of the CFSE labeled monoclonal $CD8^+$ T cells showed that CFSE dilution was characterized by broadly varying patterns from highly distinct peaks to poorly resolved generational clusters. We propose that an explicit consideration of the asymmetry in protein partition between the daughter cells facilitates a consistent mathematical description of CFSE histogram time series data (**Figure 1G**). The appropriate mathematical framework should describe the population of CFSE labeled T cells by the distribution of cells with respect to CFSE amount (unit of intensity, UI). The subpopulations differ in terms of completed rounds of division and are further distinguished in resting and proliferating states, with the respective notation and i standing for the generation (number of completed divisions), t – for time and x – for CFSE amount per cell. A conceptual scheme of the modeling approach is shown in **Figure 1G** suggesting that such a model can be naturally formulated as an extension of a generation- and division-structured population balance model with the cell cycle represented according to the G_0 model (47) and the division asymmetry explicitly taken into account.

Under conditions of symmetric $CD8^+$ T cell division with the difference of protein partition between the sister cells being equal to zero (i.e., every daughter cell inherits half of the fluorescently labeled proteins of the mother cell), the model should predict clearly distinct generations (**Figure 1B**, dashed red lines). If the division is "weakly" asymmetric, i.e., the protein partition between the sister cells is different, the width of the CFSE distribution of the successive generations should become broader (**Figure 1D**, dashed red lines). Further increase in the degree of the asymmetry would result in a substantial overlap of the distinct cell generations (**Figure 1F**, dashed red lines). Obviously, this type of behavior of T cells – and other cells such as tumor cells needs to be regarded as a cause of a poor resolution of the generations in CFSE histograms (**Figures 1D,F**, solid black lines) thus creating an obstacle on the application of standard CFSE analysis tools.

The fitting of mathematical models for asymmetric cell division as conceptualized in **Figure 1G** to the time series data provides a tool for the estimation of the cell physiology parameters such as: (i) the generation-specific activation and death rates (α_i, β_i); (ii) the duration of the division cycle characterized by the time-lag (τ_i); (iii) the division asymmetry factors ($m_1 + m_2 = 1$), specifying the fraction of proteins which is inherited by the first and the second daughter cells, respectively; and (iv) the natural decay of the CFSE fluorescence intensity of the labeled cells (parameterized as kx). Taken together, asymmetric cell division improves assessment of T cell performance parameters from CFSE-based proliferation assays, even under conditions of poorly separated peaks.

CONCLUDING REMARKS

It is considered that the regulation of cell expansion and differentiation can occur by modulating the degree of asymmetry of cell divisions (17). It has been clearly shown that T lymphocyte division in response to pathogen exhibits unequal partitioning of proteins that mediate signaling and cell fate determination (13). Hence, asymmetric T lymphocyte division provides an additional mechanism for generating functionally heterogeneous populations of $CD8^+$ T cells both in primary and memory adaptive immune responses (48). Since a precise mechanistic link between the quantitative differences in partitioning of specific proteins between daughter cells and the developmental path of antigen-specific T cells remains to be established (49), mathematical modeling is now a key "instrument" for understanding the regulation of individual cell fates (15, 16, 50).

The addition of asymmetric T cell division to the analysis of CFSE-based proliferation data fills important gaps as it: (i) allows one to estimate the proliferation parameters for asymmetrically dividing cells directly from CFSE histograms with poorly resolved generations peaks and (ii) introduces a quantitative parameter which characterizes the difference in the partition of the fluorescent proteins between daughter cells and can be directly estimated from the same CFSE dilution data. A further question in CFSE analyses open for examination is the interplay between experimental variability, biological variability, and model parsimony. We expect that new mathematical tools for the analysis of a fundamental property of cell division, i.e., the phenotypic identity or differences of the daughter cells known as asymmetry, will be developed and introduced into daily experimental work. Thereby, a better understanding of the diversity and mechanisms underlying activation and homeostasis of T cell responses will be achieved.

ACKNOWLEDGMENTS

This work has been supported by the Swiss National Science Foundation (130823 and 141918 to Burkhard Ludewig), the Vontobel Foundation (to Burkhard Ludewig), the Russian Foundation of Basic Research (11-01-00117a to Gennady Bocharov and Tatyana Luzyanina), and the Program of the Russian Academy of Sciences "Basic research for Medicine" (to Gennady Bocharov and Tatyana Luzyanina). We thank the reviewers and the editor for their insightful comments and the thorough work on our manuscript.

REFERENCES

1. Zinkernagel RM. Immunology taught by viruses. *Science* (1996) **271**:173–8. doi:10.1126/science.271.5246.173
2. Davenport MP, Belz GT, Ribeiro RM. The race between infection and immunity: how do pathogens set the pace? *Trends Immunol* (2009) **30**:61–6. doi:10.1016/j.it.2008.11.001
3. Lyons AB, Parish CR. Determination of lymphocyte division by flow cytometry. *J Immunol Methods* (1994) **171**:131–7. doi:10.1016/0022-1759(94)90236-4
4. Parish CR, Glidden MH, Quah BJ, Warren HS. Use of the intracellular fluorescent dye CFSE to monitor lymphocyte migration and proliferation. *Curr Protoc Immunol* (2009) **84**:4.9.1–4.9.13. doi:10.1002/0471142735.im0409s84
5. Quah BJ, Parish CR. New and improved methods for measuring lymphocyte proliferation in vitro and in vivo using CFSE-like fluorescent dyes. *J Immunol Methods* (2012) **379**:1–14. doi:10.1016/j.jim.2012.02.012
6. Nordon RE, Nakamura M, Ramirez C, Odell R. Analysis of growth kinetics by division tracking. *Immunol Cell Biol* (1999) **77**:523–9. doi:10.1046/j.1440-1711.1999.00869.x
7. De Boer RJ, Perelson AS. Quantifying T lymphocyte turnover. *J Theor Biol* (2013) **327**:45–87. doi:10.1016/j.jtbi.2012.12.025
8. Banks HT, Thompson WC. Mathematical models of dividing cell populations: application to CFSE data. *Math Model Nat Phenom* (2012) **7**:24–52. doi:10.1051/mmnp/20127504
9. Miao H, Jin X, Perelson AS, Wu H. Evaluation of multitype mathematical models for CFSE-labeling experiment data. *Bull Math Biol* (2012) **74**:300–26. doi:10.1007/s11538-011-9668-y

10. Sennerstam R. Partition of protein (mass) to sister cell pairs at mitosis: a re-evaluation. *J Cell Sci* (1988) **90**:301–6.
11. Banks HT, Choi A, Huffman T, Nardini J, Poag L, Thompson WC. Quantifying CFSE label decay in flow cytometry data. *Appl Math Lett* (2013) **26**:571–7. doi:10.1016/j.aml.2012.12.010
12. Hyrien O, Zand MS. A mixture model with dependent observations for the analysis of CFSE-labeling experiments. *J Am Stat Assoc* (2008) **103**:222–39. doi:10.1198/016214507000000194
13. Chang JT, Palanivel VR, Kinjyo I, Schambach F, Intlekofer AM, Banerjee A, et al. Asymmetric T lymphocyte division in the initiation of adaptive immune responses. *Science* (2007) **315**:1687–91. doi:10.1126/science.1139393
14. King CG, Koehli S, Hausmann B, Schmaler M, Zehn D, Palmer E. T cell affinity regulates asymmetric division, effector cell differentiation, and tissue pathology. *Immunity* (2012) **37**:709–20. doi:10.1016/j.immuni.2012.06.021
15. Buchholz VR, Flossdorf M, Hensel I, Kretschmer L, Weissbrich B, Graf P, et al. Disparate individual fates compose robust CD8+ T cell immunity. *Science* (2013) **340**:630–5. doi:10.1126/science.1235454
16. Gerlach C, Rohr JC, Perie L, van RN, van Heijst JW, Velds A, et al. Heterogeneous differentiation patterns of individual CD8+ T cells. *Science* (2013) **340**:635–9. doi:10.1126/science.1235487
17. Tajbakhsh S, Rocheteau P, Le R I. Asymmetric cell divisions and asymmetric cell fates. *Annu Rev Cell Dev Biol* (2009) **25**:671–99. doi:10.1146/annurev.cellbio.24.110707.175415
18. Ahmed R, Gray D. Immunological memory and protective immunity: understanding their relation. *Science* (1996) **272**:54–60. doi:10.1126/science.272.5258.54
19. Seder RA, Ahmed R. Similarities and differences in CD4+ and CD8+ effector and memory T cell generation. *Nat Immunol* (2003) **4**:835–42. doi:10.1038/ni969
20. Chenn A, McConnell SK. Cleavage orientation and the asymmetric inheritance of Notch1 immunoreactivity in mammalian neurogenesis. *Cell* (1995) **82**:631–41. doi:10.1016/0092-8674(95)90035-7
21. Edgar BA. Intestinal stem cells: no longer immortal but ever so clever. *EMBO J* (2012) **31**:2441–3. doi:10.1038/emboj.2012.133
22. Probst HC, Tschannen K, Gallimore A, Martinic M, Basler M, Dumrese T, et al. Immunodominance of an antiviral cytotoxic T cell response is shaped by the kinetics of viral protein expression. *J Immunol* (2003) **171**:5415–22.
23. Wherry EJ, Ahmed R. Memory CD8 T-cell differentiation during viral infection. *J Virol* (2004) **78**:5535–45. doi:10.1128/JVI.78.11.5535-5545.2004
24. Choi YS, Kageyama R, Eto D, Escobar TC, Johnston RJ, Monticelli L, et al. ICOS receptor instructs T follicular helper cell versus effector cell differentiation via induction of the transcriptional repressor Bcl6. *Immunity* (2011) **34**:932–46. doi:10.1016/j.immuni.2011.03.023
25. Barnett BE, Ciocca ML, Goenka R, Barnett LG, Wu J, Laufer TM, et al. Asymmetric B cell division in the germinal center reaction. *Science* (2012) **335**:342–4. doi:10.1126/science.1213495
26. Duffy KR, Wellard CJ, Markham JF, Zhou JH, Holmberg R, Hawkins ED, et al. Activation-induced B cell fates are selected by intracellular stochastic competition. *Science* (2012) **335**:338–41. doi:10.1126/science.1213230
27. Celli S, Garcia Z, Bousso P. CD4 T cells integrate signals delivered during successive DC encounters in vivo. *J Exp Med* (2005) **202**:1271–8. doi:10.1084/jem.20051018
28. Ganusov VV, Pilyugin SS, De Boer RJ, Murali-Krishna K, Ahmed R, Antia R. Quantifying cell turnover using CFSE data. *J Immunol Methods* (2005) **298**:183–200. doi:10.1016/j.jim.2005.01.011
29. Yates A, Chan C, Strid J, Moon S, Callard R, George AJ, et al. Reconstruction of cell population dynamics using CFSE. *BMC Bioinformatics* (2007) **8**(196):196. doi:10.1186/1471-2105-8-196
30. Lee HY, Hawkins E, Zand MS, Mosmann T, Wu H, Hodgkin PD, et al. Interpreting CFSE obtained division histories of B cells in vitro with Smith-Martin and cyton type models. *Bull Math Biol* (2009) **71**:1649–70. doi:10.1007/s11538-009-9418-6
31. Zilman A, Ganusov VV, Perelson AS. Stochastic models of lymphocyte proliferation and death. *PLoS ONE* (2010) **5**:e12775. doi:10.1371/journal.pone.0012775
32. Banks HT, Thompson WC, Peligero C, Giest S, Argilaguet J, Meyerhans A. A division-dependent compartmental model for computing cell numbers in CFSE-based lymphocyte proliferation assays. *Math Biosci Eng* (2012) **9**:699–736. doi:10.3934/mbe.2012.9.699
33. Ko KH, Odell R, Nordon RE. Analysis of cell differentiation by division tracking cytometry. *Cytometry A* (2007) **71**:773–82.
34. Deenick EK, Gett AV, Hodgkin PD. Stochastic model of T cell proliferation: a calculus revealing IL-2 regulation of precursor frequencies, cell cycle time, and survival. *J Immunol* (2003) **170**:4963–72.
35. Ganusov VV, Milutinovic D, De Boer RJ. IL-2 regulates expansion of CD4+ T cell populations by affecting cell death: insights from modeling CFSE data. *J Immunol* (2007) **179**:950–7.
36. Takizawa H, Regoes RR, Boddupalli CS, Bonhoeffer S, Manz MG. Dynamic variation in cycling of hematopoietic stem cells in steady state and inflammation. *J Exp Med* (2011) **208**:273–84. doi:10.1084/jem.20101643
37. Akbarian V, Wang W, Audet J. Measurement of generation-dependent proliferation rates and death rates during mouse erythroid progenitor cell differentiation. *Cytometry A* (2012) **81**:382–9. doi:10.1002/cyto.a.22031
38. Luzyanina T, Roose D, Schenkel T, Sester M, Ehl S, Meyerhans A, et al. Numerical modelling of label-structured cell population growth using CFSE distribution data. *Theor Biol Med Model* (2007) **4**(26):26. doi:10.1186/1742-4682-4-26
39. Banks HT, Sutton KL, Thompson WC, Bocharov G, Roose D, Schenkel T, et al. Estimation of cell proliferation dynamics using CFSE data. *Bull Math Biol* (2011) **73**:116–50. doi:10.1007/s11538-010-9524-5
40. Hasenauer J, Schittler D, Allgower F. Analysis and simulation of division- and label-structured population models: a new tool to analyze proliferation assays. *Bull Math Biol* (2012) **74**:2692–732. doi:10.1007/s11538-012-9774-5
41. Hyrien O, Chen R, Zand MS. An age-dependent branching process model for the analysis of CFSE-labeling experiments. *Biol Direct* (2010) **5**(41):41–5. doi:10.1186/1745-6150-5-41
42. Matera G, Lupi M, Ubezio P. Heterogeneous cell response to topotecan in a CFSE-based proliferation test. *Cytometry A* (2004) **62**:118–28. doi:10.1002/cyto.a.20097
43. Cervantes-Barragan L, Kalinke U, Zust R, Konig M, Reizis B, Lopez-Macias C, et al. Type I IFN-mediated protection of macrophages and dendritic cells secures control of murine coronavirus infection. *J Immunol* (2009) **182**:1099–106.
44. Perlman S, Netland J. Coronaviruses post-SARS: update on replication and pathogenesis. *Nat Rev Microbiol* (2009) **7**:439–50. doi:10.1038/nrmicro2147
45. Bergmann CC, Lane TE, Stohlman SA. Coronavirus infection of the central nervous system: host-virus stand-off. *Nat Rev Microbiol* (2006) **4**:121–32. doi:10.1038/nrmicro1343
46. Uckert W, Schumacher TN. TCR transgenes and transgene cassettes for TCR gene therapy: status in 2008. *Cancer Immunol Immunother* (2009) **58**:809–22. doi:10.1007/s00262-008-0649-4
47. Burns FJ, Tannock IF. On the existence of a G0-phase in the cell cycle. *Cell Tissue Kinet* (1970) **3**:321–34.
48. Ciocca ML, Barnett BE, Burkhardt JK, Chang JT, Reiner SL. Cutting edge: asymmetric memory T cell division in response to rechallenge. *J Immunol* (2012) **188**:4145–8. doi:10.4049/jimmunol.1200176
49. Oliaro J, Van Ham V, Sacirbegovic F, Pasam A, Bomzon Z, Pham K, et al. Asymmetric cell division of T cells upon antigen presentation uses multiple conserved mechanisms. *J Immunol* (2010) **185**:367–75. doi:10.4049/jimmunol.0903627
50. Buchholz VR, Graf P, Busch DH. The smallest unit: effector and memory CD8(+) T cell differentiation on the single cell level. *Front Immunol* (2013) **4**(31):31. doi:10.3389/fimmu.2013.00031
51. Bernard S, Pujo-Menjouet L, Mackey MC. Analysis of cell kinetics using a cell division marker: mathematical modeling of experimental data. *Biophys J* (2003) **84**:3414–24. doi:10.1016/S0006-3495(03)70063-0
52. Veiga-Fernandes H, Walter U, Bourgeois C, McLean A, Rocha B. Response of naive and memory CD8+ T cells to antigen stimulation in vivo. *Nat Immunol* (2000) **1**:47–53. doi:10.1038/76907
53. Revy P, Sospedra M, Barbour B, Trautmann A. Functional antigen-independent synapses formed between T cells and dendritic cells. *Nat Immunol* (2001) **2**:925–31. doi:10.1038/ni713

54. Hawkins ED, Turner ML, Dowling MR, van GC, Hodgkin PD. A model of immune regulation as a consequence of randomized lymphocyte division and death times. *Proc Natl Acad Sci U S A.* (2007) **104**:5032–7. doi:10.1073/pnas.0700026104
55. Smith JA, Martin L. Do cells cycle? *Proc Natl Acad Sci U S A* (1973) **70**:1263–7. doi:10.1073/pnas.70.4.1263
56. Kendall DG. On the role of variable generation time in the development of a stochastic birth process. *Biometrika* (1948) **35**:316–30. doi:10.2307/2332354

2

The protective and therapeutic function of small heat shock proteins in neurological diseases

Sara E. Brownell[1,2], Rachel A. Becker[1] and Lawrence Steinman[1]*

[1] Department of Neurology and Neurological Sciences, Stanford University, Stanford, CA, USA
[2] Department of Biology, Stanford University, Stanford, CA, USA

Edited by:
Willem Van Eden, Utrecht University, Netherlands

Reviewed by:
Ruurd Van Der Zee, Universiteit Utrecht, Netherlands
Harm Kampinga, University Medical Center Groningen, Netherlands
N. H. Lubsen, Radboud University Nijmegen, Netherlands

***Correspondence:**
Lawrence Steinman, Department of Neurology and Neurological Sciences, Beckman Center for Molecular Medicine, Campus Drive, Room B002, Stanford, CA 94305-5316, USA.
e-mail: steinman@stanford.edu

Historically, small heat shock proteins (sHSPs) have been extensively studied in the context of being intracellular molecular chaperones. However, recent studies looking at the role of sHSPs in neurological diseases have demonstrated a near universal upregulation of certain sHSPs in damaged and diseased brains. Initially, it was thought that sHSPs are pathological in these disease states because they are found in the areas of damage. However, transgenic overexpression and exogenous administration of sHSPs in various experimental disease paradigms have shown just the contrary – that sHSPs are protective, not pathological. This review examines sHSPs in neurological diseases and highlights the potential for using these neuroprotective sHSPs as novel therapeutics. It first addresses the endogenous expression of sHSPs in a variety of neurological disorders. Although many studies have examined the expression of sHSPs in neurological diseases, there are no review articles summarizing these data. Furthermore, it focuses on recent studies that have investigated the therapeutic potential of sHSPs for neurological diseases. Finally, it will explain what we think is the function of endogenous sHSPs in neurological diseases.

Keywords: small heat shock proteins, neuroinflammation, neurological diseases, HSPB1, HSPB5, sHSPs

OVERVIEW OF SMALL HEAT SHOCK PROTEINS

Small heat shock proteins (sHSPs) have molecular weights between 12 and 43 kDa, distinguishing them in size from large heat shock proteins (Ganea, 2001; Arrigo et al., 2007). There are 10 human sHSPs: HSPB1–HSPB10 (Kappé et al., 2003). They share common structural characteristics, including a highly conserved 90 amino acid long HSP20 domain, often referred to as the alpha-crystallin domain, and the capacity to form large dynamic oligomers (Poulain et al., 2010). sHSPs are intracellular molecular chaperones (Horwitz, 1992; Van Montfort et al., 2001). As chaperone proteins, sHSPs bind misfolded proteins and prevent them from aggregating. However, they are unable to actively re-fold the protein themselves due to their lack of ATPase activity. Instead, sHSPs sequester the misfolded proteins within the cell to prevent aggregation until a large heat shock protein can assist in refolding (Jakob et al., 1993).

Although sHSPs share both common structural and functional characteristics, they differ in tissue distribution and expression patterns (**Table 1**). HSPB1, HSPB5, HSPB6, HSPB7, and HSPB8 are ubiquitously expressed, and are constitutively present in the brain at low levels (Quraishe et al., 2008). HSPB4 is expressed in the lens of the eye, composing nearly 50% of the protein mass in the human lens (Andley, 2007). HSPB2 and HSPB3 are expressed in muscle and heart (Quraishe et al., 2008), although a recent study indicates that they also have some expression in the brain (Kirbach and Golenhofen, 2011). HSPB9 and HSPB10 are expressed in the testes (Quraishe et al., 2008). Notably, only three members of the sHSP family (HSPB1, HSPB5, and HSPB8) are induced in response to challenges such as heat (Morimoto and Santoro, 1998; Zhang et al., 2002), glucocorticoids (Nédellec et al., 2002), prostaglandins (Ito et al., 1997), and interferon-gamma (Oba et al., 2008), rendering them true sHSPs that are upregulated in response to cellular stress.

Biochemical, biophysical, and crystallography studies have elucidated the structure of HSPB5 and key residues important for quaternary structure and chaperone function (Bagnéris et al., 2009; Jehle et al., 2009, 2010, 2011). Naturally occurring mutations in conserved regions in several human sHSPs have functional consequences including myopathies (Vicart et al., 1998; Simon et al., 2007), cataracts (Litt et al., 1998), and Charcot Marie Tooth disease (Evgrafov et al., 2004; Ackerley et al., 2006). The crystal structures of sHSPs give us insights into understanding how some of these mutations have pathological consequences. However, mounting evidence over the past two decades suggests that sHSPs may not only play a role in maintaining a healthy body, but that they also have protective functions in disease or injury to the central nervous system (CNS; Sun and MacRae, 2005; Arrigo et al., 2007; Steinman, 2008). This insight has illuminated the possibility of using sHSPs as a novel class of neuroprotective agents.

ROLE OF ENDOGENOUS sHSPs IN NEUROLOGICAL DISEASES

Altered regulation of sHSPs has been seen in many neurodegenerative and neuroinflammatory diseases in both human and rodent brain tissue. A summary of published studies is shown in **Table 2.**

TAUOPATHIES: ALZHEIMER'S DISEASE AND PICK'S COMPLEX

Tauopathies are neurological diseases that involve abnormal aggregation of the tau protein in the brain (Ballatore et al., 2011). The healthy tau protein stabilizes microtubules, which are necessary

Table 1 | Endogenous expression of sHSPs in the brain.

sHSP	Alternate name	Constitutive expression in brain
BI	Hsp 27 (human)	Quraishe et al. (2008)
	Hsp 25 (mouse)	Armstrong et al. (2001), Kirbach and Golenhofen (2011)
B2	MKBP	Kirbach and Golenhofen (2011), limited expression
B3	–	Kirbach and Golenhofen (2011), limited expression
B4	Alpha-A crystallin (cryaa)	
B5	Alpha-B crystallin (cryab)	Quraishe et al. (2008), Kirbach and Golenhofen (2011), Dubin et al. (1989)
B6	Hsp 20	Quraishe et al. (2008), Kirbach and Golenhofen (2011)
B7	–	Quraishe et al. (2008), mRNA, not protein
B8	Hsp 22	Quraishe et al. (2008), Kirbach and Golenhofen (2011)
B9	–	
B10	–	

for the proper transportation of proteins and neurotransmitters along neuronal axons. However, when tau becomes defective and hyperphosphorylated, it can aggregate and forms neurofibrillary tangles (NFTs) that interfere with normal neuronal function and ultimately lead to cell death.

The most common tauopathy is Alzheimer's disease, a neurodegenerative disease characterized by NFTs and amyloid-rich plaques in the brain that ultimately results in cognitive decline and dementia (Ballard et al., 2011). The endogenous regulation of sHSPs in Alzheimer's disease has been well examined. HSPB1 levels are elevated in the cortex of Alzheimer's patients, with higher levels corresponding to increased severity and duration of dementia (Renkawek et al., 1994a). In fact, HSPB1 levels correlate significantly with levels of phosphorylated tau (Shimura et al., 2004; Björkdahl et al., 2008), suggesting that it may play a role in protecting the cell from the pathological effects of hyperphosphorylated tau.

HSPB5 is also upregulated in Alzheimer's disease (Iwaki et al., 1992; Shinohara et al., 1993; Renkawek et al., 1994b) and highly expressed in ballooned neurons (Lowe et al., 1992). Mao et al. (2001) found that HSPB5 is highly expressed in neurons in the vicinity of extracellular NFTs, but less so in classical senile plaques, diffuse plaques, and intracellular NFTs.

Three other sHSPs have been shown to be elevated in Alzheimer's disease: HSPB2, HSPB6, and HSPB8. Using immunohistochemistry, Wilhelmus et al. (2006b) found small, but not significant, elevations in HSPB2 and HSPB6 in Alzheimer brains. HSPB6 localizes to both diffuse and classic senile plaques, whereas HSPB2 was only present in the classic senile plaques. An additional study by Wilhelmus et al. (2006a) showed that HSPB8 is found in classic senile plaques from AD brains. These data collectively indicate that certain members of sHSPs are elevated in Alzheimer's disease, but it is unknown whether they are playing a protective or pathological role in the disease process and there are no studies to date that investigate the therapeutic potential of sHSPs in Alzheimer's disease.

Less common tauopathies include Pick's complex, which is now more commonly referred to as frontotemporal dementia (FTD; Weder et al., 2007). This collection of tauopathies includes frontotemporal lobar degeneration, corticobasal degeneration (CBD), progressive supranuclear palsy (PSP), and familial tauopathy FTD with parkinsonism linked to chromosome 17 (FTDP-17; Kertesz, 2003; Tolnay and Probst, 2003).

In many of these conditions, tau pathology is not limited to neurons and instead extends to glial cells such as astrocytes and oligodendrocytes (Komori, 1999). Both HSPB1 and HSPB5 were found to be elevated in brains of patients with olivary hypertrophy, a condition characterized by the enlargement of neurons and neuronal loss in response to a lesion in the dentatoolivary pathway. This can occur as a result of trauma, tumors, cerebrovascular disease, and PSP, a component of Pick's Complex (Hanihara et al., 1998). HSPB5 has been shown to be upregulated early in disease progression in neurons and later in astrocytes, but HSPB1 was only elevated in astrocytes later in the disease course (Fukushima et al., 2006). However, another study did not find upregulation of HSPB1 or HSPB5 in neurons, but rather that localization of these sHSPs is specific to glial cells in sporadic CBD and PSP and familial FTDP-17 (Dabir et al., 2004). The specificity to astrocytes was confirmed by a study that found elevated levels of HSPB1 in astrocytes in PSP and CBD (Schwarz et al., 2010). It is currently unknown why there are elevated levels of sHSPs in these diseases; there have been no published studies determining the effects that a loss of sHSP (i.e., using genetically deficient mice) or a gain of sHSP (i.e., exogenous administration or overexpression) would have on these diseases.

OTHER PROTEIN AGGREGATION DISEASES: PARKINSON'S AND ALS

Parkinson's disease is a neurodegenerative disease that is caused by the loss of dopamine-producing neurons in the substantia nigra. The decrease in dopamine is accompanied by an accumulation of alpha-synuclein protein, forming inclusions called Lewy bodies (Burn, 2006). Clinical features of Parkinson's disease are described by the acronym TRAP: tremor at rest, rigidity, akinesia or bradykinesia (loss of movement and slowness of movement, respectively), and postural instability (Jankovic, 2008).

HSPB1 and HSPB5 are upregulated in the cortex of Parkinson's disease patients (Renkawek et al., 1994a, 1999). These sHSPs are associated with an increased number of tangles in the hippocampus of these patients. Mouse data corroborated the human data, and showed similar elevations in both HSPB1 and HSPB5 using the transgenic Parkinson's model, alpha-SynA53T (Wang et al., 2008).

Amyotrophic lateral sclerosis (ALS), also known as Lou Gehrig's disease, is a neurodegenerative disease characterized by the progressive loss of motor neurons. ALS is associated with the formation of intraneuronal proteinaceous inclusions that are non-amyloid, many of which include hyperphosphorylated and ubiquitinated TAR DNA-binding protein 43 (TDP-43; Perry et al., 2010). Approximately 95% of ALS cases appear to be sporadic and the remaining 5% are familial (Traub et al., 2011). Twenty percent of the familial cases can be attributed to a mutation

Table 2 | Small heat shock protein expression in human and rodent models of neurological diseases.

Disease	sHSP	Model system	Regulation	
			Up	Down
Amyotrophic lateral sclerosis (ALS)	B1	Mouse	Vleminckx et al. (2002), Wang et al. (2008)	Maatkamp et al. (2004)
	B5	Mouse	Vleminckx et al. (2002), Wang et al. (2008)	–
		Human	Iwaki et al. (1992)	–
Alexander's disease	B1	Human	Head et al. (1993), Iwaki et al. (1993)	–
	B5	Human	Head et al. (1993), Iwaki et al. (1989), Iwaki et al. (1992), Iwaki et al. (1993)	–
Alzheimer's disease	B1	Human	Renkawek et al. (1994b), Björkdahl et al. (2008), Shinohara et al. (1993), Wilhelmus et al. (2006b)	–
	B2	Human	Wilhelmus et al. (2006b)	–
	B5	Human	Björkdahl et al. (2008), Shinohara et al. (1993), Lowe et al. (1992), Renkawek et al. (1994a), Iwaki et al. (1992), Wilhelmus et al. (2006b)	–
	B6	Human	Wilhelmus et al. (2006b)	–
	B8	Human	Wilhelmus et al. (2006a)	–
Epilepsy	B1	Human	Bidmon et al. (2004)	–
Huntington's disease	B5	Mouse	–	Zabel et al. (2002)
Multiple sclerosis	B1	Human	Aquino et al. (1997), Han et al. (2009)	–
	B5	Human	Sinclair et al. (2005), Bajramovic et al. (1997), Iwaki et al. (1992)	–
Other tauopathies	B1	Human	Fukushima et al. (2006), Dabir et al. (2004), Schwarz et al. (2010)	–
	B5	Human	Fukushima et al. (2006), Dabir et al. (2004), Lowe et al. (1992), Iwaki et al. (1992), Kato et al. (1992)	–
Parkinson's disease	B1	Human	Renkawek et al. (1994b), Renkawek et al. (1999)	–
		Mouse	Wang et al. (2008)	–
	B5	Human	Renkawek et al. (1999), Iwaki et al. (1992)	–
		Mouse	Wang et al. (2008)	–
Prion disease	B1	Mouse	Tortosa et al. (2008)	–
		Sheep	Vidal et al. (2009)	–
	B5	Human	Renkawek et al. (1992), Kato et al. (1992), Iwaki et al. (1992)	–
Spinocerebellar ataxias	B1	Human cell lines	Chang et al. (2005)	Tsai et al. (2005), Wen et al. (2003), Chang et al. (2005)
	B1	Mouse	Chang et al. (2005)	–
	B1	Human	Chang et al. (2005)	–
Stroke	B1	Rat	Imura et al. (1999)	–
	B5	Rat	Piao et al. (2005)	–
		Human	Minami et al. (2003), Lowe et al. (1992)	–

in the superoxide dismutase 1 (SOD1) enzyme (Rosen et al., 1993).

Iwaki et al. (1992) found that eight human ALS brains had higher immunoreactivity against HSPB5 compared with healthy brains. This result is corroborated in a study using the mutant SOD mouse model of familial ALS, in which SOD1^{G93A} mice exhibited higher levels of HSPB5 in the cytoplasm of reactive glial cells (Vleminckx et al., 2002). This study found that levels of HSPB1 were upregulated in mouse neurons and glial cells as well. However, the story is complicated by the fact that Maatkamp et al. (2004) found that protein levels of HSPB1 were downregulated just before the degeneration of motoneurons in the mutant SOD mouse model. They also found that mRNA levels of HSPB1 remained unchanged despite lower protein levels, highlighting the need for further studies to clarify what the role of sHSPs might be in ALS.

POLY-GLUTAMINE DISEASES: HUNTINGTON'S AND SPINOCEREBELLAR ATAXIAS

Poly-Q diseases are caused by genetic mutations that lead to a trinucleotide repeat of CAG, the triplet that encodes the amino acid glutamine. This increases the number of glutamines in the protein from as few as 20 to as many as 306 residues depending on the disease. These diseases are known as poly-Q diseases based on the one letter amino acid abbreviation of glutamine, and they include Huntington's disease (HD), dentatorubral-pallidoluysian atrophy (DRPLA), spinobulbar muscular atrophy (SBMA), and the spinocerebellar ataxias (SCAs; Paulson et al., 2000).

Huntington's disease is a neurodegenerative disease caused by a poly-glutamine expansion of the huntingtin (Htt) gene (Eidelberg and Surmeier, 2011). It typically appears during middle age and is characterized by chorea, or involuntary, explosive, fidgeting movements.

The SCA diseases are a group of neurodegenerative disorders that are also caused by an expanded poly-glutamine repeat. They manifest as a loss of gait and coordination difficulties. There are distinct subtypes, each caused by a specific mutation in a gene encoding an ataxin protein; around 30 different genes have been identified to date (Di Donato et al., 2001).

Contrary to findings in other protein aggregation diseases of the CNS, elevation of sHSPs have not been observed in the poly-Q diseases. One study using the R6/2 mouse model of HD found reduced levels of HSPB5 at the end of the disease course (Zabel et al., 2002). However, studies on HSPB1 in SCA found that HSPB1 is downregulated early in the disease (Wen et al., 2003; Chang et al., 2005; Tsai et al., 2005), but upregulated during later stages of the disease (Chang et al., 2005). These controversial data might uncover a dynamic property in the expression of sHSPs, indicating the need to examine sHSP expression at multiple time points in all diseases discussed above.

INFECTIOUS PROTEIN AGGREGATION DISEASE: PRIONS

Misfolded prions are infectious proteins that are responsible for the transmissible spongiform encephalopathies (Prusiner, 1998; DeArmond and Prusiner, 2003). These include bovine spongiform encephalopathy (BSE, commonly referred to as "mad cow disease") in cattle, scrapie in sheep, and Creutzfeldt–Jakob disease (CJD) in humans.

Small heat shock proteins are elevated in prion disease. HSPB1 is increased in scrapie in sheep (Vidal et al., 2009) and in a mouse model of BSE (Tortosa et al., 2008). Research on HSPB5 has been limited to humans; HSPB5 has been shown to be dramatically elevated in both glia and neurons from CJD brains (Kato et al., 1992; Renkawek et al., 1992). Given the similarities in protein aggregation between tauopathies and prions, it is likely that sHSPs are playing similar roles in both disease states.

LEUKODYSTROPHIES: ALEXANDER'S DISEASE

Alexander's disease is a rare genetic disease, a leukodystrophy with abnormal development of the myelin sheath, resulting from a mutation in the glial fibrillary acidic protein (GFAP; Messing et al., 2010). Alexander's disease is typified by the appearance of Rosenthal fibers – fibrous, eosinophilic deposits in the brain that are involved in the pathogenesis of the disease. It is a progressive, neurodegenerative disease that is usually fatal.

Both HSPB1 and HSPB5 are upregulated in Alexander's disease. Head et al. (1993) showed that both mRNA and protein levels of HSPB1 and HSPB5 were elevated in Rosenthal fibers in astrocytes taken from human patients, which was corroborated by Iwaki et al. (1989, 1993). Additionally, mouse models of Alexander's disease that lacked HSPB5 demonstrated greater mortality, indicating that the presence of alpha-B crystallin in the astrocytes is protective (Hagemann et al., 2009).

AUTOIMMUNE DISEASES: MULTIPLE SCLEROSIS

Multiple sclerosis (MS) is an autoimmune demyelinating disease of the CNS that manifests as lesions predominantly in the white matter (Rejdak et al., 2010). It is characterized by a T cell mediated attack on the myelin sheath surrounding the axons of neurons. Although protein aggregation has not been observed in MS, sHSPs are elevated and appear to play a protective role during the course of the disease.

van Noort et al. (1995) first identified that HSPB5 is involved in MS pathogenesis when they pinpointed this molecule as the most immunodominant myelin T cell antigen in this disease. These findings suggested that HSPB5 might be an autoantigen in MS and that immune cells attacked endogenous HSPB5 as part of the pathology of the disease. This theory was supported by data that showed high levels of HSPB5 in astrocytes and oligodendrocytes in MS lesions (Iwaki et al., 1992; Bajramovic et al., 1997). Although subsequent studies found that HSPB5 was the most abundant transcript in MS lesions (Chabas et al., 2001), attempts to induce experimental autoimmune encephalomyelitis (EAE), the predominant mouse model of MS, with HSPB5 as an antigen, rather than using a myelin antigen, were never successful (Verbeek et al., 2007). Further research indicated that although HSPB5 is upregulated during the course of the disease, its purpose is protective rather than pathological. A 2007 study conducted by Ousman et al. (2007) found that mice deficient in HSPB5 suffered from more severe EAE than wild type mice and that treatment with exogenous HSPB5 ameliorated EAE. This study demonstrated that the absence of HSPB5 results in a more pro-inflammatory state of immune cells and a higher level of immune cell infiltration into the brain. Furthermore, treatment of HSPB5 deficient EAE mice or WT EAE mice with exogenous HSPB5 decreases immune infiltration into the brain and shifts the phenotype of these immune cells to an anti-inflammatory state. Additional studies have validated the initial reports that HSPB5 is elevated in the MS brain (Sinclair et al., 2005) and that HSPB5 is elevated in the blood of MS patients (Rothbard et al., 2012).

HSPB1 has also been shown to be upregulated in MS. Using immunohistochemistry, HSPB1 was found to be elevated in astrocytes and oligodendrocytes in the plaques (Aquino et al., 1997). A recent study found elevated levels of HSPB1 circulating in the blood of MS patients, peaking during relapses (Ce et al., 2011).

ACUTE NEUROLOGICAL INSULT AND INFLAMMATION: STROKE AND EPILEPSY

Small heat shock proteins are not just upregulated in long-term, chronic diseases of the CNS; recent studies have shown an upregulation in acute inflammatory conditions such as stroke and epilepsy.

Stroke is the result of the lack of blood supply to the brain, leading to brain injury. The most common type is ischemic stroke, which is defined as a blocked blood vessel to the brain. Inflammatory mediators exacerbate acute stroke. These mediators infiltrate the injured area upon reperfusion. Several studies have been conducted that examine the expression of HSPB5 in human and mouse models of stroke. HSPB5 is found in ballooned neurons at the edge of cerebral infarcts (Lowe et al., 1992) and elevated in 68% of human stroke brains, specifically in the neurons (Minami et al., 2003). Studies using rodent models of cerebral ischemia indicate that HSPB5 is transiently upregulated in neurons a few hours after reperfusion and followed by gradual sustained increase in astrocytes (Piao et al., 2005). HSPB5 has also been shown to be elevated in human and mouse plasma post-stroke (Arac et al., 2011). Notably, HSPB1 is also upregulated in both rat and mouse models of ischemia (Imura et al., 1999) and overexpression of HSPB1 is neuroprotective in cerebral ischemia models (van der Weerd et al., 2010).

Epilepsy is a neurological disorder characterized by seizures. These are due to abnormal, excessive, or synchronous neuronal activity in the brain (Vezzani et al., 2011). Only one study has found that HSPB1 is elevated in epileptic human neocortex (Bidmon et al., 2004). Using immunohistochemistry, they found that HSPB1 was located in both astrocytes and the walls of blood vessels.

PROOF OF CONCEPT THERAPEUTIC EXPERIMENTS

Many studies have shown that endogenous sHSPs are elevated in neurological diseases, with some studies showing the lack of sHSPs leads to worse disease, implying a protective role for these molecules. This has led to the examination of these molecules as potential novel therapeutics with proof of concept experiments in mice using three routes of administration: transgenic overexpression, viral administration, and exogenous treatment (**Table 3**).

PARKINSON'S DISEASE AND ALS

Using a viral vector, HSPB1 has been shown to have a positive effect in an *in vitro* model of Parkinson's disease by protecting against alpha-synuclein induced cell death (Zourlidou et al., 2004). However, no studies have been conducted on the therapeutic effects of HSPB1 on *in vivo* models of PD.

Overexpression studies using transgenic mouse models of ALS have shown mixed results. One study demonstrates that overexpression of transgenic HSPB1 in the $SOD1^{G93A}$ mouse model of ALS by crossing $SOD1^{G93A}$ mice with HSPB1 overexpressing mice did not delay disease onset or decrease disease severity (Krishnan et al., 2008), despite the fact that HSPB1 overexpression was protective in acute motor neuron injury (Sharp et al., 2006). However, another study by Sharp et al. (2008) indicates that HSPB1 does have a positive effect early in the disease course in the same mouse model of ALS. They show that $SOD1^{G93A}$/HSP27 double transgenic mice had delayed decline in motor strength and increased survival of spinal motor neurons compared to $SOD1^{G93A}$ single transgenics during the early phase of disease. *In vitro* experiments using SOD1 mutant cells demonstrate that HSPB1 has an anti-apoptotic function (Patel et al., 2005). This suggests that HSPB1 does have an effect, but the levels in the overexpressing mouse may not be high enough to combat the chronic disease state. It may also suggest that the cellular upregulation of sHSPs represents only one part of the protective response and that the presence of sHSPs in the plasma may be a crucial factor in ameliorating disease.

ALEXANDER'S DISEASE

A study conducted by Hagemann et al. (2009) using a mouse model of Alexander's disease demonstrated that mice lacking HSPB5 exhibited increased mortality, but restoring HSPB5 specifically in astrocytes using a GFAP promoter reversed this effect. Additionally, transgenic overexpression of HSPB5 protects mice from death in a second model of Alexander's disease that typically causes the mice to die at one month of age (Hagemann et al., 2009).

MULTIPLE SCLEROSIS

Mice lacking HSPB5 were found to suffer from more severe disease in the experimental autoimmune encephalomyelitis (EAE) model of MS, and intravenous administration of exogenous HSPB5 ameliorated disease (Ousman et al., 2007). EAE mice treated with HSPB5 showed a dampened immune response, including less proliferation of immune cells and a lower production of pro-inflammatory cytokines (Ousman et al., 2007). Furthermore, we believe that this anti-inflammatory effect is based on HSPB5's ability to act as a chaperone extracellularly, binding pro-inflammatory molecules, including members of the acute phase, coagulation, and complement pathways (Rothbard et al., 2012). Additional experiments using other members of the sHSP family have indicated that all members are therapeutic in EAE and they act through anti-inflammatory effects (unpublished data). This further expands the research supporting the therapeutic possibilities of sHSPs in MS (Steinman, 2008).

STROKE

Transgenic mice that overexpress HSPB1 exhibited 30% smaller lesion sizes after undergoing a permanent MCAO model of stroke (van der Weerd et al., 2010). This corroborated previous work conducted in a cardiac ischemia model that showed that transgenic overexpression of HSPB1 was protective (Hollander et al., 2004). Virally administered HSPB1 was also shown to be protective in cerebral ischemia, although the mechanism was not clear (Badin et al., 2006). The researchers of that study speculated that the protective effect of HSPB1 might be due to its chaperone function. Finally, recent work has shown that HSPB5 is therapeutic when treating mouse models of stroke 12 h post-insult (Arac et al., 2011).

MECHANISMS OF sHSP NEUROPROTECTION

A substantial number of studies have indicated that endogenous sHSPs, particularly HSPB1 and HSPB5, are upregulated in CNS injury and disease. Studies investigating both sHSP deficiency and overexpression support the conclusion that these molecules are serving neuroprotective roles rather than pathological ones.

A caveat to the studies done using the HSPB5 deficient mice: these mice also lack the sHSP HSPB2. HSPB2 is not thought to be

Table 3 | Overexpression and exogenous administration of sHSPs.

Disease	sHSP	Model system	Treatment type	Therapeutic efficacy
ALS	B1	SOD1^{G93A} mouse model of ALS	Tg overexpression	No effect (Krishnan et al., 2008) Effective in early, but not late disease (Sharp et al., 2008)
		SOD1 mutant neuronal cell lines	Viral vector	Anti-apoptotic (Patel et al., 2005)
Alexander's disease	B5	GFAP^{Tg} and GFAP^{Tg}; GFAP$^{+/R236H}$ mouse models of Alexander's disease	Tg overexpression	Rescue of lethal phenotype in GFAP^{Tg}/cryab null mice by induction of Cryab under GFAP promoter (Hagemann et al., 2009)
Huntington's disease	B1	R6/2 mouse model of Huntington's disease	Tg overexpression	No effect (Zourlidou et al., 2007)
		COS-7 (monkey kidney) or SK-N-SH (human neuroblastoma) cells transfected with huntingtin exon 1 (httEx1) fused to EGFP	Cellular co-transfection	Prevented poly-Q mediated cell death, but did not prevent protein aggregation (Wyttenbach et al., 2002)
Multiple sclerosis	B5	EAE mouse model of MS	Exogenous administration	Decreased clinical score when administered at peak of disease (Ousman et al., 2007; Rothbard et al., 2012) Reduced apoptosis in CNS (Ousman et al., 2007)
Parkinson's disease	B1	Cells expressing alpha-synuclein	Viral vector	Anti-apoptotic (Zourlidou et al., 2004)
Ischemia/reperfusion (stroke)	B1	Permanent middle cerebral artery occlusion (MCAO) mouse model of cerebral ischemia	Tg overexpression	Reduced infarct size (van der Weerd et al., 2010)
			Viral vector	Reduced infarct size (Badin et al., 2006)
			Exogenous administration	Reduced infarct size (Arac et al., 2011)
Acute nerve injury	B1	Neonatal nerve injury, mouse	Tg overexpression	Rescues motor neurons 5–6 months following injury (Sharp et al., 2006)

inducible, so the levels of HSPB2 are typically not elevated in neurological diseases (for an exception see Wilhelmus et al., 2006b). Although we believe that the phenotype we see in HSPB5 deficient mice is due to the lack of HSPB5 alone, it is possible that the lack of HSPB2 is contributing to the effects observed in these mice. However, HSPB5/HSPB2 deficient mice have worse disease, which supports the idea that sHSPs are serving protective roles whether that is due to HSPB2 or HSPB5. An additional point to consider is whether the phenotype observed in HSPB5/HSPB2 deficient mice is due to the lack of the sHSPs or the altered levels of another molecule that is dependent on normal sHSP function. If isogenic mouse strains are not used as controls, then it is possible that polymorphisms in other genes could be the cause of differences seen between the WT and HSPB5/HSPB2 deficient mice.

How sHSPs are neuroprotective is still a subject of debate. It could be due to its molecular chaperone properties that prevent protein aggregation, in particular for protein aggregation diseases such as Alzheimer's or Parkinson's. However, sHSPs are also protective in non-aggregation diseases such as acute ischemia. Several studies have indicated an anti-apoptotic role for sHSPs, which might be the reason they are protective. HSPB5 and HSPB1 have been shown to be anti-apoptotic when overexpressed by either a transgene or virus (Akbar et al., 2003; Kalwy et al., 2003; Li et al., 2005). HSPB5 confers protection against apoptosis through the regulation of caspase-3, a proapoptotic factor (Shin et al., 2009) and has also been shown to sequester the p53 tumor suppressor, thus preventing apoptosis (Liu et al., 2007).

However, in light of recent studies that have indicated that sHSPs have an anti-inflammatory role (Ousman et al., 2007; Arac et al., 2011), the anti-apoptotic effects of sHSPs are unlikely to be the whole story. Although historically the brain was thought to be immune privileged, research over the past few decades has shown that the immune system is an important factor in many neurological diseases previously thought to be independent of the immune system, including Alzheimer's and stroke. Endogenously upregulated sHSPs may be playing dual roles as both anti-apoptotic and anti-inflammatory molecules in these diseases. In fact, Arac et al. (2011) investigated the relative effects of the deficiency of HSPB5 in the immune system and the brain post-stroke by doing a bone marrow chimera experiment. By irradiating WT and $HSPB5^{-/-}$ mice, depleting their immune systems, and reconstituting their immune systems with immune cells from either WT or HSPB5 deficient mice, they created four different types of mice: WT mice with WT immune cells, WT mice with $HSPB5^{-/-}$ immune cells, $HSPB5^{-/-}$ mice with WT immune cells, and $HSPB5^{-/-}$ mice with $HSPB5^{-/-}$ immune cells. After inducing stroke and comparing infarct size, they found that deficiencies of HSPB5 in either the brain or immune system alone increases infarct size and together result in a synergistic effect (Arac et al., 2011). They did not demonstrate any specificity to particular brain cells and this is an area of future investigation to fully understand the contribution of HSPB5 in the brain compared to the immune system.

The mechanism of action by which sHSPs are anti-inflammatory is currently under investigation. A study conducted by Rothbard et al. (2012) suggests that HSPB5 acts extracellularly as a molecular chaperone, binding acute inflammatory molecules. Notably, they showed that HSPB5 binding was temperature-dependent and binding increases with an increase in temperature, making HSPB5 more effective at sites of inflammation. Exactly how endogenous HSPB5 is released from cells is currently a matter of speculation. HSPB5 does not possess a signal sequence, so it is not secreted by the normal secretory pathway. However, a recent paper showed that HSPB5 could be released via exosomes (Gangalum et al., 2011). Additionally, if damage is occurring in the brain, it is very likely that cells are undergoing apoptosis or necrosis and releasing HSPB5 upon death. However, whether HSPB5 is released in a regulated manner through a specific process or leaked out of damaged or dying cells, the specific mechanism by which it becomes extracellular does not affect our interpretation that it can act as an extracellular chaperone.

Although we do see higher endogenous levels of sHSPs in neurological diseases, in particular at the site of damage, studies investigating the therapeutic effect of sHSPs using exogenous administration of sHSPs have been focused only on mouse models of MS and stroke. Using varying concentrations of human recombinant HSPB5 administered both intravenously and intraperitoneally, a therapeutic effect of HSPB5 has been shown in mouse models of MS (Ousman et al., 2007; unpublished data). This therapeutic effect has been demonstrated in EAE mice with different genetic backgrounds and we have seen a similar therapeutic effect from the administration of other members of the sHSP family (unpublished data). HSPB5 has also been shown to be therapeutic when administered intraperitoneally in a mouse model of stroke (Arac et al., 2011). We believe that it is likely that exogenous administration of HSPB5 will be therapeutic in other neurological diseases, but the experiments have yet to be done.

The vast literature indicating that endogenous sHSPs, particularly HSPB1 and HSPB5, are protective in neurological diseases opens the door for the possibility that these molecules could be developed as novel therapeutics. To date, therapeutic strategies utilizing sHSPs have been conducted solely in mice; however, the data generated from these experiments have provided the foundation to pursue this exciting avenue of therapy.

REFERENCES

Ackerley, S., James, P. A., Kalli, A., French, S., Davies, K. E., and Talbot, K. (2006). A mutation in the small heat-shock protein HSPB1 leading to distal hereditary motor neuronopathy disrupts neurofilament assembly and the axonal transport of specific cellular cargoes. *Hum. Mol. Genet.* 15, 347–354.

Akbar, M. T., Lundberg, A. M., Liu, K., Vidyadaran, S., Wells, K. E., Dolatshad, H., Wynn, S., Wells, D. J., Latchman, D. S., and de Belleroche, J. (2003). The neuroprotective effects of heat shock protein 27 overexpression in transgenic animals against kainate-induced seizures and hippocampal cell death. *J. Biol. Chem.* 278, 19956–19965.

Andley, U. P. (2007). Crystallins in the eye: function and pathology. *Prog. Retin. Eye Res.* 26, 78–98.

Aquino, D. A., Capello, E., Weisstein, J., Sanders, V., Lopez, C., Tourtellotte, W. W., Brosnan, C. F., Raine, C. S., and Norton, W. T. (1997). Multiple sclerosis: altered expression of 70- and 27-kDa heat shock proteins in lesions and myelin. *J. Neuropathol. Exp. Neurol.* 56, 664–672.

Arac, A., Brownell, S. E., Rothbard, J. B., Chen, C., Ko, R. M., Pereira, M. P., Albers, G. W., Steinman, L., and Steinberg, G. K. (2011). Systematic augmentation of alpha B crystallin, a novel immunomodulatory target, provides therapeutic benefit twelve hours post-stroke onset. *Proc. Natl. Acad. Sci. U.S.A.* 108, 13287–13292.

Armstrong, C. L., Krueger-Naug, A. M., Currie, R. W., and Hawkes, R. (2001). Constitutive expression of heat shock protein HSP25 in the central nervous system of the developing and adult mouse. *J. Comp. Neurol.* 434, 262–274.

Arrigo, A. P., Simon, S., Gibert, B., Kretz-Remy, C., Nivon, M., Czekalla, A., Guillet, D., Moulin, M., Diaz-Latoud, C., and Vicart, P. (2007). Hsp27 (HspB1) and alphaB-crystallin (HspB5) as therapeutic targets. *FEBS Lett.* 581, 3665–3674.

Badin, R. A., Lythgoe, M. F., van der Weerd, L., Thomas, D. L., Gadian, D. G., and Latchman, D. S. (2006). Neuroprotective effects of virally delivered HSPs in experimental stroke. *J. Cereb. Blood Flow Metab.* 26, 371–381.

Bagnéris, C., Bateman, O. A., Naylor, C. E., Cronin, N., Boelens, W. C., Keep, N. H., and Slingsby, C. (2009). Crystal structures of alpha-crystallin domain dimers of alphaB-crystallin and Hsp20. *J. Mol. Biol.* 392, 1242–1252.

Bajramovic, J. J., Lassmann, H., and van Noort, J. M. (1997). Expression of alphaB-crystallin in glia cells during lesional development in multiple sclerosis. *J. Neuroimmunol.* 78, 143–151.

Ballard, C., Gauthier, S., Corbett, A., Brayne, C., Aarsland, D., and Jones, E. (2011). Alzheimer's disease. *Lancet* 377, 1019–1031.

Ballatore, C., Brunden, K. R., Trojanowski, J. Q., Lee, V. M., Smith AB, I. I., and Huryn, D. M. (2011). Modulation of protein-protein interactions as a therapeutic strategy for the treatment of neurodegenerative tauopathies. *Curr. Top. Med. Chem.* 11, 317–330.

Bidmon, H. J., Görg, B., Palomero-Gallagher, N., Behne, F., Lahl, R., Pannek, H. W., Speckmann, E. J., and Zilles, K. (2004). Heat shock protein-27 is upregulated in the temporal cortex of patients with epilepsy. *Epilepsia* 45, 1549–1559.

Björkdahl, C., Sjögren, M. J., Zhou, X., Concha, H., Avila, J., Winblad, B., and Pei, J. J. (2008). Small heat shock proteins Hsp27 or alphaB-crystallin and the protein components of neurofibrillary tangles: tau and neurofilaments. *J. Neurosci. Res.* 86, 1343–1352.

Burn, D. J. (2006). Cortical Lewy body disease and Parkinson's disease dementia. *Curr. Opin. Neurol.* 19, 572–579.

Ce, P., Erkizan, O., and Gedizlioglu, M. (2011). Elevated HSP27 levels during attacks in patients with multiple sclerosis. *Acta Neurol. Scand.* 124, 317–320.

Chabas, D., Baranzini, S. E., Mitchell, D., Bernard, C. C., Rittling, S. R., Denhardt, D. T., Sobel, R. A., Lock, C., Karpuj, M., Pedotti, R., Heller, R., Oksenberg, J. R., and Steinman, L. (2001). The influence of the proinflammatory cytokine, osteopontin, on autoimmune demyelinating disease. *Science* 294, 1731–1735.

Chang, W. H., Cemal, C. K., Hsu, Y. H., Kuo, C. L., Nukina, N., Chang, M. H., Hu, H. T., Li, C., and Hsieh, M. (2005). Dynamic expression of Hsp27 in the presence of mutant ataxin-3. *Biochem. Biophys. Res. Commun.* 336, 258–267.

Dabir, D. V., Trojanowski, J. Q., Richter-Landsberg, C., Lee, V. M., and Forman, M. S. (2004). Expression of the small heat-shock protein alphaB-crystallin in tauopathies with glial pathology. *Am. J. Pathol.* 164, 155–166.

DeArmond, S. J., and Prusiner, S. B. (2003). Perspectives on prion biology, prion disease pathogenesis, and pharmacologic approaches to treatment. *Clin. Lab. Med.* 23, 1–41.

Di Donato, S., Gellera, C., and Mariotti, C. (2001). The complex clinical and genetic classification of inherited ataxias. II. Autosomal recessive ataxias. *Neurol. Sci.* 22, 219–228.

Dubin, R. A., Wawrousek, E. F., and Piatigorsky, J. (1989). Expression of the murine alpha B-crystallin gene is not restricted to the lens. *Mol. Cell. Biol.* 9, 1083–1091.

Eidelberg, D., and Surmeier, D. J. (2011). Brain networks in Huntington disease. *J. Clin. Invest.* 121, 484–492.

Evgrafov, O. V., Mersiyanova, I., Irobi, J., Van Den Bosch, L., Dierick, I., Leung, C. L., Schagina, O., Verpoorten, N., Van Impe, K., Fedotov, V., Dadali, E., Auer-Grumbach, M., Windpassinger, C., Wagner, K., Mitrovic, Z., Hilton-Jones, D., Talbot, K., Martin, J. J., Vasserman, N., Tverskaya, S., Polyakov, A., Liem, R. K., Gettemans, J., Robberecht, W., De Jonghe, P., and Timmerman, V. (2004). Mutant small heat-shock protein 27 causes axonal Charcot-Marie-tooth disease and distal hereditary motor neuropathy. *Nat. Genet.* 36, 602–606.

Fukushima, K., Mizuno, Y., Takatama, M., and Okamoto, K. (2006). Increased neuronal expression of alpha B-crystallin in human olivary hypertrophy. *Neuropathology* 26, 196–200.

Ganea, E. (2001). Chaperone-like activity of alpha-crystallin and other small heat shock proteins. *Curr. Protein Pept. Sci.* 2, 205–225.

Gangalum, R. K., Atanasov, I. C., Zhou, Z. H., and Bhat, S. P. (2011). AlphaB-crystallin is found in detergent-resistant membrane microdomains and is secreted via exosomes from human retinal pigment epithelial cells. *J. Biol. Chem.* 286, 3261–3269.

Hagemann, T. L., Boelens, W. C., Wawrousek, E. F., and Messing, A. (2009). Suppression of GFAP toxicity by alphaB-crystallin in mouse models of Alexander disease. *Hum. Mol. Genet.* 18, 1190–1199.

Han, M. H., Hwang, S. I., Roy, D. B., Lundgren, D. H., Price, J. V., Ousman, S. S., Fernald, G. H., Gerlitz, B., Robinson, W. H., Baranzini, S. E., Grinnell, B. W., Raine, C. S., Sobel, R. A., Han, D. K., and Steinman, L. (2009). Proteomic analysis of active multiple sclerosis lesions reveals therapeutic targets. *Nature* 451, 1076–1081.

Hanihara, T., Amano, N., Takahashi, T., Itoh, Y., and Yagishita, S. (1998). Hypertrophy of the inferior olivary nucleus in patients with progressive supranuclear palsy. *Eur. Neurol.* 39, 97–102.

Head, M. W., Corbin, E., and Goldman, J. E. (1993). Overexpression and abnormal modification of the stress proteins alpha B-crystallin and HSP27 in Alexander disease. *Am. J. Pathol.* 143, 1743–1753.

Hollander, J. M., Martin, J. L., Belke, D. D., Scott, B. T., Swanson, E., Krishnamoorthy, V., and Dillmann, W. H. (2004). Overexpression of wild-type heat shock protein 27 and a nonphosphorylatable heat shock protein 27 mutant protects against ischemia/reperfusion injury in a transgenic mouse model. *Circulation* 110, 3544–3552.

Horwitz, J. (1992). Alpha-crystallin can function as a molecular chaperone. *Proc. Natl. Acad. Sci. U.S.A.* 89, 10449–10453.

Imura, T., Shimohama, S., Sato, M., Nishikawa, H., Madono, K., Akaike, A., and Kimura, J. (1999). Differential expression of small heat shock proteins in reactive astrocytes after focal ischemia: possible role of beta-adrenergic receptor. *J. Neurosci.* 19, 9768–9779.

Ito, H., Okamoto, K., and Kato, K. (1997). Prostaglandins stimulate the stress-induced synthesis of hsp27 and alpha B crystallin. *J. Cell. Physiol.* 170, 255–262.

Iwaki, T., Iwaki, A., Tateishi, J., Sakaki, Y., and Goldman, J. E. (1993). Alpha B-crystallin and 27-kd heat shock protein are regulated by stress conditions in the central nervous system and accumulate in Rosenthal fibers. *Am. J. Pathol.* 143, 487–495.

Iwaki, T., Kume-Iwaki, A., Liem, R. K., and Goldman, J. E. (1989). Alpha B-crystallin is expressed in non-lenticular tissues and accumulates in Alexander's disease brain. *Cell* 57, 71–78.

Iwaki, T., Wisniewski, T., Iwaki, A., Corbin, E., Tomokane, N., Tateishi, J., and Goldman, J. E. (1992). Accumulation of alpha B-crystallin in central nervous system glia and neurons in pathologic conditions. *Am. J. Pathol.* 140, 345–356.

Jakob, U., Gaestel, M., Engel, K., and Buchner, J. (1993). Small heat shock proteins are molecular chaperones. *J. Biol. Chem.* 268, 1517–1520.

Jankovic, J. (2008). Parkinson's disease: clinical features and diagnosis. *J. Neurol. Neurosurg. Psychiatr.* 79, 368–376.

Jehle, S., Rajagopal, P., Bardiaux, B., Markovic, S., Kühne, R., Stout, J. R., Higman, V. A., Klevit, R. E., van Rossum, B. J., and Oschkinat, H. (2010). Solid-state NMR and SAXS studies provide a structural basis for the activation of alphaB-crystallin oligomers. *Nat. Struct. Mol. Biol.* 17, 1037–1042.

Jehle, S., van Rossum, B., Stout, J. R., Noguchi, S. M., Falber, K., Rehbein, K., Oschkinat, H., Klevit, R. E., and Rajagopal, P. (2009). alphaB-crystallin: a hybrid solid-state/solution-state NMR investigation reveals structural aspects of the heterogeneous oligomer. *J. Mol. Biol.* 385, 1481–1497.

Jehle, S., Vollmar, B. S., Bardiaux, B., Dove, K. K., Rajagopal, P., Gonen, T., Oschkinat, H., and Klevit, R. E. (2011). N-terminal domain of alphaB-crystallin provides a conformational switch for multimerization and structural heterogeneity. *Proc. Natl. Acad. Sci. U.S.A.* 108, 6409–6414.

Kalwy, S. A., Akbar, M. T., Coffin, R. S., de Belleroche, J., and Latchman, D. S. (2003). Heat shock protein 27 delivered via a herpes simplex virus vector can protect neurons of the hippocampus against kainic-acid-induced cell loss. *Brain Res. Mol. Brain Res.* 111, 91–103.

Kappé, G., Franck, E., Verschuure, P., Boelens, W. C., Leunissen, J. A., and de Jong, W. W. (2003). The human genome encodes 10 alpha-crystallin-related small heat shock proteins: HspB1-10. *Cell Stress Chaperones* 8, 53–61.

Kato, S., Hirano, A., Umahara, T., Kato, M., Herz, F., and Ohama, E. (1992). Comparative immunohistochemical study on the expression of alpha B crystallin, ubiquitin and stress-response protein 27 in ballooned neurons in various disorders. *Neuropathol. Appl. Neurobiol.* 18, 335–340.

Kertesz, A. (2003). Pick complex: an integrative approach to frontotemporal dementia: primary progressive aphasia, corticobasal degeneration, and progressive supranuclear palsy. *Neurologist* 9, 311–317.

Kirbach, B. B., and Golenhofen, N. (2011). Differential expression and induction of small heat shock proteins in rat brain and cultured hippocampal neurons. *J. Neurosci. Res.* 89, 162–175.

Komori, T. (1999). Tau-positive glial inclusions in progressive supranuclear palsy, corticobasal degeneration and Pick's disease. *Brain Pathol.* 9, 663–679.

Krishnan, J., Vannuvel, K., Andries, M., Waelkens, E., Robberecht, W., and Van Den Bosch, L. (2008). Over-expression of Hsp27 does not influence disease in the mutant SOD1 (G93A) mouse model of amyotrophic lateral sclerosis. *J. Neurochem.* 106, 2170–2183.

Li, D. W., Liu, J. P., Mao, Y. W., Xiang, H., Wang, J., Ma, W. Y., Dong, Z., Pike, H. M., Brown, R. E., and Reed, J. C. (2005). Calcium-activated RAF/MEK/ERK signaling pathway mediates p53-dependent apoptosis and is abrogated by alpha B-crystallin through inhibition of RAS activation. *Mol. Biol. Cell* 16, 4437–4453.

Litt, M., Kramer, P., LaMorticella, D. M., Murphey, W., Lovrien, E. W., and Weleber, R. G. (1998). Autosomal dominant congenital cataract associated with a missense mutation in the human alpha crystallin gene CRYAA. *Hum. Mol. Genet.* 7, 471–474.

Liu, S., Li, J., Tao, Y., and Xiao, X. (2007). Small heat shock protein alphaB-crystallin binds to p53 to sequester its translocation to mitochondria during hydrogen peroxide-induced apoptosis. *Biochem. Biophys. Res. Commun.* 354, 109–114.

Lowe, J., Errington, D. R., Lennox, G., Pike, I., Spendlove, I., Landon, M., and Mayer, R. J. (1992). Ballooned neurons in several neurodegenerative diseases and stroke contain alpha B crystallin. *Neuropathol. Appl. Neurobiol.* 18, 341–350.

Maatkamp, A., Vlug, A., Haasdijk, E., Troost, D., French, P. J., and Jaarsma, D. (2004). Decrease of Hsp25 protein expression precedes degeneration of motoneurons in

ALS-SOD1 mice. *Eur. J. Neurosci.* 20, 14–28.

Mao, J. J., Katayama, S., Watanabe, C., Harada, Y., Noda, K., Yamamura, Y., and Nakamura, S. (2001). The relationship between alphaB-crystallin and neurofibrillary tangles in Alzheimer's disease. *Neuropathol. Appl. Neurobiol.* 27, 180–188.

Messing, A., Daniels, C. M., and Hagemann, T. L. (2010). Strategies for treatment in Alexander disease. *Neurotherapeutics* 7, 507–515.

Minami, M., Mizutani, T., Kawanishi, R., Suzuki, Y., and Mori, H. (2003). Neuronal expression of alphaB crystallin in cerebral infarction. *Acta Neuropathol.* 105, 549–554.

Morimoto, R. I., and Santoro, M. G. (1998). Stress-inducible responses and heat shock proteins: new pharmacologic targets for cytoprotection. *Nat. Biotechnol.* 16, 833–838.

Nédellec, P., Edling, Y., Perret, E., Fardeau, M., and Vicart, P. (2002). Glucocorticoid treatment induces expression of small heat shock proteins in human satellite cell populations: consequences for a desmin-related myopathy involving the R120G alpha B-crystallin mutation. *Neuromuscul. Disord.* 12, 457–465.

Oba, M., Yano, S., Shuto, T., Suico, M. A., Eguma, A., and Kai, H. (2008). IFN-gamma down-regulates Hsp27 and enhances hyperthermia-induced tumor cell death in vitro and tumor suppression in vivo. *Int. J. Oncol.* 32, 1317–1324.

Ousman, S. S., Tomooka, B. H., van Noort, J. M., Wawrousek, E. F., O'Connor, K. C., Hafler, D. A., Sobel, R. A., Robinson, W. H., and Steinman, L. (2007). Protective and therapeutic role for alphaB-crystallin in autoimmune demyelination. *Nature* 448, 474–479.

Patel, Y. J., Payne Smith, M. D., de Belleroche, J., and Latchman, D. S. (2005). Hsp27 and Hsp70 administered in combination have a potent protective effect against FALS-associated SOD1-mutant-induced cell death in mammalian neuronal cells. *Brain Res. Mol. Brain Res.* 134, 256–274.

Paulson, H. L., Bonini, N. M., and Roth, K. A. (2000). Polyglutamine disease and neuronal cell death. *Proc. Natl. Acad. Sci. U.S.A.* 97, 12957–12958.

Perry, J., Shin, D. S., Pratt, A. J., and Getzoff, E. D. (2010). Amyotrophic lateral sclerosis. *Adv. Exp. Med. Biol.* 685, 9–20.

Piao, C. S., Kim, S. W., Kim, J. B., and Lee, J. K. (2005). Co-induction of alphaB-crystallin and MAPKAPK-2 in astrocytes in the penumbra after transient focal cerebral ischemia. *Exp. Brain Res.* 163, 421–429.

Poulain, P., Gelly, J. C., and Flatters, D. (2010). Detection and architecture of small heat shock protein monomers. *PLoS ONE* 5, e9990. doi:10.1371/journal.pone.0009990

Prusiner, S. B. (1998). Prions. *Proc. Natl. Acad. Sci. U.S.A.* 95, 13363–13383.

Quraishe, S., Asuni, A., Boelens, W. C., O'Connor, V., and Wyttenbach, A. (2008). Expression of the small heat shock protein family in the mouse CNS: differential anatomical and biochemical compartmentalization. *Neuroscience* 153, 483–491.

Rejdak, K., Jackson, S., and Giovannoni, G. (2010). Multiple sclerosis: a practical overview for clinicians. *Br. Med. Bull.* 95, 79–104.

Renkawek, K., Bosman, G. J., and de Jong, W. W. (1994a). Expression of small heat-shock protein hsp 27 in reactive gliosis in Alzheimer disease and other types of dementia. *Acta Neuropathol.* 87, 511–519.

Renkawek, K., Voorter, C. E., Bosman, G. J., van Workum, F. P., and de Jong, W. W. (1994b). Expression of alpha B-crystallin in Alzheimer's disease. *Acta Neuropathol.* 87, 155–160.

Renkawek, K., de Jong, W. W., Merck, K. B., Frenken, C. W., van Workum, F. P., and Bosman, G. J. (1992). alpha B-crystallin is present in reactive glia in Creutzfeldt-Jakob disease. *Acta Neuropathol.* 83, 324–327.

Renkawek, K., Stege, G. J., and Bosman, G. J. (1999). Dementia, gliosis and expression of the small heat shock proteins hsp27 and alpha B-crystallin in Parkinson's disease. *Neuroreport* 10, 2273–2276.

Rosen, D. R., Siddique, T., Patterson, D., Figlewicz, D. A., Sapp, P., Hentati, A., Donaldson, D., Goto, J., O'Regan, J. P., Deng, H. X., Rahmani, Z., Krizus, A., McKenna-Yasek, D., Cayabyab, A., Gaston, S. M., Berger, R., Tanzi, R. E., Halperin, J. J., Herzfeldt, B., den Bergh R, V., Hung, W.-Y., Bird, T., Deng, G., Mulder, D. W., Smyth, C., Laing, N. G., Soriano, E., Pericak–Vance, M. A., Haines, J., Rouleau, G. A., Gusella, J. S., Horvitz, H. R., and Brown, R. H. Jr. (1993). Mutations in Cu/Zn superoxide dismutase gene are associated with familial amyotrophic lateral sclerosis. *Nature* 362, 59–62.

Rothbard, J. B., Kurnellas, M. P., Brownell, S., Adams, C. M., Su, L., Axtell, R. C., Chen, R., Fathman, C. G., Robinson, W. H., and Steinman, L. (2012). Therapeutic effects of systemic administration of chaperone αB-crystallin associated with binding proinflammatory plasma proteins. *J. Biol. Chem.* 287, 9708–9721.

Schwarz, L., Vollmer, G., and Richter-Landsberg, C. (2010). The small heat shock protein HSP25/27 (HspB1) is abundant in cultured astrocytes and associated with astrocytic pathology in progressive supranuclear palsy and corticobasal degeneration. *Int. J. Cell Biol.* 2010, 717520.

Sharp, P., Krishnan, M., Pullar, O., Navarrete, R., Wells, D., and de Belleroche, J. (2006). Heat shock protein 27 rescues motor neurons following nerve injury and preserves muscle function. *Exp. Neurol.* 198, 511–518.

Sharp, P. S., Akbar, M. T., Bouri, S., Senda, A., Joshi, K., Chen, H. J., Latchman, D. S., Wells, D. J., and de Belleroche, J. (2008). Protective effects of heat shock protein 27 in a model of ALS occur in the early stages of disease progression. *Neurobiol. Dis.* 30, 42–55.

Shimura, H., Miura-Shimura, Y., and Kosik, K. S. (2004). Binding of tau to heat shock protein 27 leads to decreased concentration of hyperphosphorylated tau and enhanced cell survival. *J. Biol. Chem.* 279, 17957–17962.

Shin, J. H., Kim, S. W., Lim, C. M., Jeong, J. Y., Piao, C. S., and Lee, J. K. (2009). alphaB-crystallin suppresses oxidative stress-induced astrocyte apoptosis by inhibiting caspase-3 activation. *Neurosci. Res.* 64, 355–361.

Shinohara, H., Inaguma, Y., Goto, S., Inagaki, T., and Kato, K. (1993). Alpha B crystallin and HSP28 are enhanced in the cerebral cortex of patients with Alzheimer's disease. *J. Neurol. Sci.* 119, 203–208.

Simon, S., Fontaine, J. M., Martin, J. L., Sun, X., Hoppe, A. D., Welsh, M. J., Benndorf, R., and Vicart, P. (2007). Myopathy-associated alphaB-crystallin mutants: abnormal phosphorylation, intracellular location, and interactions with other small heat shock proteins. *J. Biol. Chem.* 282, 34276–34287.

Sinclair, C., Mirakhur, M., Kirk, J., Farrell, M., and McQuaid, S. (2005). Up-regulation of osteopontin and alpha beta-crystallin in the normal-appearing white matter of multiple sclerosis: an immunohistochemical study utilizing tissue microarrays. *Neuropathol. Appl. Neurobiol.* 31, 292–303.

Steinman, L. (2008). New targets for treatment of multiple sclerosis. *J. Neurol. Sci.* 274, 1–4.

Sun, Y., and MacRae, T. H. (2005). The small heat shock proteins and their role in human disease. *FEBS J.* 272, 2613–2627.

Tolnay, M., and Probst, A. (2003). The neuropathological spectrum of neurodegenerative tauopathies. *IUBMB Life* 55, 299–305.

Tortosa, R., Vidal, E., Costa, C., Alamillo, E., Torres, J. M., Ferrer, I., and Pumarola, M. (2008). Stress response in the central nervous system of a transgenic mouse model of bovine spongiform encephalopathy. *Vet. J.* 178, 126–129.

Traub, R., Mitsumoto, H., and Rowland, L. P. (2011). Research advances in amyotrophic lateral sclerosis, 2009 to 2010. *Curr. Neurol. Neurosci. Rep.* 11, 67–77.

Tsai, H. F., Lin, S. J., Li, C., and Hsieh, M. (2005). Decreased expression of Hsp27 and Hsp70 in transformed lymphoblastoid cells from patients with spinocerebellar ataxia type 7. *Biochem. Biophys. Res. Commun.* 334, 1279–1286.

van der Weerd, L., Tariq Akbar, M., Aron Badin, R., Valentim, L. M., Thomas, D. L., Wells, D. J., Latchman, D. S., Gadian, D. G., Lythgoe, M. F., and de Belleroche, J. S. (2010). Overexpression of heat shock protein 27 reduces cortical damage after cerebral ischemia. *J. Cereb. Blood Flow Metab.* 30, 849–856.

Van Montfort, R., Slingsby, C., and Vierling, E. (2001). Structure and function of the small heat shock protein/alpha-crystallin family of molecular chaperones. *Adv. Protein Chem.* 59, 105–156.

van Noort, J. M., van Sechel, A. C., Bajramovic, J. J., el Ouagmiri, M., Polman, C. H., Lassmann, H., and Ravid, R. (1995). The small heat-shock protein alpha B-crystallin as candidate autoantigen in multiple sclerosis. *Nature* 375, 798–801.

Verbeek, R., van Dongen, H., Wawrousek, E. F., Amor, S., and van Noort, J. M. (2007). Induction of EAE by T cells specific for alpha B-crystallin depends on prior viral infection in the CNS. *Int. Immunol.* 19, 277–285.

Vezzani, A., French, J., Bartfai, T., and Baram, T. Z. (2011). The role of inflammation in epilepsy. *Nat. Rev. Neurol.* 7, 31–40.

Vicart, P., Caron, A., Guicheney, P., Li, Z., Prévost, M. C., Faure, A., Chateau, D., Chapon, F., Tomé, F., Dupret, J. M., Paulin, D., and Fardeau, M. (1998). A missense mutation in the alphaB-crystallin chaperone gene causes a desmin-related myopathy. *Nat. Genet.* 20, 92–95.

Vidal, E., Acín, C., Foradada, L., Monzón, M., Márquez, M., Monleón, E., Pumarola, M., Badiola, J. J., and Bolea, R. (2009). Immunohistochemical characterisation of classical scrapie neuropathology in sheep. *J. Comp. Pathol.* 141, 135–146.

Vleminckx, V., Van Damme, P., Goffin, K., Delye, H., Van Den Bosch, L., and Robberecht, W. (2002). Upregulation of HSP27 in a transgenic model of ALS. *J. Neuropathol. Exp. Neurol.* 61, 968–974.

Wang, J., Martin, E., Gonzales, V., Borchelt, D. R., and Lee, M. K. (2008). Differential regulation of small heat shock proteins in transgenic mouse models of neurodegenerative diseases. *Neurobiol. Aging* 29, 586–597.

Weder, N. D., Aziz, R., Wilkins, K., and Tampi, R. R. (2007). Frontotemporal dementias: a review. *Ann. Gen. Psychiatry* 6, 15.

Wen, F. C., Li, Y. H., Tsai, H. F., Lin, C. H., Li, C., Liu, C. S., Lii, C. K., Nukina, N., and Hsieh, M. (2003). Down-regulation of heat shock protein 27 in neuronal cells and non-neuronal cells expressing mutant ataxin-3. *FEBS Lett.* 546, 307–314.

Wilhelmus, M. M., Boelens, W. C., Otte-Höller, I., Kamps, B., Kusters, B., Maat-Schieman, M. L., de Waal, R. M., and Verbeek, M. M. (2006a). Small heat shock protein HspB8: its distribution in Alzheimer's disease brains and its inhibition of amyloid-beta protein aggregation and cerebrovascular amyloid-beta toxicity. *Acta Neuropathol.* 111, 139–149.

Wilhelmus, M. M., Otte-Höller, I., Wesseling, P., de Waal, R. M., Boelens, W. C., and Verbeek, M. M. (2006b). Specific association of small heat shock proteins with the pathological hallmarks of Alzheimer's disease brains. *Neuropathol. Appl. Neurobiol.* 32, 119–130.

Wyttenbach, A., Sauvageot, O., Carmichael, J., Diaz-Latoud, C., Arrigo, A. P., and Rubinsztein, D. C. (2002). Heat shock protein 27 prevents cellular polyglutamine toxicity and suppresses the increase of reactive oxygen species caused by huntingtin. *Hum. Mol. Genet.* 11, 1137–1151.

Zabel, C., Chamrad, D. C., Priller, J., Woodman, B., Meyer, H. E., Bates, G. P., and Klose, J. (2002). Alterations in the mouse and human proteosome caused by Huntington's disease. *Mol. Cell Proteomics* 1, 366–375.

Zhang, Y., Huang, L., Zhang, J., Moskophidis, D., and Mivechi, N. F. (2002). Targeted disruption of hsf1 leads to lack of thermotolerance and defines tissue-specific regulation for stress-inducible Hsp molecular chaperones. *J. Cell. Biochem.* 86, 376–393.

Zourlidou, A., Gidalevitz, T., Kristiansen, M., Landles, C., Woodman, B., Wells, D. J., Latchman, D. S., de Belleroche, J., Tabrizi, S. J., Morimoto, R. I., and Bates, G. P. (2007). Hsp27 overexpression in the R6/2 mouse model of Huntington's disease: chronic neurodegeneration does not induce Hsp27 activation. *Hum. Mol. Genet.* 16, 1078–1090.

Zourlidou, A., Payne Smith, M. D., and Latchman, D. S. (2004). HSP27 but not HSP70 has a potent protective effect against alpha-synuclein-induced cell death in mammalian neuronal cells. *J. Neurochem.* 88, 1439–1448.

3

Inferring HIV escape rates from multi-locus genotype data

Taylor A. Kessinger[1], *Alan S. Perelson*[2] *and Richard A. Neher*[1*]

[2] *Evolutionary Dynamics and Biophysics, Max Planck Institute for Developmental Biology, Tübingen, Germany*
Theoretical Biology and Biophysics, Los Alamos National Laboratory, Los Alamos, NM, USA

Edited by:
Rob J. De Boer, Utrecht University, Netherlands

Reviewed by:
Viktor Müller, Hungarian Academy of Sciences and Eötvös Loránd University, Hungary
Vitaly V. Ganusov, University of Tennessee, USA
Aridaman Pandit, Utrecht University, Netherlands

***Correspondence:**
Richard A. Neher, Evolutionary Dynamics and Biophysics, Max Planck Institute for Developmental Biology, Spemannstraße 35, 72076 Tübingen, Germany
e-mail: richard.neher@tuebingen.mpg.de

Cytotoxic T-lymphocytes (CTLs) recognize viral protein fragments displayed by major histocompatibility complex molecules on the surface of virally infected cells and generate an anti-viral response that can kill the infected cells. Virus variants whose protein fragments are not efficiently presented on infected cells or whose fragments are presented but not recognized by CTLs therefore have a competitive advantage and spread rapidly through the population. We present a method that allows a more robust estimation of these escape rates from serially sampled sequence data. The proposed method accounts for competition between multiple escapes by explicitly modeling the accumulation of escape mutations and the stochastic effects of rare multiple mutants. Applying our method to serially sampled HIV sequence data, we estimate rates of HIV escape that are substantially larger than those previously reported. The method can be extended to complex escapes that require compensatory mutations. We expect our method to be applicable in other contexts such as cancer evolution where time series data is also available.

Keywords: HIV, CTL escape, cytotoxic T-lymphocytes, HIV evolution, viral dynamics, selection coefficient

INTRODUCTION

During the first few months of HIV infection, the HIV genome typically undergoes a series of rapid amino acid substitutions that reduce immune pressure by cytotoxic T-lymphocytes (CTLs); this process is referred to as CTL escape (1). The substitutions arise by random mutation and spread through the viral population by impairing either the presentation of viral epitopes on the cell surface or the recognition of the viral epitope by T-cell receptors. Avoiding recognition is an obvious benefit to the mutant virus, but escape mutations can interfere with processes necessary for virus replication and infection and thereby reduce the virus' intrinsic fitness (2–5). The rate at which escape variants displace the founder sequences depends on both "avoided killing" and the fitness cost. To quantify the role of individual CTL clones in controlling the viral population and the fitness costs associated with escape mutations, one would like to infer the escape rate associated with the individual mutations from serially sampled sequence data (4, 6).

With a single escape mutation and dense, deeply sampled data, the escape rate can simply be estimated by fitting a logistic curve to the time course of the mutation's frequency (4, 6). The logistic curve has two parameters: the growth or escape rate and the frequency at the initial time point. In many cases, however, the data obtained from infected patients are scarce, and estimating two parameters reliably from the data is not possible since one needs at least two time points at which the mutation is at intermediate frequency between 0 and 1 (4). **Figure 1** shows an example of such time series sequence data from CTL escape during early HIV infection. Time points are far apart and the sampling depth is low. Furthermore, it is not the case that only a single escape mutation is observed; rather, several mutations rapidly emerge in different places in the viral genome (7, 8). Multiple escapes imply immune pressure on many epitopes. Since the viral population and its mutation rate are large (9, 10), these different escape mutations will arise almost simultaneously. Initially, these escape mutations exist in the population as single mutant genomes until they are combined into multiple mutants by recurrent mutation or recombination (11, 12). The competition between viral variants affects the trajectories of individual escape mutations, so estimating their intrinsic growth rate by logistic fitting is not accurate. This competition is known as "clonal interference" in population genetics. The degree of competition between genotypes depends on the population size, the mutation rate, and the recombination rate in HIV populations. The latter-most is rather low (13, 14), and two strongly selected mutations in a large population are more likely to be combined by additional *de novo* mutation than recombination with another rare single mutation.

Here, we develop a strategy for inference that allows one to obtain robust escape rate estimates from the scarce data typical of studies of CTL escape. The inference is based on explicit modeling of the process of mutation accumulation in the founder sequence. Thereby, we exploit constraints imposed by the underlying dynamics of mutation and selection in the high dimensional space of possible genotypes.

Despite the large number of possible genomes that can be formed from different combinations of escape mutations, we typically observe one or two dominant genotypes at a time – at least during the first few months of the infection. Furthermore, these genotypes dominate only transiently and are quickly displaced by genotypes with an even greater number of escape mutations; see **Figure 1**. These observations agree with results from ref. (15), where a model of acute HIV infection was used to show

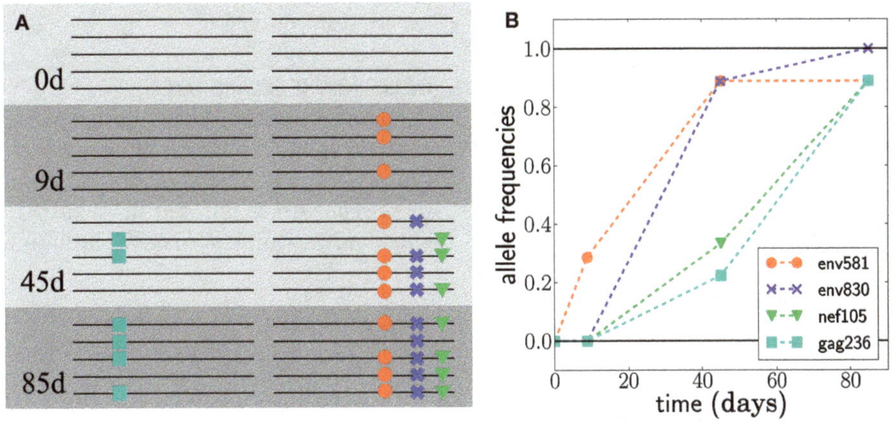

FIGURE 1 | Escape from T-cell mediated immunity. The virus population in patient CH58 quickly acquires four substitutions. **(A)** shows a sketch of genotypes at the first 4 escape mutations, observed at different times; see (7, 8) for the actual data. **(B)** shows the frequencies of the mutations in samples of size 7 at day 9 and size 9 at days 45 and 85.

that strongly selected escape mutations fix sequentially. Note that we don't assume a particular sequence of dominant genotypes *a priori*. Instead, we observe a sequence of dominant genotypes and try to infer the evolutionary scenario that most likely gave rise to this sequence of genotypes. While we model only these genotypes, many minor variants certainly exist. But only those dominant variants that are likely to give rise to the future populations need to be modeled accurately. Later in infection, the viral population is very diverse and cannot be analyzed using our method.

Given a data set from early infection, it is typically straightforward to define a series of dominant genotypes that likely have arisen through step-wise accumulation of mutations. Note that most likely all escape mutations constantly arise in different combinations, but typically only one combination rises quickly enough to dominate the population. This dominant genotype is then in most cases the source for the next dominant genotype. Later in infection, however, recombination is sufficiently frequent that no dominant genotype exists and mutations can spread simultaneously.

In Ganusov et al. (11), a framework for multi-locus modeling of CTL escape is presented. Building on this framework, we explicitly model the transition from one dominant genotype to another, which is a good approximation of the dynamics for rapid CTL escape in acute infection. The restriction to dominant genotypes captures the interference between escapes at different epitopes while avoiding the need to solve the full multi-locus problem.

We will first define a model of the dynamics of escape mutations. This model serves a twofold purpose: it defines the parameters we would like to estimate from the data and provides us with a computational tool to investigate how the accuracy of the inference depends on sampling depth and frequency, as well as how sensitively it depends on the values of parameters such as mutation rates or the population size. We reanalyze existing CTL escape data and find that accounting for multi-locus effects in a finite population results in higher estimates of the escape rates.

RESULTS

MODEL

In the majority of sexually transmitted HIV infections, a single "transmitted/founder" virus initiates the new infection resulting in an initially homogeneous viral population (8, 16). However, as HIV replicates in its new host, mutations accumulate. Mutations within or in proximity to CTL epitopes can reduce immune pressure by facilitating the avoidance of CTL recognition. While one often observes several escape mutations within a single epitope (17, 18), we do not differentiate between different mutations within the same epitope and model L epitopes that can be either be mutant or wild-type. Assuming that the escape at multiple epitopes has additive effects, ε_j, the growth rate (birth rate minus death rate) of a genotype is given by

$$F(g, t) = F_0(t) + \sum_i \varepsilon_i s_i \tag{1}$$

where $g = \{s_1, \ldots, s_L\}$ specifies the genotype. Here, $s_i = 0$ corresponds to a wild-type epitope at locus i, whereas $s_i = 1$ signifies escape at that epitope. $F_0(t)$ accounts for a genotype independent modulation of the growth rate. The latter could, for example, be due to variable numbers of target cells (19, 20). $F_0(t)$ controls the total population size, while the differences between genotypes are accounted for by $\sum_i \varepsilon_i s_i$ and result in differential amplification of some genotypes over others. The ε_i are the escape rates that we would like to estimate from the data and should be interpreted as the net effect of avoided killing and the possible fitness costs associated with the mutation; see e.g., Ganusov et al. (11). The fitness costs are modulated by the overall growth rate of the viral population and could therefore be slightly time dependent. We neglect this complication. Within our model, mutations arise at a rate μ per base per generation. This rate can be epitope dependent. Motivated by the frequent template switching of HIV reverse transcriptase (21), our general model of the HIV population includes recombination, which is assumed to occur with rate r. In the event of recombination, all L epitopes are reassorted, but an explicit genetic map could be implemented as well.

We implemented our model as a computer simulation in Python using the population genetic library FFPopSim (22). The simulation stores the population $n(g, t)$ of each of the 2^L possible genotypes. In each generation, the expected changes of the $n(g, t)$ due to mutation, selection, and recombination are calculated. The population of the next generation is then sampled from the expected genotype frequencies $\gamma(g, t) = n(g, t)/N$. The size of the population, N, can be set at will each generation. In this way, up to 15 epitopes can be simulated for 1000 generations within seconds to minutes.

A typical realization of the population dynamics is shown in **Figure 2**, where we have assumed a generation time of 1 day. As expected, the population is dominated by one genotype at a time. Furthermore, the mutations accumulate in decreasing order of escape rate, and the new dominant genotype arises from the previous by incorporation of the mutation with the largest escape rate available. There are, however, many minority genotypes which are rarely observed. **Figure 2C** shows the frequencies on a logarithmic scale, where the minor variants are visible. We use these simulations to test the accuracy and robustness of the inference procedure developed below.

Of the many possible genotypes that are present at any moment, only a small fraction is likely to be observed in a small sample and to be relevant in the future. Simulations and data suggest that the dominant genotypes accumulate mutations one by one – this greatly simplifies the task of estimating escape rates from the data. Instead of considering the dynamics of all possible genotypes (2^L), we will restrict the inference to a chain of genotypes, each containing one additional mutation compared to its predecessor.

The best estimate for the HIV generation time is $d = 2$ days (23), while estimates of escape rates are typically given in units of inverse days rather than generations. For simplicity, we simulate our model assuming one generation per day and state all rates in units of 1/day. Our results are insensitive to the choice of the generation time. Doubling the generation time has similar effects to dividing the population size by 2, as this keeps the strength of genetic drift constant.

INFERRING THE ESCAPE RATES

Suppose we have obtained sequence samples of size n_i at different time points t_i and each of these samples consists of different genotypes g present in $k(g, t_i)$ copies. If the actual frequencies of those genotypes at different times are $\gamma(g, t_i)$, the probability of obtaining the sample at t_i is given by the multinomial distribution

$$P\left(\text{sample}\right) = \frac{n_i!}{\prod_g k\left(g, t_i\right)!} \prod_g \gamma\left(g, t_i\right)^{k(g, t_i)} \qquad (2)$$

If the underlying dynamics was deterministic, the frequencies $\gamma(g, t)$ would be unique functions of the model parameters we want to estimate. In that case we could use Bayes' theorem, choose suitable priors, and determine the posterior distribution of the parameter values. However, both the model and the actual viral dynamics are stochastic, and "replaying" the history would result in different trajectories. Furthermore, most of the 2^L possible genotypes remain unobserved. This leaves us with the choice of either some type of approximate Bayesian computation that compares repeated simulations of the model with appropriate summary statistics (24) or a reduced description of only the observed genotypes, with the stochasticity captured by nuisance parameters (25).

We opt for the latter and model only those genotypes that dominate the population. We label these genotypes by the number of escape mutations they carry, e.g., g_1 carries the first escape mutations, g_2 the first and the second, and so forth. The frequency of a genotype is affected by stochastic forces only while it is very rare. If the genotype is favored, it will rapidly rise to high frequency, and the stochastic effects will no longer be relevant. It is therefore convenient to summarize the stochastic behavior by the time, τ, at which its frequency crosses the threshold to essentially deterministic dynamics. Since the dynamics is deterministic after this "seed

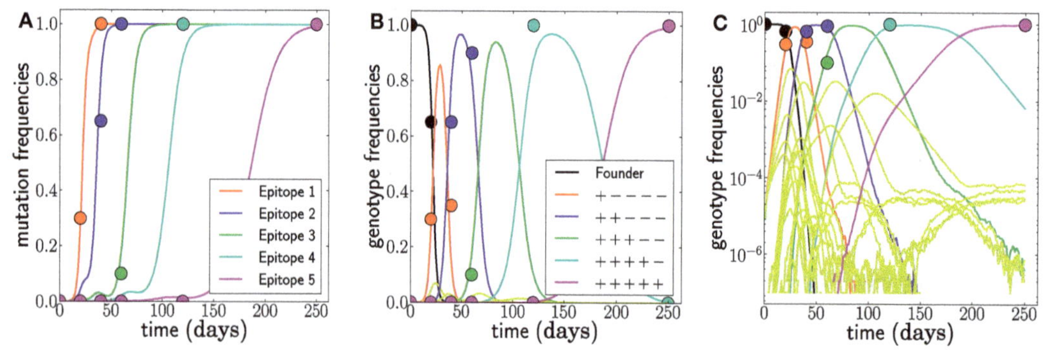

FIGURE 2 | Example of simulated escape mutations spreading through the population. **(A)** Even though all epitopes are targeted from $t = 0$, escape mutations spread sequentially. The mutation frequency in a sample of size 20 at different time points is indicated by colored dots. **(B)** The rising mutation frequencies are associated with the rise and fall of multi-locus genotypes. The founder virus is first replaced by a dominant single mutant, which itself is replaced by a double mutant and so forth. Note, however, that the virus population explores many combinations of mutations but that these minor variants never reach appreciable frequency. This is best seen in **(C)**, where all 32 genotype frequencies are shown on a logarithmic scale. These rare variants are rarely sampled, and their noisy dynamics suggests that little information can be gained from them. Here, $N = 10^7$, $\mu = 10^{-5}$, and $r = 0$, and escape rates are $\varepsilon_i = 0.5, 0.4, 0.25, 0.15, 0.08$ per day.

time," all the (unobserved) stochasticity can be accounted for by an appropriate choice of the seed time (26, 27). For each of the dominant escape variants, g_j, with $j = 1$ to $j = L$ escaped epitopes, we define a seed time τ_j to accommodate the stochastic aspects of the escape dynamics.

After crossing the deterministic threshold, the population frequencies of the dominant genotypes evolve according to

$$\dot{\gamma}_j(t) = F(g_j, t)\,\gamma_j(t) + \mu\left[\gamma_{j-1}(t) - \gamma_j(t)\right] \qquad (3)$$

if $t > \tau_j$. Conversely, $\gamma_j(t) = 0$ for $t < \tau_j$. The growth rate $F(g_j, t)$ of genotype j is the sum of the escape rates ε_k of the epitopes $k = 1, \ldots, j$ and the density regulating part $F_0(t)$; compare to equation (1). The escape rates are what we would like to estimate. The seed time, τ_j, corresponds to the time at which a genotype with all escape mutations up to mutation j first establishes[1]. At the seed time, we initialize the genotype frequency at $\gamma_j(\tau_j) = N^{-1}$. If seed times are chosen appropriately, this model provides a very accurate description of the frequency dynamics of the dominant genotypes in the full stochastic model; see **Figure 3**.

At face value, the deterministic model has two parameters per epitope – one escape rate and one seed time. The seed times, however, are quite strongly constrained by basic facts of the evolutionary dynamics. The genotype g_j carrying mutations $i = 1, \ldots, j$ arises with rate $\mu N(t)\gamma_{j-1}(t)$ from the genotype g_{j-1} carrying only $j - 1$ mutations. This means it is unlikely that genotype j arises early while $\gamma_{j-1}(t)$ is still very small. However, once the previous genotype $j - 1$ is common, genotype j is produced frequently. The distribution of the time at which the first copy of genotype j arises is given by the product of the rate of production and the probability that it has not yet been produced. The latter is the negative exponential of the integral of the production rate up to this point. Hence, the distribution of the seed time τ_j, given the trajectory of the previous genotype γ_{j-1}, is given by

$$Q(\tau_j|\gamma_{j-1}(t)) \approx \mu N(\tau_j)\gamma_{j-1}(\tau_j)e^{-\mu\int_0^{\tau_j} N(t)\gamma_{j-1}(t)\,dt}. \qquad (4)$$

Since the $\gamma_j(t)$ are uniquely specified by $\{\tau_k, \varepsilon_k\}_{k=1,\ldots,L}$, we can write the posterior probability of the parameters as

$$P(\{\varepsilon_j, \tau_j\}) \propto \prod_i P(\text{sample}_i|\Theta) \prod_j Q(\tau_j|\Theta)\, U(\varepsilon_j), \qquad (5)$$

where $\Theta = \{\varepsilon_k, \tau_k\}_{k=1\ldots L}$ and $U(\varepsilon_j)$ is our prior on the escape rates. We employ a Laplace prior $U(\varepsilon) = \exp(-\Phi\varepsilon)$ parameterized by Φ favoring small escape rates. The prior regularizes the search for the minimum and results in conservative estimates of escape rates.

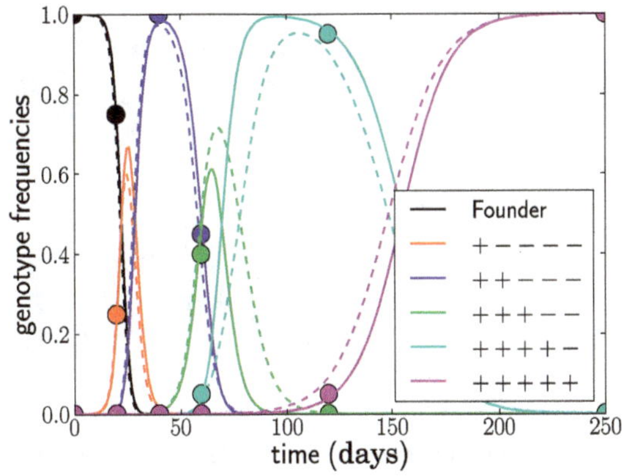

FIGURE 3 | The deterministic model parameterized by seed times τ_j for the L dominant genotypes and the escape rates of epitopes ε_i (solid lines) captures the dynamics of the stochastic model accurately (dashed lines). The trajectories (and seed times) vary from run to run. In this run, $N = 10^7$, $\mu = 10^{-5}$, and $r = 0$ and the escape rates are $\varepsilon_i = 0.5$, 0.4, 0.25, 0.15, 0.08 per day.

OBTAINING MAXIMUM LIKELIHOOD ESTIMATES

Finding the set of escape rates and seed times that maximizes the posterior probability can be difficult due to multiple maxima and ridges in the high dimensional search space, and uncertainty remains. To ensure that the global optimum will be reliably discovered, we exploit the sequential nature of the dynamics and use the fact that earlier escapes strongly affect the timing of the later ones, but not vice versa. Thus adding genotypes with an increasing number of mutations one at a time results in a reasonable initial guess on top of which a global true multi-locus search can be performed.

We have implemented such a search in Python, and the computationally expensive calculation of the posterior probability is implemented in C. The code infers parameters as follows:

- Fit the first escape assuming $\tau_1 = 0$ by a simple one dimensional minimization. This assumes that single mutants are already present in the population, consistent with the large viral population size present by the time a patient has been identified as HIV-1 infected (28, 29).
- Add additional epitopes successively by mapping the entire two-dimensional posterior distribution $P(\varepsilon_j, \tau_j)$ at fixed $\{\varepsilon_k, \tau_k\}$ for $k < j$. This step is illustrated in **Figure 4A**.
- Refine the estimates through local optimization via gradient descent, Monte Carlo methods, or local exhaustive search. The resulting parameters and trajectories are shown for one example in **Figure 4B**.
- Generate posterior distributions by Markov chain Monte Carlo (MCMC).

This procedure is described in more detail in the Section "Materials and Methods." Fitting five epitopes takes on the order of a minute on one 2011 desktop machine (Apple iMac i7 2.93 GHz). Generating the local posterior distribution by MCMC takes roughly 20 min for 10^6 steps.

COMPARISON TO SIMULATED DATA

To evaluate the accuracy and reliability of our inference scheme, we performed true multi-locus stochastic simulations using

[1]There is a brief period after the initial production of the mutation during which the dynamics is stochastic and the initial mutant establishes only with a probability roughly equal to εd, where $d = 2$ days is the generation time (23). However, we find $\varepsilon d \approx 1$ and ignore this complication.

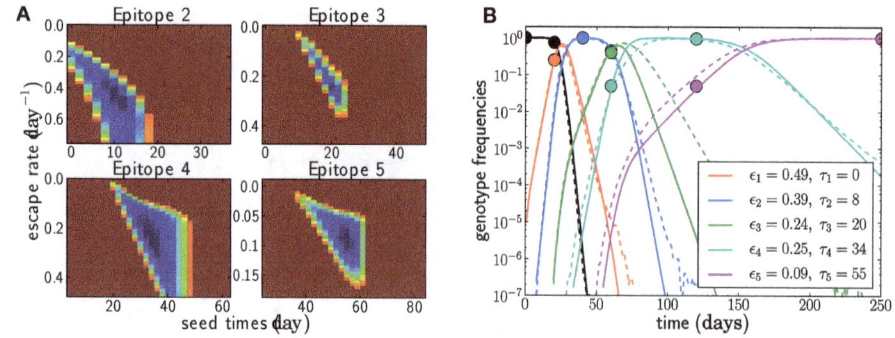

FIGURE 4 | Adding epitopes one by one is a feasible and reliable fitting strategy. Assuming we know the population was homogeneous at $t = 0$, there is only one free parameter for the first epitope, which is easily determined. For all subsequent epitopes, we need to determine the seed time τ_j and the escape rate ε_j. In **(A)**, the negative log posterior probability of these parameters is shown for each of the epitopes. The surface typically exhibits a single minimum. **(B)** shows the genotype frequencies of the founder virus and the dominant escape variants (solid lines: model fit, dashed lines: actual simulated trajectories). The estimated escape rates of individual epitopes and the seed times of genotypes containing all escape mutations up to j are given in the legend. Only the samples indicated by balls (20 sequences at each time point) were used for the estimation. In this run, $N = 10^7$, $\mu = 10^{-5}$, $r = 0$, and the escape rates $\varepsilon_j = 0.5, 0.4, 0.25, 0.15, 0.08$ per day.

FFPopSim (see Materials and Methods) and sampled genotypes from the simulation at a small number of time points. Time points and sample sizes were chosen to mimic patient data. We then inferred parameters from this "toy" data set and compared the result to the actual values. When interpreting these comparisons, it is important to distinguish two sources of error. First, limited sample size and sampling frequency will incur errors due to inaccurate estimates of the actual genotype frequencies from the sample. The second source of uncertainty is an inappropriate choice of model or model parameters. Such inappropriate model choices might include wrong estimates of the population size or mutation rates, the presence or absence of recombination, or time variable CTL activity.

We generate data assuming escape rates $\varepsilon_j = 0.5, 0.4, 0.25, 0.15, 0.08$ per day and sample the population on days $t_i = 0, 20, 40, 60, 120, 250$. An example of such samples is shown in **Figure 2**. Note that each genotype is typically only sampled at a single data point; it easily happens that a genotype is hardly seen at all. We therefore expect all inferences to be quite noisy as is the case with patient data.

Sample size and sampling frequency dependence

With more frequent and deeper sampling, inferring the model parameters is expected to become simpler. Indeed, as soon as each genotype is sampled more than once at intermediate frequency, one can estimate its growth advantage simply from its rate of increase. This is the rationale behind previous studies such as (4, 6). In many data sets, however, this condition is not met. By constraining the seed time based on the evolutionary trajectory of the previous escape, our method is able to produce a more accurate reconstruction of parameters with less data.

Figure 5 shows the estimates obtained as a function of the sampling frequency and sample size. Increasing the sample size improves the estimates only moderately, whereas increasing the sampling frequency leads to substantial improvements.

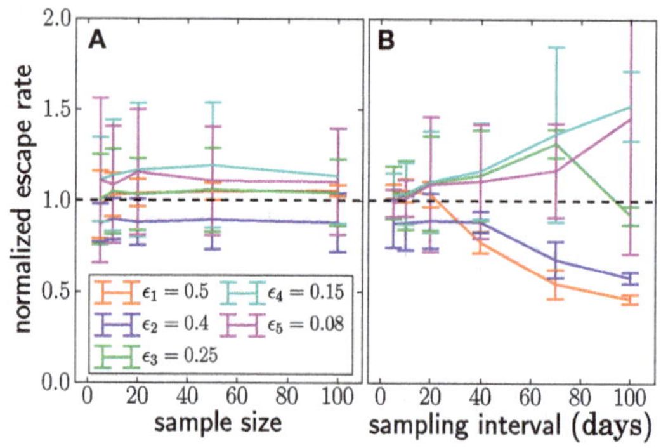

FIGURE 5 | The dependence of the accuracy of inference on sample sizes (A) and sampling intervals (B). The actual normalized escape rate is 1.0 and is shown by the dashed line. Sample size only moderately affects the accuracy, while sparse sampling (every 40 days in this example) leads to serious loss of accuracy. Sample size is $n = 20$ when sample intervals are varied, and sampling times are as illustrated in **Figure 2** when sample size is varied. The plots show the mean ± one standard deviation. The actual values of the escape rates simulated are shown in the legend (same on both panels). In each run, $N = 10^7$, $\mu = 10^{-5}$, and $r = 0$. Mean and standard deviation at each point are calculated from 100 independent simulations.

Model deviations

The population size and the mutation rate explicitly enter our model through the seed time prior, but we rarely know these numbers accurately. Hence we need to understand how inaccurate assumptions affect our estimates. If we assume that $N\mu$ is larger than it really is, our inference method will favor seeding subsequent genotypes too early, which in turn results in erroneously small estimates of escape rates. We varied N and μ and observed the expected effect on the estimates as shown in **Figure 6**. The dependence on μ is stronger than that on N, since the effect of a larger population size is partly canceled by the longer time necessary to amplify the novel mutation to macroscopic numbers.

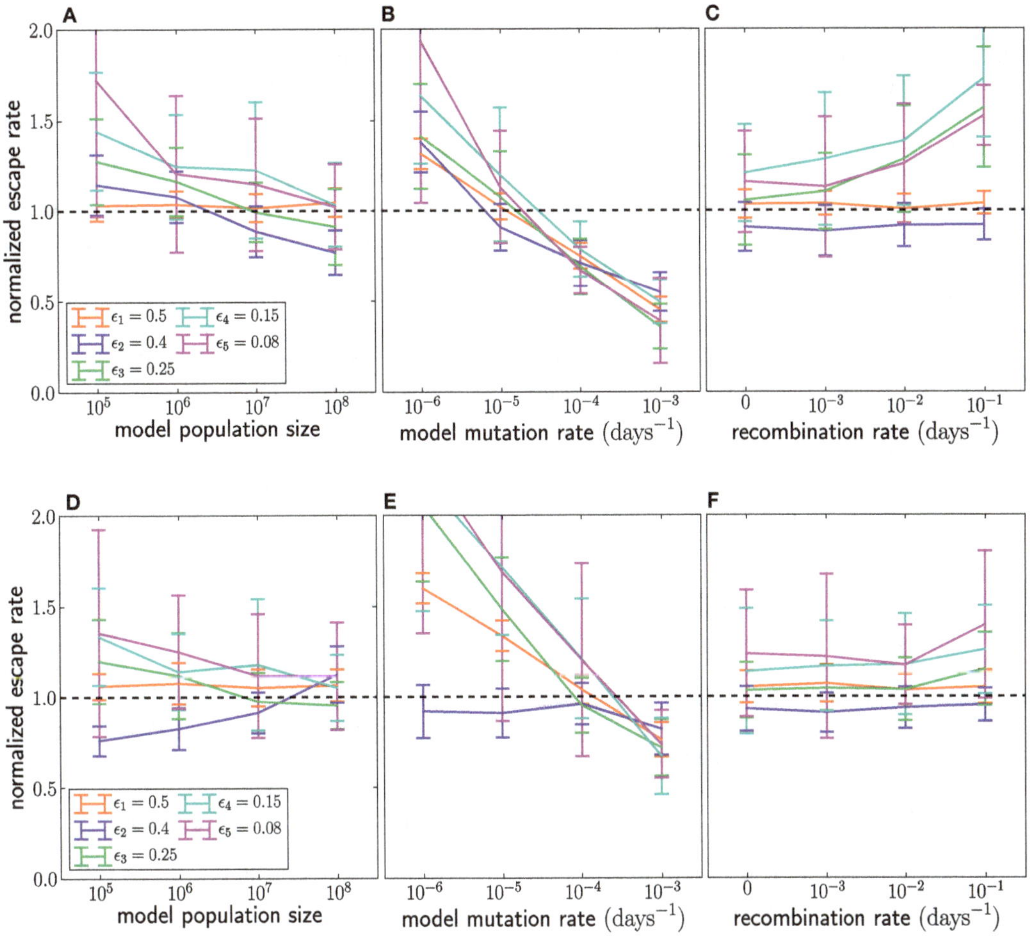

FIGURE 6 | The effect of assuming the wrong population parameters on the escape rate estimates. To quantify the robustness against wrong assumptions, we simulate escape dynamics with parameters different from those assumed in the escape rate estimation. **(A–C)** show simulations with $N = 10^7$ and $\mu = 10^{-5}$ per day, while **(D–F)** use a 10-fold higher mutation rate $\mu = 10^{-4}$. In **(C,F)**, the simulated recombination rate varies as shown. **(A,D)** Assuming a too small population size results in estimates that are too large. The effect is more pronounced at lower mutations rates. **(B)** Similarly, if the mutation rate is assumed too large, the estimated seeding of multiple mutants occurs too early and the estimates of escape rates are too low. Note that assuming the correct rates [$\mu = 10^{-5}$ in **(B)** and $\mu = 10^{-4}$ in **(F)**] results in unbiased estimates. **(C,F)** If the population recombines, the actual seed times are smaller than those estimated by the fitting routine. To compensate for the shorter time interval during which the escape variant rises, the estimates of escape rates are larger than the actual escape rates, at least at low mutation rates. For high mutation rates, recombination is less important because additional mutations are more efficient at producing multiple mutants than recombination. Mean and standard deviation at each point are calculated from 100 independent simulations.

However, even the dependence on μ is rather weak, and changing μ 10-fold only changes estimates of escape rates by $\pm 50\%$. The underlying reason is that the seed times depend primarily on the logarithm of $N\mu \cdot Q(\tau_j|\gamma_{j-1}(t))$ (see equation (4)), which peaks when $N\mu\gamma_{j-1}(t) \approx 1$. Because $\gamma_{j-1}(t)$ is growing exponentially, the position of the peak changes only logarithmically with the prefactor $N\mu$. Changes in μ also affect the dynamics through the initial rise in frequency of novel genotypes due to recurrent mutations; see equation (3).

Another factor that affects seed times is recombination. HIV recombines via template switching following the coinfection of one target cell by several virus particles (21). In chronic infection, coinfection occurs with a frequency of about 1% (13, 14). Recombination is not modeled in the seed time prior of our inference method but can speed up escape by combining escape mutations at different epitopes. As a result, if recombination is present, seeding tends to happen earlier than our prior would suggest. If the model assumes that seeding occurs later than in reality, there is less time for an escape variant to grow to its observed frequency. Hence the estimated escape rate (growth rate) is larger than the actual escape rate to compensate for the shorter time. In **Figure 6**, we compare the estimates obtained by applying our inference method to simulation data with recombination. Recombination starts to have substantial effects once coinfection exceeds a few percent. Recombination primarily affects the incorporation of more weakly selected mutations and can be ignored for very strongly selected CTL escape mutations. Recombination also has negligible effects if the mutation rate is large as is seen in **Figure 6F**.

Unobserved intermediates and compensatory mutations

The time intervals between successive samples are sometimes too large to observe the accumulation of single mutations, so the dominant genotype at one time point differs by more than one mutation from the previous. This can arise for two reasons. First, one or several unobserved genotypes may have transiently been at high frequency but been out-competed by later genotypes before the next sample was taken. Second, one escape might have required more than one mutation, for example because single mutants are not viable and a compensatory mutation is needed (30). Both scenarios can be accounted for in our scheme and are illustrated in **Figure 7**.

Unobserved, but individually beneficial, intermediate genotypes can be included by assuming they all have the same escape rate and were seeded one from the other. There is not sufficient information to estimate more than an average escape rate for all of them. For a given set of sampled frequencies, the estimated escape rates increase as more and more intermediates are assumed. Such unobserved intermediates are common in the data from infected individuals analyzed below.

Compensatory mutations and "multiple-hit" escapes can be accounted for by replacing the single site mutation rate in equation (4) by the effective rate at which the viable escape mutant appears. In the simplest case where all intermediate states are lethal and mutations are independent, this rate is simply the probability μ^k, where k is the number of mutations needed. In other cases, the rates to multiple hits can be calculated using branching process approximations (31, 32). The choice of the relevant effective mutation rate for complex escapes must be made on a case-by-case basis. The effective mutation rate of a multiple-hit escape will often be low enough that its seed time is not very well constrained. If, for example, the population size is $N = 10^8$ and the effective mutation rate is 10^{-10}, the seed time distribution has a width of more than 100 days. Given this weak constraint, more data are required in order to estimate the escape rate accurately; see **Figure 7**.

IMMUNE ESCAPE IN HIV-INFECTED PATIENTS

Cytotoxic T-lymphocyte escape was characterized in detail in the patients CH58, CH40, and CH77 (7, 8) and further analyzed in Ganusov et al. (4). Sequences were obtained by single genome amplification followed by traditional sequencing. The data are sparser and less densely sampled than most of the artificial examples analyzed above, so any estimates are necessarily rather imprecise. Furthermore, we do not know exactly when infection occurred or CTL selection started. The days given in the above papers are relative to the date of identification of the patient as HIV infected. It has been estimated that in a chronically infected patient, there are a total of around 4×10^7 infected cells (33). Hence, the population size is $N \approx 10^7$ but might be larger during peak viremia or smaller due to bottleneck effects or the myriad of factors influencing patient-to-patient variation in viral load. We determined posterior distributions for population sizes ranging from $N = 10^5$ to $N = 10^8$. The mutation rate was set to 10^{-5} per day (10). This value is appropriate if only one escape mutation per epitope is available. If escape can happen in many different ways, a higher rate of about $\mu = 10^{-4}$ per day should be used, so we repeated the estimation with $\mu = 10^{-4}$ finding similar results; see below. Both of these scenarios are observed (18). Recombination in HIV occurs but is not modeled here because its rate is low (13, 14), and it is expected to be less relevant for the strong escapes in large populations. In large populations, recurrent mutation is often more effective at accumulating escape mutations than recombination between two rare variants. Nevertheless, the neglect of recombination can lead to overestimation of escape rates; see above. Lastly, we assume that infection occurred $\tau = 20$ days before the patient was identified and the viral population sampled (7).

For each patient, we initially considered all non-synonymous mutations that are eventually sampled at high frequency as potential candidates for sequential escape mutants. Nearby mutations in the same epitope were combined into one escape. We refined this list of candidates by considering only time points early in infection

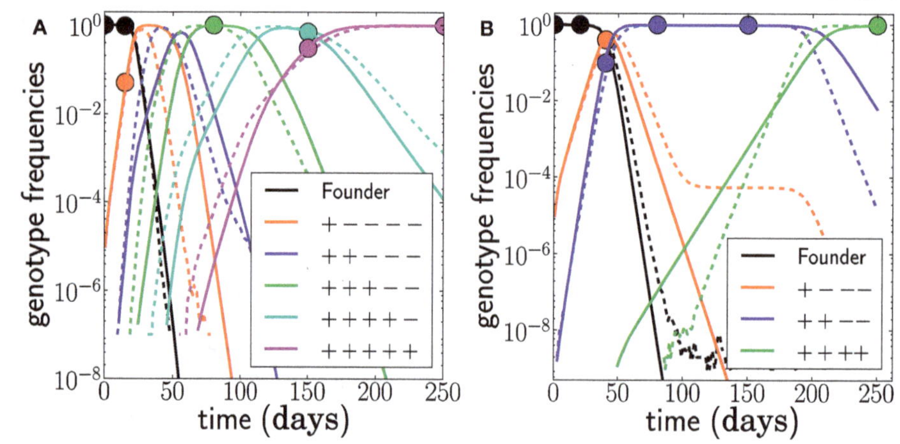

FIGURE 7 | Unobserved intermediates and compensatory mutations. **(A)** shows a scenario where the genotype with only 2 escape mutations (blue) was not observed even though this genotype was transiently at high frequencies. We fit this scenario by assuming both mutations have the same escape rate but occur sequentially ($N = 10^7$, $r = 0$, $\mu = 10^{-5}$). **(B)** shows a scenario where escape mutations 3 and 4 only occur together and any genotype containing only one of the two mutations is not viable. Hence the effective mutation rate into the genotype is $\mu^2 = 10^{-10}$ and the waiting time for this genotype is longer. Note that the population size is $N = 10^9$ in this example ($r = 0$, $\mu = 10^{-5}$). The last escape only appears once the previous escape mutations have reached frequency one, and the seeding time is quite variable.

that were sampled with more than 5 genomes per time point and only the earliest 3-6 strong escapes. All samples used had between 7 and 15 sequences. The frequencies of these escape mutations and their linkage into multi-locus genotypes in the 5′ and 3′ half of the genome, which were sequenced independently, can be easily determined from the alignment provided in Salazar-Gonzales et al. (8). Linkage information between the 5′ and 3′ half genomes is missing but can in all cases be imputed using the assumption of sequential escapes. We ignored mutations whose frequency does not increase monotonically such as pol80 in subject CH40. Later in infection, there is extensive non-synonymous diversity and it is not feasible to fit a time course for most of these mutations.

In CH40 we considered samples at time points $t = 0, 16, 45, 111$, and 181 days and identified escape in six epitopes; the first escape occurs in nef185, followed by three indistinguishable escapes at gag113, gag389, and vpr74 and two additional escapes in vif161 and env145. Following Ganusov et al. (4) the number in the epitope name refers to the beginning of the 18-mer peptide covering the epitope. The mutation at env145 was not analyzed in Ganusov et al. (4), and 145 is simply the number of the mutated amino acid in gp120. The indistinguishable escapes gag113, gag389, and vpr74 are treated as described in the section on unobserved intermediates (all three escapes are assumed to have identical escape rates and only their seed times are varied). Note that the fifth escape at epitope vif161 shows almost the same escape pattern as the three indistinguishable escapes preceding it. The escape rates of gag113, gag389, vpr74, and vif161 should therefore be interpreted with care. In CH58 we considered samples at time points $t = 0$, 9, 45, and 85 days and identified four escapes; the first escape is at env581 and the second at env830, followed by nef105 and gag236. In CH77 we considered samples at time points $t = 0$, 14, and 32 days and identified four escapes, namely the first escape in tat55 and subsequent escapes in env350, nef17, and nef73.

Given the above assumptions, we obtained estimates for the seed time and escape rate of each mutation. For each patient, we obtained initial estimates using a naïve single epitope fit for each mutation; then, we iterated our multi-epitope fitting model five times. Next, we obtained posterior distributions for the escape rates, all shown in **Figure 8**, by performing a MCMC simulation using the likelihood function given in equation (5). After obtaining our estimates, we randomly changed the escape rates in increments of ± 0.01 and the seed times by ± 1, reevaluated the likelihood, and accepted the change with probability $\min(1, \exp(\Delta))$, where Δ is the change in log-likelihood. The resulting Markov chain was run for 10^6 steps with samples taken every 1000 steps.

Figure 8 shows the posterior distributions of the escape rates for different epitopes in the three patients evaluated assuming a mutation rate $\mu = 10^{-5}$ per day. Larger population sizes result in smaller estimates of the escape rates, as expected from **Figure 6A**. The posterior distributions for the first escapes are often very tight, but they depend on the time of the onset of CTL selection, which we have set here to $T = 20$ days prior to the first sample. If we assume that the time of the onset of CTL selection coincided with the first sample (i.e., $T = 0$), the estimates of escape rates of the first epitope ε_1 are around 0.9, while later escapes are almost not sensitive to the choice of T.

While the posterior distributions of escape rates of subsequent escape rates are quite broad, they nevertheless suggest that escape rates can be substantially higher than previously estimated (4, 6). Furthermore, the escape rate is not obviously negatively correlated with the time of emergence during acute infection with HIV-1, at least for the earliest four to six escapes. The underlying reason for this is that selection on a late escape is only active after the successful multiple mutant has been produced. In previous single epitope estimates, selection was allowed to act on the mutant frequency from the very beginning, resulting in a reduced estimate of the escape rate. **Figure 8** also shows the inferred trajectories for the most likely parameter combination for patient CH40. One clearly sees the rapid rise and fall of multiple genotypes between the second and third time point. Given the large number of genotypes involved and the little data available, the escape rates estimated for this case are rather noisy. But this analysis clearly shows that strong selection is necessary to bring four mutations to fixation in just a few weeks. We repeated the analysis of the patient data assuming a mutation rate of $\mu = 10^{-4}$ and show the results in **Figure 9**. The overall picture is similar to what we found for $\mu = 10^{-5}$ per day, but escape rates tend to be lower.

DISCUSSION

We have suggested a way to infer viral escape rates from time series data sparsely sampled from the evolutionary dynamics of asexual or rarely sexual populations such as HIV. We exploit the sequential manner in which escape mutations accumulate, which allows us to constrain the times at which new escape mutations arose. These constraints regularize the inference to a large extent, but additional stability is gained by prioritizing small escape rates through an exponential prior.

Escape rates of single escape mutations have so far been estimated by comparing the time series data to a model that assumes logistic growth of the mutation with a constant rate. This approach has been used to analyze the intra-patient dynamics of recombinant HIV (34), drug resistance (35, 36), and CTL escape dynamics (4, 6, 20, 37, 38). While these methods work well if each mutation is sampled multiple times at intermediate frequencies, they provide very conservative lower bounds when data are sparse. Furthermore, they ignore the effects of competition between escapes at different epitopes and assume that each epitope can be treated independently. Since the recombination frequency in HIV is low (13, 14, 39), this can be a poor approximation. Our method improves on previous methods on both of these counts. We explicitly model the competition between escape mutations. This competition places constraints on the times at which genotypes with multiple escapes first arise (double mutants arise only after the single mutants), which makes the inference more robust and the lower bound tighter.

A related method to estimate CTL escape rates has been proposed by Leviyang (12), who modeled multiple escape mutations by an escape graph that is traversed by the viral population. Combining these two approaches, intra-epitope competition as modeled in (12) and the between epitope competition studied here, would be an interesting extension. Similar ideas have been developed in the context of mutations in cancer or evolution experiments (40).

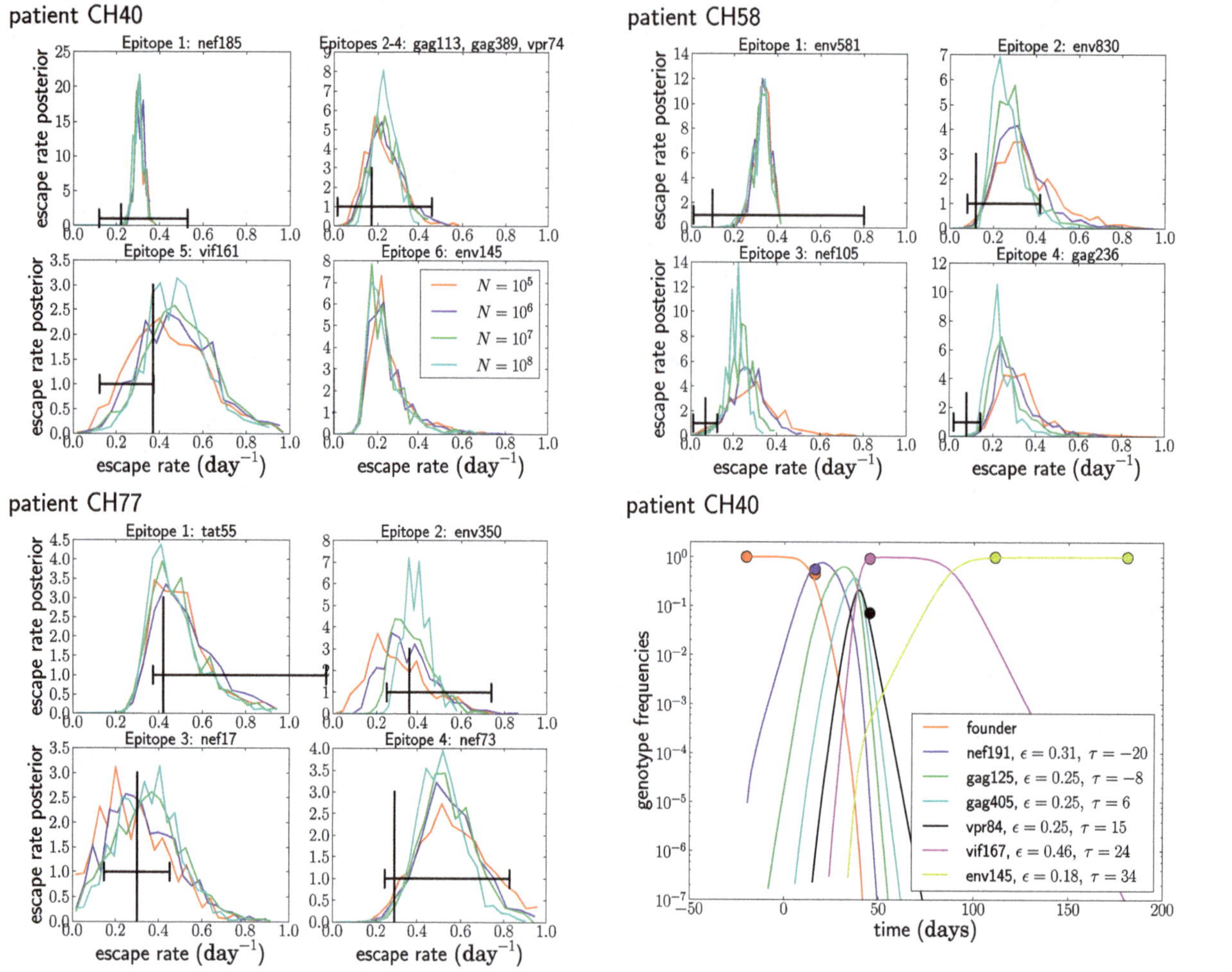

FIGURE 8 | The posterior distribution of the escape rates for different population sizes. It is assumed that CTL selection starts 20 days prior to the date of identification, and the fitness prior has weight $\Phi = 10$. The black vertical and horizontal lines indicate the estimates and confidence intervals obtained in Ganusov et al. (4). Note that the mutation env145 in CH40 was not analyzed in Ganusov et al. (4). The lower right panel shows the most likely genotype trajectories for patient CH40 with parameters $N = 10^7$ and $\mu = 10^{-5}$. Each curve is labeled by an epitope but should be understood as the frequency of the genotype that has escaped at this and all previous epitopes. Note that no data are available to differentiate epitopes gag113, gag389, and vpr74. For those, we assume an arbitrary order and equal escape rates as explained in the section on unobserved intermediates.

While previous methods neglect interactions between epitopes altogether – equivalent to assuming very rapid recombination – our method ignores recombination during the inference. By comparison with simulations that include recombination, we have shown that neglecting recombination can result in overestimation of the escape rates by roughly 30% at plausible recombination rates of 1% (13, 14). We also show that neglecting recombination is less of a problem at higher mutation rates. Note that neglecting recombination cannot explain the larger escape estimates compared to previous studies. For patient CH58 we find escape rates that are up to threefold higher than earlier estimates (4), while we never see such a large deviation in our sensitivity analysis. Furthermore, the errors made when neglecting recombination for rapid early escapes are comparable to the uncertainties that result from infrequent sampling or more severe deviations of the model from reality, such as time variable CTL activity.

Reanalysis of CTL escape data from HIV using our method suggests that CTL escapes are substantially more rapid than previously thought. Even with a large prior against high escape rates ($\Phi = 10$), we estimate that the escape rates of the first 4–6 escapes are on the order of 0.3-0.4 per day. The estimates at large population sizes are fairly insensitive to the prior for population sizes of 10^6 or larger. Early in infection, it is plausible to assume that the relevant size is $N = 10^7$ (28, 29, 41). If population sizes are small, relaxing the prior against high escape rates results in larger estimates, which further supports our finding that escape rates are often large and competition between escapes needs to be modeled. Given the sparse data, we can only estimate parameters of simple models and have to neglect many complicating features of HIV biology. Among other factors, the rate at which escape mutations are selected depends on the overall R_0 of the infection, and CTL selection is probably time variable (4). The

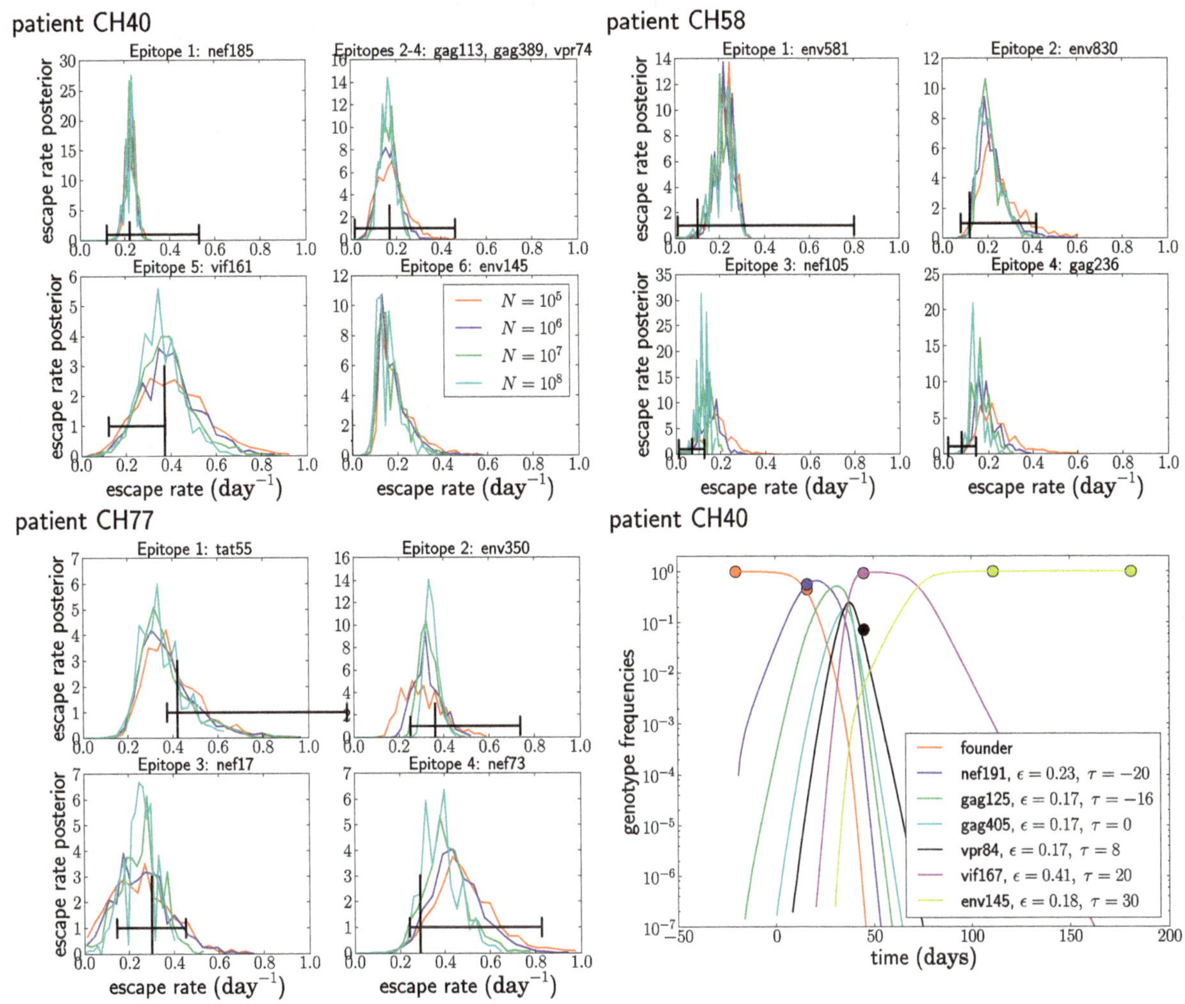

FIGURE 9 | Posterior distributions of escape rate assuming a mutation rate $\mu = 10^{-4}$ per day. See **Figure 8** for other details.

estimated parameters therefore represent time averaged effective escape rates.

The timing of escape has been shown to depend on epitope entropy and immunodominance (42). However, we modeled only the first four to six escapes in each patient, from which rather little information about differential timing can be obtained. In the case of CH77, the first four escapes occurred within a month from the identification of the patient. In patient CH58, it took roughly 3 months for four escapes to spread and the estimated escape rates are lower as expected. In the case of CH40, four of the six escapes show almost or completely indistinguishable escape patterns and we have little power to differentiate the escape rates at epitopes gag113, gag389, vpr74, and vif161. Hence any meaningful correlation with immunological features and epitope sequence conservation, i.e., low entropy, requires more data.

The proposed method to analyze multi-locus time series of adaptive evolution could be useful in many context where the genotypic compositions of large populations of viruses or cells can be monitored over time. Whenever mutations occur rapidly enough that they compete which each other, this competition has to be accounted for in the analysis. Outside of virus evolution, possible applications include the development of cancer and microbial evolution experiments.

MATERIALS AND METHODS

DATA PREPARATION

Our fitting method uses counts k_{ij} of genotypes g_j at time points t_i to infer escape rates of individual mutations. The procedure used to obtain successive genotype counts from sequence data sampled from patients is outlined in the text. As input data, our analysis scripts expect a white-space delimited text file with a format shown in **Table 1**. In addition, a separate file with the total number of sequences at each time point can be provided. This file is expected to have the same format as the matrix with the genotype counts; see **Table 1**. In absence of such a file, the sample sizes at each time point are obtained by summing the genotype counts.

To test our method, artificial data $k_{ij} = k(g_j, t_i)$ were obtained from simulated trajectories (generated by FFPopSim) by binomial sampling (with size n_i) at specified time points t_i. Trajectory generation and sampling are implemented in the

Table 1 | Format of input data: the escape mutations are ordered first by the time of first observation and then by abundance.

Time (days)	Founder	Env581	Env830	Nef105	Gag236
9	5	2	0	0	0
45	0	0	5	3	0
85	0	0	0	0	8

Each entry in the table in a particular column reports the number of times a sequence is observed containing the escape of that column and all previous escape mutations.

file `model_fit/ctlutils.py` at http://git.tuebingen.mpg.de/ctlfit; see below.

Sequence data

The HIV sequences for patients CH40, CH58, and CH77 where downloaded from http://www.hiv.lanl.gov/content/sequence/HIV/USER_ALIGNMENTS/Salazar.html (8).

INFERENCE

The inference procedure consists of *initial guessing, sequential addition of escapes, multi-dimensional refinement,* and estimation of *posterior distributions.* The implementation can be found in `src/ctl_fit.py`, with the C code for the likelihood calculation in `src/cfit.cpp`.

Initial guesses

We produce initial guesses by single epitope modeling. The frequency of each escape mutation, ν_j, grows logistically with the escape rate (11). We expect that only the frequency of the first escape mutation is significantly affected by mutational input, because it receives input from the abundant founder sequence, whereas the later escapes only receive mutational input from the previously escaped genotype, which is still rare when the novel escape arises. Hence we only model the mutational dynamics of the first escape. In a single epitope model, the frequency of the founder variant is one minus the frequency of the escape variant. The frequency of the escape variant increases by $\mu(1-\nu_1)$ per day due to mutations from the founder and decreases by $\mu\nu_1$ due to further mutations to additional escapes. Combined with the logistic growth, the dynamics of ν_1 is described by

$$\dot{\nu}_1(t) = \varepsilon_1\nu_1(1-\nu_1) + \mu\left[1-2\nu_1\right]. \qquad (6)$$

with initial condition $\nu_1(0)=0$. Note the difference between the allele frequency ν, which refers to a particular escape mutation, and γ, which corresponds to frequencies of particular multi-epitope genotypes. The above ODE has the solution

$$\nu_1(t) = \frac{1}{2\varepsilon_1}\left[\varepsilon_1 - 2\mu + R\tanh\left(\frac{\alpha+t}{2}R\right)\right] \qquad (7)$$

where $R=\sqrt{\varepsilon_1^2+4\mu^2}$ and $\alpha=\frac{4\mu-2\varepsilon_1}{4\mu^2+\varepsilon_1^2}$ (11). The escape rate ε_1 is determined by maximizing the likelihood (equation (5)) using `fmin` from `scipy` (43).

The seed time τ_j of subsequent escape mutants g_j is determined by maximizing the seed time prior $Q(\tau_j|\gamma_{j-1})$ defined in equation (4) using the previously determined γ_{j-1}. The frequencies of mutations are assumed to follow a logistic trajectory since the genotype from which they receive mutational input is itself still at low frequency:

$$\nu_j(t) = \frac{e^{\varepsilon_j(t-\tau_j)}}{e^{\varepsilon_j(t-\tau_j)} + N\varepsilon_j} \quad j>1. \qquad (8)$$

Again, we maximize the posterior probability, equation (5), to obtain an initial estimate of ε_j.

Sequential addition of escapes

Given the initial estimates for the first escape, we now add subsequent escapes to the multi-epitope model, which is formulated in terms of genotype counts k_{ij} and frequencies $\gamma_j(t)$. Note that the interpretation of genotype counts depends on how many epitopes are modeled. For example, if we model epitopes $1,\ldots,j$ out of a total of L epitopes, counts for genotype j are $k_{ij}=\sum_{l=j}^{L}k_{il}$, i.e., we ignore all later escapes.

If the added escape is unique, i.e., no other escape mutation has the exact same temporal pattern, we calculate the likelihood on a 21×31 grid of escape rates and seed times; comp. **Figure 4**. The grid spans values between 0 and twice the initial estimate for both the seed time and the escape rate. The most likely combination of seed time and escape rate is chosen, and the procedure is repeated with the next epitope.

If multiple epitopes exhibit the same temporal pattern, we add them all at once, constrain their escape rates to be equal, and assume they emerged in the order listed in the genotype matrix. Since we now have to optimize one joint escape rate and multiple seed times, we do not map the likelihood surface exhaustively but rather perform a greedy search. We examine next-neighbor moves with steps $\delta\tau=\pm1$ day and $\delta\varepsilon=\pm0.02$ per day, moves which change all seed times by $\delta\tau$, and 20 moves in which all seed times and escape rates are changed by $\delta\tau$ and $\delta\varepsilon$ with random sign; the step that maximizes the likelihood is accepted. This is repeated until no favorable move is found and further repeated with $\delta\varepsilon=\pm0.01$ and ±0.001 per day.

Refinement

We then iterate sequentially over every epitope and optimize its seed time and escape rate as described above, but with all other epitopes part of the multi-epitope model. This typically leads to rather small adjustments and converges rapidly.

Posterior distributions

To determine the posterior distribution of the escape rates, we attempt to change all seed times and escape rates by $\delta\tau=\pm1$ day and $\delta\varepsilon=\pm0.01$ per day with random sign. The move is accepted with probability $\min(1,\exp(\Delta))$, where Δ is the difference in log-likelihood before and after the change. We sample this Markov chain every 1000 moves and thereby map the posterior distribution of seed times and escape rates.

USAGE

All source code and scripts are available at http://git.tuebingen.mpg.de/ctlfit.

Building

The part of our method that is implemented in C and the python bindings can be built using `make` and the Makefile provided in the `src` directory. Prerequisites for building are `python2.7`, `scipy`, `numpy`, `swig`, and a `gcc` compiler.

Fitting

Given a text file with genotype counts specified as shown in **Table 1**, fitting is performed by calling the script `fit_escapes.py` with Python. Parameters can be set via command line arguments:

```
python fit_escapes.py --input datafile        (9)
```

where `--input` specifies the file with the genotype counts. Other parameters can be modified in a similar manner. Running the script with the option `--help` prints a list of all parameters. The estimated escape rates and seed times as well as the sampled posterior distribution will be saved in the directory `fit_escapes_output`, unless otherwise specified.

ACKNOWLEDGMENTS

We are grateful for stimulating discussions with F. Zanini. This work is supported by the ERC starting Grant HIVEVO 260686 (Richard A. Neher) and in part by the National Science Foundation under Grant No. NSF PHY11-25915. This work was performed under the auspices of the US Department of Energy under contract DE-AC52-06NA25396 and supported by NIH grants R01-AI028433, UM1-AI100645-01, and the National Center for Research Resources and the Office of Research Infrastructure Programs (ORIP) through grant R01-OD011095 (Alan S. Perelson).

REFERENCES

1. McMichael AJ, Borrow P, Tomaras GD, Goonetilleke N, Haynes BF. The immune response during acute HIV-1 infection: clues for vaccine development. *Nat Rev Immunol* (2009) **10**(1):11. doi:10.1038/nri2674
2. Fernandez CS, Stratov I, De Rose R, Walsh K, Dale CJ, Smith MZ, et al. Rapid viral escape at an immunodominant simian-human immunodeficiency virus cytotoxic T-lymphocyte epitope exacts a dramatic fitness cost. *J Virol* (2005) **79**(9):5721–31. doi:10.1128/JVI.79.9.5721-5731.2005
3. Li B, Gladden AD, Altfeld M, Kaldor JM, Cooper DA, Kelleher AD, et al. Rapid reversion of sequence polymorphisms dominates early human immunodeficiency virus type 1 evolution. *J Virol* (2007) **81**(1):193–201. doi:10.1128/JVI.01231-06
4. Ganusov VV, Goonetilleke N, Liu MKP, Ferrari G, Shaw GM, McMichael AJ, et al. Fitness costs and diversity of the cytotoxic T lymphocyte (CTL) response determine the rate of CTL escape during acute and chronic phases of HIV infection. *J Virol* (2011) **85**(20):10518–28. doi:10.1128/JVI.00655-11
5. Seki S, Matano T. CTL escape and viral fitness in HIV/SIV infection. *Front Microbiol* (2012) **2**:267. doi:10.3389/fmicb.2011.00267
6. Asquith B, Edwards CTT, Lipsitch M, McLean AR. Inefficient cytotoxic T lymphocyte-mediated killing of HIV-1-infected cells in vivo. *PLoS Biol* (2006) **4**(4):e90. doi:10.1371/journal.pbio.0040090
7. Goonetilleke N, Liu MKP, Salazar-Gonzalez JF, Ferrari G, Giorgi E, Ganusov VV, et al. The first T cell response to transmitted/founder virus contributes to the control of acute viremia in HIV-1 infection. *J Exp Med* (2009) **206**(6):1253–72. doi:10.1084/jem.20090365
8. Salazar-Gonzalez JF, Salazar MG, Keele BF, Learn GH, Giorgi EE, Li H, et al. Genetic identity, biological phenotype, and evolutionary pathways of transmitted/founder viruses in acute and early HIV-1 infection. *J Exp Med* (2009) **206**(6):1273–89. doi:10.1084/jem.20090378
9. Perelson AS, Neumann AU, Markowitz M, Leonard JM, Ho DD. HIV-1 dynamics in vivo: virion clearance rate, infected cell life-span, and viral generation time. *Science* (1996) **271**(5255):1582–6. doi:10.1126/science.271.5255.1582
10. Mansky LM, Temin HM. Lower in vivo mutation rate of human immunodeficiency virus type 1 than that predicted from the fidelity of purified reverse transcriptase. *J Virol* (1995) **69**(8):5087–94.
11. Ganusov VV, Neher RA, Perelson AS. Mathematical modeling of escape of HIV from cytotoxic T lymphocyte responses. *J Stat Mech* (2013) **2013**(1):P01010. doi:10.1088/1742-5468/2013/01/P01010
12. Leviyang S. Computational inference methods for selective sweeps arising in acute HIV infection. *Genetics* (2013) **194**:737–52. doi:10.1534/genetics.113.150862
13. Neher RA, Leitner T. Recombination rate and selection strength in HIV intra-patient evolution. *PLoS Comput Biol* (2010) **6**(1):e1000660. doi:10.1371/journal.pcbi.1000660
14. Batorsky R, Kearney MF, Palmer SE, Maldarelli F, Rouzine IM, Coffin JM. Estimate of effective recombination rate and average selection coefficient for HIV in chronic infection. *Proc Natl Acad Sci U S A* (2011) **108**(14):5661–6. doi:10.1073/pnas.1102036108
15. da Silva J. The dynamics of HIV-1 adaptation in early infection. *Genetics* (2012) **190**(3):1087–99. doi:10.1534/genetics.111.136366
16. Keele BF, Giorgi EE, Salazar-Gonzalez JF, Decker JM, Pham KT, Salazar MG, et al. Identification and characterization of transmitted and early founder virus envelopes in primary HIV-1 infection. *Proc Natl Acad Sci U S A* (2008) **105**(21):7552–7. doi:10.1073/pnas.0802203105
17. Fischer W, Ganusov VV, Giorgi EE, Hraber PT, Keele BF, Leitner T, et al. Transmission of single HIV-1 genomes and dynamics of early immune escape revealed by ultra-deep sequencing. *PLoS ONE* (2010) **5**(8):e12303. doi:10.1371/journal.pone.0012303
18. Henn MR, Boutwell CL, Charlebois P, Lennon NJ, Power KA, Macalalad AR, et al. Whole genome deep sequencing of HIV-1 reveals the impact of early minor variants upon immune recognition during acute infection. *PLoS Pathog* (2012) **8**(3):e1002529. doi:10.1371/journal.ppat.1002529
19. Petravic J, Loh L, Kent SJ, Davenport MP. CD4+ target cell availability determines the dynamics of immune escape and reversion in vivo. *J Virol* (2008) **82**(8):4091–101. doi:10.1128/JVI.02552-07
20. Ganusov VV, De Boer RJ. Estimating costs and benefits of CTL escape mutations in SIV/HIV infection. *PLoS Comput Biol* (2006) **2**(3):e24. doi:10.1371/journal.pcbi.0020024
21. Levy DN, Aldrovandi GM, Kutsch O, Shaw GM. Dynamics of HIV-1 recombination in its natural target cells. *Proc Natl Acad Sci U S A* (2004) **101**(12):4204–9. doi:10.1073/pnas.0306764101
22. Zanini F, Neher RA. FFPopSim: an efficient forward simulation package for the evolution of large populations. *Bioinformatics* (2012) **28**(24):3332–3. doi:10.1093/bioinformatics/bts633
23. Markowitz M, Louie M, Hurley A, Sun E, Di Mascio M, Perelson AS, et al. A novel antiviral intervention results in more accurate assessment of human immunodeficiency virus type 1 replication dynamics and T-cell decay in vivo. *J Virol* (2003) **77**(8):5037–8. doi:10.1128/JVI.77.8.5037-5038.2003
24. Sunnker M, Busetto AG, Numminen E, Corander J, Foll M, Dessimoz C. Approximate Bayesian computation. *PLoS Comput Biol* (2013) **9**(1):e1002803. doi:10.1371/journal.pcbi.1002803
25. Basu D. On the elimination of nuisance parameters. *J Am Stat Assoc* (1977) **72**(358):355–66. doi:10.1080/01621459.1977.10481002
26. Kepler TB, Perelson AS. Modeling and optimization of populations subject to time-dependent mutation. *Proc Natl Acad Sci U S A* (1995) **92**(18):8219–23. doi:10.1073/pnas.92.18.8219
27. Desai MM, Fisher DS. Beneficial mutation selection balance and the effect of linkage on positive selection. *Genetics* (2007) **176**(3):1759–98. doi:10.1534/genetics.106.067678
28. Coffin JM. HIV population dynamics in vivo: implications for genetic variation, pathogenesis, and therapy. *Science* (1995) **267**(5197):483–9. doi:10.1126/science.7824947

29. Perelson AS, Essunger P, Ho DD. Dynamics of HIV-1 and CD4+ lymphocytes in vivo. *AIDS* (1997) **11**(Suppl A):S17–24.
30. Read EL, Tovo-Dwyer AA, Chakraborty AK. Stochastic effects are important in intrahost HIV evolution even when viral loads are high. *Proc Natl Acad Sci U S A* (2012) **109**(48):19727–32. doi:10.1073/pnas.1206940109
31. Weissman DB, Desai MM, Fisher DS, Feldman MW. The rate at which asexual populations cross fitness valleys. *Theor Popul Biol* (2009) **75**(4):286–300. doi:10.1016/j.tpb.2009.02.006
32. Neher RA, Shraiman BI. Genetic draft and quasi-neutrality in large facultatively sexual populations. *Genetics* (2011) **188**:975–96. doi:10.1534/genetics.111.128876
33. Haase AT, Henry K, Zupancic M, Sedgewick G, Faust RA, Melroe H, et al. Quantitative image analysis of HIV-1 infection in lymphoid tissue. *Science* (1996) **274**(5289):985–9. doi:10.1126/science.274.5289.985
34. Liu S-L, Mittler JE, Nickle DC, Mulvania TM, Shriner D, Rodrigo AG, et al. Selection for human immunodeficiency virus type 1 recombinants in a patient with rapid progression to AIDS. *J Virol* (2002) **76**(21):10674–84. doi:10.1128/JVI.76.21.10674-10684.2002
35. Paredes R, Sagar M, Marconi VC, Hoh R, Martin JN, Parkin NT, et al. In vivo fitness cost of the m184v mutation in multidrug-resistant human immunodeficiency virus type 1 in the absence of lamivudine. *J Virol* (2009) **83**(4):2038–43. doi:10.1128/JVI.02154-08
36. Bonhoeffer S, Barbour AD, De Boer RJ. Procedures for reliable estimation of viral fitness from time-series data. *Proc Biol Sci* (2002) **269**(1503):1887–93. doi:10.1098/rspb.2002.2097
37. Asquith B, McLean AR. In vivo CD8+ T cell control of immunodeficiency virus infection in humans and macaques. *Proc Natl Acad Sci U S A* (2007) **104**(15):6365–70. doi:10.1073/pnas.0700666104
38. Petravic J, Ribeiro RM, Casimiro DR, Mattapallil JJ, Roederer M, Shiver JW, et al. Estimating the impact of vaccination on acute simian-human immunodeficiency virus/simian immunodeficiency virus infections. *J Virol* (2008) **82**(23):11589–98. doi:10.1128/JVI.01596-08
39. Josefsson L, King MS, Makitalo B, Brännström J, Shao W, Maldarelli F, et al. Majority of CD4+ T cells from peripheral blood of HIV-1-infected individuals contain only one HIV DNA molecule. *Proc Natl Acad Sci U S A* (2011) **108**(27):11199–204. doi:10.1073/pnas.1107729108
40. Illingworth CJR, Mustonen V. A method to infer positive selection from marker dynamics in an asexual population. *Bioinformatics* (2012) **28**(6):831–7. doi:10.1093/bioinformatics/btr722
41. Boltz VF, Ambrose Z, Kearney MF, Shao W, Ramani VNK, Maldarelli F, et al. Ultrasensitive allele-specific PCR reveals rare preexisting drug-resistant variants and a large replicating virus population in macaques infected with a simian immunodeficiency virus containing human immunodeficiency virus reverse transcriptase. *J Virol* (2012) **86**(23):12525–30. doi:10.1128/JVI.01963-12
42. Liu MKP, Hawkins N, Ritchie AJ, Ganusov VV, Whale V, Brackenridge S, et al. Vertical T cell immunodominance and epitope entropy determine HIV-1 escape. *J Clin Invest* (2013) **123**(1):380–93. doi:10.1172/JCI65330
43. Oliphant T. Python for scientific computing. *Comput Sci Eng* (2007) **9**(3):10–20. doi:10.1109/MCSE.2007.58

4

Chronic inflammation in cancer development

Gabriele Multhoff [1,2]*, _Michael Molls_ [1] and _Jürgen Radons_ [3]

[1] *Department of Radiation Oncology, Klinikum rechts der Isar, Technische Universität München, Munich, Germany*
[2] *Clinical Cooperation Group Innate Immunity in Tumor Biology, Helmholtz Zentrum München, Munich, Germany*
[3] *multimmune GmbH, Munich, Germany*

Edited by:
Cristina Bonorino, Pontificia Universidade Catolica do Rio Grande do Sul, Brazil

Reviewed by:
Lidija Klampfer, Montefiore Medical Center and Albert Einstein Cancer Center, USA
Ana Paula Souza, Pontificia Universidade Católica do Rio Grande do Sul, Brazil

****Correspondence:***
Gabriele Multhoff, Department of Radiation Oncology, Klinikum rechts der Isar, Technische Universität München, Ismaningerstr. 22, D-81675 Munich, Germany.
e-mail: gabriele.multhoff@lrz.tu-muenchen.de

Chronic inflammatory mediators exert pleiotropic effects in the development of cancer. On the one hand, inflammation favors carcinogenesis, malignant transformation, tumor growth, invasion, and metastatic spread; on the other hand inflammation can stimulate immune effector mechanisms that might limit tumor growth. The link between cancer and inflammation depends on intrinsic and extrinsic pathways. Both pathways result in the activation of transcription factors such as NF-κB, STAT-3, and HIF-1 and in accumulation of tumorigenic factors in tumor and microenvironment. STAT-3 and NF-κB interact at multiple levels and thereby boost tumor-associated inflammation which can suppress anti-tumor immune responses. These factors also promote tumor growth, progression, and metastatic spread. IL-1, IL-6, TNF, and PGHS-2 are key mediators of an inflammatory milieu by modulating the expression of tumor-promoting factors. In this review we concentrate on the crucial role of pro-inflammatory mediators in inflammation-driven carcinogenesis and outline molecular mechanisms of IL-1 signaling in tumors. In addition, we elucidate the dual roles of stress proteins as danger signals in the development of anti-cancer immunity and anti-apoptotic functions.

Keywords: inflammation, carcinogenesis, tumorigenic factors, heat shock proteins, NF-κB, STAT-3, IL-1

INTRODUCTION

Based on the presence of leukocytes in cancerous lesions, Rudolf Virchow, the founder of cellular pathology, speculated about an association between chronic inflammation and development of cancer already in 1863 (Virchow, 1863). In line with this observation, epidemiological studies indicate that apart from hereditary predisposition, inflammation serves as a potential risk factor for the development of cancer. Nowadays it is generally accepted that up to 25% of human malignancies are related to chronic inflammation and to viral and bacterial infections (Hussain and Harris, 2007). **Table 1** provides an overview on inflammatory and pathogenic conditions that are considered to be associated with malignant transformation.

Cancer-related chronic inflammation facilitates unlimited replicative potential, independence of growth factors, resistance to growth inhibition, escape of programmed cell death, enhanced angiogenesis, tumor extravasation, and metastasis (Hanahan and Weinberg, 2000). Cancer-related inflammation represents the seventh hallmark in the development of cancer (Colotta et al., 2009). Persistent microbial infections induced by parasites, bacteria, and viruses and physical and/or chemical stimuli can cause inflammation (Coussens and Werb, 2002). Bacterial infections following surgical removal of primary tumors can promote metastatic growth in mice (Pidgeon et al., 1999) and humans (Taketomi et al., 1997). This process is mediated most likely by endotoxins altering the critical balance between cell growth and angiogenesis (Pidgeon et al., 1999). Moreover, chronic inflammation induced by non-infectious agents can also contribute to carcinogenesis and act as a driving force in tumor development. Apart from toxins, oncoproteins and growth factors can affect the host via an activation of pattern recognition receptors (PRR) that interact with pathogen-associated molecular patterns (PAMP). These receptors comprise to members of the Toll-like receptor (TLR) family, nucleotide-binding oligomerization domain-like (NOD-like) receptors (NLR), C-type lectin receptors (CLR), triggering receptors on myeloid cells (TREM), and retinoic acid inducible gene-I-like receptors (RLR; Kawai and Akira, 2011). Binding of PAMP to these receptors leads to an initiation of the host's immune response by activation of inflammatory cells. The engagement of PRR triggers the induction of intracellular signaling pathways that induce the activation of numerous transcription factors such as NF-κB, STAT, and FOXO. These factors regulate the expression of several genes involved in the innate and adaptive immunity (Akira et al., 2006; Karin et al., 2006). Inadequate pathogen eradication, recurring tissue injury, prolonged inflammatory signaling, and failure of anti-inflammatory mechanisms can cause chronic inflammation which as a result supports tumorigenesis.

IMPACT OF INFLAMMATION IN TUMORIGENESIS

Numerous studies provide evidence that chronic inflammation increases the risk of cancer, promotes tumor progression, and supports metastatic spread (Mantovani et al., 2008; Aggarwal and Gehlot, 2009). In the initial phase of tumor development, inflammatory mediators such as cytokines, reactive oxygen species (ROS), and reactive nitrogen species (RNS) derived from tumor-infiltrating immune cells induce epigenetic alterations in premalignant lesions and silence tumor suppressor genes (Grivennikov and Karin, 2010). During tumor promotion, immune cells secrete cytokines and chemokines that act as survival and proliferation factors for malignant cells. The angiogenic switch is critical for

Table 1 | Inflammation and their related cancers.

Inductor	Inflammation	Cancer
Gut pathogens	Inflammatory bowel disease	Colorectal cancer
Tobacco smoke	Bronchitis	Bronchial lung cancer
Helicobacter pylori	Gastritis	Gastric cancer
Human papilloma virus	Cervicitis	Cervical cancer
Hepatitic B/C virus	Hepatitis	Hepatocellular carcinoma
Bacteria, gall bladder stones	Cholecystitis	Gall bladder cancer
Tobacco, genetics, alcohol	Pancreatitis	Pancreatic cancer
Epstein-Barr virus	Mononucleosis	Burkitt's lymphoma
Ultraviolet light	Sunburn	Melanoma
Asbestos fibers	Asbestosis	Mesothelioma
Gram-uropathogens	Schistosomiasis (Bilharzia)	Bladder cancer
Gastric acid, alcohol, tobacco	Esophagitis	Esophageal adenocarcinoma

an adequate supply of tumor cells with oxygen, nutrition, growth, and survival factors (Zumsteg and Christofori, 2009). During tumor progression and metastasis, both tumor and immune cells produce cytokines and chemokines leading to an increase in cell survival, motility, and invasiveness (DeNardo et al., 2008). Epithelial–mesenchymal transition (EMT), a crucial process in tumor invasiveness and metastasis, is also promoted (Yang and Weinberg, 2008). EMT refers to the loss of carcinoma epithelial phenotype and the acquisition of mesenchymal features (Zeisberg and Neilson, 2009). The group of Mehta recently found that aberrant tissue transglutaminase (TG2) expression induces EMT in epithelial cells (Kumar et al., 2010). This finding, in conjunction with the observation that inflammatory signals (e.g., TGF-β, TNF, and NF-κB) which induce EMT, also induce TG2 expression (Kawata et al., 2011), suggests a possible link between TG2, inflammation, and cancer progression presumably yielding novel therapeutic targets for improved patient outcomes. Other typical markers of EMT are cadherin-11 and fibroblast-specific protein (FSP)-1 which are associated with an increased motility (Zeisberg and Neilson, 2009). Twist is necessary to repress the transcription of E-cadherin (Thiery et al., 2009; Zeisberg and Neilson, 2009).

PATHWAYS CONNECTING INFLAMMATION AND CANCER

According to Mantovani et al. (2008), the connection between tumorigenesis and inflammation is mediated via intrinsic and extrinsic pathways. The intrinsic pathway is activated by genetic alterations causing inflammation and neoplasia. These alterations comprise mutation-driven proto-oncogene activation, chromosomal rearrangement/amplification, and inactivation of tumor suppressor genes. Transformed cells secrete inflammatory mediators and thus generate an inflammatory microenvironment. The extrinsic pathway is driven by inflammation or infections that increase the risk for the development of cancer in organs at risk such as the prostate, pancreas, colon, lung, and skin. Both pathways interfere in tumor cells and induce the activation of several transcription factors such as NF-κB, STAT-3, and HIF-1 that result in the formation of pro-inflammatory factors including chemokines, cytokines, and PGHS-2. These molecules recruit and activate various leukocyte populations such as macrophages, mast cells, eosinophils, and neutrophils into the tumor microenvironment like stromal and endothelial cells as well as infiltrating cells. This concerted action of tumor and micromilieu results in a more pronounced generation of inflammatory mediators that drives the progression of a positive amplification loop which further triggers tumor growth and invasiveness.

Proto-oncogene activation represents a critical component in the intrinsic pathway of cancer-related inflammation. In this context, mutations in *RAS* genes play an important role in tumorigenesis. Overall, up to 30% of all human tumors harbor mutations in canonical *RAS* genes (*KRAS, HRAS, NRAS*). Remarkably, these oncogenic mutations predominantly affect the *KRAS* locus, with oncogenic *KRAS* mutations being detected in 25–30% of all screened tumor samples (Forbes et al., 2011). The high frequency of *KRAS* mutations and their appearance in early tumor stages argue for a causative role of the K-Ras protein in human tumorigenesis (Fernandez-Medarde and Santos, 2011). More than 30 years ago the founding members of the *RAS* gene superfamily (*HRAS, NRAS, KRAS)* were discovered in human tumors as the first proto-oncogenes. Members of the RAS family are crucial for the connection of up-stream signals to down-stream effector pathways that are functionally related to cell cycle progression, growth, migration, cytoskeletal changes, apoptosis, and senescence. In tumor cells, activation of mutated RAS is followed by the induction of several intracellular signaling pathways. Signaling cascades induced by mutated RAS comprise the RAF/MEK/ERK kinase cascade, the PI3K/AKT pathway, and RalGDS proteins (Downward, 2009), the latter belonging to the family of nucleotide-exchange factors activating small GTPases such as RalB. Via the exocyst complex, an octameric protein complex implicated in tethering of vesicles to membranes (Yamashita et al., 2010), RalB stimulates the TANK-binding kinase-1 (TBK-1) resulting in NF-κB activation by IκBα phosphorylation. In cancer cells, a constitutive activation of this pathway, via chronic RalB activation, restricts the initiation of apoptosis after oncogenic stress (Chien et al., 2006). Beside NF-κB activation, TBK-1 activates the transcription factors IRF-3 and IRF-7 (Hacker and Karin, 2006) leading to the production of growth and inflammatory mediators. Previously it has been shown that K-Ras is a direct inducer of pro-inflammatory IL-6 and pro-angiogenic IL-8 required for the initiation of tumor-associated inflammation and neovascularization and promoting tumor growth. In these studies knock-down of *IL6*, genetic ablation of the *IL6* gene, or treatment with a neutralizing IL-6 antibody retarded K-Ras-driven tumorigenesis (Ancrile et al., 2007). Overexpression of oncogenic K-Ras in tumorigenic HeLa cells induced IL-8 secretion, while IL-8 inhibition reduced growth of these cells and the number of CD31+ cells in a xenograft tumor model (Sparmann and Bar-Sagi, 2004). Moreover, TBK-1 and NF-κB signaling have been identified as being essential in K-Ras mutant tumors (Barbie et al., 2009). Regarding these observations it was assumed that targeting the NF-κB signaling pathway might be effective in treating RAS-mutated tumors (Downward, 2009). Meylan et al. (2009) demonstrated that inhibition of the NF-κB pathway in lung tumors resulted in significantly reduced tumor growth.

CRITICAL MOLECULES IN CANCER-RELATED INFLAMMATION

Tumor-associated inflammation requires the presence and activation of inflammatory cells such as macrophages and granulocytes in the tumor microenvironment, formation of inflammatory mediators by tumor and stromal cells, tumor remodeling, and angiogenesis (Kundu and Surh, 2008; Colotta et al., 2009). Accumulation of microbial pathogens and tissue necrosis activate transcription factors that are necessary for the expression of, e.g., pro-angiogenic factors (IL-8, VEGF), growth factors (IL-6, GM-CSF), anti-apoptotic factors (Bcl-X_L, c-FLIP), invasion-promoting factors (MMP-2, MMP-7, MMP-9, uPA), inflammatory enzymes (PGHS-2, LOX), prostaglandins, iNOS, chemokines (CCL2, CCL20, IL-8), and pro-inflammatory cytokines (IL-1, IL-6, IL-23, TNF, TGF-β, EGF) that support the malignant phenotype. All molecules mentioned above are regulated by the transcription factor NF-κB, a key orchestrator in innate immunity and inflammation that has emerged as a crucial tumor promoter (Karin, 2006). The presence of constitutively active NF-κB was found to be associated with poor clinical outcome (for an overview see Aggarwal and Gehlot, 2009). NF-κB activation in inflammatory cells in response to infectious pathogens, pro-inflammatory mediators as well as necrotic cell products results in the generation of secretable factors that support growth, survival, and vascularization of pre-malignant and malignant cells (Karin, 2006). Activation of NF-κB up-regulates cell cycle mediators (cyclin D1, c-Myc), anti-apoptotic (c-FLIP, survivin, Bcl-X_L) and adhesion molecules (ICAM-1, ELAM-1, VCAM-17), proteolytic enzymes (e.g., MMP, uPA), and pro-inflammatory factors (PGHS-2, cytokines) that promote an invasive phenotype (Aggarwal and Gehlot, 2009). iNOS is another important inflammatory mediator that causes the production of NO by macrophages that links chronic inflammation and tumorigenesis. Elevated levels of NO have been found in numerous pre-cancerous and malignant lesions such as Barrett's mucosa (Wilson et al., 1998), prostate cancer (Aaltoma et al., 2001), breast cancer (De Paepe et al., 2002), and gastrointestinal carcinomas (Wink et al., 1998; Jaiswal et al., 2001). The iNOS product NO contributes to inflammation-associated tumorigenesis by inducing DNA damage, suppression of DNA repair, modification of oncoproteins, inhibition of apoptosis, promotion of tumor growth, angiogenesis, and metastasis as well as suppression of anti-tumor immunity (De Paepe et al., 2002). The NO-mediated inhibition of DNA repair enables cells harboring epigenetic alterations to escape from apoptosis. This results in clonal expansion of pre-malignant cells and subsequently to carcinogenesis (Sawa and Ohshima, 2006). Furthermore, NO promotes tumor growth by a transactivation of HIF-1α (Sandau et al., 2000), induces the expression of pro-angiogenic VEGF (Ravi et al., 2000), and down-regulates the tumor suppressor protein p53 (Ambs et al., 1998).

RANKL

RANKL, a member of the TNF superfamily of cytokines, was originally found in T and dendritic cells (DC). RANKL supports differentiation and survival of effector cells (Anderson et al., 1997). Moreover, it is essential for the differentiation of bone-resorbing osteoclasts derived from monocyte–macrophage precursors, and enables survival and function of mature osteoclasts (Li et al., 2000; Teitelbaum, 2000). Recent studies documented an expression of RANKL in a variety of other cell types, including tumor cells. Breast cancer cells are able to produce RANKL (Park et al., 2003; Cross et al., 2006) and stimulate osteoclast differentiation when co-cultured with bone marrow stromal cells (Park et al., 2003). HIF-1α-induced expression of RANKL initiates an increased migration of breast cancer cells via the PI3K/AKT pathway (Tang et al., 2011). The expression of RANKL in prostate cancer cells was found to be associated with an increased appearance of bone metastases (Brown et al., 2001; Chen et al., 2006). In head and neck squamous cell carcinoma RANKL expression promotes EMT and tumor progression by inducing VEGF-independent angiogenesis (Yamada et al., 2011). Moreover, the activity of RANKL was found to be involved in the pathophysiology of osteosarcoma (Mori et al., 2007a,b), giant cell tumors of the bone (Ng et al., 2010), Paget's sarcomas (Sun et al., 2006), and vascular diseases (Hofbauer and Schoppet, 2004). The expression of RANKL increases in response to pro-inflammatory mediators, such as IL-1 (Fernandez et al., 2010; Jurado et al., 2010). In fibroblast-like synoviocytes, murine osteoblastic, and fibroblastic cells, IL-23 was found to induce an up-regulation of RANKL via STAT-3 and NF-κB signaling pathways (Li et al., 2010; Mori et al., 2011). An exposure of these cells to pro-inflammatory cytokines such as IL-1, TNF, and IL-6 resulted into a direct or indirect activation of STAT-3 in a feed-forward loop. Further evidence for a crucial role of STAT-3 in the regulation of RANKL is shown by Schulze et al. (2010) who found that osteolytic prostate cancer cells induce the expression of RANKL in a STAT-3/5-dependent manner. Together these data highlight the significance of a STAT-3/5-mediated cytokine production in tumor cell migration and the formation of distant metastases.

IL-1 AND TNF

Elevated levels of IL-1 have been identified in several human tumor entities such as melanoma, head and neck, colon, lung, and breast cancer. Overall, patients harboring IL-1-positive tumors have markedly worse prognoses (Lewis et al., 2006). Due to its pleiotropic nature, IL-1 promotes tumor growth and metastasis in an autocrine/paracrine manner. IL-1 is produced by tumor, stromal and endothelial cells, and the host's infiltrating immune cells (Lewis et al., 2006). Depending on its subcellular location, different IL-1 isoforms mediate different functions. Membrane-bound IL-1α which is expressed on malignant cells induces anti-tumor immune responses, whereas, intracellular residing precursors of IL-1α control homeostatic functions including gene expression, differentiation, and cell growth. In contrast, low concentrations of secreted IL-1β down-regulate inflammatory responses and immune mechanisms, whereas high concentrations promote inflammation-associated tissue damage and tumor invasiveness (Apte et al., 2006). IL-1 can stimulate other cell types to produce pro-angiogenic and pro-metastatic mediators and thus plays an important role in inflammation-associated carcinogenesis (Lin and Karin, 2007; Voronov et al., 2007). In pancreatic cancer IL-1 confers chemoresistance via an up-regulation of PGHS-2 (Angst et al., 2008) and promotes angiogenesis during tumor progression (Shchors et al., 2006).

IL-1α and IL-1β exert identical agonist actions by binding to the IL-1 receptor type I (IL-1RI). After ligation, IL-1/IL-1RI associates with the IL-1 receptor accessory protein (IL-1RAcP) leading to activation of intracellular signal transduction cascades. This complex recruits a number of intracellular adapter molecules including MyD88 (Watters et al., 2007; Gay et al., 2011) to activate signal transduction pathways such as AP-1, p38MAPK, JNK, and NF-κB (**Figure 1**). In particular NF-κB provides a mechanistic link between inflammation and tumorigenesis. NF-κB is a major factor which controls apoptosis-based tumor immune surveillance mechanisms of pre-neoplastic and malignant cells. NF-κB also regulates tumor angiogenesis and invasiveness (Karin, 2006), and may contribute to chemoresistance of tumor cells (Fahy et al., 2004). A detailed description of the IL-1 signaling pathway is visualized schematically in **Figure 1**.

A third ligand, the naturally occurring IL-1 receptor antagonist (IL-1Ra), also binds to IL-1RI and acts as a true receptor antagonist. Because of its collagenase and prostaglandin-inhibiting properties, IL-1Ra (anakinra™) is approved for the treatment of chronic inflammatory diseases including rheumatoid arthritis (Dinarello, 1996) and systemic onset juvenile idiopathic arthritis (Hedrich et al., 2011). It has also been identified as being powerful in reverting IL-1 effects in numerous pathological settings (Dinarello, 1996). Actually, anakinra was successfully used in treating the rare lymphoproliferative disorder Castleman's disease (El-Osta et al., 2010) as well as in myeloma (Lust et al., 2009) rendering the use of anakinra and other IL-1-blocking agents such as canakinumab™(anti-IL-1β antibody) or rilonacept™(construct of the two extracellular chains of IL-1RI/IL-1RAcP complex fused to the Fc segment of IgG) promising therapeutic approaches in human metastatic diseases. The last two agents have been approved for the treatment of the cryopyrin-associated periodic syndrome (CAPS; Hoffman et al., 2008; Lachmann et al., 2009a), a grouping of familial cold auto-inflammatory syndrome, Muckle–Wells syndrome, and neonatal onset multi-inflammatory disease. As summarized by Dinarello (2010), there are two meaningful reasons for the use of IL-1-blocking agents in the treatment of metastatic diseases. On the one hand, none of the above mentioned agents have been found as being associated with any organ toxicities, gastrointestinal, or hematological abnormalities. On the other hand, unlike TNF-blocking agents IL-1-inhibiting treatments lack opportunistic infections although routine bacterial and upper airway infections are observed. Due to the safety of IL-1 blockage and the availability of the three therapeutics in limiting IL-1 actions, clinical trials are encouraged. An NIH trial of anakinra in the treatment of cutaneous melanoma is ongoing because IL-1 plays a pivotal role in angiogenesis by inducing/up-regulating pro-angiogenic IL-8 and VEGF contributing to the pathogenesis of, e.g., multiple melanoma (Dinarello, 2010).

As a pleiotropic cytokine, IL-1 harbors numerous intensifying effects on the physiological functions of diverse innate and immunocompetent cells (Mizel, 1982), IL-12-mediated induction of Th1 development (Weaver et al., 1988), and induction of Th17 cells (Sutton et al., 2006). IL-1 effects on immune tolerance are also reported (Nakata et al., 1995). For instance, IL-1β stimulates function of memory T cells and impairs that of Treg cells (O'Sullivan et al., 2006). This brief overview highlights the complexity of the mechanisms by which IL-1 regulates all types of immune responses including tumor cell eradication.

IL-1β is first synthesized as biologically inactive precursor (pro-IL-1β) that is further processed by caspase-1, also known as IL-1-converting enzyme (ICE), to the mature form, while pro-IL-1α is cleaved by calpain. Although IL-1β contributes to growth and metastatic spread in experimental and human cancers, the molecular mechanisms regulating the conversion of pro-IL-1β to the secreted and active cytokine remains to be elucidated.

An elaborate multi-protein complex, the so-called "inflammasome," is responsible for the recruitment and activation of caspase-1 (Martinon et al., 2002). Each inflammasome consists of different members of the nucleotide oligomerization domain-like receptor (NLR) family of proteins. Two of the best characterized human inflammasomes are NALP (NACHT, LRR, and pyrin domain-containing protein) 1 inflammasome and NALP2/3 inflammasome (Franchi et al., 2009). It was shown previously that in several auto-inflammatory diseases constitutive activation of NALP3 inflammasome leads to sustained local and systemic inflammation mediated by IL-1β (Goldbach-Mansky et al., 2006; Lachmann et al., 2009b). Recently, constitutively activated inflammasome was found in human melanoma cells (Okamoto et al., 2010). In this study human melanoma cells from the late stage of the disease spontaneously secrete biologically active IL-1β in the absence of exogenous stimuli because of constitutive activation of the inflammasome and IL-1 receptor (IL-1R) signaling. From these findings it can be concluded that IL-1-mediated autoinflammation contributes to the development and progression of human melanoma suggesting that inhibiting the inflammasome pathway or reducing IL-1 activity can be a therapeutic option for melanoma patients. The inflammasome also plays a substantial role in environmental cancer. It has been shown previously that silica and asbestos both activate the NALP3 inflammasome resulting in an increased IL-1β production and causing lung inflammation (Dostert et al., 2008). Chronic exposure to asbestos has been identified as being a high-risk factor for the development of mesothelioma implying a crucial contribution of inflammasome-mediated inflammation to the pathogenesis of mesothelioma. Controversely, in an animal model of colitis-associated cancer (CAC) the NALP3 inflammasome was found to be protective against CAC (Allen et al., 2010). The NALP3 inflammasome in DC obviously plays a crucial role by linking innate and adaptive immune responses against dying tumors (Ghiringhelli et al., 2009). Based on these observations one can hypothesize that constitutively active NALP3 inflammasome as can be found in certain tumors produces large amounts of IL-1 contributing to cancer-related inflammation and thus promoting tumor growth and invasiveness, whereas activation of the inflammasome in tumor-infiltrating immune cells might be beneficial in inducing anti-tumor immunity. According to Menu and Vince (2011), the NALP3 inflammasome can be considered as a triple-function agent ("the good, the bad, and the ugly") in human malignancies.

The pleiotropic cytokine TNF plays a dual role in tumorigenesis. At high concentrations TNF is destructive to tumor vasculature and induces necrosis. On the other hand, its critical role in chronic inflammation and its tumor-promoting capacity are well documented (Lin and Yeh, 2005; Mocellin et al., 2005). An increased expression of TNF was found in human bladder, breast, colorectal,

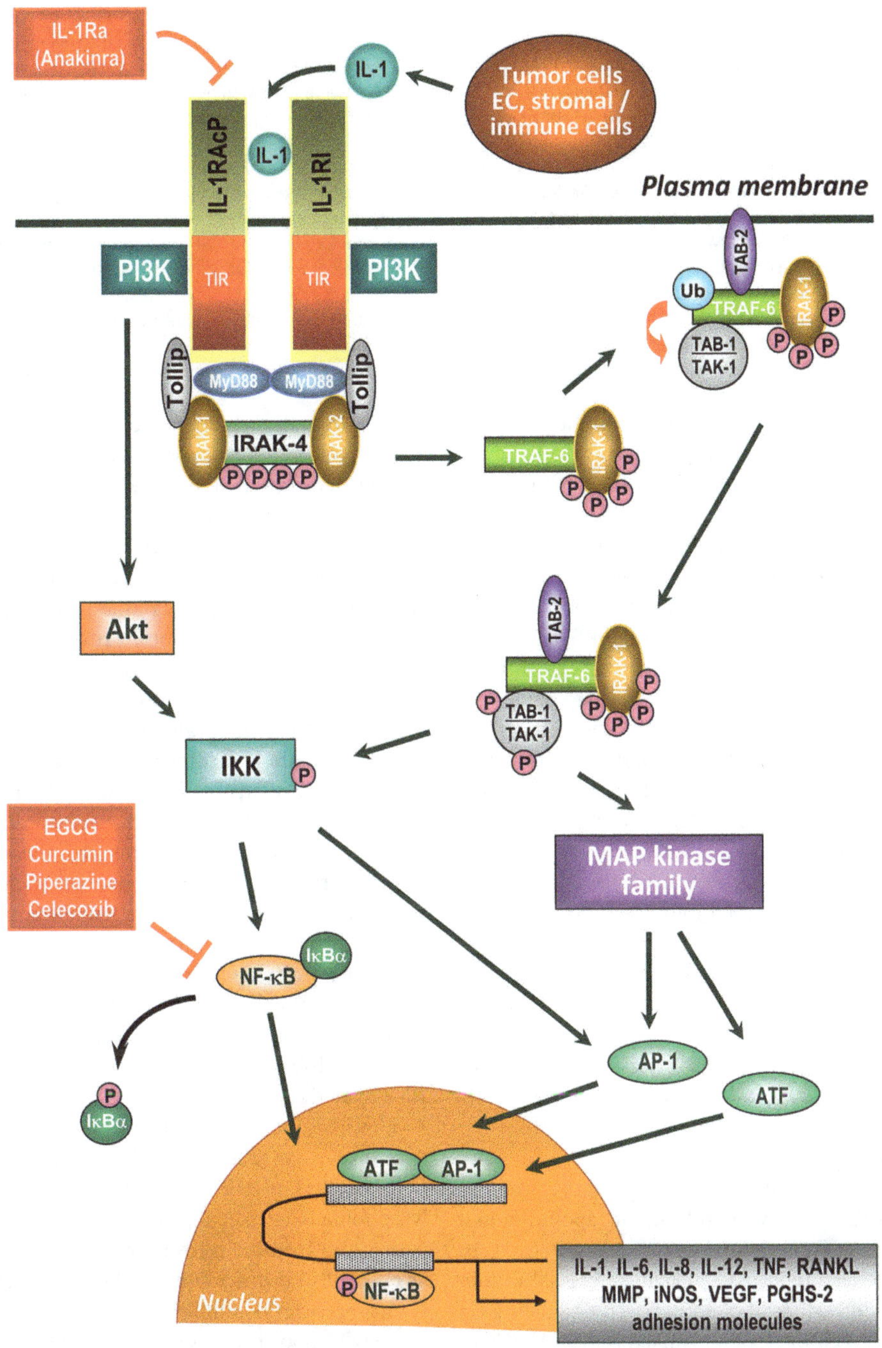

FIGURE 1 | IL-1 signaling in the tumor microenvironment. IL-1 is a critical molecule in inflammation-associated carcinogenesis produced directly by tumor cells or cells of the tumor microenvironment. IL-1 signal transduction is initiated by binding of either form of IL-1 to IL-1 receptor type I (IL-1RI), which undergoes a conformational change allowing the IL-1 receptor accessory protein (IL-1RAcP) to recognize the ligated IL-1RI. IL-1RAcP does not recognize IL-1 but represents an essential component in the IL-1 signaling pathway (Wesche et al., 1997b; Radons et al., 2002). The naturally occurring IL-1 receptor antagonist (IL-1Ra) also binds to IL-1RI without leading to its activation. Ligand-mediated heterodimerization of the receptor complex leads to recruitment of dimeric myeloid differentiation protein 88 (MyD88) via its TIR domain (Muzio et al., 1997; Wesche et al., 1997a; Radons et al., 2003) followed by complex formation between IRAK-4, MyD88, and IL-1RAcP and subsequent phosphorylation of IRAK-4 (Cahill and Rogers, 2008). After recruitment of IRAK-1/Tollip to the complex, IRAK-1 is initially phosphorylated by IRAK-4 (Born et al., 1998; Dunne and O'Neill, 2003). Subsequently, IRAK-1 (and possibly IRAK-2) becomes hyperphosphorylated and dissociates into the cytoplasm where it binds TNF receptor-associated factor 6 (TRAF-6; Cao et al., 1996). IRAK-1 interacts with membrane-bound TAK-binding protein 2 (TAB-2) as well as TAK-1/TAB-1 complex (Dower and Qwarnstrom, 2003) followed by translocation of TAB-2 from the plasma membrane to the signalosome and subsequent partial activation of TAK-1 by TAB-2. IRAK-1, presumably as dimer or oligomer, enables dimerization of TRAF-6 resulting in its ubiquitination and activation. In close proximity to TAB-2, TAK-1 is partially activated followed by complete activation through polyubiquitinated TRAF-6 (Kishimoto et al., 2000;

(continued)

FIGURE 1 | Continued
Martin and Wesche, 2002) enabling activation of numerous signaling cascades. Polyubiquitination of TRAF-6 obviously occurs through IRAK-2 (Keating et al., 2007). On the one hand, TAK-1 activates certain members of the MAP kinase family leading to activation of AP-1 and ATF (Ninomiya-Tsuji et al., 1999; O'Neill, 2000; Hefler et al., 2005; Blanco et al., 2008) the latter augmenting NF-κB-mediated transcription via transactivation (Jefferies and O'Neill, 2000; Cahill and Rogers, 2008). On the other hand, TAK-1 phosphorylates and activates IKK resulting in phosphorylation and inactivation of IκBα (Wang et al., 2001). Afterward, IκBα dissociates from the complex with NF-κB and undergoes proteasomal degradation. After phosphorylation, NF-κB translocates to the nucleus and activates NF-κB-dependent gene transcription (Chen and Greene, 2004). Inhibitors of NF-κB activation are indicated that suppress the inflammatory network in cancer development. IL-1 signaling also involves recruitment of PI3-kinase (PI3K) to the IL-1 receptor complex via the p85 regulatory subunit of PI3K (Reddy et al., 1997) and subsequent activation of AKT/PKB leading to IKK-dependent activation of NF-κB and AP-1 (Cahill and Rogers, 2008). Receptor ligation can also activate numerous G proteins resulting in activation of AP-1 and ATF mediated by several MAP kinases and an IκBα-independent transactivation of NF-κB (Singh et al., 1999; Jefferies and O'Neill, 2000). IL-1 signaling finally regulates gene expression of a great variety of tumorigenic factors including pro-angiogenic factors (IL-8, VEGF), growth factors (IL-6, GM-CSF), anti-apoptotic factors (Bcl-X_L, c-FLIP), invasion-promoting factors (MMP-2, MMP-7, MMP-9, uPA), inflammatory enzymes (PGHS-2, LOX), prostaglandins, iNOS, chemokines (CCL2, CCL20, IL-8), and pro-inflammatory cytokines (IL-1, IL-6, IL-23, TNF, TGF-β, EGF, RANKL).

and prostate cancer as well as in leukemia and lymphoma (Balkwill and Mantovani, 2001). TNF is also produced by cells of the tumor microenvironment. Binding of TNF to the TNF receptor 1 (TNFR1) activates signaling cascades of NF-κB and c-Jun N-terminal kinase (JNK) which lead to an up-regulation of several pro-inflammatory, pro-angiogenic and invasiveness-promoting factors, and to the induction of anti-apoptotic molecules such as the caspase-8 inhibitor c-FLIP. Activation of NF-κB in response to TNFR1 terminates the activity of JNK (Kamata et al., 2005). The ubiquitin ligase Itch is a substrate of JNK that enables the degradation of c-FLIP (Chang et al., 2006). Inhibition of JNK via NF-κB-mediated blockage leads to an inactivation of Itch. This prevents degradation of c-FLIP and ensures tumor cell survival. Apart from its role in tumor initiation, TNF promotes angiogenesis and impairs immune surveillance by affecting T cell responses and the activity of macrophages (Elgert et al., 1998). The tumor-promoting role of TNF was confirmed in animal models. In the absence of TNF mice do not develop hepatocellular carcinoma in response to cholestatic hepatitis (Pikarsky et al., 2004). TNF and TNFR-deficient mice were also found to be resistant to chemically induced carcinogenesis of the skin (Arnott et al., 2004). These findings indicate that pro-inflammatory activity of TNF functions as a pivotal mediator in tumorigenesis (Lin and Karin, 2007).

IL-6 AND PGHS-2 (COX-2)

IL-6 is another NF-κB-regulated pleiotropic pro-inflammatory mediator that enables tumor growth and inhibits apoptosis in a variety of human tumors (Rose-John and Schooltink, 2007). In contrast, IL-6 has also been reported as playing a crucial role in terminating inflammation (Hudson et al., 2008). IL-6 signaling via the membrane-bound receptor IL-6Ra is linked to the JAK/STAT pathway (predominantly through activation of STAT-3) and leads to the expression of genes encoding for anti-apoptotic cell cycle progression molecules (Lin and Karin, 2007). In contrast, a soluble form of the IL-6R can bind IL-6 with the same affinity as the membrane-bound form and the complex of IL-6 and the soluble IL-6R (sIL6R) can induce signaling in a process called IL-6 trans-signaling (Peters et al., 1998). Because the IL-6R is only sparely expressed, IL-6 trans-signaling dramatically increases the number of potential IL-6 target cells (Rose-John et al., 2006). Animal models of inflammatory colon cancer suggest that IL-6 trans-signaling serves as the major pro-inflammatory paradigm of IL-6 signaling under pathophysiologic conditions (Becker et al., 2004). It turns out that regenerative or anti-inflammatory activities of IL-6 are mediated by classic signaling whereas pro-inflammatory responses of interleukin-6 are rather mediated by trans-signaling (Rabe et al., 2008). This is important since therapeutic blockade of IL-6 by the neutralizing anti-IL-6 receptor monoclonal antibody tocilizumab™ has recently been approved for the treatment of inflammatory diseases. A recently performed clinical trial revealed that IL-6 inhibition by tocilizumab retards joint damage progression in patients with rheumatoid arthritis (Smolen et al., 2011). Interestingly, inhibition of IL-6R-mediated signaling using tocilizumab in a xenograft model of oral squamous cell carcinoma (OSCC) suppressed tumor growth and angiogenesis by down-regulating VEGF mRNA expression (Shinriki et al., 2009). Clinical studies inclusive those mentioned above have shown that inhibition of IL-6 signaling by tocilizumab is therapeutically effective not only in chronic inflammatory diseases such as rheumatoid arthritis (Nishimoto et al., 2004), juvenile idiopathic arthritis (Yokota et al., 2004), and Crohn's disease (Ito et al., 2004) but also in Castleman's disease (Nishimoto et al., 2005). In all of these diseases, tocilizumab ameliorates inflammatory manifestations, and normalizes acute phase protein levels. Given its success in treating these diseases, tocilizumab may also prove useful in treating IL-6-related cancers.

Elevated IL-6 levels are found in numerous tumors such as multiple myeloma (Klein et al., 1992), colorectal cancer (Chung and Chang, 2003), gastric carcinoma (Kai et al., 2005), and Hodgkin lymphoma (Cozen et al., 2004). Moreover, malignant ascites from patients with epithelial ovarian cancer was found to contain high levels of IL-6 (Offner et al., 1995). In breast cancer patients high IL-6 concentrations induced by an *IL6* gene polymorphism correlate with poor prognosis (Berger, 2004). A comparison of non-metastasizing pancreatic cancer, benign prostatic hyperplasia, and metastasized pancreatic cancer revealed elevated levels of IL-6 in the latter, more aggressive tumor (Weiss et al., 2011). In this study it was shown that IL-6 leads to an increased expression of uPA and VEGF which implies a crucial role of IL-6 in angiogenesis of pancreatic tumors. In OSCC lysophosphatidic acid (LPA), a bioactive lipid with a growth factor-like activity induces the secretion of IL-6 and IL-8 in an NF-κB- and AP-1-dependent manner (Hwang et al., 2011). Direct stimulation of human osteoblasts with IL-6 and IL-8 induced the expression of RANKL and thereby promotes osteoclast formation. From these findings it can be concluded that IL-6 and IL-8 derived from LPA-stimulated OSCC play a crucial role in osteogenesis and bone resorption. Inhibition of IL-6 signaling in colon cancer resulted in a reduced tumor growth in mice (Becker et al., 2004; Greten et al., 2004). Incubation of cholangiocarcinoma cells with an anti-IL-6-neutralizing antiserum reduced AKT phosphorylation and down-regulated the expression of Mcl-1. This indicates a contribution of IL-6 in the AKT-mediated survival mechanisms (Kobayashi et al., 2005).

PGHS-2, formerly termed as COX-2, has emerged as another pro-inflammatory mediator in tumorigenesis whose expression is mediated by NF-κB. The expression of PGHS-2 is inducible in response to stimuli such as mitogens, cytokines, growth factors, or hormones. PGHS-2 is the rate-limiting enzyme involved in the conversion of arachidonic acid to prostanoids acting as key mediators of inflammation. Aberrant or increased expression of PGHS-2 has been shown to be involved in the pathogenesis of breast, gastric, colorectal, lung, prostate, head/neck, and pancreatic cancer. PGHS-2 affects cell proliferation, apoptosis, angiogenesis, and metastasis (Lu et al., 2006; Aggarwal and Gehlot, 2009). Overexpression of PGHS-2 results in the secretion of large amounts of VEGF and therefore, is associated with increased tumor cell invasion and poor prognosis (Raut et al., 2004; Ladetto et al., 2005). In human basal cell carcinoma cells elevated levels of PGHS-2 led to an up-regulated expression of the anti-apoptotic molecules Mcl-1 and Bcl-2, VEGF and basic fibroblast growth factor (bFGF; Tjiu et al., 2006). In chronic inflammation, endothelial cells express both, acute phase genes and adhesion molecules that enable recruitment of leukocytes to the site of tissue damage. Moreover, an enhanced production of prostaglandins mediated by PGHS-2 augments vasopermeability leading to a more pronounced recruitment of leukocytes (Jura et al., 2005). Leukocytes are the main source of RNS and ROS acting as chemical effectors in inflammation-driven carcinogenesis (Kundu and Surh, 2008). We identified a constitutively enhanced expression of PGHS-2 in human pancreatic adenocarcinoma cells that is further increased in the presence of IL-1 (Bauer et al., 2009; Hoffmann et al., 2011). The constitutive production of PGHS-2 and its key product PGE_2 in the microenvironment of pancreatic carcinomas accounts for an enhanced malignancy of pancreatic tumor cells which is caused by inhibition of apoptosis, increase in cell proliferation, induction of angiogenesis, and invasion of malignant cells into surrounding tissue (Merati et al., 2001; Kong et al., 2002; Garcea et al., 2005). PGHS-2 also induces the expression of MMP-2 (Surh et al., 2001; Sansone et al., 2009; Wang et al., 2009b) and pro-inflammatory IL-6 and IL-1 via PGE_2 (Takahashi et al., 2008). PGHS-2-mediated effects on growth, angiogenesis, invasiveness, and metastasis are augmented by the IL-1-induced up-regulation of the enzyme by forcing the progression of a positive amplification loop triggered by PGE_2 and IL-6. Of note, it was demonstrated that PGE_2 contributes to cancer progression by inhibiting DC differentiation and function, acting paradoxically as an immunosuppressive factor (Muthuswamy et al., 2010; Stock et al., 2011). In cervical cancer, PGE_2 was found to induce a cytokine production profile and phenotypical features of tolerogenic DC suggesting that the altered expression of PGE_2 might promote carcinogenesis by favoring (pre)cancer immunotolerance (Herfs et al., 2009). In addition, IL-6 derived from tumor cells or cells of the tumor microenvironment was shown to polarize DC toward immune tolerance through the induction of STAT-3 activation (Alshamsan, 2011). Therefore, tumor-induced p-STAT-3 in DC can be seen as a promising target for colon cancer immunotherapy. In this context, knocking-down the IL-6 receptor α-chain of DC vaccines significantly enhanced the frequency of tumor-specific CD8+ CTL-producing effector molecules such as IFN-γ, TNF, FasL, perforin, and granzyme B, and generated more CD8+ memory T cells, leading to the substantially prolonged survival of cytotoxic lymphocytes (Tc1) tumor-bearing mice (Hwang et al., 2010).

Most of the PGHS-2-induced effects are mediated through its product PGE_2 (Yoshimatsu et al., 2001a,b). Thus, down-regulation of prostaglandins in tumor tissues by PGHS-2 inhibition blocks several neoplastic pathways leading to the suppression of tumor growth (Maier et al., 2004). In this context, PGHS-2 inhibitors hold promise for cancer chemoprevention. Among them, the non-steroidal anti-inflammatory drug (NSAID) celecoxib constitutes a potent and specific inhibitor of the inducible human PGHS-2. Celecoxib interferes with tumor initiation and tumor cell growth *in vitro* and *in vivo*. Preclinical studies demonstrate promising anti-cancer effects of celecoxib in colorectal, pancreatic as well as head and neck carcinomas. Additionally, celecoxib was found to increase tumor cell sensitivity toward radiochemotherapy (reviewed by Jendrossek, 2011). Celecoxib has also been found to impair tissue expression of VEGF, tumor angiogenesis, and metastasis in an experimental model of pancreatic cancer (Wei et al., 2004). Thus, modulation of PGHS-2 expression may be a promising approach in cancer therapy (Jimeno et al., 2006). However, due to the high toxicity of PGHS-2 inhibitors, the development of novel components is necessary (Spektor and Fuster, 2005; Lee et al., 2007). Randomized clinical trials and meta-analyses reported on an increased risk for cardiovascular diseases in patients receiving long-term treatment with PGHS-2 inhibitors. These cardiovascular adverse effects include myocardial infarction, stroke, and cardiovascular death/heart failure (summarized by Trelle et al., 2011). This increased rate of life-threatening cardiovascular side effects led to the withdrawal of the PGHS-2 inhibitors valdecoxib and rofecoxib from the market that had been approved by the United States Food and Drug Association. A patient-pooled analysis of adjudicated data from 7,950 patients in six placebo-controlled trials demonstrated a dose regimen-related increase in the risk of serious cardiovascular events after a daily administration of 400 and 800 mg celecoxib (Solomon et al., 2008). Although long-term treatment with high-dose celecoxib can enhance the risk for cardiovascular diseases, the drug is still used at lower doses in the United States since it is less toxic compared to other PGHS-2 inhibitors (Solomon et al., 2008; Trelle et al., 2011).

A novel approach to overcome the limitations associated with the toxicity of PGHS-2 inhibitors is to combine chemical PGHS-2 inhibitors at low doses with naturally occurring compounds such as the catechin EGCG which is a promising chemopreventive agent derived from green tea (summarized by Cerella et al., 2010). Our group investigated the effects of a combinatorial treatment with celecoxib and EGCG on the expression of IL-1-induced tumorigenic factors in human pancreatic adenocarcinoma cells. We found that the combined administration of celecoxib and EGCG can induce synergistic cancer preventive effects in pancreatic cancer cells by down-regulating tumorigenic factors and inducing apoptosis (Härdtner et al., 2009). Previous investigations of our group and others revealed anti-proliferative and apoptosis-inducing effects of EGCG and celecoxib in pancreatic cancer cells (Chen and Zhang, 2007; Inaba et al., 2008; Xu et al., 2008; Hoffmann et al., 2011). The anti-proliferative properties of NSAID such as celecoxib are related to effects on the cell cycle (Xiong, 2004) including changes in gene expression that favor cell cycle arrest (Yip-Schneider et al., 2001; Tseng et al., 2002). Interestingly, several studies revealed an anti-proliferative effect of PGHS-2-selective inhibitors not only in PGHS-2-positive but also in PGHS-2-negative pancreatic tumor cells implying that the inhibitory action of NSAID on cell proliferation can affect both, PGHS-2-dependent and -independent pathways (Molina et al., 1999; Yip-Schneider et al., 2001). Numerous investigations also documented an apoptosis-inducing potential of NSAID (Maier et al., 2004; Suganuma et al., 2011). Celecoxib targets several proteins distinct from PGHS-2 that are involved in the control of cell survival and cell death including the anti-apoptotic proteins survivin, Mcl-1, and Bcl-2 (Sakoguchi-Okada et al., 2007; Rudner et al., 2010). Further, PGHS-2-independent molecular targets of celecoxib comprise the survival kinase AKT/PKB and its up-stream regulator 3-phosphoinositide-dependent kinase-1 (PDK-1; Belham et al., 1999; Kulp et al., 2004), cyclin-dependent kinase inhibitors, and cyclins (Grosch et al., 2006), as well as the sarcoplasmic/endoplasmic reticulum calcium ATPase SERCA (Johnson et al., 2002). By counteracting these molecules celecoxib interferes with the activation status of caspases and finally induces apoptosis.

EGCG-mediated effects on apoptosis include caspase-3/-9 activation, PARP cleavage, Bax oligomerization, mitochondrial membrane depolarization, direct interaction with anti-apoptotic members of the Bcl-2 family as well as NF-κB inhibition (Lambert et al., 2005; Shimizu et al., 2005; Inaba et al., 2008). Celecoxib is reported to interfere, among others, with the NF-κB signaling pathway (Niederberger et al., 2001; Shirode and Sylvester, 2010) providing the basis for the synergism with EGCG. Based on these findings one can hypothesize that celecoxib in combination with EGCG may promote apoptosis directly or indirectly thus altering the cellular death threshold in tumor cells (Jendrossek, 2011). In previous studies EGCG has been shown to synergistically enhance the effects of TRAIL (Siddiqui et al., 2008) and PGHS-2 inhibitors NS-398 (Adhami et al., 2007) and celecoxib (Basu and Haldar, 2009). In a human lung (Suganuma et al., 2011) and prostate cancer (Adhami et al., 2007) model the combination of celecoxib and EGCG increased tumor cell apoptosis and decreased inflammation. Other natural compounds affecting the PGHS-2 expression include the non-flavonoid polyphenols curcumin from turmeric *Curcuma longa,* resveratrol from red wine, isoflavone genistein from lupin as well as omega-3 fatty acids from oily fish flaxseeds. Such a combinatory administration might have future clinical implications with respect to an adjuvant therapy in cancer patients, since it might reduce the adverse effects of high-dose celecoxib as a monotherapy.

INTERACTIONS OF NF-κB AND STAT-3

Both, STAT-3 and NF-κB are crucial for cancer-related inflammation. NF-κB does not only mediate tumorigenesis but also exerts anti-tumorigenic effects in tumor cells and in the tumor microenvironment (for a review see Ben-Neriah and Karin, 2011). Evidence for a positive association of NF-κB activation with tumor-associated inflammation came from colitis-associated colon cancer (Greten et al., 2004; Pikarsky et al., 2004) and hepatitis-associated hepatocellular carcinoma (Pikarsky et al., 2004). Colitis-associated colon cancer represents a classical example for an inflammation-triggered malignancy. NF-κB activation in intestinal epithelial cells of this cancer model was found to enhance the survival of pre-malignant progenitor cells by inducing anti-apoptotic Bcl-X_L (Greten et al., 2004; Pikarsky et al., 2004). NF-κB activation in cancer seems to be related, at least in part, by mutations in components of the signaling cascade or effects of inflammatory factors in the tumor microenvironment that accumulate after NF-κB activation (Karin et al., 2002). Transcriptional activation of NF-κB leads to the induction of pro-inflammatory cytokines (e.g., IL-1, IL-6, TNF), chemokines (IL-8), PGHS-2, MMP, and adhesion molecules (ICAM-1, VCAM-1). The presence of constitutively active NF-κB in most tumors correlate with a poor clinical outcome (Weichert et al., 2007). Moreover, most chemopreventive agents including nutraceuticals derived from different sources have the potential to suppress constitutive and inducible NF-κB activation pathways (Aggarwal and Gehlot, 2009) in order to block chronic inflammation.

Whilst NF-κB signaling contributes to both, inflammation-driven carcinogenesis and anti-tumor immunity, STAT-3 induces cancer-promoting inflammation and restrains anti-tumor immune responses by counteracting NF-κB-induced expression of anti-tumor Th1 cytokines (IL-12, IFN-γ; Kortylewski et al., 2005; Yu et al., 2007). Furthermore, STAT-3 contributes to the expansion and development of Treg and Th17 cells (Wang et al., 2009a; Wu et al., 2009). STAT-3 also induces the expression of tumorigenic mediators (cytokines, pro-angiogenic, and growth factors) and their corresponding receptors that in turn activate a STAT-3 mediated immunoregulatory circuit in the tumor microenvironment (Yu et al., 2007). Thus, the constitutive activation of STAT-3, does not only promote cancer-related inflammation but also suppresses anti-tumor immune responses (Yu et al., 2009).

As already mentioned, the association of cancer with chronic inflammation is related to intrinsic and extrinsic pathways, both leading to activation of NF-κB and STAT-3. Similarly to NF-κB, constitutively active STAT-3 is found in breast, ovarian, prostate, and brain tumors, leukemia, lymphoma, and multiple myeloma. STAT-3 activation results in the modulation of the expression of numerous genes that are crucial for maintaining/amplifying tumor-associated inflammation and promoting tumor growth and progression (Yu et al., 2009). The NF-κB family comprises homo- and heterodimeric transcription factors consisting of RelA, c-Rel, RelB, NF-κB1 (p50 and its precursor p105), and NF-κB2 (p52 and its precursor p100) with RelA-p50 as being the most prominent NF-κB transcription factor (Vallabhapurapu and Karin, 2009). Physiologically, NF-κB is sequestered in the cytosol by its inhibitory component, IκBα. Upon phosphorylation by the IκB kinase complex (IKK), IκBα is degraded in an ubiquitin-dependent manner in the proteasome. Then NF-κB translocates into the nucleus where predominantly RelA-p50 up-regulates the expression of Th1 immunostimulatory genes (IL-12, CD40, CD80) that are important for the control of microbial infections and tumor cells (Yu et al., 2007, 2009). STAT-3 opposes the anti-tumor immune responses mediated by NF-κB within a cell. On the one hand, STAT-3 is able to inhibit IKK during acute inflammation and thus attenuates Th1 immune responses (Lee et al., 2009). On the other hand, STAT-3 prolongs the nuclear retention of RelA during oncogenic and chronic inflammation by acting as a co-transcription factor for RelA thus contributing to the persistent activation of NF-κB during chronic inflammation and the malignant process (Yu et al., 2009). It has been shown previously that STAT-3 promotes nuclear localization of RelA by acetyltransferase p300-mediated acetylation affecting the NF-κB/IκBα interaction and avoiding its nuclear export (Chen and Greene, 2004). Since STAT-3 is a prerequisite for p300-mediated acetylation of RelA, constitutive activity of RelA in tumors requires continuous STAT-3 signaling (Lee et al., 2009). Accordingly, increased STAT-3 activity found in tumors preferentially leads to an association of NF-κB with STAT-3 via p300. Due to the NF-κB activating capacity of STAT-3 in malignancies constitutive activity of STAT-3 found in tumors preferentially requires RelA (Yu et al., 2009). As stated by the authors, this reciprocal relationship is related to the fact that numerous RelA-encoded target gene products function as STAT-3 activators (e.g., IL-6, IL-11, IL-17, IL-21, IL-23, PGHS-2). Remarkably, expression of IL-6, IL-17, IL-23, and PGHS-2 (all of them activating STAT-3) depends on STAT-3 as co-transcription factor for NF-κB. As a consequence, STAT-3 and NF-κB interact at multiple levels and thereby boost tumor-associated inflammation.

HEAT SHOCK PROTEINS AND TUMORIGENESIS

Heat shock proteins (HSP) are highly conserved proteins expressed in a wide range of species where they inhabit nearly all cellular and subcellular compartments. Environmental stress (e.g., heat, hypoxia, bacterial infections, heavy metals, oxidative stress, inflammation) as well as physiological processes (differentiation, proliferation, maturation) result in an increased HSP synthesis (Lindquist and Craig, 1988; DeNagel and Pierce, 1992). Intracellular residing HSP protect cells against lethal damage induced by environmental stress, and support folding and transport of newly produced polypeptides and aberrant proteins (Hartl, 1996). Depending on their intra-/extracellular localization HSP mediate different functions. On the one hand, up-regulated intracellular HSP levels protect tumor cells from lethal damage induced by environmental stress. On the other hand, membrane-bound and extracellular residing HSP with molecular weights of 70 and 90 kDa were identified as key regulators of the host's immune system.

A variety of HSP were found on the plasma membrane of tumor cell lines as determined by selective cell surface protein profiling (Shin et al., 2003). These findings were confirmed by a broad screening program of human tumor biopsies in our laboratory using cmHsp70.1 mAb (Stangl et al., 2011). Phenotypic analyses revealed that Hsp70, the major stress-inducible member of the HSP70 group, is found on the plasma membrane in 50–70% of colon, lung, pancreas, mammary, head and neck, lung, and urogenital carcinomas (Multhoff et al., 1995a,b; Chen et al., 2002). Metastases exhibit an elevated Hsp70 membrane density compared to primary tumors in humans (unpublished observation). These data were confirmed in a xenograft tumor mouse model. After orthotopic injection of human tumor cells into immunodeficient animals the cell surface density of Hsp70 was greater on metastases than on primary tumors (Multhoff et al., 2000; Stangl et al., 2006). Interestingly, the corresponding normal tissue of the mice was always found to be membrane Hsp70-negative (Stangl et al., 2011). These findings might be explained by the fact that membrane Hsp70 might facilitate metastases, support adherence of tumor cells to endothelial cells and organs, or might confer resistance to an unfavorable milieu during metastasis. In line with these findings we could show that overall survival of patients with membrane Hsp70-positive squamous cell carcinomas of the lung and lower rectal carcinomas was significantly reduced compared to those patients with membrane Hsp70-negative tumors (Pfister et al., 2007). Apart from solid tumors also bone marrow samples of patients suffering from acute (AML) and chronic (CML) myeloid leukemia are frequently membrane Hsp70-positive (Gehrmann et al., 2003). Quantitative analysis revealed that ~15–20% of the total Hsp70 is present in tumor cell membranes (Gehrmann et al., 2008). The anchorage of Hsp70 within the plasma membrane is most likely mediated by the tumor-specific glycosphingolipid Gb3 (Gehrmann et al., 2008). This led us to the hypothesis that membrane Hsp70 might provide an ideal tumor-specific molecule for a targeted immunotherapeutic approach.

Even in the absence of immunogenic peptides, Hsp70, or a peptide derived thereof in combination with pro-inflammatory cytokines such as IL-2 and IL-15 has the capacity to stimulate the cytolytic activity of NK cells against membrane Hsp70-positive tumor cells (Multhoff et al., 1997, 2001). The mechanism of tumor cell killing has been identified as perforin-independent granzyme B-mediated apoptosis (Gross et al., 2003b). Granzyme B derived from activated NK cells specifically binds to membrane Hsp70 on tumor cells and following Hsp70-mediated endocytosis, apoptosis is induced (Gross et al., 2003a,b). Hsp70 also has been detected on tumor-derived exosomes of membrane Hsp70-positive tumors (Gastpar et al., 2005). These data suggest that NK cells might be attracted to membrane Hsp70-positive tumors *in vivo* via the secretion of Hsp70 surface-positive exosomes. Incubation of NK cells with Hsp70 protein or a 14mer-peptide derived from the C-terminus of Hsp70 is accompanied by an up-regulation of activating receptors on NK cells such as CD94/NKG2C, NKG2D, NKp30, NKp44, and NKp46 (Gross et al., 2003b,c). Hsp70 membrane-positive tumors are thus efficiently eliminated by NK cells that had been pre-stimulated with low dose IL-2 plus Hsp70 peptide (Multhoff et al., 1999). Adoptive transfer of these TKD-stimulated NK cells in tumor-bearing mice revealed identical results *in vivo* (Botzler et al., 1998; Multhoff et al., 2000; Moser et al., 2002). It is known that IL-2-activated NK cells are able to induce regression of established lung and liver tumors (Schwarz et al., 1989; Yasumura et al., 1994; Vujanovic et al., 1995; Whiteside et al., 1998). Our group identified a specific migratory capacity of NK cells toward Hsp70-postive tumor cells and supernatants derived thereof. The same effect could be observed for the Hsp70 peptide TKD (Gastpar et al., 2004). From these results we speculated that killing of Hsp70-positive tumors *in vivo* might be related to an enhanced migratory and cytolytic capacity of pre-activated NK cells.

The rapid induction of HSP in response to environmental stress is based on a variety of genetic and biochemical processes referred to as the heat shock response (HSR; Shamovsky and Nudler, 2008). The link between HSR and cancer development has been emerging since more than 20 years. HSR is regulated mainly at the transcription level by heat shock factors (HSF). Among them, HSF-1 is considered as being the key transcription factor of stress-inducible HSP (Pirkkala et al., 2001; Akerfelt et al., 2010). As a consequence, HSP are over-expressed in a wide spectrum of human malignancies contributing to tumor growth, differentiation, invasiveness, and metastasis and being associated with poor prognosis in certain cancer types (Ciocca and Calderwood, 2005). HSP over-expression in tumor cells plays a pivotal role in tumorigenesis by inhibiting apoptosis and senescence. In breast cancer, transformation-induced activation of HSF-1 results in an up-regulated expression of Hsp27 and Hsp70 which in turn results in protection against apoptosis (Calderwood, 2010). HSF-1 also triggers expression of Hsp90, an essential factor in tumor growth due to its ability to chaperone a variety of oncogenic signaling proteins including Her-2/neu and c-Src (Kamal et al., 2003; Neckers and Lee, 2003; Calderwood, 2010). Several studies have shown that Her-2/neu (c-ErbB-2) is amplified and over-expressed in many tumors such as breast, ovarian, and gastric adenocarcinoma (Hynes and Stern, 1994). Since HSP over-expression also protects from drug-related apoptosis (Khaleque et al., 2005), these mechanisms highlight the role of HSP in tumor progression and therapy resistance.

Recent studies indicate an involvement of HSP such as Hsp70/Hsp72 and Hsp90 in the recognition of PAMP by binding to TLR-4 within lipid rafts (Triantafilou and Triantafilou, 2004; Wheeler et al., 2009). Since extracellular residing Hsp70 acts as a danger signal for the immune system (Matzinger, 1998), this stress protein has been added to the list of "alarmins." Endogenous alarmins and exogenous PAMP both comprise the group of danger-associated molecular patterns (DAMP; Bianchi, 2007). Hsp70, added exogenously to cells stimulates the production of pro-inflammatory cytokines TNF, IL-1β, and IL-6 by antigen presenting cells (Asea et al., 2000a,b, 2002). Extracellular Hsp70 has also been found to induce IL-8 production in human bronchial epithelial cells (Chase et al., 2007). *In vitro* co-culturing of colon tumor cell spheroids with normal cells caused a significant tumor grade-dependent increase in IL-6 production thereby altering Hsp70 expression (Paduch et al., 2009). From these observations it can be concluded that Hsp70 may enhance the impact of tumorigenic mediators in the tumor microenvironment.

CONCLUDING REMARKS

Cancer-related inflammation has emerged as one of the hallmarks of cancer (Hanahan and Weinberg, 2011). In the last two decades, several tumorigenic factors have been identified as being implicated in inflammation-associated carcinogenesis. These factors are released by tumor cells or cells of the tumor microenvironment such as stromal cells, endothelial cells, or host infiltrating cells, respectively, and include pro-inflammatory cytokines, pro-angiogenic and growth-promoting factors, anti-apoptotic and invasion-promoting factors, inflammatory enzymes, prostaglandins, iNOS as well as chemokines. Among them, IL-1, TNF, and IL-6 act as crucial mediators of inflammation-driven tumorigenesis forming an inflammatory network in cancer as outlined in **Figure 2.** These mediators activate the key transcription factors in tumor-associated inflammation: NF-κB, STAT-3, and HIF-1 impacting any stage of tumorigenesis such as initiation, promotion as well as progression, and metastasis. It is noteworthy that NF-κB might be the central player in tumorigenesis. NF-κB is activated by a great variety of lifestyle-related factors including infectious agents, irradiation, environmental stimuli, tobacco, stress, dietary agents, obesity, and alcohol accounting for almost 95% of all cancers (Aggarwal and Gehlot, 2009). Modern anti-tumor therapies thus aim to suppress NF-κB activation. Most of the chemopreventive agents have been found as being able to suppress NF-κB activation like the selective PGHS-2 inhibitor celecoxib. Moreover, lifestyle-related agents derived from different sources including fruits, legumes, vegetables, grains, spices, and exercise are also able to inhibit NF-κB leading to suppression of the inflammatory network (Aggarwal and Gehlot, 2009). Clinical and pre-clinical studies are conducted to suppress the inflammatory network by the use of, e.g., steroids (dexamethasone, prednisolone), TNF inhibitors (thalidomide = thalomid™, anti-TNF antibodies such as infliximab = remicade™, etanercept = enbrel™, adalimumab = humira™), IL-1 inhibitors (anakinra™ = IL-1 receptor antagonist), PGHS-2 inhibitors (celecoxib), NF-κB inhibitors (curcumin, EGCG, piperazine), and RANKL inhibitors (denosumab™ = fully human monoclonal anti-RANKL antibody). A promising approach in cancer therapy also might be targeting HSP, because up-regulated Hsp90 and Hsp70 in cancer cells have

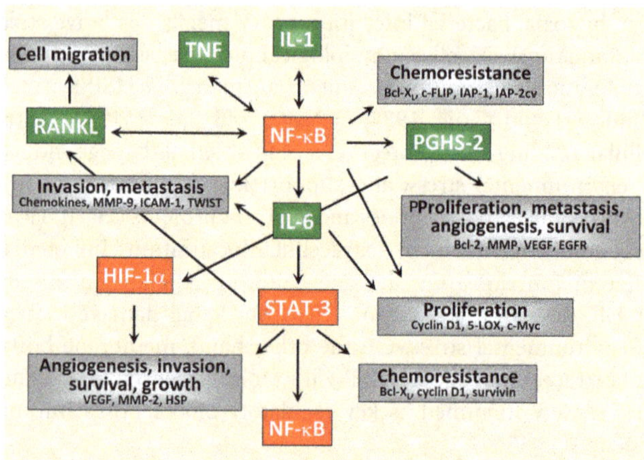

FIGURE 2 | Interactions of inflammatory mediators in tumor cells. Schematical simplified representation of the complex intracellular signaling network in cancer. Among the tumorigenic factors produced by tumor cells or cells of the tumor microenvironment, IL-1, TNF, and IL-6 act as crucial mediators of inflammation-driven tumorigenesis. In particular IL-1 and TNF are major pleiotropic cytokines involved in tumor/host interactions. Nevertheless, these cytokines function as autocrine growth factors and modulate the expression of several tumorigenic factors at any stage of tumorigenesis not only affecting proliferation, migration, and survival of tumor cells but also angiogenesis, invasiveness, metastasis as well as chemoresistance of tumors.

been recognized as important drug targets and are under intensive studies in recent years. HSP are currently being targeted in the therapy of breast cancer and other carcinomas and effective drugs for Hsp90 (e.g., geldanamycin and its analogs) have been synthesized and evaluated in clinical trials (Calderwood and Gong, 2011; Kim and Kim, 2011). HSP vaccines have been intensively studied in the preceding two decades, proving to be safe and effective in treating a number of malignancies (Murshid et al., 2011). However, therapeutical approaches that completely block one tumorigenic factor should be avoided, since it might also interfere with the physiological anti-tumor immune response and could therefore prove to be harmful. Instead, partial inhibition of numerous factors is preferred resulting in an enhanced efficacy thereby being less toxic to the patient.

ACKNOWLEDGMENTS

The authors want to thank Anett Lange for excellent editorial assistance. The work was supported by the Deutsche Forschungsgemeinschaft (DFG) SFB-824, DFG-Cluster of Excellence: Munich Advanced Photonics, Bundesministerium für Bildung und Forschung (BMBF) MOBITUM (01EZ0826) Innovative Therapies (01GU0823), m^4 – Personalized Medicine and Targeted Therapies (01EX1021C), Kompetenzverbund Strahlenforschung (03NUK007E), and multimmune GmbH.

REFERENCES

Aaltoma, S. H., Lipponen, P. K., and Kosma, V. M. (2001). Inducible nitric oxide synthase (iNOS) expression and its prognostic value in prostate cancer. *Anticancer Res.* 21, 3101–3106.

Adhami, V. M., Malik, A., Zaman, N., Sarfaraz, S., Siddiqui, I. A., Syed, D. N., Afaq, F., Pasha, F. S., Saleem, M., and Mukhtar, H. (2007). Combined inhibitory effects of green tea polyphenols and selective cyclooxygenase-2 inhibitors on the growth of human prostate cancer cells both *in vitro* and *in vivo*. *Clin. Cancer Res.* 13, 1611–1619.

Aggarwal, B. B., and Gehlot, P. (2009). Inflammation and cancer: how friendly is the relationship for cancer patients? *Curr. Opin. Pharmacol.* 9, 351–369.

Akerfelt, M., Morimoto, R. I., and Sistonen, L. (2010). Heat shock factors: integrators of cell stress, development and lifespan. *Nat. Rev. Mol. Cell Biol.* 11, 545–555.

Akira, S., Uematsu, S., and Takeuchi, O. (2006). Pathogen recognition and innate immunity. *Cell* 124, 783–801.

Allen, I. C., TeKippe, E. M., Woodford, R. M., Uronis, J. M., Holl, E. K., Rogers, A. B., Herfarth, H. H., Jobin, C., and Ting, J. P. (2010). The NLRP3 inflammasome functions as a negative regulator of tumorigenesis during colitis-associated cancer. *J. Exp. Med.* 207, 1045–1056.

Alshamsan, A. (2011). Induction of tolerogenic dendritic cells by IL-6-secreting CT26 colon carcinoma. *Immunopharmacol. Immunotoxicol.* doi: 10.3109/08923973.2011.625034. [Epub ahead of print].

Ambs, S., Merriam, W. G., Ogunfusika, M. O., Bennett, W. P., Ishibe, N., Hussain, S. P., Tzeng, E. E., Geller, D. A., Billiar, T. R., and Harris, C. C. (1998). p53 and vascular endothelial growth factor regulate tumor growth of NOS2-expressing human carcinoma cells. *Nat. Med.* 4, 1371–1376.

Ancrile, B., Lim, K. H., and Counter, C. M. (2007). Oncogenic Ras-induced secretion of IL6 is required for tumorigenesis. *Genes Dev.* 21, 1714–1719.

Anderson, D. M., Maraskovsky, E., Billingsley, W. L., Dougall, W. C., Tometsko, M. E., Roux, E. R., Teepe, M. C., DuBose, R. F., Cosman, D., and Galibert, L. (1997). A homologue of the TNF receptor and its ligand enhance T-cell growth and dendritic-cell function. *Nature* 390, 175–179.

Angst, E., Reber, H. A., Hines, O. J., and Eibl, G. (2008). Mononuclear cell-derived interleukin-1 beta confers chemoresistance in pancreatic cancer cells by upregulation of cyclooxygenase-2. *Surgery* 144, 57–65.

Apte, R. N., Krelin, Y., Song, X., Dotan, S., Recih, E., Elkabets, M., Carmi, Y., Dvorkin, T., White, R. M., Gayvoronsky, L., Segal, S., and Voronov, E. (2006). Effects of micro-environment- and malignant cell-derived interleukin-1 in carcinogenesis, tumour invasiveness and tumour-host interactions. *Eur. J. Cancer* 42, 751–759.

Arnott, C. H., Scott, K. A., Moore, R. J., Robinson, S. C., Thompson, R. G., and Balkwill, F. R. (2004). Expression of both TNF-alpha receptor subtypes is essential for optimal skin tumour development. *Oncogene* 23, 1902–1910.

Asea, A., Kabingu, E., Stevenson, M. A., and Calderwood, S. K. (2000a). HSP70 peptidembearing and peptide-negative preparations act as chaperokines. *Cell Stress Chaperones* 5, 425–431.

Asea, A., Kraeft, S. K., Kurt-Jones, E. A., Stevenson, M. A., Chen, L. B., Finberg, R. W., Koo, G. C., and Calderwood, S. K. (2000b). HSP70 stimulates cytokine production through a CD14-dependant pathway, demonstrating its dual role as a chaperone and cytokine. *Nat. Med.* 6, 435–442.

Asea, A., Rehli, M., Kabingu, E., Boch, J. A., Bare, O., Auron, P. E., Stevenson, M. A., and Calderwood, S. K. (2002). Novel signal transduction pathway utilized by extracellular HSP70: role of toll-like receptor (TLR) 2 and TLR4. *J. Biol. Chem.* 277, 15028–15034.

Balkwill, F., and Mantovani, A. (2001). Inflammation and cancer: back to Virchow? *Lancet* 357, 539–545.

Barbie, D. A., Tamayo, P., Boehm, J. S., Kim, S. Y., Moody, S. E., Dunn, I. F., Schinzel, A. C., Sandy, P., Meylan, E., Scholl, C., Frohling, S., Chan, E. M., Sos, M. L., Michel, K., Mermel, C., Silver, S. J., Weir, B. A., Reiling, J. H., Sheng, Q., Gupta, P. B., Wadlow, R. C., Le, H., Hoersch, S., Wittner, B. S., Ramaswamy, S., Livingston, D. M., Sabatini, D. M., Meyerson, M., Thomas, R. K., Lander, E. S., Mesirov, J. P., Root, D. E., Gilliland, D. G., Jacks, T., and Hahn, W. C. (2009). Systematic RNA interference reveals that oncogenic KRAS-driven cancers require TBK1. *Nature* 462, 108–112.

Basu, A., and Haldar, S. (2009). Combinatorial effect of epigallocatechin-3-gallate and TRAIL on pancreatic cancer cell death. *Int. J. Oncol.* 34, 281–286.

Bauer, L., Venz, S., Junker, H., Brandt, R., and Radons, J. (2009). Nicotinamide phosphoribosyltransferase and prostaglandin H2 synthase 2 are up-regulated in human pancreatic adenocarcinoma cells after stimulation with interleukin-1. *Int. J. Oncol.* 35, 97–107.

Becker, C., Fantini, M. C., Schramm, C., Lehr, H. A., Wirtz, S., Nikolaev, A., Burg, J., Strand, S., Kiesslich, R., Huber, S., Ito, H., Nishimoto, N., Yoshizaki, K., Kishimoto, T., Galle, P. R., Blessing, M., Rose-John, S., and Neurath, M. F. (2004). TGF-beta suppresses tumor progression in colon cancer by inhibition of IL-6 trans-signaling. *Immunity* 21, 491–501.

Belham, C., Wu, S., and Avruch, J. (1999). Intracellular signalling: PDK1 – a kinase at the hub of things. *Curr. Biol.* 9, R93–R96.

Ben-Neriah, Y., and Karin, M. (2011). Inflammation meets cancer, with NF-kappaB as the matchmaker. *Nat. Immunol.* 12, 715–723.

Berger, F. G. (2004). The interleukin-6 gene: a susceptibility factor that may contribute to racial and ethnic disparities in breast cancer mortality. *Breast Cancer Res. Treat.* 88, 281–285.

Bianchi, M. E. (2007). DAMPs, PAMPs and alarmins: all we need to know about danger. *J. Leukoc. Biol.* 81, 1–5.

Blanco, S., Sanz-Garcia, M., Santos, C. R., and Lazo, P. A. (2008). Modulation of interleukin-1 transcriptional response by the interaction between VRK2 and the JIP1 scaffold protein. *PLoS ONE* 3, e1660. doi:10.1371/journal.pone.0001660

Born, T. L., Thomassen, E., Bird, T. A., and Sims, J. E. (1998). Cloning of a novel receptor subunit, AcPL, required for interleukin-18 signaling. *J. Biol. Chem.* 273, 29445–29450.

Botzler, C., Schmidt, J., Luz, A., Jennen, L., Issels, R., and Multhoff, G. (1998). Differential Hsp70 plasma-membrane expression on primary human tumors and metastases in mice with severe combined immunodeficiency. *Int. J. Cancer* 77, 942–948.

Brown, J. M., Corey, E., Lee, Z. D., True, L. D., Yun, T. J., Tondravi, M., and Vessella, R. L. (2001). Osteoprotegerin and rank ligand expression in prostate cancer. *Urology* 57, 611–616.

Cahill, C. M., and Rogers, J. T. (2008). Interleukin (IL) 1beta induction of IL-6 is mediated by a novel phosphatidylinositol 3-kinase-dependent AKT/IkappaB kinase alpha pathway targeting activator protein-1. *J. Biol. Chem.* 283, 25900–25912.

Calderwood, S. K. (2010). Heat shock proteins in breast cancer progression - a suitable case for treatment? *Int. J. Hyperthermia* 26, 681–685.

Calderwood, S. K., and Gong, J. (2011). Molecular chaperones in mammary cancer growth and breast tumor therapy. *J. Cell Biochem.* doi: 10.1002/jcb.23461. [Epub ahead of print].

Cao, Z., Xiong, J., Takeuchi, M., Kurama, T., and Goeddel, D. V. (1996). TRAF6 is a signal transducer for interleukin-1. *Nature* 383, 443–446.

Cerella, C., Sobolewski, C., Dicato, M., and Diederich, M. (2010). Targeting COX-2 expression by natural compounds: a promising alternative strategy to synthetic COX-2 inhibitors for cancer chemoprevention and therapy. *Biochem. Pharmacol.* 80, 1801–1815.

Chang, L., Kamata, H., Solinas, G., Luo, J. L., Maeda, S., Venuprasad, K., Liu, Y. C., and Karin, M. (2006). The E3 ubiquitin ligase itch couples JNK activation to TNFalpha-induced cell death by inducing c-FLIP(L) turnover. *Cell* 124, 601–613.

Chase, M. A., Wheeler, D. S., Lierl, K. M., Hughes, V. S., Wong, H. R., and Page, K. (2007). Hsp72 induces inflammation and regulates cytokine production in airway epithelium through a TLR4- and NF-kappaB-dependent mechanism. *J. Immunol.* 179, 6318–6324.

Chen, G., Sircar, K., Aprikian, A., Potti, A., Goltzman, D., and Rabbani, S. A. (2006). Expression of RANKL/RANK/OPG in primary and metastatic human prostate cancer as markers of disease stage and functional regulation. *Cancer* 107, 289–298.

Chen, L., and Zhang, H. Y. (2007). Cancer preventive mechanisms of the green tea polyphenol (-)-epigallocatechin-3-gallate. *Molecules* 12, 946–957.

Chen, L. F., and Greene, W. C. (2004). Shaping the nuclear action of NF-kappaB. *Nat. Rev. Mol. Cell Biol.* 5, 392–401.

Chen, X., Tao, Q., Yu, H., Zhang, L., and Cao, X. (2002). Tumor cell membrane-bound heat shock protein 70 elicits antitumor immunity. *Immunol. Lett.* 84, 81–87.

Chien, Y., Kim, S., Bumeister, R., Loo, Y. M., Kwon, S. W., Johnson, C. L., Balakireva, M. G., Romeo, Y., Kopelovich, L., Gale, M. Jr., Yeaman, C., Camonis, J. H., Zhao, Y., and White, M. A. (2006). RalB GTPase-mediated activation of the IkappaB family kinase TBK1 couples innate immune signaling to tumor cell survival. *Cell* 127, 157–170.

Chung, Y. C., and Chang, Y. F. (2003). Serum interleukin-6 levels reflect the disease status of colorectal cancer. *J. Surg. Oncol.* 83, 222–226.

Ciocca, D. R., and Calderwood, S. K. (2005). Heat shock proteins in cancer: diagnostic, prognostic, predictive, and treatment implications. *Cell Stress Chaperones* 10, 86–103.

Colotta, F., Allavena, P., Sica, A., Garlanda, C., and Mantovani, A. (2009). Cancer-related inflammation, the seventh hallmark of cancer: links to genetic instability. *Carcinogenesis* 30, 1073–1081.

Coussens, L. M., and Werb, Z. (2002). Inflammation and cancer. *Nature* 420, 860–867.

Cozen, W., Gill, P. S., Ingles, S. A., Masood, R., Martinez-Maza, O., Cockburn, M. G., Gauderman, W. J., Pike, M. C., Bernstein, L., Nathwani, B. N., Salam, M. T., Danley, K. L., Wang, W., Gage, J., Gundell-Miller, S., and Mack, T. M. (2004). IL-6 levels and genotype are associated with risk of young adult Hodgkin lymphoma. *Blood* 103, 3216–3221.

Cross, S. S., Harrison, R. F., Balasubramanian, S. P., Lippitt, J. M., Evans, C. A., Reed, M. W., and Holen, I. (2006). Expression of receptor activator of nuclear factor kappabeta ligand (RANKL) and tumour necrosis factor related, apoptosis inducing ligand (TRAIL) in breast cancer, and their relations with osteoprotegerin, oestrogen receptor, and clinicopathological variables. *J. Clin. Pathol.* 59, 716–720.

De Paepe, B., Verstraeten, V. M., De Potter, C. R., and Bullock, G. R. (2002). Increased angiotensin II type-2 receptor density in hyperplasia, DCIS and invasive carcinoma of the breast is paralleled with increased iNOS expression. *Histochem. Cell Biol.* 117, 13–19.

DeNagel, D. C., and Pierce, S. K. (1992). A case for chaperones in antigen processing. *Immunol. Today* 13, 86–89.

DeNardo, D. G., Johansson, M., and Coussens, L. M. (2008). Immune cells as mediators of solid tumor metastasis. *Cancer Metastasis Rev.* 27, 11–18.

Dinarello, C. A. (1996). Biologic basis for interleukin-1 in disease. *Blood* 87, 2095–2147.

Dinarello, C. A. (2010). Why not treat human cancer with interleukin-1 blockade? *Cancer Metastasis Rev.* 29, 317–329.

Dostert, C., Petrilli, V., Van, B. R., Steele, C., Mossman, B. T., and Tschopp, J. (2008). Innate immune activation through Nalp3 inflammasome sensing of asbestos and silica. *Science* 320, 674–677.

Dower, S. K., and Qwarnstrom, E. E. (2003). Signalling networks, inflammation and innate immunity. *Biochem. Soc. Trans.* 31, 1462–1471.

Downward, J. (2009). Cancer: a tumour gene's fatal flaws. *Nature* 462, 44–45.

Dunne, A., and O'Neill, L. A. (2003). The interleukin-1 receptor/Toll-like receptor superfamily: signal transduction during inflammation and host defense. *Sci. STKE* 2003, re3.

Elgert, K. D., Alleva, D. G., and Mullins, D. W. (1998). Tumor-induced immune dysfunction: the macrophage connection. *J. Leukoc. Biol.* 64, 275–290.

El-Osta, H., Janku, F., and Kurzrock, R. (2010). Successful treatment of Castleman's disease with interleukin-1 receptor antagonist (Anakinra). *Mol. Cancer Ther.* 9, 1485–1488.

Fahy, B. N., Schlieman, M. G., Virudachalam, S., and Bold, R. J. (2004). Inhibition of AKT abrogates chemotherapy-induced NF-kappaB survival mechanisms: implications for therapy in pancreatic cancer. *J. Am. Coll. Surg.* 198, 591–599.

Fernandez, M., Pino, A. M., Figueroa, P., and Rodriguez, J. P. (2010). The increased expression of receptor activator of nuclear-kappaB ligand (RANKL) of multiple myeloma bone marrow stromal cells is inhibited by the bisphosphonate ibandronate. *J. Cell. Biochem.* 111, 130–137.

Fernandez-Medarde, A., and Santos, E. (2011). Ras in cancer and developmental diseases. *Genes Cancer* 2, 344–358.

Forbes, S. A., Bindal, N., Bamford, S., Cole, C., Kok, C. Y., Beare, D., Jia, M., Shepherd, R., Leung, K., Menzies, A., Teague, J. W., Campbell, P. J., Stratton, M. R., and Futreal, P. A. (2011). COSMIC: mining complete cancer genomes in the Catalogue of Somatic Mutations in Cancer. *Nucleic Acids Res.* 39, D945–D950.

Franchi, L., Eigenbrod, T., Munoz-Planillo, R., and Nunez, G. (2009). The inflammasome: a caspase-1-activation platform that regulates immune responses and disease pathogenesis. *Nat. Immunol.* 10, 241–247.

Garcea, G., Dennison, A. R., Steward, W. P., and Berry, D. P. (2005). Role of inflammation in pancreatic carcinogenesis and the implications for future therapy. *Pancreatology* 5, 514–529.

Gastpar, R., Gehrmann, M., Bausero, M. A., Asea, A., Gross, C., Schroeder, J. A., and Multhoff, G. (2005). Heat shock protein 70 surface-positive tumor exosomes stimulate migratory and cytolytic activity of natural killer cells. *Cancer Res.* 65, 5238–5247.

Gastpar, R., Gross, C., Rossbacher, L., Ellwart, J., Riegger, J., and Multhoff, G. (2004). The cell surface-localized heat shock protein 70 epitope TKD induces migration and cytolytic activity selectively in human NK cells. *J. Immunol.* 172, 972–980.

Gay, N. J., Gangloff, M., and O'Neill, L. A. (2011). What the Myddosome structure tells us about the initiation of innate immunity. *Trends Immunol.* 32, 104–109.

Gehrmann, M., Liebisch, G., Schmitz, G., Anderson, R., Steinem, C., De Maio, A., Pockley, G., and Multhoff, G. (2008). Tumor-specific Hsp70 plasma membrane localization is enabled by the glycosphingolipid Gb3. *PLoS ONE* 3, e1925. doi:10.1371/journal.pone.0001925

Gehrmann, M., Schmetzer, H., Eissner, G., Haferlach, T., Hiddemann, W., and Multhoff, G. (2003). Membrane-bound heat shock protein 70 (Hsp70) in acute myeloid leukemia: a tumor specific recognition structure for the cytolytic activity of autologous NK cells. *Haematologica* 88, 474–476.

Ghiringhelli, F., Apetoh, L., Tesniere, A., Aymeric, L., Ma, Y., Ortiz, C., Vermaelen, K., Panaretakis, T., Mignot, G., Ullrich, E., Perfettini, J. L., Schlemmer, F., Tasdemir, E., Uhl, M., Genin, P., Civas, A., Ryffel, B., Kanellopoulos, J., Tschopp, J., Andre, F., Lidereau, R., McLaughlin, N. M., Haynes, N. M., Smyth, M. J., Kroemer, G., and Zitvogel, L. (2009). Activation of the NLRP3 inflammasome in dendritic cells induces IL-1beta-dependent adaptive immunity against tumors. *Nat. Med.* 15, 1170–1178.

Goldbach-Mansky, R., Dailey, N. J., Canna, S. W., Gelabert, A., Jones, J., Rubin, B. I., Kim, H. J., Brewer, C., Zalewski, C., Wiggs, E., Hill, S., Turner, M. L., Karp, B. I., Aksentijevich, I., Pucino, F., Penzak, S. R., Haverkamp, M. H., Stein, L., Adams, B. S., Moore, T. L., Fuhlbrigge, R. C., Shaham, B., Jarvis, J. N., O'Neil, K., Vehe, R. K., Beitz, L. O., Gardner, G., Hannan, W. P., Warren, R. W., Horn, W., Cole, J. L., Paul, S. M., Hawkins,

P. N., Pham, T. H., Snyder, C., Wesley, R. A., Hoffmann, S. C., Holland, S. M., Butman, J. A., and Kastner, D. L. (2006). Neonatal-onset multisystem inflammatory disease responsive to interleukin-1beta inhibition. *N. Engl. J. Med.* 355, 581–592.

Greten, F. R., Eckmann, L., Greten, T. F., Park, J. M., Li, Z. W., Egan, L. J., Kagnoff, M. F., and Karin, M. (2004). IKKbeta links inflammation and tumorigenesis in a mouse model of colitis-associated cancer. *Cell* 118, 285–296.

Grivennikov, S. I., and Karin, M. (2010). Inflammation and oncogenesis: a vicious connection. *Curr. Opin. Genet. Dev.* 20, 65–71.

Grosch, S., Maier, T. J., Schiffmann, S., and Geisslinger, G. (2006). Cyclooxygenase-2 (COX-2)-independent anticarcinogenic effects of selective COX-2 inhibitors. *J. Natl. Cancer Inst.* 98, 736–747.

Gross, C., Hansch, D., Gastpar, R., and Multhoff, G. (2003a). Interaction of heat shock protein 70 peptide with NK cells involves the NK receptor CD94. *Biol. Chem.* 384, 267–279.

Gross, C., Koelch, W., DeMaio, A., Arispe, N., and Multhoff, G. (2003b). Cell surface-bound heat shock protein 70 (Hsp70) mediates perforin-independent apoptosis by specific binding and uptake of granzyme B. *J. Biol. Chem.* 278, 41173–41181.

Gross, C., Schmidt-Wolf, I. G., Nagaraj, S., Gastpar, R., Ellwart, J., Kunz-Schughart, L. A., and Multhoff, G. (2003c). Heat shock protein 70-reactivity is associated with increased cell surface density of CD94/CD56 on primary natural killer cells. *Cell Stress Chaperones* 8, 348–360.

Hacker, H., and Karin, M. (2006). Regulation and function of IKK and IKK-related kinases. *Sci. STKE* 2006, re13.

Hanahan, D., and Weinberg, R. A. (2000). The hallmarks of cancer. *Cell* 100, 57–70.

Hanahan, D., and Weinberg, R. A. (2011). Hallmarks of cancer: the next generation. *Cell* 144, 646–674.

Härdtner, C., Brandt, R., Multhoff, G., and Radons, J. (2009). (-)-Epigallocatechin-3-gallate compensates for celecoxib-mediated upregulation of PGHS-2 expression in human pancreatic adenocarcinoma cells under tumor-associated inflammatory conditions. *Eur. J. Immunol.* 39(Suppl. 1/09), 530–531.

Hartl, F. U. (1996). Molecular chaperones in cellular protein folding. *Nature* 381, 571–579.

Hedrich, C. M., Bruck, N., Fiebig, B., and Gahr, M. (2011). Anakinra: a safe and effective first-line treatment in systemic onset juvenile idiopathic arthritis (SoJIA). *Rheumatol. Int.* doi: 10.1007/s00296-011-2249-4. [Epub ahead of print].

Hefler, L. A., Grimm, C., Lantzsch, T., Lampe, D., Leodolter, S., Koelbl, H., Heinze, G., Reinthaller, A., Tong-Cacsire, D., Tempfer, C., and Zeillinger, R. (2005). Interleukin-1 and interleukin-6 gene polymorphisms and the risk of breast cancer in caucasian women. *Clin. Cancer Res.* 11, 5718–5721.

Herfs, M., Herman, L., Hubert, P., Minner, F., Arafa, M., Roncarati, P., Henrotin, Y., Boniver, J., and Delvenne, P. (2009). High expression of PGE2 enzymatic pathways in cervical (pre)neoplastic lesions and functional consequences for antigen-presenting cells. *Cancer Immunol. Immunother.* 58, 603–614.

Hofbauer, L. C., and Schoppet, M. (2004). Clinical implications of the osteoprotegerin/RANKL/RANK system for bone and vascular diseases. *JAMA* 292, 490–495.

Hoffman, H. M., Throne, M. L., Amar, N. J., Sebai, M., Kivitz, A. J., Kavanaugh, A., Weinstein, S. P., Belomestnov, P., Yancopoulos, G. D., Stahl, N., and Mellis, S. J. (2008). Efficacy and safety of rilonacept (interleukin-1 Trap) in patients with cryopyrin-associated periodic syndromes: results from two sequential placebo-controlled studies. *Arthritis Rheum.* 58, 2443–2452.

Hoffmann, J., Junker, H., Schmieder, A., Venz, S., Brandt, R., Multhoff, G., Falk, W., and Radons, J. (2011). EGCG downregulates IL-1RI expression and suppresses IL-1-induced tumorigenic factors in human pancreatic adenocarcinoma cells. *Biochem. Pharmacol.* 82, 1153–1162.

Hudson, B. I., Carter, A. M., Harja, E., Kalea, A. Z., Arriero, M., Yang, H., Grant, P. J., and Schmidt, A. M. (2008). Identification, classification, and expression of RAGE gene splice variants. *FASEB J.* 22, 1572–1580.

Hussain, S. P., and Harris, C. C. (2007). Inflammation and cancer: an ancient link with novel potentials. *Int. J. Cancer* 121, 2373–2380.

Hwang, W., Jung, K., Jeon, Y., Yun, S., Kim, T. W., and Choi, I. (2010). Knockdown of the interleukin-6 receptor alpha chain of dendritic cell vaccines enhances the therapeutic potential against IL-6 producing tumors. *Vaccine* 29, 34–44.

Hwang, Y. S., Lee, S. K., Park, K. K., and Chung, W. Y. (2011). Secretion of IL-6 and IL-8 from lysophosphatidic acid-stimulated oral squamous cell carcinoma promotes osteoclastogenesis and bone resorption. *Oral Oncol.* doi:10.1016/j.oraloncology.2011.08.022. [Epub ahead of print].

Hynes, N. E., and Stern, D. F. (1994). The biology of erbB-2/neu/HER-2 and its role in cancer. *Biochim. Biophys. Acta* 1198, 165–184.

Inaba, H., Nagaoka, Y., Kushima, Y., Kumagai, A., Matsumoto, Y., Sakaguchi, M., Baba, K., and Uesato, S. (2008). Comparative examination of anti-proliferative activities of (-)-epigallocatechin gallate and (-)-epigallocatechin against HCT116 colorectal carcinoma cells. *Biol. Pharm. Bull.* 31, 79–84.

Ito, H., Takazoe, M., Fukuda, Y., Hibi, T., Kusugami, K., Andoh, A., Matsumoto, T., Yamamura, T., Azuma, J., Nishimoto, N., Yoshizaki, K., Shimoyama, T., and Kishimoto, T. (2004). A pilot randomized trial of a human anti-interleukin-6 receptor monoclonal antibody in active Crohn's disease. *Gastroenterology* 126, 989–996.

Jaiswal, M., LaRusso, N. F., and Gores, G. J. (2001). Nitric oxide in gastrointestinal epithelial cell carcinogenesis: linking inflammation to oncogenesis. *Am. J. Physiol. Gastrointest. Liver Physiol.* 281, G626–G634.

Jefferies, C. A., and O'Neill, L. A. (2000). Rac1 regulates interleukin 1-induced nuclear factor kappaB activation in an inhibitory protein kappaBalpha-independent manner by enhancing the ability of the p65 subunit to transactivate gene expression. *J. Biol. Chem.* 275, 3114–3120.

Jendrossek, V. (2011). Targeting apoptosis pathways by celecoxib in cancer. *Cancer Lett.* doi: 10.1016/j.canlet.2011.01.012. [Epub ahead of print].

Jimeno, A., Amador, M. L., Kulesza, P., Wang, X., Rubio-Viqueira, B., Zhang, X., Chan, A., Wheelhouse, J., Kuramochi, H., Tanaka, K., Danenberg, K., Messersmith, W. A., Almuete, V., Hruban, R. H., Maitra, A., Yeo, C. J., and Hidalgo, M. (2006). Assessment of celecoxib pharmacodynamics in pancreatic cancer. *Mol. Cancer Ther.* 5, 3240–3247.

Johnson, A. J., Hsu, A. L., Lin, H. P., Song, X., and Chen, C. S. (2002). The cyclo-oxygenase-2 inhibitor celecoxib perturbs intracellular calcium by inhibiting endoplasmic reticulum Ca^{2+}-ATPases: a plausible link with its anti-tumour effect and cardiovascular risks. *Biochem. J.* 366, 831–837.

Jura, N., Archer, H., and Bar-Sagi, D. (2005). Chronic pancreatitis, pancreatic adenocarcinoma and the black box in-between. *Cell Res.* 15, 72–77.

Jurado, S., Garcia-Giralt, N., Diez-Perez, A., Esbrit, P., Yoskovitz, G., Agueda, L., Urreizti, R., Perez-Edo, L., Salo, G., Mellibovsky, L., Balcells, S., Grinberg, D., and Nogues, X. (2010). Effect of IL-1beta, PGE(2), and TGF-beta1 on the expression of OPG and RANKL in normal and osteoporotic primary human osteoblasts. *J. Cell. Biochem.* 110, 304–310.

Kai, H., Kitadai, Y., Kodama, M., Cho, S., Kuroda, T., Ito, M., Tanaka, S., Ohmoto, Y., and Chayama, K. (2005). Involvement of proinflammatory cytokines IL-1beta and IL-6 in progression of human gastric carcinoma. *Anticancer Res.* 25, 709–713.

Kamal, A., Thao, L., Sensintaffar, J., Zhang, L., Boehm, M. F., Fritz, L. C., and Burrows, F. J. (2003). A high-affinity conformation of Hsp90 confers tumour selectivity on Hsp90 inhibitors. *Nature* 425, 407–410.

Kamata, H., Honda, S., Maeda, S., Chang, L., Hirata, H., and Karin, M. (2005). Reactive oxygen species promote TNFalpha-induced death and sustained JNK activation by inhibiting MAP kinase phosphatases. *Cell* 120, 649–661.

Karin, M. (2006). Nuclear factor-kappaB in cancer development and progression. *Nature* 441, 431–436.

Karin, M., Cao, Y., Greten, F. R., and Li, Z. W. (2002). NF-kappaB in cancer: from innocent bystander to major culprit. *Nat. Rev. Cancer* 2, 301–310.

Karin, M., Lawrence, T., and Nizet, V. (2006). Innate immunity gone awry: linking microbial infections to chronic inflammation and cancer. *Cell* 124, 823–835.

Kawai, T., and Akira, S. (2011). Toll-like receptors and their crosstalk with other innate receptors in infection and immunity. *Immunity* 34, 637–650.

Kawata, M., Koinuma, D., Ogami, T., Umezawa, K., Iwata, C., Watabe, T., and Miyazono, K. (2011). TGF-beta-induced epithelial-mesenchymal transition of A549 lung adenocarcinoma cells is enhanced by proinflammatory cytokines derived from RAW 264.7 macrophage cells. *J. Biochem.* doi: 10.1093/jb/mvr136. [Epub ahead of print].

Keating, S. E., Maloney, G. M., Moran, E. M., and Bowie, A. G. (2007).

IRAK-2 participates in multiple toll-like receptor signaling pathways to NFkappaB via activation of TRAF6 ubiquitination. *J. Biol. Chem.* 282, 33435–33443.

Khaleque, M. A., Bharti, A., Sawyer, D., Gong, J., Benjamin, I. J., Stevenson, M. A., and Calderwood, S. K. (2005). Induction of heat shock proteins by heregulin beta1 leads to protection from apoptosis and anchorage-independent growth. *Oncogene* 24, 6564–6573.

Kim, L. S., and Kim, J. H. (2011). Heat shock protein as molecular targets for breast cancer therapeutics. *J. Breast Cancer* 14, 167–174.

Kishimoto, K., Matsumoto, K., and Ninomiya-Tsuji, J. (2000). TAK1 mitogen-activated protein kinase kinase kinase is activated by autophosphorylation within its activation loop. *J. Biol. Chem.* 275, 7359–7364.

Klein, B., Lu, Z. Y., Gaillard, J. P., Harousseau, J. L., and Bataille, R. (1992). Inhibiting IL-6 in human multiple myeloma. *Curr. Top. Microbiol. Immunol.* 182, 237–244.

Kobayashi, S., Werneburg, N. W., Bronk, S. F., Kaufmann, S. H., and Gores, G. J. (2005). Interleukin-6 contributes to Mcl-1 up-regulation and TRAIL resistance via an Akt-signaling pathway in cholangiocarcinoma cells. *Gastroenterology* 128, 2054–2065.

Kong, G., Kim, E. K., Kim, W. S., Lee, K. T., Lee, Y. W., Lee, J. K., Paik, S. W., and Rhee, J. C. (2002). Role of cyclooxygenase-2 and inducible nitric oxide synthase in pancreatic cancer. *J. Gastroenterol. Hepatol.* 17, 914–921.

Kortylewski, M., Kujawski, M., Wang, T., Wei, S., Zhang, S., Pilon-Thomas, S., Niu, G., Kay, H., Mule, J., Kerr, W. G., Jove, R., Pardoll, D., and Yu, H. (2005). Inhibiting Stat3 signaling in the hematopoietic system elicits multicomponent antitumor immunity. *Nat. Med.* 11, 1314–1321.

Kulp, S. K., Yang, Y. T., Hung, C. C., Chen, K. F., Lai, J. P., Tseng, P. H., Fowble, J. W., Ward, P. J., and Chen, C. S. (2004). 3-phosphoinositide-dependent protein kinase-1/Akt signaling represents a major cyclooxygenase-2-independent target for celecoxib in prostate cancer cells. *Cancer Res.* 64, 1444–1451.

Kumar, A., Xu, J., Brady, S., Gao, H., Yu, D., Reuben, J., and Mehta, K. (2010). Tissue transglutaminase promotes drug resistance and invasion by inducing mesenchymal transition in mammary epithelial cells. *PLoS ONE* 5, e13390. doi:10.1371/journal.pone.0013390

Kundu, J. K., and Surh, Y. J. (2008). Inflammation: gearing the journey to cancer. *Mutat. Res.* 659, 15–30.

Lachmann, H. J., Kone-Paut, I., Kuemmerle-Deschner, J. B., Leslie, K. S., Hachulla, E., Quartier, P., Gitton, X., Widmer, A., Patel, N., and Hawkins, P. N. (2009a). Use of canakinumab in the cryopyrin-associated periodic syndrome. *N. Engl. J. Med.* 360, 2416–2425.

Lachmann, H. J., Lowe, P., Felix, S. D., Rordorf, C., Leslie, K., Madhoo, S., Wittkowski, H., Bek, S., Hartmann, N., Bosset, S., Hawkins, P. N., and Jung, T. (2009b). In vivo regulation of interleukin 1beta in patients with cryopyrin-associated periodic syndromes. *J. Exp. Med.* 206, 1029–1036.

Ladetto, M., Vallet, S., Trojan, A., Dell'Aquila, M., Monitillo, L., Rosato, R., Santo, L., Drandi, D., Bertola, A., Falco, P., Cavallo, F., Ricca, I., De, M. F., Mantoan, B., Bode-Lesniewska, B., Pagliano, G., Francese, R., Rocci, A., Astolfi, M., Compagno, M., Mariani, S., Godio, L., Marino, L., Ruggeri, M., Omede, P., Palumbo, A., and Boccadoro, M. (2005). Cyclooxygenase-2 (COX-2) is frequently expressed in multiple myeloma and is an independent predictor of poor outcome. *Blood* 105, 4784–4791.

Lambert, J. D., Hong, J., Yang, G. Y., Liao, J., and Yang, C. S. (2005). Inhibition of carcinogenesis by polyphenols: evidence from laboratory investigations. *Am. J. Clin. Nutr.* 81, 284S–291S.

Lee, H., Herrmann, A., Deng, J. H., Kujawski, M., Niu, G., Li, Z., Forman, S., Jove, R., Pardoll, D. M., and Yu, H. (2009). Persistently activated Stat3 maintains constitutive NF-kappaB activity in tumors. *Cancer Cell* 15, 283–293.

Lee, Y. H., Ji, J. D., and Song, G. G. (2007). Adjusted indirect comparison of celecoxib versus rofecoxib on cardiovascular risk. *Rheumatol. Int.* 27, 477–482.

Lewis, A. M., Varghese, S., Xu, H., and Alexander, H. R. (2006). Interleukin-1 and cancer progression: the emerging role of interleukin-1 receptor antagonist as a novel therapeutic agent in cancer treatment. *J. Transl. Med.* 4, 48.

Li, J., Sarosi, I., Yan, X. Q., Morony, S., Capparelli, C., Tan, H. L., McCabe, S., Elliott, R., Scully, S., Van, G., Kaufman, S., Juan, S. C., Sun, Y., Tarpley, J., Martin, L., Christensen, K., McCabe, J., Kostenuik, P., Hsu, H., Fletcher, F., Dunstan, C. R., Lacey, D. L., and Boyle, W. J. (2000). RANK is the intrinsic hematopoietic cell surface receptor that controls osteoclastogenesis and regulation of bone mass and calcium metabolism. *Proc. Natl. Acad. Sci. U.S.A.* 97, 1566–1571.

Li, X., Kim, K. W., Cho, M. L., Ju, J. H., Kang, C. M., Oh, H. J., Min, J. K., Lee, S. H., Park, S. H., and Kim, H. Y. (2010). IL-23 induces receptor activator of NF-kappaB ligand expression in fibroblast-like synoviocytes via STAT3 and NF-kappaB signal pathways. *Immunol. Lett.* 127, 100–107.

Lin, W. J., and Yeh, W. C. (2005). Implication of Toll-like receptor and tumor necrosis factor alpha signaling in septic shock. *Shock* 24, 206–209.

Lin, W. W., and Karin, M. (2007). A cytokine-mediated link between innate immunity, inflammation, and cancer. *J. Clin. Invest.* 117, 1175–1183.

Lindquist, S., and Craig, E. A. (1988). The heat-shock proteins. *Annu. Rev. Genet.* 22, 631–677.

Lu, H., Ouyang, W., and Huang, C. (2006). Inflammation, a key event in cancer development. *Mol. Cancer Res.* 4, 221–233.

Lust, J. A., Lacy, M. Q., Zeldenrust, S. R., Dispenzieri, A., Gertz, M. A., Witzig, T. E., Kumar, S., Hayman, S. R., Russell, S. J., Buadi, F. K., Geyer, S. M., Campbell, M. E., Kyle, R. A., Rajkumar, S. V., Greipp, P. R., Kline, M. P., Xiong, Y., Moon-Tasson, L. L., and Donovan, K. A. (2009). Induction of a chronic disease state in patients with smoldering or indolent multiple myeloma by targeting interleukin 1{beta}-induced interleukin 6 production and the myeloma proliferative component. *Mayo Clin. Proc.* 84, 114–122.

Maier, T. J., Schilling, K., Schmidt, R., Geisslinger, G., and Grosch, S. (2004). Cyclooxygenase-2 (COX-2)-dependent and -independent anticarcinogenic effects of celecoxib in human colon carcinoma cells. *Biochem. Pharmacol.* 67, 1469–1478.

Mantovani, A., Allavena, P., Sica, A., and Balkwill, F. (2008). Cancer-related inflammation. *Nature* 454, 436–444.

Martin, M. U., and Wesche, H. (2002). Summary and comparison of the signaling mechanisms of the Toll/interleukin-1 receptor family. *Biochim. Biophys. Acta* 1592, 265–280.

Martinon, F., Burns, K., and Tschopp, J. (2002). The inflammasome: a molecular platform triggering activation of inflammatory caspases and processing of proIL-beta. *Mol. Cell* 10, 417–426.

Matzinger, P. (1998). An innate sense of danger. *Semin. Immunol.* 10, 399–415.

Menu, P., and Vince, J. E. (2011). The NLRP3 inflammasome in health and disease: the good, the bad and the ugly. *Clin. Exp. Immunol.* 166, 1–15.

Merati, K., said, S. M., Andea, A., Sarkar, F., Ben-Josef, E., Mohammad, R., Philip, P., Shields, A. F., Vaitkevicius, V., Grignon, D. J., and Adsay, N. V. (2001). Expression of inflammatory modulator COX-2 in pancreatic ductal adenocarcinoma and its relationship to pathologic and clinical parameters. *Am. J. Clin. Oncol.* 24, 447–452.

Meylan, E., Dooley, A. L., Feldser, D. M., Shen, L., Turk, E., Ouyang, C., and Jacks, T. (2009). Requirement for NF-kappaB signalling in a mouse model of lung adenocarcinoma. *Nature* 462, 104–107.

Mizel, S. B. (1982). Interleukin 1 and T cell activation. *Immunol. Rev.* 63, 51–72.

Mocellin, S., Rossi, C. R., Pilati, P., and Nitti, D. (2005). Tumor necrosis factor, cancer and anticancer therapy. *Cytokine Growth Factor Rev.* 16, 35–53.

Molina, M. A., Sitja-Arnau, M., Lemoine, M. G., Frazier, M. L., and Sinicrope, F. A. (1999). Increased cyclooxygenase-2 expression in human pancreatic carcinomas and cell lines: growth inhibition by nonsteroidal anti-inflammatory drugs. *Cancer Res.* 59, 4356–4362.

Mori, K., Berreur, M., Blanchard, F., Chevalier, C., Guisle-Marsollier, I., Masson, M., Redini, F., and Heymann, D. (2007a). Receptor activator of nuclear factor-kappaB ligand (RANKL) directly modulates the gene expression profile of RANK-positive Saos-2 human osteosarcoma cells. *Oncol. Rep.* 18, 1365–1371.

Mori, K., Le Goff, B., Berreur, M., Riet, A., Moreau, A., Blanchard, F., Chevalier, C., Guisle-Marsollier, I., Leger, J., Guicheux, J., Masson, M., Gouin, F., Redini, F., and Heymann, D. (2007b). Human osteosarcoma cells express functional receptor activator of nuclear factor-kappa B. *J. Pathol.* 211, 555–562.

Mori, T., Miyamoto, T., Yoshida, H., Asakawa, M., Kawasumi, M., Kobayashi, T., Morioka, H., Chiba, K., Toyama, Y., and Yoshimura, A. (2011). IL-1β and TNFα-initiated IL-6-STAT3 pathway is critical in mediating inflammatory cytokines and RANKL expression in inflammatory arthritis. *Int. Immunol.* 23, 701–712.

Moser, C., Schmidbauer, C., Gurtler, U., Gross, C., Gehrmann, M., Thonigs, G., Pfister, K., and Multhoff, G. (2002). Inhibition of tumor growth in mice with severe combined immunodeficiency is mediated by heat shock protein 70 (Hsp70)-peptide-activated, CD94 positive natural killer cells. *Cell Stress Chaperones* 7, 365–373.

Multhoff, G., Botzler, C., Jennen, L., Schmidt, J., Ellwart, J., and Issels, R. (1997). Heat shock protein 72 on tumor cells: a recognition structure for natural killer cells. *J. Immunol.* 158, 4341–4350.

Multhoff, G., Botzler, C., Wiesnet, M., Eissner, G., and Issels, R. (1995a). CD3- large granular lymphocytes recognize a heat-inducible immunogenic determinant associated with the 72-kD heat shock protein on human sarcoma cells. *Blood* 86, 1374–1382.

Multhoff, G., Botzler, C., Wiesnet, M., Muller, E., Meier, T., Wilmanns, W., and Issels, R. D. (1995b). A stress-inducible 72-kDa heat-shock protein (HSP72) is expressed on the surface of human tumor cells, but not on normal cells. *Int. J. Cancer* 61, 272–279.

Multhoff, G., Mizzen, L., Winchester, C. C., Milner, C. M., Wenk, S., Eissner, G., Kampinga, H. H., Laumbacher, B., and Johnson, J. (1999). Heat shock protein 70 (Hsp70) stimulates proliferation and cytolytic activity of natural killer cells. *Exp. Hematol.* 27, 1627–1636.

Multhoff, G., Pfister, K., Botzler, C., Jordan, A., Scholz, R., Schmetzer, H., Burgstahler, R., and Hiddemann, W. (2000). Adoptive transfer of human natural killer cells in mice with severe combined immunodeficiency inhibits growth of Hsp70-expressing tumors. *Int. J. Cancer* 88, 791–797.

Multhoff, G., Pfister, K., Gehrmann, M., Hantschel, M., Gross, C., Hafner, M., and Hiddemann, W. (2001). A 14-mer Hsp70 peptide stimulates natural killer (NK) cell activity. *Cell Stress Chaperones* 6, 337–344.

Murshid, A., Gong, J., Stevenson, M. A., and Calderwood, S. K. (2011). Heat shock proteins and cancer vaccines: developments in the past decade and chaperoning in the decade to come. *Expert Rev. Vaccines* 10, 1553–1568.

Muthuswamy, R., Mueller-Berghaus, J., Haberkorn, U., Reinhart, T. A., Schadendorf, D., and Kalinski, P. (2010). PGE(2) transiently enhances DC expression of CCR7 but inhibits the ability of DCs to produce CCL19 and attract naive T cells. *Blood* 116, 1454–1459.

Muzio, M., Ni, J., Feng, P., and Dixit, V. M. (1997). IRAK (Pelle) family member IRAK-2 and MyD88 as proximal mediators of IL-1 signaling. *Science* 278, 1612–1615.

Nakata, Y., Matsuda, K., Uzawa, A., Nomura, M., Akashi, M., and Suzuki, G. (1995). Administration of recombinant human IL-1 by Staphylococcus enterotoxin B prevents tolerance induction in vivo. *J. Immunol.* 155, 4231–4235.

Neckers, L., and Lee, Y. S. (2003). Cancer: the rules of attraction. *Nature* 425, 357–359.

Ng, P. K., Tsui, S. K., Lau, C. P., Wong, C. H., Wong, W. H., Huang, L., and Kumta, S. M. (2010). CCAAT/enhancer binding protein beta is up-regulated in giant cell tumor of bone and regulates RANKL expression. *J. Cell. Biochem.* 110, 438–446.

Niederberger, E., Tegeder, I., Vetter, G., Schmidtko, A., Schmidt, H., Euchenhofer, C., Brautigam, L., Grosch, S., and Geisslinger, G. (2001). Celecoxib loses its anti-inflammatory efficacy at high doses through activation of NF-kappaB. *FASEB J.* 15, 1622–1624.

Ninomiya-Tsuji, J., Kishimoto, K., Hiyama, A., Inoue, J., Cao, Z., and Matsumoto, K. (1999). The kinase TAK1 can activate the NIK-I kappaB as well as the MAP kinase cascade in the IL-1 signalling pathway. *Nature* 398, 252–256.

Nishimoto, N., Kanakura, Y., Aozasa, K., Johkoh, T., Nakamura, M., Nakano, S., Nakano, N., Ikeda, Y., Sasaki, T., Nishioka, K., Hara, M., Taguchi, H., Kimura, Y., Kato, Y., Asaoku, H., Kumagai, S., Kodama, F., Nakahara, H., Hagihara, K., Yoshizaki, K., and Kishimoto, T. (2005). Humanized anti-interleukin-6 receptor antibody treatment of multicentric Castleman disease. *Blood* 106, 2627–2632.

Nishimoto, N., Yoshizaki, K., Miyasaka, N., Yamamoto, K., Kawai, S., Takeuchi, T., Hashimoto, J., Azuma, J., and Kishimoto, T. (2004). Treatment of rheumatoid arthritis with humanized anti-interleukin-6 receptor antibody: a multicenter, double-blind, placebo-controlled trial. *Arthritis Rheum.* 50, 1761–1769.

Offner, F. A., Obrist, P., Stadlmann, S., Feichtinger, H., Klingler, P., Herold, M., Zwierzina, H., Hittmair, A., Mikuz, G., and Abendstein, B. (1995). IL-6 secretion by human peritoneal mesothelial and ovarian cancer cells. *Cytokine* 7, 542–547.

Okamoto, M., Liu, W., Luo, Y., Tanaka, A., Cai, X., Norris, D. A., Dinarello, C. A., and Fujita, M. (2010). Constitutively active inflammasome in human melanoma cells mediating autoinflammation via caspase-1 processing and secretion of interleukin-1beta. *J. Biol. Chem.* 285, 6477–6488.

O'Neill, L. A. (2000). The interleukin-1 receptor/Toll-like receptor superfamily: signal transduction during inflammation and host defense. *Sci. STKE* 2000, re1.

O'Sullivan, B. J., Thomas, H. E., Pai, S., Santamaria, P., Iwakura, Y., Steptoe, R. J., Kay, T. W., and Thomas, R. (2006). IL-1 beta breaks tolerance through expansion of CD25+ effector T cells. *J. Immunol.* 176, 7278–7287.

Paduch, R., Jakubowicz-Gil, J., and Kandefer-Szerszen, M. (2009). Expression of HSP27, HSP72 and MRP proteins in in vitro co-culture of colon tumour cell spheroids with normal cells after incubation with rhTGF- beta1 and/or CPT-11. *J. Biosci.* 34, 927–940.

Park, H. R., Min, S. K., Cho, H. D., Kim, D. H., Shin, H. S., and Park, Y. E. (2003). Expression of osteoprotegerin and RANK ligand in breast cancer bone metastasis. *J. Korean Med. Sci.* 18, 541–546.

Peters, M., Muller, A. M., and Rose-John, S. (1998). Interleukin-6 and soluble interleukin-6 receptor: direct stimulation of gp130 and hematopoiesis. *Blood* 92, 3495–3504.

Pfister, K., Radons, J., Busch, R., Tidball, J. G., Pfeifer, M., Freitag, L., Feldmann, H. J., Milani, V., Issels, R., and Multhoff, G. (2007). Patient survival by Hsp70 membrane phenotype: association with different routes of metastasis. *Cancer* 110, 926–935.

Pidgeon, G. P., Harmey, J. H., Kay, E., Da Costa, M., Redmond, H. P., and Bouchier-Hayes, D. J. (1999). The role of endotoxin/lipopolysaccharide in surgically induced tumour growth in a murine model of metastatic disease. *Br. J. Cancer* 81, 1311–1317.

Pikarsky, E., Porat, R. M., Stein, I., Abramovitch, R., Amit, S., Kasem, S., Gutkovich-Pyest, E., Urieli-Shoval, S., Galun, E., and Ben-Neriah, Y. (2004). NF-kappaB functions as a tumour promoter in inflammation-associated cancer. *Nature* 431, 461–466.

Pirkkala, L., Nykanen, P., and Sistonen, L. (2001). Roles of the heat shock transcription factors in regulation of the heat shock response and beyond. *FASEB J.* 15, 1118–1131.

Rabe, B., Chalaris, A., May, U., Waetzig, G. H., Seegert, D., Williams, A. S., Jones, S. A., Rose-John, S., and Scheller, J. (2008). Transgenic blockade of interleukin 6 transsignaling abrogates inflammation. *Blood* 111, 1021–1028.

Radons, J., Dove, S., Neumann, D., Altmann, R., Botzki, A., Martin, M. U., and Falk, W. (2003). The interleukin 1 (IL-1) receptor accessory protein Toll/IL-1 receptor domain: analysis of putative interaction sites in vitro mutagenesis and molecular modeling. *J. Biol. Chem.* 278, 49145–49153.

Radons, J., Gabler, S., Wesche, H., Korherr, C., Hofmeister, R., and Falk, W. (2002). Identification of essential regions in the cytoplasmic tail of interleukin-1 receptor accessory protein critical for interleukin-1 signaling. *J. Biol. Chem.* 277, 16456–16463.

Raut, C. P., Nawrocki, S., Lashinger, L. M., Davis, D. W., Khanbolooki, S., Xiong, H., Ellis, L. M., and McConkey, D. J. (2004). Celecoxib inhibits angiogenesis by inducing endothelial cell apoptosis in human pancreatic tumor xenografts. *Cancer Biol. Ther.* 3, 1217–1224.

Ravi, R., Mookerjee, B., Bhujwalla, Z. M., Sutter, C. H., Artemov, D., Zeng, Q., Dillehay, L. E., Madan, A., Semenza, G. L., and Bedi, A. (2000). Regulation of tumor angiogenesis by p53-induced degradation of hypoxia-inducible factor 1alpha. *Genes Dev.* 14, 34–44.

Reddy, S. A., Huang, J. H., and Liao, W. S. (1997). Phosphatidylinositol 3-kinase in interleukin 1 signaling. Physical interaction with the interleukin 1 receptor and requirement in NFkappaB and AP-1 activation. *J. Biol. Chem.* 272, 29167–29173.

Rose-John, S., Scheller, J., Elson, G., and Jones, S. A. (2006). Interleukin-6 biology is coordinated by membrane-bound and soluble receptors: role in inflammation and cancer. *J. Leukoc. Biol.* 80, 227–236.

Rose-John, S., and Schooltink, H. (2007). Cytokines are a therapeutic target for the prevention of inflammation-induced cancers. *Recent Results Cancer Res.* 174, 57–66.

Rudner, J., Elsaesser, S. J., Muller, A. C., Belka, C., and Jendrossek, V. (2010). Differential effects of anti-apoptotic Bcl-2 family members Mcl-1, Bcl-2, and Bcl-xL on celecoxib-induced apoptosis. *Biochem. Pharmacol.* 79, 10–20.

Sakoguchi-Okada, N., Takahashi-Yanaga, F., Fukada, K., Shiraishi, F., Taba, Y., Miwa, Y., Morimoto, S., Iida, M., and Sasaguri, T. (2007). Celecoxib inhibits the expression of survivin via the suppression of promoter activity in human colon cancer cells. *Biochem. Pharmacol.* 73, 1318–1329.

Sandau, K. B., Faus, H. G., and Brune, B. (2000). Induction of hypoxia-inducible-factor 1 by nitric oxide is mediated via the PI 3K pathway. *Biochem. Biophys. Res. Commun.* 278, 263–267.

Sansone, P., Piazzi, G., Paterini, P., Strillacci, A., Ceccarelli, C., Minni, F., Biasco, G., Chieco, P., and Bonafe, M. (2009). Cyclooxygenase-2/carbonic anhydrase-IX up-regulation promotes invasive potential and hypoxia survival in colorectal cancer cells. *J. Cell. Mol. Med.* 13, 3876–3887.

Sawa, T., and Ohshima, H. (2006). Nitrative DNA damage in inflammation and its possible role in carcinogenesis. *Nitric Oxide* 14, 91–100.

Schulze, J., Albers, J., Baranowsky, A., Keller, J., Spiro, A., Streichert, T., Zustin, J., Amling, M., and Schinke, T. (2010). Osteolytic prostate cancer cells induce the expression of specific cytokines in bone-forming osteoblasts through a Stat3/5-dependent mechanism. *Bone* 46, 524–533.

Schwarz, R. E., Vujanovic, N. L., and Hiserodt, J. C. (1989). Enhanced antimetastatic activity of lymphokine-activated killer cells purified and expanded by their adherence to plastic. *Cancer Res.* 49, 1441–1446.

Shamovsky, I., and Nudler, E. (2008). New insights into the mechanism of heat shock response activation. *Cell. Mol. Life Sci.* 65, 855–861.

Shchors, K., Shchors, E., Rostker, F., Lawlor, E. R., Brown-Swigart, L., and Evan, G. I. (2006). The Myc-dependent angiogenic switch in tumors is mediated by interleukin 1beta. *Genes Dev.* 20, 2527–2538.

Shimizu, M., Deguchi, A., Lim, J. T., Moriwaki, H., Kopelovich, L., and Weinstein, I. B. (2005). (-)-Epigallocatechin gallate and polyphenon E inhibit growth and activation of the epidermal growth factor receptor and human epidermal growth factor receptor-2 signaling pathways in human colon cancer cells. *Clin. Cancer Res.* 11, 2735–2746.

Shin, B. K., Wang, H., Yim, A. M., Le Naour, F., Brichory, F., Jang, J. H., Zhao, R., Puravs, E., Tra, J., Michael, C. W., Misek, D. E., and Hanash, S. M. (2003). Global profiling of the cell surface proteome of cancer cells uncovers an abundance of proteins with chaperone function. *J. Biol. Chem.* 278, 7607–7616.

Shinriki, S., Jono, H., Ota, K., Ueda, M., Kudo, M., Ota, T., Oike, Y., Endo, M., Ibusuki, M., Hiraki, A., Nakayama, H., Yoshitake, Y., Shinohara, M., and Ando, Y. (2009). Humanized anti-interleukin-6 receptor antibody suppresses tumor angiogenesis and in vivo growth of human oral squamous cell carcinoma. *Clin. Cancer Res.* 15, 5426–5434.

Shirode, A. B., and Sylvester, P. W. (2010). Synergistic anticancer effects of combined gamma-tocotrienol and celecoxib treatment are associated with suppression in Akt and NFkappaB signaling. *Biomed. Pharmacother.* 64, 327–332.

Siddiqui, I. A., Malik, A., Adhami, V. M., Asim, M., Hafeez, B. B., Sarfaraz, S., and Mukhtar, H. (2008). Green tea polyphenol EGCG sensitizes human prostate carcinoma LNCaP cells to TRAIL-mediated apoptosis and synergistically inhibits biomarkers associated with angiogenesis and metastasis. *Oncogene* 27, 2055–2063.

Singh, R., Wang, B., Shirvaikar, A., Khan, S., Kamat, S., Schelling, J. R., Konieczkowski, M., and Sedor, J. R. (1999). The IL-1 receptor and Rho directly associate to drive cell activation in inflammation. *J. Clin. Invest.* 103, 1561–1570.

Smolen, J. S., Avila, J. C., and Aletaha, D. (2011). Tocilizumab inhibits progression of joint damage in rheumatoid arthritis irrespective of its anti-inflammatory effects: disassociation of the link between inflammation and destruction. *Ann. Rheum. Dis.* doi: 10.1136/annrheumdis-2011-200395. [Epub ahead of print].

Solomon, S. D., Wittes, J., Finn, P. V., Fowler, R., Viner, J., Bertagnolli, M. M., Arber, N., Levin, B., Meinert, C. L., Martin, B., Pater, J. L., Goss, P. E., Lance, P., Obara, S., Chew, E. Y., Kim, J., Arndt, G., and Hawk, E. (2008). Cardiovascular risk of celecoxib in 6 randomized placebo-controlled trials: the cross trial safety analysis. *Circulation* 117, 2104–2113.

Sparmann, A., and Bar-Sagi, D. (2004). Ras-induced interleukin-8 expression plays a critical role in tumor growth and angiogenesis. *Cancer Cell* 6, 447–458.

Spektor, G., and Fuster, V. (2005). Drug insight: cyclo-oxygenase 2 inhibitors and cardiovascular risk-where are we now? *Nat. Clin. Pract. Cardiovasc. Med.* 2, 290–300.

Stangl, S., Gehrmann, M., Riegger, J., Kuhs, K., Riederer, I., Sievert, W., Hube, K., Mocikat, R., Dressel, R., Kremmer, E., Pockley, A.G., Friedrich, L., Vigh, L., Skerra, A., and Multhoff, G. (2011). Targeting membrane heat-shock protein 70 (Hsp70) on tumors by cmHsp70.1 antibody. *Proc. Natl. Acad. Sci. U.S.A.* 108, 733–738.

Stangl, S., Wortmann, A., Guertler, U., and Multhoff, G. (2006). Control of metastasized pancreatic carcinomas in SCID/beige mice with human IL-2/TKD-activated NK cells. *J. Immunol.* 176, 6270–6276.

Stock, A., Booth, S., and Cerundolo, V. (2011). Prostaglandin E2 suppresses the differentiation of retinoic acid-producing dendritic cells in mice and humans. *J. Exp. Med.* 208, 761–773.

Suganuma, M., Saha, A., and Fujiki, H. (2011). New cancer treatment strategy using combination of green tea catechins and anticancer drugs. *Cancer Sci.* 102, 317–323.

Sun, S. G., Lau, Y. S., Itonaga, I., Sabokbar, A., and Athanasou, N. A. (2006). Bone stromal cells in pagetic bone and Paget's sarcoma express RANKL and support human osteoclast formation. *J. Pathol.* 209, 114–120.

Surh, Y. J., Chun, K. S., Cha, H. H., Han, S. S., Keum, Y. S., Park, K. K., and Lee, S. S. (2001). Molecular mechanisms underlying chemopreventive activities of anti-inflammatory phytochemicals: down-regulation of COX-2 and iNOS through suppression of NF-kappa B activation. *Mutat. Res.* 480–481, 243–268.

Sutton, C., Brereton, C., Keogh, B., Mills, K. H., and Lavelle, E. C. (2006). A crucial role for interleukin (IL)-1 in the induction of IL-17-producing T cells that mediate autoimmune encephalomyelitis. *J. Exp. Med.* 203, 1685–1691.

Takahashi, T., Uehara, H., Bando, Y., and Izumi, K. (2008). Soluble EP2 neutralizes prostaglandin E2-induced cell signaling and inhibits osteolytic tumor growth. *Mol. Cancer Ther.* 7, 2807–2816.

Taketomi, A., Takenaka, K., Matsumata, T., Shimada, M., Higashi, H., Shirabe, K., Itasaka, H., Adachi, E., Maeda, T., and Sugimachi, K. (1997). Circulating intercellular adhesion molecule-1 in patients with hepatocellular carcinoma before and after hepatic resection. *Hepatogastroenterology* 44, 477–483.

Tang, Z. N., Zhang, F., Tang, P., Qi, X. W., and Jiang, J. (2011). Hypoxia induces RANK and RANKL expression by activating HIF-1alpha in breast cancer cells. *Biochem. Biophys. Res. Commun.* 408, 411–416.

Teitelbaum, S. L. (2000). Bone resorption by osteoclasts. *Science* 289, 1504–1508.

Thiery, J. P., Acloque, H., Huang, R. Y., and Nieto, M. A. (2009). Epithelial-mesenchymal transitions in development and disease. *Cell* 139, 871–890.

Tjiu, J. W., Liao, Y. H., Lin, S. J., Huang, Y. L., Tsai, W. L., Chu, C. Y., Kuo, M. L., and Jee, S. H. (2006). Cyclooxygenase-2 overexpression in human basal cell carcinoma cell line increases antiapoptosis, angiogenesis, and tumorigenesis. *J. Invest. Dermatol.* 126, 1143–1151.

Trelle, S., Reichenbach, S., Wandel, S., Hildebrand, P., Tschannen, B., Villiger, P. M., Egger, M., and Juni, P. (2011). Cardiovascular safety of non-steroidal anti-inflammatory drugs: network meta-analysis. *BMJ* 342, c7086.

Triantafilou, M., and Triantafilou, K. (2004). Heat-shock protein 70 and heat-shock protein 90 associate with Toll-like receptor 4 in response to bacterial lipopolysaccharide. *Biochem. Soc. Trans.* 32, 636–639.

Tseng, W. W., Deganutti, A., Chen, M. N., Saxton, R. E., and Liu, C. D. (2002). Selective cyclooxygenase-2 inhibitor rofecoxib (Vioxx) induces expression of cell cycle arrest genes and slows tumor growth in human pancreatic cancer. *J. Gastrointest. Surg.* 6, 838–843.

Vallabhapurapu, S., and Karin, M. (2009). Regulation and function of NF-kappaB transcription factors in the immune system. *Annu. Rev. Immunol.* 27, 693–733.

Virchow, R. (1863). *Die krankhaften Geschwülste.* Berlin: August Hirschwald.

Voronov, E., Carmi, Y., and Apte, R. N. (2007). Role of IL-1-mediated inflammation in tumor angiogenesis. *Adv. Exp. Med. Biol.* 601, 265–270.

Vujanovic, N. L., Yasumura, S., Hirabayashi, H., Lin, W. C., Watkins, S., Herberman, R. B., and Whiteside, T. L. (1995). Antitumor activities of subsets of human IL-2-activated natural killer cells in solid tissues. *J. Immunol.* 154, 281–289.

Wang, C., Deng, L., Hong, M., Akkaraju, G. R., Inoue, J., and Chen, Z. J. (2001). TAK1 is a

ubiquitin-dependent kinase of MKK and IKK. *Nature* 412, 346–351.
Wang, L., Yi, T., Kortylewski, M., Pardoll, D. M., Zeng, D., and Yu, H. (2009a). IL-17 can promote tumor growth through an IL-6-Stat3 signaling pathway. *J. Exp. Med.* 206, 1457–1464.
Wang, S., Liu, Q., Zhang, Y., Liu, K., Yu, P., Liu, K., Luan, J., Duan, H., Lu, Z., Wang, F., Wu, E., Yagasaki, K., and Zhang, G. (2009b). Suppression of growth, migration and invasion of highly-metastatic human breast cancer cells by berbamine and its molecular mechanisms of action. *Mol. Cancer* 8, 81.
Watters, T. M., Kenny, E. F., and O'Neill, L. A. (2007). Structure, function and regulation of the Toll/IL-1 receptor adaptor proteins. *Immunol. Cell Biol.* 85, 411–419.
Weaver, C. T., Hawrylowicz, C. M., and Unanue, E. R. (1988). T helper cell subsets require the expression of distinct costimulatory signals by antigen-presenting cells. *Proc. Natl. Acad. Sci. U.S.A.* 85, 8181–8185.
Wei, D., Wang, L., He, Y., Xiong, H. Q., Abbruzzese, J. L., and Xie, K. (2004). Celecoxib inhibits vascular endothelial growth factor expression in and reduces angiogenesis and metastasis of human pancreatic cancer via suppression of Sp1 transcription factor activity. *Cancer Res.* 64, 2030–2038.
Weichert, W., Boehm, M., Gekeler, V., Bahra, M., Langrehr, J., Neuhaus, P., Denkert, C., Imre, G., Weller, C., Hofmann, H. P., Niesporek, S., Jacob, J., Dietel, M., Scheidereit, C., and Kristiansen, G. (2007). High expression of RelA/p65 is associated with activation of nuclear factor-kappaB-dependent signaling in pancreatic cancer and marks a patient population with poor prognosis. *Br. J. Cancer* 97, 523–530.
Weiss, T. W., Simak, R., Kaun, C., Rega, G., Pfluger, H., Maurer, G., Huber, K., and Wojta, J. (2011). Oncostatin M and IL-6 induce u-PA and VEGF in prostate cancer cells and correlate in vivo. *Anticancer Res.* 31, 3273–3278.
Wesche, H., Henzel, W. J., Shillinglaw, W., Li, S., and Cao, Z. (1997a). MyD88: an adapter that recruits IRAK to the IL-1 receptor complex. *Immunity* 7, 837–847.
Wesche, H., Korherr, C., Kracht, M., Falk, W., Resch, K., and Martin, M. U. (1997b). The interleukin-1 receptor accessory protein (IL-1RAcP) is essential for IL-1-induced activation of interleukin-1 receptor-associated kinase (IRAK) and stress-activated protein kinases (SAP kinases). *J. Biol. Chem.* 272, 7727–7731.
Wheeler, D. S., Chase, M. A., Senft, A. P., Poynter, S. E., Wong, H. R., and Page, K. (2009). Extracellular Hsp72, an endogenous DAMP, is released by virally infected airway epithelial cells and activates neutrophils via Toll-like receptor (TLR)-4. *Respir. Res.* 10, 31.
Whiteside, T. L., Vujanovic, N. L., and Herberman, R. B. (1998). Natural killer cells and tumor therapy. *Curr. Top. Microbiol. Immunol.* 230, 221–244.
Wilson, K. T., Fu, S., Ramanujam, K. S., and Meltzer, S. J. (1998). Increased expression of inducible nitric oxide synthase and cyclooxygenase-2 in Barrett's esophagus and associated adenocarcinomas. *Cancer Res.* 58, 2929–2934.
Wink, D. A., Vodovotz, Y., Laval, J., Laval, F., Dewhirst, M. W., and Mitchell, J. B. (1998). The multifaceted roles of nitric oxide in cancer. *Carcinogenesis* 19, 711–721.
Wu, S., Rhee, K. J., Albesiano, E., Rabizadeh, S., Wu, X., Yen, H. R., Huso, D. L., Brancati, F. L., Wick, E., McAllister, F., Housseau, F., Pardoll, D. M., and Sears, C. L. (2009). A human colonic commensal promotes colon tumorigenesis via activation of T helper type 17 T cell responses. *Nat. Med.* 15, 1016–1022.
Xiong, H. Q. (2004). Molecular targeting therapy for pancreatic cancer. *Cancer Chemother. Pharmacol.* 54(Suppl. 1), S69–S77.
Xu, X. F., Xie, C. G., Wang, X. P., Liu, J., Yu, Y. C., Hu, H. L., and Guo, C. Y. (2008). Selective inhibition of cyclooxygenase-2 suppresses the growth of pancreatic cancer cells in vitro and in vivo. *Tohoku J. Exp. Med.* 215, 149–157.
Yamada, T., Tsuda, M., Takahashi, T., Totsuka, Y., Shindoh, M., and Ohba, Y. (2011). RANKL expression specifically observed in vivo promotes epithelial mesenchymal transition and tumor progression. *Am. J. Pathol.* 178, 2845–2856.
Yamashita, M., Kurokawa, K., Sato, Y., Yamagata, A., Mimura, H., Yoshikawa, A., Sato, K., Nakano, A., and Fukai, S. (2010). Structural basis for the Rho- and phosphoinositide-dependent localization of the exocyst subunit Sec3. *Nat. Struct. Mol. Biol.* 17, 180–186.
Yang, J., and Weinberg, R. A. (2008). Epithelial-mesenchymal transition: at the crossroads of development and tumor metastasis. *Dev. Cell* 14, 818–829.
Yasumura, S., Lin, W. C., Hirabayashi, H., Vujanovic, N. L., Herberman, R. B., and Whiteside, T. L. (1994). Immunotherapy of liver metastases of human gastric carcinoma with interleukin 2-activated natural killer cells. *Cancer Res.* 54, 3808–3816.
Yip-Schneider, M. T., Sweeney, C. J., Jung, S. H., Crowell, P. L., and Marshall, M. S. (2001). Cell cycle effects of nonsteroidal anti-inflammatory drugs and enhanced growth inhibition in combination with gemcitabine in pancreatic carcinoma cells. *J. Pharmacol. Exp. Ther.* 298, 976–985.
Yokota, S., Miyamae, T., Imagawa, T., Iwata, N., Katakura, S., and Mori, M. (2004). Inflammatory cytokines and systemic-onset juvenile idiopathic arthritis. *Mod. Rheumatol.* 14, 12–17.
Yoshimatsu, K., Altorki, N. K., Golijanin, D., Zhang, F., Jakobsson, P. J., Dannenberg, A. J., and Subbaramaiah, K. (2001a). Inducible prostaglandin E synthase is overexpressed in non-small cell lung cancer. *Clin. Cancer Res.* 7, 2669–2674.
Yoshimatsu, K., Golijanin, D., Paty, P. B., Soslow, R. A., Jakobsson, P. J., DeLellis, R. A., Subbaramaiah, K., and Dannenberg, A. J. (2001b). Inducible microsomal prostaglandin E synthase is overexpressed in colorectal adenomas and cancer. *Clin. Cancer Res.* 7, 3971–3976.
Yu, H., Kortylewski, M., and Pardoll, D. (2007). Crosstalk between cancer and immune cells: role of STAT3 in the tumour microenvironment. *Nat. Rev. Immunol.* 7, 41–51.
Yu, H., Pardoll, D., and Jove, R. (2009). STATs in cancer inflammation and immunity: a leading role for STAT3. *Nat. Rev. Cancer* 9, 798–809.
Zeisberg, M., and Neilson, E. G. (2009). Biomarkers for epithelial-mesenchymal transitions. *J. Clin. Invest.* 119, 1429–1437.
Zumsteg, A., and Christofori, G. (2009). Corrupt policemen: inflammatory cells promote tumor angiogenesis. *Curr. Opin. Oncol.* 21, 60–70.

5

The shape of the lymphocyte receptor repertoire: lessons from the B cell receptor

Katherine J. L. Jackson*, Marie J. Kidd, Yan Wang and Andrew M. Collins

School of Biotechnology and Biomolecular Sciences, University of New South Wales, Sydney, NSW, Australia

Edited by:
Ramit Mehr, Bar-Ilan University, Israel

Reviewed by:
Ramit Mehr, Bar-Ilan University, Israel
Gur Yaari, Yale University, USA
Nir Friedman, Weizmann Institute of Science, Israel

****Correspondence:***
Katherine J. L. Jackson, School of Biotechnology and Biomolecular Sciences, University of New South Wales, Sydney, NSW 2052, Australia
e-mail: katherine.jackson@unsw.edu.au

Both the B cell receptor (BCR) and the T cell receptor (TCR) repertoires are generated through essentially identical processes of V(D)J recombination, exonuclease trimming of germline genes, and the random addition of non-template encoded nucleotides. The naïve TCR repertoire is constrained by thymic selection, and TCR repertoire studies have therefore focused strongly on the diversity of MHC-binding complementarity determining region (CDR) CDR3. The process of somatic point mutations has given B cell studies a major focus on variable (IGHV, IGLV, and IGKV) genes. This in turn has influenced how both the naïve and memory BCR repertoires have been studied. Diversity (D) genes are also more easily identified in BCR VDJ rearrangements than in TCR VDJ rearrangements, and this has allowed the processes and elements that contribute to the incredible diversity of the immunoglobulin heavy chain CDR3 to be analyzed in detail. This diversity can be contrasted with that of the light chain where a small number of polypeptide sequences dominate the repertoire. Biases in the use of different germline genes, in gene processing, and in the addition of non-template encoded nucleotides appear to be intrinsic to the recombination process, imparting "shape" to the repertoire of rearranged genes as a result of differences spanning many orders of magnitude in the probabilities that different BCRs will be generated. This may function to increase the precursor frequency of naïve B cells with important specificities, and the likely emergence of such B cell lineages upon antigen exposure is discussed with reference to public and private T cell clonotypes.

Keywords: BCR repertoire, TCR repertoire, V(D)J recombination, public clonotypes, private clonotypes, combinatorial diversity, junctional diversity

GERMLINE GENES AND LYMPHOCYTE DIVERSITY

The mammalian immune system has the ability to respond to almost any antigen to which it is exposed because of the incredible diversity of lymphocyte receptor molecules. The diversity of both the B cell receptor (BCR) repertoire and the T cell receptor (TCR) repertoire is made possible by multiple sets of highly similar genes that recombine to form functional genes. Immunoglobulin heavy chains are encoded by recombined VDJ genes that are formed from sets of Variable (V), Diversity (D), and Joining (J) genes (IGHV, IGHJ, IGHD), while VJ rearrangements of kappa and lambda chain V genes (IGKV, IGLV) and J genes (IGKJ, IGLJ) encode the immunoglobulin light chains (1, 2). TCR β-chains and δ-chains are similarly encoded by distinct sets of V, D, and J genes (TRBV, TRBD, TRBJ; TRDV, TRDD, TRDJ), while α-chains and γ-chains are encoded by additional sets of V and J genes (TRAV, TRAJ; TRGV, TRGJ) (3–5). The resulting combinatorial diversity is expanded still further by junctional diversification arising from exonuclease trimming of the recombining gene ends and from the essentially random addition of nucleotides, between the recombining genes, by the enzyme terminal deoxynucleotidyl transferase (TdT) (6). Together, combinatorial diversity and junctional diversity create the diversity of the naïve T cell and B cell repertoires. Limitations to diversity may however be a feature of V(D)J rearrangement that is as significant to immune function as the bewildering number of lymphocyte specificities that can theoretically be generated.

This review will present evidence that biases in the processes that generate combinatorial and junctional diversity are such that the probabilities of different BCRs and TCRs being generated is highly variable. This results in B and T cells of some specificities being present within the naïve repertoire at high frequency, while other specificities may or may not be present at all. The unevenness of the receptor abundance distribution can be said to give "shape" to the naïve B and T lymphocyte repertoires. This distribution may be further shaped by processes including positive and negative selection, clonal expansion and, in the case of immunoglobulin genes, by somatic hypermutation, however this review will focus upon recombination and gene processing.

As the shape of the naïve human B and T cell lymphocyte repertoire is an outcome of the evolution of genetically determined biases, this should ensure the presence of critical rearrangements in the repertoire of all individuals. It should also ensure that these critical rearrangements are carried by multiple naïve cells (see **Figure 1**). Such populations of specific naïve lymphocytes will have a competitive advantage during antigen-driven clonal selection, and any discussion of repertoire diversity that is limited to the size of the population of unique receptors will therefore be ignoring a parameter of likely biological significance. In this review, we

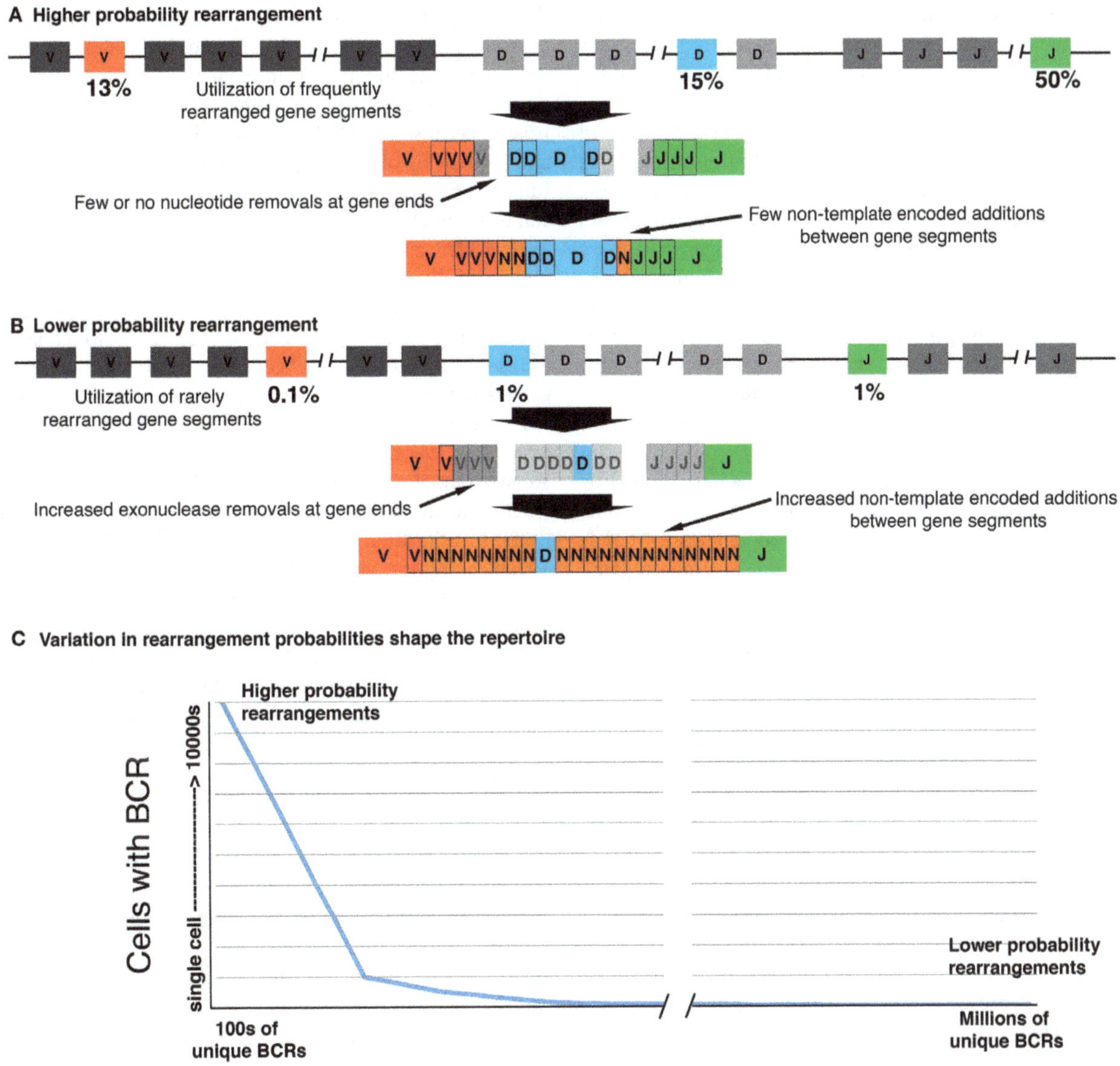

FIGURE 1 | The receptor repertoire has "shape," as biases and constraints in the recombination process vary the probabilities of generating particular V(D)J rearrangements. **(A)** Higher probability rearrangements are generated through utilization of more frequently rearranged gene segments. These segments are joined with minimal gene processing and N-addition, increasing the chance of independent rearrangements with identical or near identical CDR3s. **(B)** Lower probability rearrangements utilize rarely rearranged germline gene segments and the CDR3s are more diverse owing to increased nucleotide removals and additions at the joins. **(C)** The many order of magnitude differences in the likelihood of generating particular rearrangements shape the repertoire, with higher probability rearrangements being frequently generated and as a consequence being carried by many identical B-cells. Only a relatively small number of unique rearrangements will be generated with probabilities high enough to be carried by a large number of B cells, but this should ensure that they are always present in the repertoire at significant levels. Conversely, lower probability rearrangements may be so rare that they are carried only by a single B cell, or are entirely absent from the repertoire. The lower probability rearrangements that are carried by just one or at most a few B-cells likely represent many millions of unique rearrangements.

will use the term "repertoire" to refer to the complete set of receptors that are carried by an individual, including multiple copies of particular sequences. The number of unique sequences that are found within an individual's repertoire will be described as the "diversity" of the repertoire.

The size of the sets of germline genes make a major contribution to lymphocyte diversity, but surprisingly, our knowledge of these germline genes is far from complete. In part this is the result of the complexity of the loci, for they feature numerous highly similar genes that are thought to have evolved via gene conversion (7), and duplication and divergence (8). These genes are interspersed with many pseudogenes and repetitive elements (8). Sequencing and annotation of the loci is therefore challenging. These complexities also mean that SNPs arising from short read-length sequences generated in studies such as the HapMap and 1000 Genomes projects, cannot be used for the imputation of full-length allelic variants. In fact, these projects utilize polyclonal lymphoblastoid cells lines in which the immunoglobulin loci have undergone somatic recombination, and the rearranged genes may have been affected by somatic point mutation. This makes these cell lines unsuited to the study of immunoglobulin genes (9).

Arguably, it is the BCR germline genes that are best known, and paradoxically, this is because of their transformation through the process of somatic hypermutation, during an immune response. IGHV genes are by far the longest of the recombining IGH genes, and they are the principal targets of the mutational machinery (10, 11). Many studies of the immunogenetics of immunoglobulin have therefore concentrated upon the IGHV genes. As it is necessary to be certain of the germline origin of mutated sequences, if accurate studies of point mutations are to be conducted, the complete and accurate definition of the set of germline immunoglobulin IGHV genes and allelic variants has been and should remain a focus of research.

The official human IGHV germline gene dataset, curated by the ImMunoGeneTics (IMGT) group, includes 129 functional genes, open reading frames (ORF), and pseudogenes, as well as over 200 allelic variants (12). Interest in these germline genes has increased in recent years, resulting in 40 new allelic variants being reported since 2005 (13–17). Many additional IGHV allelic variants have also been identified in recent high-throughput sequencing studies, through analysis of cDNA-derived VDJ gene rearrangements (18, 19), but these have not been accepted as part of the official IGHV dataset. We have designated alleles identified in this way with unofficial allele names using an indicator ("p") of their "putative" nature (e.g., IGHV3-9*p03) (15), and these additional alleles can be found in the UNSWIg repertoire (http://www.ihmmune.unsw.edu.au/unswig.php).

The official human light chain V gene datasets appear to be relatively complete and accurate, though few allelic variants have been reported (20). Nevertheless these few variants appear to be of functional and clinical significance. For example, a variant kappa gene allele was identified within the Navajo population and has been reported to account for the susceptibility of this population to infections (21).

The human IGH germline genes receive continuing attention while the IMGT human TCR germline gene datasets have barely changed since the complete sequences of the TCR gene loci were first described (22, 23). The IMGT TRBV dataset includes 65 functional genes, ORFs and pseudogenes, and just 13 allelic variants, and no new TRBV sequence has been added to the dataset since the publication of the complete sequence of the TRB locus in 1996 (22). Only three TRAV/TRDV sequences (24) in the IMGT dataset are derived from studies published since the reporting of the complete sequence of the TRAV/TRDV locus (23), and some variants that were described soon afterward still remain officially unrecognized (25). The incomplete nature of the IMGT TRBV, and TRAV datasets in particular are clearly highlighted in the literature, for sequencing studies have reported many SNPs in the coding regions of these genes. Subramanyan and colleagues reported 279 SNPs in a study of 63 TRBV genes in 10 individuals from each of four human populations (26). Of these reported SNPs, 114 were located in coding regions of functional TRBV genes (26). A similar study of 57 TRAV/TRDV genes in the same 40 individuals resulted in the discovery of 284 SNPs, 51 of which encode amino acid changes in the coding regions of the gene sequences (27). The allelic variants associated with these TRAV/TRDV and TRBV SNPs have not been reported in the literature or in sequence databases, and they have not been incorporated into the official gene datasets. This is surprising because the SNPs were identified through amplification and sequencing of full-length genomic sequences. It is also unfortunate, for studies of TCR polymorphisms have shown that they can be of functional significance (28, 29).

The BCR and TCR D loci contribute differently to the generation of diversity, and the differences in the nature of the loci have influenced BCR and TCR research directions. The 27 human IGHD genes include 25 functional genes, 23 of which are unique (30). Although some IGHD genes, especially those of the IGHD1 gene family, are very similar, there is considerable sequence diversity amongst the genes. The lengths of the IGHD genes vary from 11 nucleotides to 37 nucleotides, and almost all of them are substantially longer than the TRBD and TRDD genes. This length and the IGHD gene variability have made improvement in the identification of IGHD genes within VDJ rearrangements a challenging but achievable research goal. Pursuit of this goal has driven the development of immunoglobulin gene alignment utilities including SODA2 (31), IgBLAST (32), and iHMMune-align (33). The objective measurement of the performance of these utilities is made difficult, however, by a lack of appropriate data sets. Ideally, performance would be measured using rearranged sequences of known composition. As such sets are unavailable, clonally related sequences can be used (32, 33). We have also compared the performance of different utilities using a set of long-read pyrosequenced (Roche 454) IGH rearrangements from an individual with a homozygous deletion of six IGHD genes (34). This test measures performance by the number of VDJ rearrangements in the dataset that are said to include the absent IGHD genes. Together these studies demonstrate that IGHD genes can now be identified with confidence, and as a consequence, analysis of the BCR heavy chain complementarity determining region (CDR) 3 can include detailed analysis of IGHD gene usage, gene processing, and N nucleotide addition.

Analysis of the TCR CDR3 is not so easy. The two human TRBD genes are both short (12 and 16 nucleotides) and highly similar at their 5′ ends (22). This makes their identification in VDJ rearrangements particularly difficult. The TRBD genes within a VDJ rearrangement are likely to be flanked by N-REGIONS of non-template encoded nucleotides. These nucleotides are introduced through the action of the TdT enzyme, which is biased to the addition of guanine (G) nucleotides (35) and to the addition of homopolymer tracts (36, 37). Distinguishing TRBD gene ends from G-rich N nucleotides is difficult because the TRBD genes are G-rich at both their 5′ and 3′ ends. A final complication is that the two alleles of TRBD2 differ by just a single nucleotide. This critical nucleotide is flanked on both sides, in both alleles, by GGG motifs. For these reasons, few TCR studies have included detailed analysis of TRBD genes and their processing, or of the N-REGIONS that can only be defined after the identification of a TRBD gene segment within the CDR3. Even the most recently developed TCR alignment utility excludes identification of TRBD genes from its output (38).

Analysis of the VDJ junction in TRD rearrangements is equally difficult. The three human TRDD genes are just 8, 9, and 13 nucleotides in length (4). This makes their reliable identification within VDJ rearrangements especially problematic if nucleotides have been lost through exonuclease activity. Application of an approach previously used in the analysis of BCR sequences (37) suggests that eight nucleotides is the minimum D gene length that will allow TRDD genes to be reliably distinguished from N-REGIONS within a junction of 12 or fewer nucleotides, while 9 nucleotides are needed for regions from 13 to 15 nucleotides and 10 nucleotides for junctions greater than 15 nucleotides (Jackson, unpublished data). It is therefore no surprise that few studies have reported the partitioning of TRD junctions as two of the three TRDD genes can only be confidently delineated from N-additions in their unprocessed form.

The J loci of the human BCR and TCR also include important differences. The IGHJ locus includes six functional genes, which are all found downstream of the IGHD locus in a single cluster. Allelic variants have been reported for IGHJ3, IGHJ4, IGHJ5, and IGHJ6, though there is reason to doubt the existence of the reported allelic variants of IGHJ3 and IGHJ5 (39). TCR J genes are more numerous and are differently organized. The TRBJ genes are found as a block of six genes located downstream from the TRDB1 gene, and a block of seven genes located downstream from the TRDB2 gene. The TRDB1 gene can pair with all J genes, but the TRDB2 gene is strongly biased toward pairing with its associated J genes (40). There are also four functional J genes in the TRDJ locus. Functional allelic variants have only been reported for the TRBJ1-6 gene.

BIASES IN COMBINATORIAL DIVERSITY AND THE SHAPING OF THE REPERTOIRE

Combinatorial diversity is that part of repertoire diversity that results from the fact that functional receptor genes form by the recombination of members of the sets of germline V, D, and J genes. This diversity is usually calculated by simply multiplying together the number of functional V, D, and J genes that are available within the genome. Such calculations, however, may promote misunderstandings, for they encourage the view that "all genes are equal," and that all combinations are equally likely. TCR studies have paid considerable attention to capturing an unbiased sampling of the repertoire, for example using 5′ RACE to amplify TCR transcripts from the constant region gene. Such studies have shown that TCR genes are highly biased in their usage (41–43). In contrast, many BCR repertoire studies have amplified both mRNA and genomic rearrangements, often using IGHV gene family-targeting primer sets that were developed for the detection of malignancies rather than for the investigation of the repertoire (44, 45). Such primers almost certainly lead to some distortions in the relative abundances of different sequences that are seen. Nevertheless, BCR studies utilizing different primer sets, and amplifying different source material are surprisingly consistent, and the B cell literature provides unequivocal evidence of strong gene utilization biases.

Different IGHV genes are used at frequencies that range from as little as 0.1% to more than 10% of all rearrangements in an individual's naïve B cell repertoire (18, 46). Utilization frequencies also vary between alleles. For example, analysis of VDJ recombination in different individuals has shown that IGHV1-2*02 is used approximately three times as often as IGHV1-2*04, in individuals who carry both these alleles (18). IGHV utilization frequencies are surprisingly constant between individuals (47). Examples of such consistency include IGHV1-46 which varies from 2 to 3.1% in different individuals (average 2.65%), IGHV3-21 which varies from 3.5 to 6.3% (average 4.59%), and IGHV3-49 which varies from 0.8 to 1.3% (average 1.0%) (18). This is not true for all genes, with different individuals utilizing IGHV1-69 at frequencies that range from 3.1 to 9.1% (average 6.2%) (18). IGHV3-23, which is typically the most utilized IGHV gene, was seen on average in 6.7% of all VDJ sequences, but its utilization frequency in one individual was 13.7% (18).

Biased gene usage is not confined to the IGHV genes. IGHD gene usage varies from less than 1% (IGHD4-4/11) to over 15% (IGHD3-22) of total rearrangements. Biases in the resulting amino acid sequences of the CDR3 junction are even greater. IGHD segments can be utilized in all three reading frames, and each IGHD gene is therefore able to encode three distinct amino acid sequences. Analysis of IGH rearrangements in which the IGHJ is out-of-frame, and which are therefore non-productive, shows each IGHD gene rearranges at equal frequency in each of the three RFs, however among productive rearrangements there is a strong skewing of the utilization of each gene toward a dominant RF (48). This dominance is constant between individuals, and the preferred RF is gene family dependent. Analysis of in-frame and out-of-frame IGH rearrangements sequenced using the Illumina platform suggests that the underlying rearrangement processes have no reading frame bias, but that bias emerges from stronger negative selection of sequences in certain reading frames (48). Such negative selection particularly focuses on non-productive sequences that result from the presence of stop codons within the junction region. These are seen when many IGHD genes are translated in the non-dominant reading frame, and such genes can only be utilized in those reading frames if the stop codons are removed by exonuclease trimming. When analysis of IGHD usage in the expressed repertoire factors in the three RFs, the IGHD gene utilization frequencies span three orders of magnitude. There is also considerable variation between the utilization frequencies of IGHJ genes. The IGHJ4 gene is present in approximately 45–50% of rearrangements, while IGHJ6 accounts for a further 20–25% of VDJ rearrangements (49, 50). IGHJ1, on the other hand, is utilized by only 1% of all rearrangements (39).

Biases in light chain gene usage are just as strong. For IGK rearrangements, preferential inclusion of IGKV3-20 was noted in early studies of the expressed IGK repertoire of both adults and neonates (51–53), while single cell PCR (54) and bioinformatics analysis of IGK rearrangements from sequence databases showed IGKV3-15, IGKV3-11, IGKV1-5, IGKV2-30, and IGKV1-30/IGKV1D-39 to also display preferential rearrangement (20). These biases were confirmed again recently in a high-throughput sequencing study which also highlighted similarities in usage between individuals, including similarities between individuals from geographically distant and ethnically distinct populations (55). Under-utilization and over-utilization of the J gene segments have been reported. IGKJ1 and IGKJ2 appear more frequently, while there is under-utilization of IGKJ3 and IGKJ5 (20, 53, 54). This skewing of IGKJ usage toward the genes located 5′ in the IGKJ locus is seen despite the necessity for selection of more 3′ IGKJ genes during secondary IGK rearrangements (56, 57). A similar bias toward 5′ IGKJ genes is also seen in the mouse, and modeling of mouse light chain rearrangement supports the strong underlying tendency toward the initial rearrangement of IGKJ1 or IGKJ2 (58). The IGLV usage is strongly skewed toward a limited number of the functional V segments with 3 of the 30 IGLVs accounting for more than 50% of expressed rearrangements, and with individual IGLV segment frequencies ranging from 0.02 to 27% (59). Only four of the seven IGLJ are considered functional (60). The four IGLJ range from almost 55% utilization in the expressed B cell repertoire for IGLJ7, to just 5.5% for IGLJ1 (61).

Although bias in the reading frame of the IGHD gene is the result of selection, other biases appear to be intrinsic to the recombination process, for when analysis is confined to non-productive rearrangements which carry an out-of-frame J-REGION, preferential gene usage is still seen (48). Such sequences are not subject to positive or negative selection. The same biases have been observed among transcripts generated from transgenic mice that carry a human heavy chain mini-locus (62), while in NOD-scid-IL2Rγ null mice that had been reconstituted with human hematopoietic stem cells, typical patterns of biased usage were seen amongst the expressed light chain genes (63). Recent studies in monozygotic twins show that they share utilization frequencies for both the heavy and light chain genes (46, 63), with correlations in a similar range to replicate biological samples. When one twin was investigated following lymphocyte ablation therapy, the reconstituted repertoire showed the same utilization patterns (46). Unrelated individuals did not share this degree of correlation. The biases in utilization frequencies of different V, D, and J genes therefore appear to be genetically determined, and when acted upon by the recombination machinery, the biases in that process give rise to an individual's distinct repertoire. Repertoire shape is therefore directly linked to the genotype of an individual's immunoglobulin gene loci. This has become even clearer since high-throughput sequencing has allowed analysis to focus upon individual chromosomes.

The large datasets that are now being generated by high-throughput sequencing from single individuals are facilitating analysis of the processes that shape the repertoire, but each dataset still represents a mixture of rearrangements from two independently recombining chromosomes. The fact that V(D)J rearrangement is an intra-chromosomal event, however, means that every V(D)J gene rearrangement provides information about the association of different genes on a chromosome. Any heterozygous locus allows each chromosome to be associated with one or the other allele at that gene locus, and large sets of V(D)J rearrangements can be analyzed to determine all the V, D, and J genes that rearrange on each chromosome. This allows the determination of inferred haplotypes (see **Figure 2**).

In practice, the complete inference of V, D, and J gene haplotypes by the analysis of V(D)J rearrangements is only likely to be possible in the case of the IGH locus. Approximately 40% of individuals are heterozygous at the IGHJ6 locus, and the IGHJ6 gene is present in nearly 25% of all rearrangements. It therefore provides an ideal "anchor-point" from which to haplotype the IGH locus. Using this approach, we recently investigated the IGH locus in nine individuals, and showed that all 18 IGH variable region gene

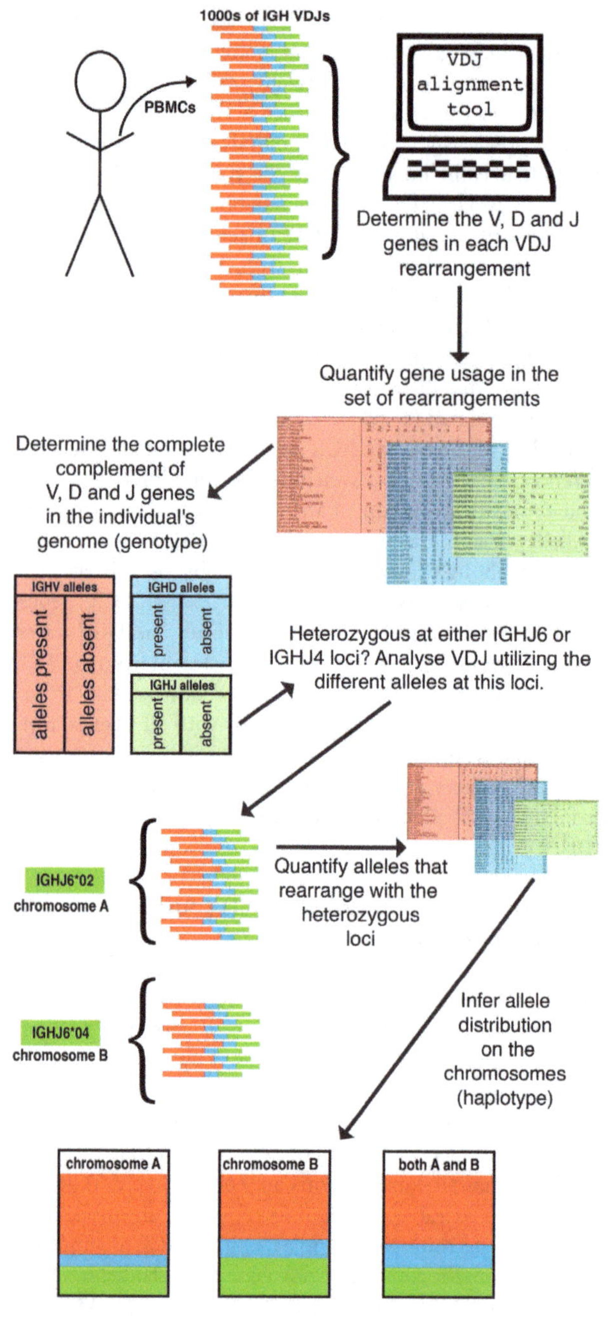

FIGURE 2 | Inference of IGH haplotypes from VDJ rearrangements. The availability of large datasets of VDJ rearrangements from single individuals permit the inference of all germline V, D, and J genes within the genome, from analysis of apparent gene utilization within a dataset. As IGH VDJ rearrangement is an intra-chromosomal event, gene pairing in VDJ rearrangements can be used to infer which gene segments are carried by the same chromosome. Leveraging the heterozygous IGHJ6 or IGHJ4 locus allows the reconstruction of IGH gene segments on each chromosome and for the IGH haplotype to be inferred.

haplotypes were unique (19). In addition to allelic variants, many IGHV and IGHD gene deletions and IGHV gene duplications were evident. The definition of haplotypes in this way is allowing IGH gene usage frequencies to be studied with unprecedented accuracy, but unfortunately no locus as appropriate as the IGHJ6 anchor-point exists amongst the light chain genes or amongst TCR genes. Limited investigations in the past have highlighted TCR haplotypic variation in the human population (64, 65), but the extent of variation within the IGH locus suggests that considerably more TCR variation may await discovery.

Many factors have been explored to explain biases in chromosomal recombination patterns. Variations in enhancers (66) have been implicated in biased murine TCR gene usage. Variations in recombination signal sequences (RSS) also influence utilization frequencies of both human BCR (67, 68) and TCR (69) genes. The IGKV polymorphism that has been linked to increased susceptibility to *Haemophilus influenzae* in the Navajo population includes a single nucleotide change in the heptamer sequence of the RSS, and it reduces recombination by 4.5-fold relative to the common allelic variant (21). The non-amer and heptamer sequences of the RSS are separated by either a 12 or 23 base pair spacer. Spacers also show sequence variation, and there has been debate about the impact this has on recombination efficiency. While some studies did not observe any impact when the regular spacer sequence was replaced with runs of GC pairs (70), competition assays using extra chromosomal substrates suggest differences in spacer sequence can result in differences in recombination efficiency that mirror differential gene usage in the V(D)J repertoire (67, 68). However, RSS variation cannot explain all differences in allele utilization. The recent re-sequencing of the complete IGH locus found that the IGHV-associated RSS were the same as those earlier reported by Matsuda (71) even where different alleles of the gene were present (17).

Some variation in the frequency with which particular gene sequences are seen in the repertoire may be explained by copy-number variations (CNV). The presence of CNV within the IG variable gene locus was first determined using sequence-specific RFLP analysis to determine gene copy-number (72), and the affect of CNV on expression levels was investigated through the examination of the binding of an anti-idiotypic monoclonal antibody (G6) to tonsillar IgD + B-cells (73). An examination of 35 individuals found that they carried between 0 and 4 copies of the IGHV1-69 gene. Linear regression determined that for each allele copy, approximately 3% of B-cells were G6 reactive. Individual differences in the IGHV1-69 copy-number could therefore result in the contribution that this single gene makes varying from being totally absent (0 copies) to being present in as many as 12% of rearrangements in individuals with four available copies.

Sequencing of single chromosomes of an individual's IGH locus has now demonstrated that insertions, deletions, and complex events have altered the copy-number of IGHV genes, including the IGHV1-69 and IGHV3-23 genes (17). The duplicate IGHV3-23 genes remain within the genome as absolutely identical sequences. The presence of these and other CNVs has also been highlighted in bioinformatic studies of immunoglobulin genotypes (18) and haplotypes (19), where sequence data from single individuals clearly demonstrated that some individuals had more than two "alleles" of a single IGHV gene. Genes were also found to be absent from the genome of some individuals. A limitation of these bioinformatics studies was that gene duplications could only be detected if two distinct "allelic variants" were carried on a single chromosome.

In addition to the underlying biases in utilization of germline genes, a final bias has been identified that affects the contribution of recombination frequencies to repertoire diversity. For reasons that are presently unclear, there appear to be pairing preferences for some IGHD and IGHJ genes that increase the frequency of particular IGHD-IGHJ pairs within the repertoire. Biases were first observed in a small set of 59 non-productive rearrangements (74). Later analysis of 6,500 IGH VDJ sequences collected from public databases led to the observation that 5′ IGHD genes paired with increased frequency to the most 3′ IGHJ (J5/J6) and with decreased frequency to the 5′ IGHJ (J1–J4) (50). In contrast, 3′ IGHD tended to preferentially pair with 5′ IGHJ rather than 3′ IGHJ (50). This observation is also supported by analysis of very large datasets generated by pyrosequencing of VDJ rearrangements from three healthy subjects (75). Significantly more pairings were seen of IGHD2-2 and IGHD3-3 with IGHJ6, and of IGHD3-22 and IGHJ3 than would be predicted from the frequencies of these genes in the overall dataset (75).

The bias in D-J pairing also extends to the TCRB loci where the application of HTS approaches to murine TCRB repertoires has revealed a pattern of TRBD to TRBJ pairing that correlates to the genomic distance between rearranged genes (40). The TRBV and TRBJ gene usage in the mice was biased toward particular genes, but the pairings of TRBV and TRBJ were independent. The physical chromatin structure of the TRBD and TRBJ loci was investigated using a biophysical model of the chromatin conformation. The biases in TRBD to TRBJ pairing appeared to be better explained by this mechanical model than previously proposed genetic models based on RSSs (40). The model was also extended to human TRBJ usage with favorable evidence that chromatin conformation determines TRJB gene usage.

Biases in the pairing of heavy and light chains have also been reported. The existence of forbidden or unfavorable pairings of germline heavy and light chain genes was described in the early literature (76). This was not supported by later studies (77, 78), nor was it supported by a recent study that applied high-throughput sequencing to generate thousands of linked heavy and light chain genes (79).

BIASES IN JUNCTIONAL DIVERSITY AND THE SHAPING OF THE REPERTOIRE

Both the naive B cell and T cell repertoires are limited in the periphery by processes of selection. However T cell selection within the thymus is a particularly rigorous process, and it leads to dramatic differences between the potential and the observed repertoire diversity. The idiosyncratic nature of TCR selection in a human population with abundant MHC diversity also means that analysis of the processes that contribute to TCR diversity will be difficult using datasets comprising sequences from multiple individuals. Sufficiently large datasets from single individuals with a specific MHC profile finally became available with the application of high-throughput sequencing to repertoire studies. However, the continuing difficulties involved with the identification of TCR

D genes and hence the other constituent elements within the TCR CDR3 still discourage analysis of the genetic elements and processes that contribute to this region. It is therefore studies of BCR genes that provide the clearest insights into the processes that contribute palindromic P nucleotides and non-template encoded N nucleotides to the V(D)J junction, and into the process of exonuclease trimming that depletes the ends of recombining genes. A recent study of BCR CDR3 suggested that as a result of these processes, the circulating B cell population in a typical adult human includes 3–9 × 10^6 unique heavy chain CDR3 (80).

Palindromic or P nucleotides are formed by the asymmetric opening of hairpin loops that form at gene ends during the rearrangement process (81). In the absence of exonuclease activity, the opening of the hairpins can add short, self-complementary single stranded extensions into the junctions. P nucleotide addition was first recognized as a process that can contribute to TCR CDR3 (82, 83), however the contributions of P nucleotides to the BCR repertoire have been more precisely quantified (84, 85). Similarly, it is recognized that N nucleotides make a major contribution to the diversity of both the TCR and BCR repertoire (86), but only BCR N-REGIONS have been subjected to detailed analysis (37). Where BCR studies have investigated the kinds of amino acids that are likely within N-REGIONS, studies of TCR N-REGIONS have focused upon analysis of the overall contribution of N-REGIONS to αβ TCR diversity. This has been studied in a comparison of wild-type mice with mice carrying homozygous null alleles for TdT (86). N-addition was estimated to contribute to 90% of the diversity of the αβ TCR repertoire (86). Diversity could be estimated in this and other studies because of the development of "spectratyping" techniques, which is the analysis of the CDR3 length distribution in PCR amplicons. It permitted some of the first explorations of the T cell repertoire, however it only allowed detailed analysis of N-REGIONS if further sequencing was undertaken. Until the advent of high-throughput sequencing, such analysis was usually compromised by the restricted number of sequences that could be generated from any individual, and by the challenges associated with D gene identification.

Non-template encoded N-additions are intrinsically biased owing to the preference of TdT toward the incorporation of G nucleotides. This is manifested in G/C-rich additions when viewing the N-REGIONS of the coding strand, as additions may be made to both the coding and non-coding strands during recombination. This has been demonstrated through analysis of extrachromosomal substrates transfected into human cell lines (36), as well as by analysis of human BCR (37) and TCR (87) VDJ rearrangements. The G/C bias is coupled with an apparent interdependence of the additions, which leads to the formation of homopolymer tracts (36, 37, 87). Together these biases ensure that the germline gene-encoded regions of the CDR3 are frequently flanked by amino acids such as glycine, that are encoded by G-rich codons (88). It has been proposed that the inclusion of small amino acids such as glycine, which has only a single side chain, promotes flexibility of the CDR3 loop (88).

Exonuclease trimming is perhaps the least understood process that contributes to the BCR and TCR repertoires. The mechanisms responsible for the loss of nucleotides from the coding ends of the genes during rearrangement remains to be determined, but a number of features of the process have been described, and intrinsic biases have been identified. The extent of processing from each gene end involved in a join (VD or DJ) is independent (87). That is, we do not see more processing on one side of the join to compensate for reduced processing of the gene on the other side. The processing differs for V, D, and J genes and for gene families. Removals may therefore be impacted by the sequence of the gene ends. Sequences with high A/T content appear more susceptible to nucleotide loss, while sequences with high G/C content appear resistant to processing (36, 84, 89, 90). This bias is still seen after controlling for the G/C bias of N-REGIONS.

The gene sequence ends that remain after exonuclease processing provide a final bias that shapes the repertoire. The gene ends are constrained by the genetic code, to favor the formation of codons for a surprisingly limited number of amino acids. This is best illustrated in the case of the many IGHD genes that have the nucleotide sequence TAC at their 3′ end (see **Figure 3**). In the dominant reading frame, these nucleotides encode tyrosine. Removal of a single nucleotide creates a situation where only provision of a T or C (from N-addition or from the 5′ end of the IGHJ gene) will result in a functional sequence, for TAA and TAG are stop codons. Addition of C returns the sequence to its original state, while addition of T results in an alternative tyrosine codon. In this and other cases, the nucleotide sequences of the gene ends limit the diversity that results from exonuclease removals.

B CELL LINEAGES AND T CELL CLONOTYPES IN THE ANTIGEN-SPECIFIC RESPONSE

Biases that we have described in immunoglobulin V, D, and J gene usage mean that at least seven orders of magnitude separate the probabilities that the most likely and the least likely combinations of recombining genes will be generated in the bone marrow. Many additional orders of magnitude separate the most likely from the

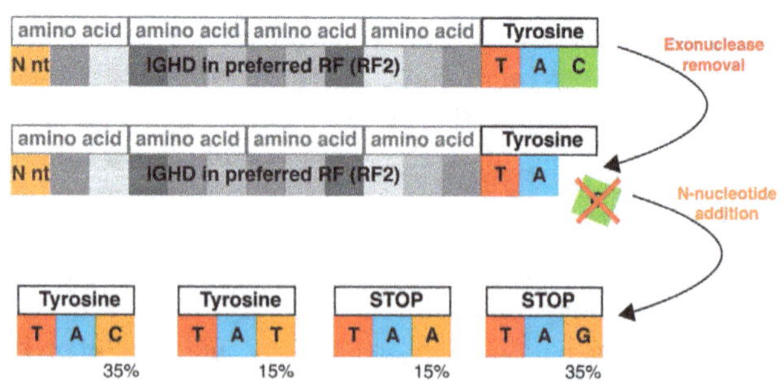

FIGURE 3 | Germline gene segment sequences constrain junctional diversity. This is illustrated by processing of the codon TAC, which encodes tyrosine as the most 3′ amino acid in the preferred reading frame of many IGHD genes. A highly probable outcome of the VDJ rearrangement process is the loss of a single nucleotide from the IGHD coding end. If this occurs, the productive repertoire for these Ds is strongly skewed toward tyrosine, as two of the four possible nucleotide replacement events generate stop codons, and the other two ensure the maintenance of tyrosine. These nucleotides may be sourced from either N-addition or from the 5′ end of an IGHJ segment. The outcome of N-addition is depicted in the bottom panel. N-additions are colored in orange and below each of the four possible outcomes is shown the likelihood of the enzyme TdT adding each nucleotide base.

least likely heavy and light chain pairs. The least likely BCRs are so unlikely to be generated in the bone marrow that they almost certainly will never be seen in an individual's lifetime. The most likely BCRs, on the other hand, may be so readily generated that they are always present within the repertoire at high copy number. These high copy-number sequences are likely to utilize a relative handful of the available germline genes, and to have been subject to minimal processing. TdT adds, on average, around 6 nucleotides between joining genes, and 30 or more nucleotides may occasionally be added to the VD, DJ, and VJ junctions, but it is highly likely that no more than two nucleotides will be added. Even long heavy chain CDR3 are likely to be the result of long germline sequences rather than the result of long N-REGIONS (47). Six or more nucleotides may be removed from the 3′ end of the IGHV gene, but most sequences lose no more than two or three IGHV nucleotides, and many sequences lose no nucleotides at all.

Without the added diversity that comes from D genes, the kappa and lambda repertoires are strongly shaped by biased gene usage and minimal processing and the diversity of the repertoires is surprisingly limited. The light chain repertoires are dominated by a very small number of amino acid sequences, and this dominance is so extreme that even in the days of Sanger sequencing, identical light chain gene rearrangements were reported by separate studies from independent laboratories (20). The theoretical diversity of the kappa repertoire has been estimated to be as high as 4×10^{24} unique nucleotide sequences (91). However analysis of kappa sequences generated from single individuals by high-throughput sequencing suggest the repertoire may include less than 10^4 unique amino acid sequences (55), and some of these sequences may be seen in over 1% of all kappa-bearing BCR (55). The diversity of the expressed lambda repertoire has recently been shown to be similarly restricted (63).

Although the heavy chain repertoire has much greater diversity then the light chain repertoire, repertoire shaping may be sufficiently extreme that some heavy chain sequences, and even some BCR will be present at high copy number in the repertoire of every individual. We are not aware of identical heavy chain sequences being amplified from multiple individuals, but highly similar "stereotypical" sequences have been found amongst leukemic clones of individuals with chronic lymphocytic leukemia (92). These stereotypical sequences differ through the stochastic processes of somatic hypermutation, but they appear to have evolved from cells expressing highly similar BCR within the naïve B cell repertoires of different individuals. Antigen selection, which may be associated with the pathogenesis of this condition (93), could be selecting and therefore revealing high copy-number heavy chain sequences.

The antigen specificity of most heavy and light chain sequences remain unclear, for it is only very recently that antigen-specific human B cells have been isolated and their BCRs investigated. The isolation of antigen-specific plasmablasts from the peripheral blood shortly after vaccination was first used to produce monoclonal human antibodies (94). These cells express BCR genes that are at once similar, as a consequence of their shared origins, yet highly divergent, as a result of the process of somatic point mutation. Together they make up a B cell clone lineage. High-throughput sequencing has since been used to identify clone lineages after booster shots with the influenza vaccine (95) and the pneumococcal vaccine (96). B cell lineages producing broadly neutralizing antibodies to HIV have also been identified using high-throughput sequencing (97). However this handful of studies of antigen-specific B cells in humans has not identified lineages that are shared between individuals. Highly similar BCR heavy chain sequences have recently been identified using high-throughput sequencing of PBMC from multiple individuals with acute symptomatic dengue (98). Although the specificities of these sequences were not determined, such lineages were not identified in uninfected individuals. These may therefore be the first antigen-specific heavy chain "public lineages" to be identified. The extent to which the response to specific antigen more generally involves such "public lineages" remains to be determined.

In contrast to the paucity of studies of antigen-specific B cells, antigen-specific TCRs have been investigated in the human repertoire for over 20 years. Early studies revealed that the immune response to specific antigen, in HLA-matched individuals, can include sets of T cells sharing identical or highly similar TCR α- and β-chains (99–101). The development of techniques for the creation of MHC peptide tetramer complexes has facilitated the identification of antigen-specific T cells by flow cytometry (102). This has allowed the detailed investigation of dominant sequence sets and these studies gave rise to the notions of public and private T cell "clonotypes." Public clonotypes are defined as VDJ amino acid sequences that are dominant and identical, or nearly identical, in multiple individuals. Private clonotypes, in contrast, are idiosyncratic. The apparently antigen-driven emergence of public B cell lineages in chronic lymphocytic B cell leukemia also has parallels amongst T cell leukemias. Studies of T cell large granular lymphocyte leukemias have identified a public clonotype in individuals with the shared DRB1*0701 HLA type (103). This same clonotype was independently identified in DRB1*0701$^+$ individuals who were infected with human cytomegalovirus (104), suggesting that antigen-driven pathogenesis may be expanding and revealing this public clonotype.

To understand the reasons for the emergence of particular clonotypes, the naïve repertoire must be better understood. Enrichment techniques have recently been developed which when combined with MHC peptide tetramer technology allows extremely rare peptide-specific naïve murine T cells to be identified (105). Using this approach in humans, naïve CD8$^+$ T cells specific for peptide-MHC have been shown to range from 0.6 to 500 cells per million cells (106, 107) and CD4+ T cells to range from 0.2 to 10 per million cells (107). Most of the cells within identified sets of antigen-specific murine T cells express unique TCRs (105), but clonal diversity within identified human cell populations remains unclear. It is likely though that in the much larger human T cell compartment, many circulating T cells could carry identical TCRs. This should ensure that early adaptive responses to these antigens are robust, for the strength of the response to antigen has been shown to reflect the size of the antigen-specific naïve T cell population (105).

The presence of particular public TCR clonotypes have not yet been reported within the naïve human TCR repertoire. Discussion of the emergence of such TCR clonotypes in an antigen-specific response has therefore been driven principally by analyses of their nucleotide and amino acid features, and the phenomenon of convergent recombination has been invoked to explain public clonotypes (108, 109). Many public TCR clonotypes are divergent at the nucleotide level, but identical at the amino acid level. This results from the fact that particular amino acid sequences can arise from multiple, variant nucleotide sequences, and that these nucleotide sequences in turn can sometimes be formed by different genes with varying levels of gene processing and nucleotide addition. Such convergent recombination will certainly contribute to the presence of multiple copies of particular amino acid clonotypes within an individual's repertoire, but arguably, it is unlikely to increase the likelihood of one clonotype over another by more than one or two orders of magnitude.

More recently the role of biases in gene usage and in the recombination process have been identified as an alternative source of public clonotypes (110). The biases in the usage of TCR V, D, and J genes are less pronounced than is the case for the BCR genes. This is the result of the lack of substantial germline diversity within the sets of TRBD and TRDD genes, and because the TRBJ and TRDJ genes lack the strong usage biases that are seen amongst the IGHJ genes. Nevertheless biases in the usage of TCR genes are still likely to ensure that the probabilities of the generation of the least likely and the most likely V(D)J combination seen in αβ and γδ TCR differ by many orders of magnitude. It has also been pointed out that many public clonotypes have short CDR3 loops that are mainly encoded by germline-derived nucleotides rather then TdT-derived nucleotides (110). The contribution this may make to the formation of T cell clonotypes is harder to judge, because of the lack of detailed analysis of these processes, in the context of the TCR repertoire. However lessons from analysis of the BCR repertoire give strong credence to this hypothesis.

Both the BCR and the TCR repertoires have been the subject of considerable study and even greater speculation over many decades. High-throughput sequencing is now revealing their separate secrets at a gratifying rate. Our understanding of the shaping of the BCR and TCR repertoires will now surely move faster if a greater dialog commences between researchers on the two sides of the lymphocyte divide. BCR repertoire studies will be transformed when greater attention is paid to antigen-specific lineages. TCR repertoire studies, in turn, could benefit from the lessons of the BCR repertoire, which suggest that the analysis of full-length V(D)J rearrangements, and detailed analysis of the nucleotide elements within the CDR3, can help explain the shaping of the repertoire.

ACKNOWLEDGMENTS

This work was made possible by a grant from the National Health and Medical Research Council.

REFERENCES

1. Tonegawa S. Somatic generation of antibody diversity. *Nature* (1983) **302**:575–81. doi:10.1038/302575a0
2. Schroeder HW Jr, Cavacini L. Structure and function of immunoglobulins. *J Allergy Clin Immunol* (2010) **125**:S41–52. doi:10.1016/j.jaci.2009.09.046
3. Davis MM, Bjorkman PJ. T-cell antigen receptor genes and T-cell recognition. *Nature* (1988) **334**:395–402. doi:10.1038/334395a0
4. Takihara Y, Tkachuk D, Michalopoulos E, Champagne E, Reimann J, Minden M, et al. Sequence and organization of the diversity, joining, and constant region genes of the human T-cell delta-chain locus. *Proc Natl Acad Sci U S A* (1988) **85**:6097–101. doi:10.1073/pnas.85.16.6097
5. Nikolich-Zugich J, Slifka MK, Messaoudi I. The many important facets of T-cell repertoire diversity. *Nat Rev Immunol* (2004) **4**:123–32. doi:10.1038/nri1292
6. Desiderio SV, Yancopoulos GD, Paskind M, Thomas E, Boss MA, Landau N, et al. Insertion of N regions into heavy-chain genes is correlated with expression of terminal deoxytransferase in B cells. *Nature* (1984) **311**:752–5.
7. Davies JM, Platts-Mills TA, Aalberse RC. The enigma of IgE+ B-cell memory in human subjects. *J Allergy Clin Immunol* (2013) **131**:972–6. doi:10.1016/j.jaci.2012.12.1569
8. Fukui K, Noma T, Takeuchi K, Kobayashi N, Hatanaka M, Honjo T. Origin of adult T-cell leukemia virus. Implication for its zoonosis. *Mol Biol Med* (1983) **1**:447–56.
9. Watson CT, Breden F. The immunoglobulin heavy chain locus: genetic variation, missing data, and implications for human disease. *Genes Immun* (2012) **13**:363–73. doi:10.1038/gene.2012.12
10. Rada C, Milstein C. The intrinsic hypermutability of antibody heavy and light chain genes decays exponentially. *EMBO J* (2001) **20**:4570–6. doi:10.1093/emboj/20.16.4570
11. Odegard VH, Schatz DG. Targeting of somatic hypermutation. *Nat Rev Immunol* (2006) **6**:573–83. doi:10.1038/nri1896
12. Pallares N, Lefebvre S, Contet V, Matsuda F, Lefranc MP. The human immunoglobulin heavy variable genes. *Exp Clin Immunogenet* (1999) **16**:36–60. doi:10.1159/000019095
13. Ohm-Laursen L, Larsen SR, Barington T. Identification of two new alleles, IGHV3-23*04 and IGHJ6*04, and the complete sequence of the IGHV3-h pseudogene in the human immunoglobulin locus and their prevalences in Danish Caucasians. *Immunogenetics* (2005) **57**:621–7. doi:10.1007/s00251-005-0035-8
14. Romo-Gonzalez T, Morales-Montor J, Rodriguez-Dorantes M, Vargas-Madrazo E. Novel substitution polymorphisms of human immunoglobulin VH genes in Mexicans. *Hum Immunol* (2005) **66**:732–40. doi:10.1016/j.humimm.2005.03.002
15. Wang Y, Jackson KJ, Sewell WA, Collins AM. Many human immunoglobulin heavy-chain IGHV gene polymorphisms have been reported in error. *Immunol Cell Biol* (2008) **86**:111–5.
16. Wang Y, Jackson KJ, Gaeta B, Pomat W, Siba P, Sewell WA, et al. Genomic screening by 454 pyrosequencing identifies a new human IGHV gene and sixteen other new IGHV allelic variants. *Immunogenetics* (2011) **63**:259–65. doi:10.1007/s00251-010-0510-8
17. Watson CT, Steinberg KM, Huddleston J, Warren RL, Malig M, Schein J, et al. Complete haplotype sequence of the human immunoglobulin heavy-chain variable, diversity, and joining genes and characterization of allelic and copy-number variation. *Am J Hum Genet* (2013) **92**:530–46. doi:10.1016/j.ajhg.2013.03.004
18. Boyd SD, Gaeta BA, Jackson KJ, Fire AZ, Marshall EL, Merker JD, et al. Individual variation in the germline Ig gene repertoire inferred from variable region gene rearrangements. *J Immunol* (2010) **184**:6986–92. doi:10.4049/jimmunol.1000445
19. Kidd MJ, Chen Z, Wang Y, Jackson KJ, Zhang L, Boyd SD, et al. The inference of phased haplotypes for the immunoglobulin H chain V region gene loci by analysis of VDJ gene rearrangements. *J Immunol* (2012) **188**:1333–40. doi:10.4049/jimmunol.1102097
20. Collins AM, Wang Y, Singh V, Yu P, Jackson KJ, Sewell WA. The reported germline repertoire of human immunoglobulin kappa chain genes is relatively complete and accurate. *Immunogenetics* (2008) **60**:669–76. doi:10.1007/s00251-008-0325-z
21. Feeney AJ, Atkinson MJ, Cowan MJ, Escuro G, Lugo G. A defective Vkappa A2 allele in Navajos which may play a role in increased susceptibility to *Haemophilus influenzae* type b disease. *J Clin Invest* (1996) **97**:2277–82. doi:10.1172/JCI118669
22. Rowen L, Koop BF, Hood L. The complete 685-kilobase DNA sequence of the human beta T cell receptor locus. *Science* (1996) **272**:1755–62. doi:10.1126/science.272.5269.1755

23. Boysen C, Simon MI, Hood L. Analysis of the 1.1-Mb human alpha/delta T-cell receptor locus with bacterial artificial chromosome clones. *Genome Res* (1997) **7**:330–8.
24. Ibberson MR, Copier JP, Llop E, Navarrete C, Hill AV, Cruickshank JK, et al. T-cell receptor variable alpha (TCRAV) polymorphisms in European, Chinese, South American, AfroCaribbean, and Gambian populations. *Immunogenetics* (1998) **47**:124–30. doi:10.1007/s002510050337
25. Moody AM, Reyburn H, Willcox N, Newsom-Davis J. New polymorphism of the human T-cell receptor AV28S1 gene segment. *Immunogenetics* (1998) **48**:62–4. doi:10.1007/s002510050401
26. Subrahmanyan L, Eberle MA, Clark AG, Kruglyak L, Nickerson DA. Sequence variation and linkage disequilibrium in the human T-cell receptor beta (TCRB) locus. *Am J Hum Genet* (2001) **69**:381–95. doi:10.1086/321297
27. Mackelprang R, Livingston RJ, Eberle MA, Carlson CS, Yi Q, Akey JM, et al. Sequence diversity, natural selection and linkage disequilibrium in the human T cell receptor alpha/delta locus. *Hum Genet* (2006) **119**:255–66. doi:10.1007/s00439-005-0111-z
28. Vessey SJ, Bell JI, Jakobsen BK. A functionally significant allelic polymorphism in a T cell receptor V beta gene segment. *Eur J Immunol* (1996) **26**:1660–3. doi:10.1002/eji.1830260739
29. Gras S, Chen Z, Miles JJ, Liu YC, Bell MJ, Sullivan LC, et al. Allelic polymorphism in the T cell receptor and its impact on immune responses. *J Exp Med* (2010) **207**:1555–67. doi:10.1084/jem.20100603
30. Corbett SJ, Tomlinson IM, Sonnhammer EL, Buck D, Winter G. Sequence of the human immunoglobulin diversity (D) segment locus: a systematic analysis provides no evidence for the use of DIR segments, inverted D segments, "minor" D segments or D-D recombination. *J Mol Biol* (1997) **270**:587–97. doi:10.1006/jmbi.1997.1141
31. Munshaw S, Kepler TB. SoDA2: a Hidden Markov Model approach for identification of immunoglobulin rearrangements. *Bioinformatics* (2010) **26**:867–72. doi:10.1093/bioinformatics/btq056
32. Ye J, Ma N, Madden TL, Ostell JM. IgBLAST: an immunoglobulin variable domain sequence analysis tool. *Nucleic Acids Res* (2013). doi:10.1093/nar/gkt382
33. Gaeta BA, Malming HR, Jackson KJ, Bain ME, Wilson P, Collins AM. iHMMune-align: hidden Markov model-based alignment and identification of germline genes in rearranged immunoglobulin gene sequences. *Bioinformatics* (2007) **23**:1580–7. doi:10.1093/bioinformatics/btm147
34. Jackson KJ, Boyd S, Gaeta BA, Collins AM. Benchmarking the performance of human antibody gene alignment utilities using a 454 sequence dataset. *Bioinformatics* (2010) **26**:3129–30. doi:10.1093/bioinformatics/btq604
35. Basu M, Hegde MV, Modak MJ. Synthesis of compositionally unique DNA by terminal deoxynucleotidyl transferase. *Biochem Biophys Res Commun* (1983) **111**:1105–12. doi:10.1016/0006-291X(83)91413-4
36. Gauss GH, Lieber MR. Mechanistic constraints on diversity in human V(D)J recombination. *Mol Cell Biol* (1996) **16**:258–69.
37. Jackson KJ, Gaeta BA, Collins AM. Identifying highly mutated IGHD genes in the junctions of rearranged human immunoglobulin heavy chain genes. *J Immunol Methods* (2007) **324**:26–37. doi:10.1016/j.jim.2007.04.011
38. Thomas N, Heather J, Ndifon W, Shawe-Taylor J, Chain B. Decombinator: a tool for fast, efficient gene assignment in T-cell receptor sequences using a finite state machine. *Bioinformatics* (2013) **29**:542–50. doi:10.1093/bioinformatics/btt004
39. Lee CE, Jackson KJ, Sewell WA, Collins AM. Use of IGHJ and IGHD gene mutations in analysis of immunoglobulin sequences for the prognosis of chronic lymphocytic leukemia. *Leuk Res* (2007) **31**:1247–52. doi:10.1016/j.leukres.2006.10.013
40. Ndifon W, Gal H, Shifrut E, Aharoni R, Yissachar N, Waysbort N, et al. Chromatin conformation governs T-cell receptor Jbeta gene segment usage. *Proc Natl Acad Sci U S A* (2012) **109**:15865–70. doi:10.1073/pnas.1203916109
41. Quiros Roldan E, Sottini A, Bettinardi A, Albertini A, Imberti L, Primi D. Different TCRBV genes generate biased patterns of V-D-J diversity in human T cells. *Immunogenetics* (1995) **41**:91–100.
42. Livak F, Burtrum DB, Rowen L, Schatz DG, Petrie HT. Genetic modulation of T cell receptor gene segment usage during somatic recombination. *J Exp Med* (2000) **192**:1191–6. doi:10.1084/jem.192.8.1191
43. Warren RL, Freeman JD, Zeng T, Choe G, Munro S, Moore R, et al. Exhaustive T-cell repertoire sequencing of human peripheral blood samples reveals signatures of antigen selection and a directly measured repertoire size of at least 1 million clonotypes. *Genome Res* (2011) **21**:790–7. doi:10.1101/gr.115428.110
44. van Dongen JJ, Langerak AW, Bruggemann M, Evans PA, Hummel M, Lavender FL, et al. Design and standardization of PCR primers and protocols for detection of clonal immunoglobulin and T-cell receptor gene recombinations in suspect lymphoproliferations: report of the BIOMED-2 Concerted Action BMH4-CT98-3936. *Leukemia* (2003) **17**:2257–317. doi:10.1038/sj.leu.2403202
45. Matthews C, Catherwood M, Morris TC, Alexander HD. Routine analysis of IgVH mutational status in CLL patients using BIOMED-2 standardized primers and protocols. *Leuk Lymphoma* (2004) **45**:1899–904. doi:10.1080/10428190410001710812
46. Glanville J, Kuo TC, Von Büdingen H-C, Guey L, Berka J, Sundar PD, et al. Naive antibody gene-segment frequencies are heritable and unaltered by chronic lymphocyte ablation. *Proc Natl Acad Sci U S A* (2011) **108**:20066–71. doi:10.1073/pnas.1107498108
47. Briney BS, Willis JR, Mckinney BA, Crowe JE Jr. High-throughput antibody sequencing reveals genetic evidence of global regulation of the naive and memory repertoires that extends across individuals. *Genes Immun* (2012) **13**:469–73. doi:10.1038/gene.2012.20
48. Benichou J, Glanville J, Prak ET, Azran R, Kuo TC, Pons J, et al. The restricted DH gene reading frame usage in the expressed human antibody repertoire is selected based upon its amino acid content. *J Immunol* (2013) **190**:5567–77. doi:10.4049/jimmunol.1201929
49. Yamada M, Wasserman R, Reichard BA, Shane S, Caton AJ, Rovera G. Preferential utilization of specific immunoglobulin heavy chain diversity and joining segments in adult human peripheral blood B lymphocytes. *J Exp Med* (1991) **173**:395–407. doi:10.1084/jem.173.2.395
50. Volpe JM, Kepler TB. Large-scale analysis of human heavy chain V(D)J recombination patterns. *Immunome Res* (2008) **4**:3. doi:10.1186/1745-7580-4-3
51. Klein R, Jaenichen R, Zachau HG. Expressed human immunoglobulin kappa genes and their hypermutation. *Eur J Immunol* (1993) **23**:3248–62. doi:10.1002/eji.1830231231
52. Cox JP, Tomlinson IM, Winter G. A directory of human germ-line V kappa segments reveals a strong bias in their usage. *Eur J Immunol* (1994) **24**:827–36. doi:10.1002/eji.1830240409
53. Weber JC, Blaison G, Martin T, Knapp AM, Pasquali JL. Evidence that the V kappa III gene usage is nonstochastic in both adult and newborn peripheral B cells and that peripheral CD5+ adult B cells are oligoclonal. *J Clin Invest* (1994) **93**:2093–105. doi:10.1172/JCI117204
54. Foster SJ, Brezinschek HP, Brezinschek RI, Lipsky PE. Molecular mechanisms and selective influences that shape the kappa gene repertoire of IgM+ B cells. *J Clin Invest* (1997) **99**:1614–27. doi:10.1172/JCI119324
55. Jackson KJ, Wang Y, Gaeta BA, Pomat W, Siba P, Rimmer J, et al. Divergent human populations show extensive shared IGK rearrangements in peripheral blood B cells. *Immunogenetics* (2012) **64**:3–14. doi:10.1007/s00251-011-0559-z
56. Gay D, Saunders T, Camper S, Weigert M. Receptor editing: an approach by autoreactive B cells to escape tolerance. *J Exp Med* (1993) **177**:999–1008. doi:10.1084/jem.177.4.999
57. Tiegs SL, Russell DM, Nemazee D. Receptor editing in self-reactive bone marrow B cells. *J Exp Med* (1993) **177**:1009–20. doi:10.1084/jem.177.4.1009
58. Mehr R, Shannon M, Litwin S. Models for antigen receptor gene rearrangement. I. Biased receptor editing in B cells: implications for allelic exclusion. *J Immunol* (1999) **163**:1793–8.
59. Ignatovich O, Tomlinson IM, Jones PT, Winter G. The creation of diversity in the human immunoglobulin V(lambda) repertoire. *J*

Mol Biol (1997) **268**:69–77. doi:10.1006/jmbi.1997.0956
60. Vasicek TJ, Leder P. Structure and expression of the human immunoglobulin lambda genes. *J Exp Med* (1990) **172**:609–20. doi: 10.1084/jem.172.2.609
61. Farner NL, Dorner T, Lipsky PE. Molecular mechanisms and selection influence the generation of the human V lambda J lambda repertoire. *J Immunol* (1999) **162**:2137–45.
62. Tuaillon N, Taylor LD, Lonberg N, Tucker PW, Capra JD. Human immunoglobulin heavy-chain minilocus recombination in transgenic mice: gene-segment use in mu and gamma transcripts *Proc Natl Acad Sci U S A* (1993) **90**:3720–4. doi:10.1073/pnas.90.8.3720
63. Hoi KH, Ippolito GC. Intrinsic bias and public rearrangements in the human immunoglobulin Vlambda light chain repertoire. *Genes Immun* (2013) **14**:271–6. doi:10.1038/gene.2013.10
64. Craddock TP, Zumla AM, Ollier WE, Chintu CZ, Muyinda GP, Lancaster FC, et al. Predominance of one T-cell antigen receptor BV haplotype in African populations. *Immunogenetics* (2000) **51**:231–7. doi:10.1007/s002510050036
65. Donaldson IJ, Shefta J, Lawson CA, Bushnell JR, Morgan AW, Isaacs JD, et al. Unique TCR beta-subunit variable gene haplotypes in Africans. *Immunogenetics* (2002) **53**:884–93. doi:10.1007/s00251-001-0406-8
66. McMurry MT, Hernandez-Munain C, Lauzurica P, Krangel MS. Enhancer control of local accessibility to V(D)J recombinase. *Mol Cell Biol* (1997) **17**:4553–61.
67. Nadel B, Tang A, Escuro G, Lugo G, Feeney AJ. Sequence of the spacer in the recombination signal sequence affects V(D)J rearrangement frequency and correlates with nonrandom Vkappa usage in vivo. *J Exp Med* (1998) **187**:1495–503. doi:10.1084/jem.187.9.1495
68. Feeney AJ, Tang A, Ogwaro KM. B-cell repertoire formation: role of the recombination signal sequence in non-random V segment utilization. *Immunol Rev* (2000) **175**:59–69. doi:10.1111/j.1600-065X.2000.imr017508.x
69. Posnett DN, Vissinga CS, Pambuccian C, Wei S, Robinson MA, Kostyu D, et al. Level of human TCRBV3S1 (V beta 3) expression correlates with allelic polymorphism in the spacer region of the recombination signal sequence. *J Exp Med* (1994) **179**:1707–11. doi:10.1084/jem.179.5.1707
70. Wei Z, Lieber MR. Lymphoid V(D)J recombination. Functional analysis of the spacer sequence within the recombination signal. *J Biol Chem* (1993) **268**:3180–3.
71. Matsuda F, Ishii K, Bourvagnet P, Kuma K, Hayashida H, Miyata T, et al. The complete nucleotide sequence of the human immunoglobulin heavy chain variable region locus. *J Exp Med* (1998) **188**:2151–62. doi:10.1084/jem.188.11.2151
72. Sasso EH, Willems Van Dijk K, Bull A, Van Der Maarel SM, Milner EC. VH genes in tandem array comprise a repeated germline motif. *J Immunol* (1992) **149**:1230–6.
73. Sasso EH, Johnson T, Kipps TJ. Expression of the immunoglobulin VH gene 51p1 is proportional to its germline gene copy number. *J Clin Invest* (1996) **97**:2074–80. doi:10.1172/JCI118644
74. Souto-Carneiro MM, Longo NS, Russ DE, Sun HW, Lipsky PE. Characterization of the human Ig heavy chain antigen binding complementarity determining region 3 using a newly developed software algorithm, JOINSOLVER. *J Immunol* (2004) **172**:6790–802.
75. Boyd SD, Marshall EL, Merker JD, Maniar JM, Zhang LN, Sahaf B, et al. Measurement and clinical monitoring of human lymphocyte clonality by massively parallel VDJ pyrosequencing. *Sci Transl Med* (2009) **1**:12ra23. doi:10.1126/scitranslmed.3000540
76. De Preval C, Fougereau M. Specific interaction between VH and VL regions of human monoclonal immunoglobulins. *J Mol Biol* (1976) **102**:657–78. doi:10.1016/0022-2836(76)90340-5
77. Brezinschek HP, Foster SJ, Dorner T, Brezinschek RI, Lipsky PE. Pairing of variable heavy and variable kappa chains in individual naive and memory B cells. *J Immunol* (1998) **160**:4762–7.
78. de Wildt RM, Hoet RM, Van Venrooij WJ, Tomlinson IM, Winter G. Analysis of heavy and light chain pairings indicates that receptor editing shapes the human antibody repertoire. *J Mol Biol* (1999) **285**:895–901. doi:10.1006/jmbi.1998.2396
79. DeKosky BJ, Ippolito GC, Deschner RP, Lavinder JJ, Wine Y, Rawlings BM, et al. High-throughput sequencing of the paired human immunoglobulin heavy and light chain repertoire. *Nat Biotechnol* (2013) **31**:166–9. doi:10.1038/nbt.2492
80. Arnaout R, Lee W, Cahill P, Honan T, Sparrow T, Weiand M, et al. High-resolution description of antibody heavy-chain repertoires in humans. *PLoS ONE* (2011) **6**:e22365. doi:10.1371/journal.pone.0022365
81. Roth DB, Menetski JP, Nakajima PB, Bosma MJ, Gellert M. V(D)J recombination: broken DNA molecules with covalently sealed (hairpin) coding ends in scid mouse thymocytes. *Cell* (1992) **70**:983–91. doi:10.1016/0092-8674(92)90248-B
82. Lafaille JJ, Decloux A, Bonneville M, Takagaki Y, Tonegawa S. Junctional sequences of T cell receptor gamma delta genes: implications for gamma delta T cell lineages and for a novel intermediate of V-(D)-J joining. *Cell* (1989) **59**:859–70. doi:10.1016/0092-8674(89)90609-0
83. Tian C, Luskin GK, Dischert KM, Higginbotham JN, Shepherd BE, Crowe JE Jr. Evidence for preferential Ig gene usage and differential TdT and exonuclease activities in human naive and memory B cells. *Mol Immunol* (2007) **44**:2173–83. doi:10.1016/j.molimm.2006.11.020
84. Jackson KJ, Gaeta B, Sewell W, Collins AM. Exonuclease activity and P nucleotide addition in the generation of the expressed immunoglobulin repertoire. *BMC Immunol* (2004) **5**:19. doi:10.1186/1471-2172-5-19
85. Lu H, Schwarz K, Lieber MR. Extent to which hairpin opening by the Artemis:DNA-PKcs complex can contribute to junctional diversity in V(D)J recombination. *Nucleic Acids Res* (2007) **35**:6917–23. doi:10.1093/nar/gkm823
86. Cabaniols JP, Fazilleau N, Casrouge A, Kourilsky P, Kanellopoulos JM. Most alpha/beta T cell receptor diversity is due to terminal deoxynucleotidyl transferase. *J Exp Med* (2001) **194**:1385–90. doi:10.1084/jem.194.9.1385
87. Murugan A, Mora T, Walczak AM, Callan CG. Statistical inference of the generation probability of T-cell receptors from sequence repertoires. *Proc Natl Acad Sci USA* (2012) **109**:16161–6. doi:10.1073/pnas.1212755109
88. Hofle M, Linthicum DS, Ioerger T. Analysis of diversity of nucleotide and amino acid distributions in the VD and DJ joining regions in Ig heavy chains. *Mol Immunol* (2000) **37**:827–35. doi:10.1016/S0161-5890(00)00110-3
89. Boubnov NV, Wills ZP, Weaver DT. V(D)J recombination coding junction formation without DNA homology: processing of coding termini. *Mol Cell Biol* (1993) **13**:6957–68.
90. Nadel B, Feeney AJ. Influence of coding-end sequence on coding-end processing in V(D)J recombination. *J Immunol* (1995) **155**:4322–9.
91. Saada R, Weinberger M, Shahaf G, Mehr R. Models for antigen receptor gene rearrangement: CDR3 length. *Immunol Cell Biol* (2007) **85**:323–32. doi:10.1038/sj.icb.7100055
92. Agathangelidis A, Darzentas N, Hadzidimitriou A, Brochet X, Murray F, Yan XJ, et al. Stereotyped B-cell receptors in one-third of chronic lymphocytic leukemia: a molecular classification with implications for targeted therapies. *Blood* (2012) **119**:4467–75. doi:10.1182/blood-2011-11-393694
93. Hoogeboom R, Van Kessel KP, Hochstenbach F, Wormhoudt TA, Reinten RJ, Wagner K, et al. A mutated B cell chronic lymphocytic leukemia subset that recognizes and responds to fungi. *J Exp Med* (2013) **210**:59–70. doi:10.1084/jem.20121801
94. Smith K, Garman L, Wrammert J, Zheng NY, Capra JD, Ahmed R, et al. Rapid generation of fully human monoclonal antibodies specific to a vaccinating antigen. *Nat Protoc* (2009) **4**:372–84. doi:10.1038/nprot.2009.3
95. Jiang N, He J, Weinstein JA, Penland L, Sasaki S, He XS, et al. Lineage structure of the human antibody repertoire in response to influenza vaccination. *Sci Transl Med* (2013) **5**:171ra119. doi:10.1126/scitranslmed.3004794
96. Wu YC, Kipling D, Dunn-Walters DK. Age-related changes in human peripheral blood IGH repertoire following vaccination. *Front Immunol* (2012) **3**:193. doi:10.3389/fimmu.2012.00193
97. Wu X, Zhou T, Zhu J, Zhang B, Georgiev I, Wang C, et al. Focused evolution of HIV-1 neutralizing antibodies revealed by structures and deep sequencing. *Science* (2011) **333**:1593–602. doi:10.1126/science.1207532

98. Parameswaran P, Yi Liu Q, Roskin KM, Jackson KK, Dixit VP, Lee J-Y, et al. Coherent immune repertoire signatures in human dengue. *Cell Host Microbe* (Forthcoming 2013).
99. Moss PA, Moots RJ, Rosenberg WM, Rowland-Jones SJ, Bodmer HC, Mcmichael AJ, et al. Extensive conservation of alpha and beta chains of the human T-cell antigen receptor recognizing HLA-A2 and influenza A matrix peptide. *Proc Natl Acad Sci U S A* (1991) **88**:8987–90. doi:10.1073/pnas.88.20.8987
100. Argaet VP, Schmidt CW, Burrows SR, Silins SL, Kurilla MG, Doolan DL, et al. Dominant selection of an invariant T cell antigen receptor in response to persistent infection by Epstein-Barr virus. *J Exp Med* (1994) **180**:2335–40. doi:10.1084/jem.180.6.2335
101. Pannetier C, Even J, Kourilsky P. T-cell repertoire diversity and clonal expansions in normal and clinical samples. *Immunol Today* (1995) **16**:176–81. doi:10.1016/0167-5699(95)80117-0
102. Altman JD, Moss PA, Goulder PJ, Barouch DH, Mcheyzer-Williams MG, Bell JI, et al. Phenotypic analysis of antigen-specific T lymphocytes. *Science* (1996) **274**:94–6. doi:10.1126/science.274.5284.94
103. Garrido P, Ruiz-Cabello F, Barcena P, Sandberg Y, Canton J, Lima M, et al. Monoclonal TCR-Vbeta13.1+/CD4+/NKa+/CD8-/+dim T-LGL lymphocytosis: evidence for an antigen-driven chronic T-cell stimulation origin. *Blood* (2007) **109**:4890–8. doi:10.1182/blood-2006-05-022277
104. Crompton L, Khan N, Khanna R, Nayak L, Moss PA. CD4+ T cells specific for glycoprotein B from cytomegalovirus exhibit extreme conservation of T-cell receptor usage between different individuals. *Blood* (2008) **111**:2053–61. doi:10.1182/blood-2007-04-079863
105. Moon JJ, Chu HH, Pepper M, Mcsorley SJ, Jameson SC, Kedl RM, et al. Naive CD4(+) T cell frequency varies for different epitopes and predicts repertoire diversity and response magnitude. *Immunity* (2007) **27**:203–13. doi:10.1016/j.immuni.2007.07.007
106. Alanio C, Lemaitre F, Law HK, Hasan M, Albert ML. Enumeration of human antigen-specific naive CD8+ T cells reveals conserved precursor frequencies. *Blood* (2010) **115**:3718–25. doi:10.1182/blood-2009-10-251124
107. Kwok WW, Tan V, Gillette L, Littell CT, Soltis MA, Lafond RB, et al. Frequency of epitope-specific naive CD4(+) T cells correlates with immunodominance in the human memory repertoire. *J Immunol* (2012) **188**:2537–44. doi:10.4049/jimmunol.1102190
108. Venturi V, Kedzierska K, Price DA, Doherty PC, Douek DC, Turner SJ, et al. Sharing of T cell receptors in antigen-specific responses is driven by convergent recombination. *Proc Natl Acad Sci USA* (2006) **103**:18691–6. doi:10.1073/pnas.0608907103
109. Quigley MF, Greenaway HY, Venturi V, Lindsay R, Quinn KM, Seder RA, et al. Convergent recombination shapes the clonotypic landscape of the naive T-cell repertoire. *Proc Natl Acad Sci USA* (2010) **107**:19414–9. doi:10.1073/pnas.1010586107
110. Miles JJ, Douek DC, Price DA. Bias in the alphabeta T-cell repertoire: implications for disease pathogenesis and vaccination. *Immunol Cell Biol* (2011) **89**:375–87. doi:10.1038/icb.2010.139

6

The porcine antibody repertoire: variations on the textbook theme

John E. Butler* and Nancy Wertz

Department of Microbiology, Carver College of Medicine, University of Iowa, Iowa City, IA, USA

Edited by:
Harry W. Schroeder, University of Alabama at Birmingham, USA

Reviewed by:
Patrick C. Wilson, University of Chicago, USA
John D. Colgan, University of Iowa, USA

***Correspondence:**
John E. Butler, Department of Microbiology, Carver College of Medicine, University of Iowa, 3-501 BSB, 51 Newton Road, Iowa City, IA 52242, USA.
e-mail: john-butler@uiowa.edu

The genes encoding the heavy and light chains of swine antibodies are organized in the same manner as in other eutherian mammals. There are ~30 VH genes, two functional DH genes and one functional JH gene, 14–60 Vκ genes, 5 Jκ segments, 12–13 functional Vλ genes, and two functional Jλ genes. The heavy chain constant regions encode the same repertoire of isotypes common to other eutherian mammals. The piglet models offers advantage over rodent models since the fetal repertoire develops without maternal influences and the precocial nature of their multiple offspring allows the experimenter to control the influences of environmental and maternal factors on repertoire development postnatally. B cell lymphogenesis in swine begins in the fetal yolk sac at 20 days of gestation (DG), moves to the fetal liver at 30 DG and eventually to the bone marrow which dominates until birth (114 DG) and to at least 5 weeks postpartum. There is no evidence that the ileal Peyers patches are a site of B cell lymphogenesis or are required for B cell maintenance. Unlike rodents and humans, light chain rearrangement begins first in the lambda locus; kappa rearrangements are not seen until late gestation. Dissimilar to lab rodents and more in the direction of the rabbit, swine utilize a small number of VH genes to form >90% of their pre-immune repertoire. Diversification in response to environmental antigen does not alter this pattern and is achieved by somatic hypermutation (SHM) of the same small number of VH genes. The situation for light chains is less well studied, but certain Vκ and Jκ and Vλ and Jλ are dominant in transcripts and in contrast to rearranged heavy chains, there is little junctional diversity, less SHM, and mutations are not concentrated in CDR regions. The transcribed and secreted pre-immune antibodies of the fetus include mainly IgM, IgA, and IgG3; this last isotype may provide a type of first responder mucosal immunity. Development of functional adaptive immunity is dependent on bacterial MAMPs or MAMPs provided by viral infections, indicating the importance of innate immunity for development of adaptive immunity. The structural analysis of Ig genes of this species indicate that especially the VH and Cγ gene are the result of tandem gene duplication in the context of genomic gene conversion. Since only a few of these duplicated VH genes substantially contribute to the antibody repertoire, polygeny may be a vestige from a time before somatic processes became prominently evolved to generate the antibody repertoire. In swine we believe such duplications within the genome have very limited functional significance and their occurrence is therefore overrated.

Keywords: antibody repertoire, swine, gene duplication, development

THE GENOMIC POTENTIAL FOR THE ANTIBODY REPERTOIRE IN SWINE

The heavy and light chain genome of swine is organized in the familiar translocon fashion of other eutherian mammals, i.e., placental mammals versus egg-layers. The heavy chain locus contains ~30 VH genes, all members of the same VH3 family (Sun et al., 1994). There are five DH segments and five JH segments. However only two DH segments and a single JH are functional (Butler et al., 1996; Eguchi-Ogawa et al., 2010; **Table 1**). Downstream, there are genes encoding Cμ, Cδ, six subclasses of Cγ, Cε, and Cα. Like cattle, Cδ is also associated with a small switch region which may or may not be regularly functional (Zhao et al., 2003; **Figure 1A**). Putative enhancer and promoter elements and switch regions similar to those described in other mammals have been reported (Sun and Butler, 1997; Eguchi-Ogawa et al., 2010).

The kappa locus is comprised of 14–60 Vκ genes in two families, five Jκ segments and a single Cκ (**Figure 1B**; Butler et al., 2004; Schwartz et al., 2012a; **Table 1**). The lambda locus is comprised of 22 Vλ genes, 13 that appear potentially functional and four Jλ genes (**Figure 1B**; Schwartz et al., 2012b). Usage of kappa and lambda gene elements is discussed in Section "The Pre-Immune Antibody Repertoire of Swine." The organization of these loci is generally conserved among eutherian mammals although the kappa locus is duplicated in rabbits (**Table 1**). It is not the purpose of this article to provide a phylogenetic review of the Ig loci of mammals and other vertebrates. We mention only selected

Table 1 | Diversity in genomic potential for antibody diversity in common mammals.

Species	V_H (F^a)	D_H	J_H	V_λ (F)	J_λ	C_λ[b]	V_κ (F)	J_κ	C_κ	κ:λ[c]
Human	87 (7)	30	9	70 (7)	7	7	66 (7)	5	1	60:40
Mouse	>100 (14)	11	4	3 (3)	4	4	140 (4)	4	1	95:5
Rabbit	>100 (1)	11	6	? (?)	2	2	>36 (?)	8	2[d]	95:5
Horse	>10 (2)	>7	>5	25 (3)	4	4	>20 (?)	5	1	5:95
Cattle	>15 (2)	3	5	83 (8)	>2	4	? (?)	?	1	5:95
Swine	>20 (1)	2[e]	1[e]	22(>2)	>4	4	14–60 (5)	5	1	50:50
Bat	>250 (>5)	?	13	? (?)	?	?	? (?)	?	?	?:?

[a] *Number of families (F) of variable region genes.*
[b] *J_λ-C_λ duplicons are the common motif in most mammals.*
[c] *Ratio of expressed light chain in adults expressed as percent.*
[d] *Rabbits have a duplicate of the entire kappa locus.*
[e] *Functional D_H and J_H genes.*
?, Number is unknown.

species as a reference to help readers less familiar with comparative immunology.

THE PIGLET MODEL FOR STUDIES OF ANTIBODY REPERTOIRE DEVELOPMENT

The piglet provides an ideal model for studies on antibody repertoire development for a number of important reasons. First, swine are members of the hoofed mammal group, i.e., Ungulates, which have a form of placentation that, unlike that in rodents, primates, and rabbits, does not allow transport of maternal antibodies and other proteins *in utero* to the developing fetus (Brambell, 1970; Butler, 1974). Gestation is 114 days which allows 84 days from the time that VDJ rearrangements first appear to study the development of B cells and the antibody repertoire during fetal life in their multiple large fetuses. Because of the placentation described, development during this period is considered intrinsic and not regulated by maternal factors transmitted *in utero.* Second, the offspring of swine and all Ungulates are Precocial. In the context of development, this refers to the ability of newborn Ungulates to be born totally mobile, with fully functional eyes and protective fur/hair and the ability to immediately forage. Thus piglets can be recovered by Caesarian surgery and reared separately from their mothers in germfree isolators or SPF autosows (Butler et al., 2009a). This allows the experimenter to control the exposure of the postnatal offspring to maternal factors, commensal flora, certain dietary regimes, and infectious agents.

The swine has another major advantage; seven major VH genes, all of the same family, two DH segments and a single JH account for >90% of the VDJ repertoire (Butler et al., 1996; Sun et al., 1998). This is true in the yolk sac (YS) at 20 days of gestation (DG) and continues into adulthood (Butler et al., 2006a, 2011a). Thus all VDJ rearrangements can be recovered from DNA or from transcripts using a single PCR primer set. Cloning these rearrangements and using probes that recognize the CDR regions of each major gene as well as sequence analysis allows vertical studies on the developing repertoire and for its quantification according to a repertoire diversification index (RDI; Butler et al., 2006a, 2011a).

These features collectively allow factors that act during the "critical window" of immune development to be addressed (**Figure 2**). The critical window in the swine system is the period when innate immunity, "natural antibodies" and passive immunity gain the help of the developing adaptive immune response system to allow offspring survival. Survival of the newborn through this critical period when adaptive responses are poorly developed depends on passive immunity in which the systemic humoral experience of the mother is transmitted via IgG and the mucosal experience by IgA. This is also the time when neonatal tolerance to non-threatening dietary antigens and commensal gut flora become established. These topics are discussed in detail in other reviews (Butler, 1983; Butler and Kehrle, 2005). Relevant to the theme of this chapter is the role played by colonizing gut flora on the development of adaptive immunity and on the diversification of the antibody repertoire.

B CELL DEVELOPMENT IN SWINE

Any discussion of antibody repertoire development requires some mention of the B cell lineage from which antibodies are derived. In the fetus, VDJ rearrangements are first seen in YS at 20 DG (Sinkora et al., 2003; Sun et al., 2012a). However signal joint circles (SJC) are difficult to recover at this time, probably because of the slow rate of B cell lymphogenesis at this early time and the rapid rate of their degradation (**Figure 3**). TdT is expressed and active at this time but N region additions and CDR3 diversity is low compared to older fetuses and young piglets (Sinkora et al., 2003; Butler et al., 2007; Sun et al., 2012a). B cell lymphogenesis moves to the fetal liver at 30 DG and remains active in this organ until the bone marrow (BM) develops at ~65 DG. SJC are readily detectable at all these sites indicating that it unlikely the B cells found in these sites are immigrants. An interesting feature of heavy chain rearrangements in early B cell lymphogenesis is the unexpected high frequency (>85%) of in-frame rearrangement (Sinkora et al., 2003), suggesting that the rearrangement and selection processes differs between early fetal stages of B cell lymphogenesis and those which occurs later in fetal and adult BM. However, evidence for B-1 and B-2 subpopulations as reported in mice (Herzenberg et al., 1986) has so far not been obtained. We also found no evidence that the ileal Peyer patches (IPP) are a site of B cell lymphogenesis or that they are needed for B cell

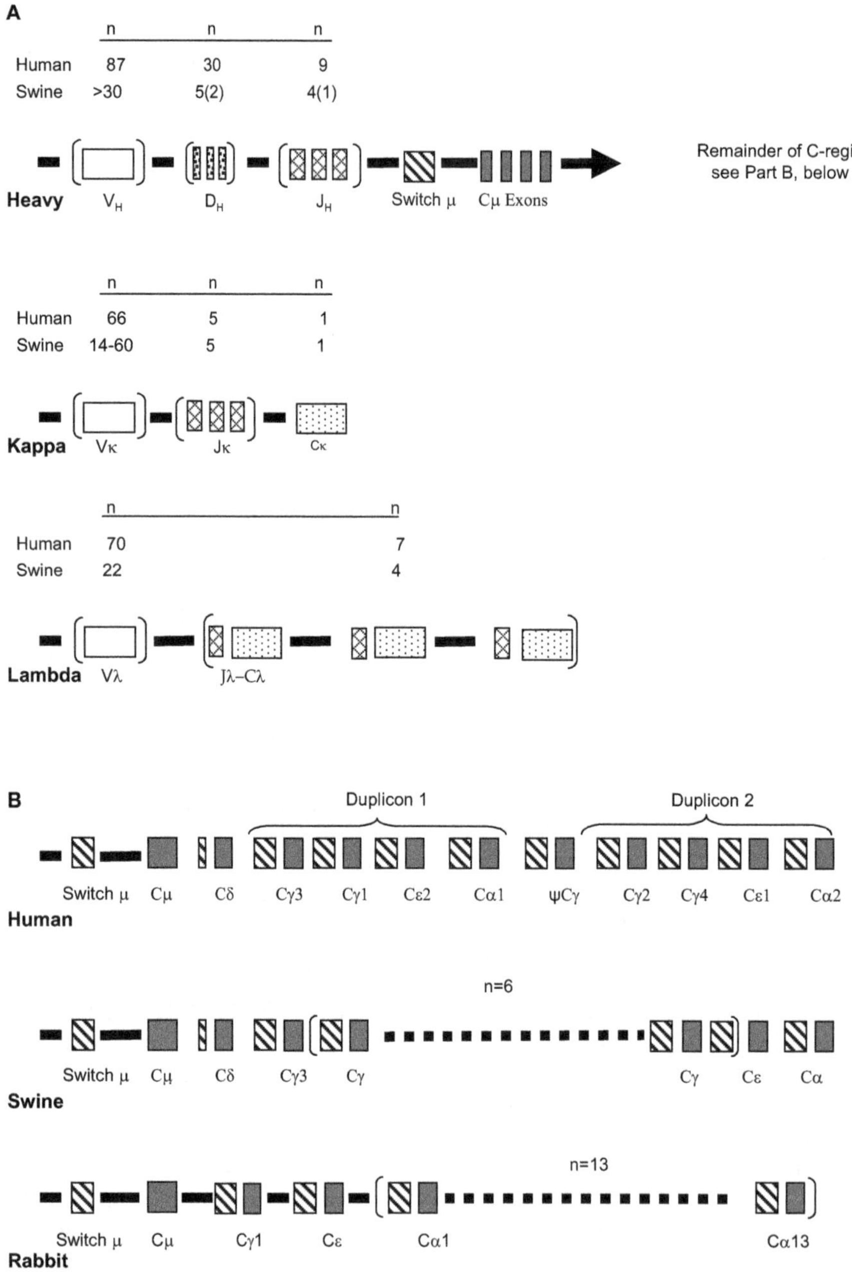

FIGURE 1 | The genomic repertoire of heavy and light chain genes of swine. (A) The light chain and heavy chain variable gene loci compared to humans. Duplicons are illustrated in parentheses with the actual number given in the mini-table above designated as "*n*." This includes duplicons of cassettes as in the lambda locus. In the swine only two DH and one JH gene segments are functional (given in parenthesis). **(B)** Variation in the organization of the heavy chain constant region among human, swine, and rabbit. Modified from Butler et al. (2011c).

maintenance (Butler et al., 2011b; Sinkora et al., 2011; Sun et al., 2012a).

A major departure from the pattern seen in lab rodents and humans is the order of light chain rearrangement. Rearrangement begins in the lambda locus at 20 DG in YS and is dominant until in late gestation when kappa rearrangements first appear (**Figure 3**; Sun et al., 2012a). This may not be unusual given that in Ungulates, lambda usage dominates the repertoire; in cattle, sheep, and horse and it can exceed >90% (Butler, 1997; **Table 1**). However usage of light chain isotypes in young pigs and adults is roughly equal, similar to humans (Hood et al., 1967; Skvaril et al., 1976; Butler et al., 2005a; Sun et al., 2012a; **Table 1**). The order of light chain gene segment usage during development has been poorly studied in any Ungulate. However, the IGLV8 (Vλ8) family is exclusively used at early sites of B cell lymphogenesis (Vazquez et al., 2012).

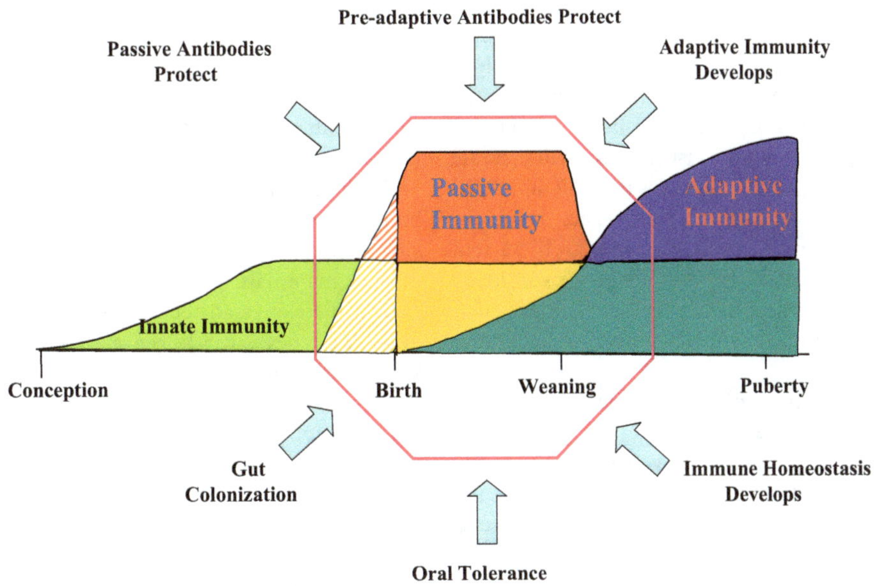

FIGURE 2 | The critical window of immunological development. The factor affecting events in the "window" are indicated. There are a number of cases of superimposing events; e.g., Passive immunity (red) superimposed on innate immunity (green) produces yellow. The "lined section" prepartum applies only to species, e.g., mice and humans, in which passive immunity also takes place *in utero*. In Ungulates like swine there is no transfer of passive antibodies *in utero*. Modified from Butler et al. (2006b).

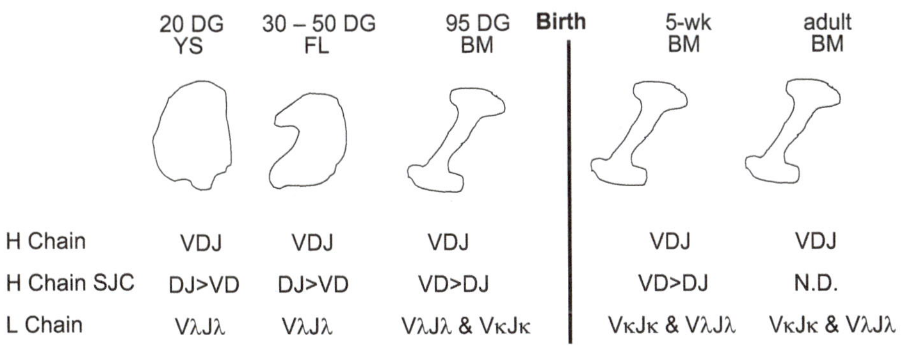

FIGURE 3 | B cell lymphogenesis in swine. Heavy and light chain rearrangements and signal joint circles (SJC) recovered from. YS, yolk sac; FL, fetal liver, BM, bone marrow; DG, day of gestation; N.D., not detected.

It has been proposed that B cell development among higher vertebrates places species into groups (Lanning et al., 2004). In rodents and primates the BM is the major site of B cell development and diversification whereas in rabbit and sheep, gut associated lymphoid tissues (GALT) are believed to be critical (Lanning et al., 2004; Mage et al., 2006). However, recent findings indicate that swine do not belong to the GALT group (Butler et al., 2011b; Sinkora et al., 2011). This is based on surgical resection of IPP, which did not affect B cell lymphogenesis, repertoire diversification and maintenance of either B or T cell levels. The swine IPP appears to be merely a type of mucosal immune tissue.

Some level of class-switch recombination (CSR) occurs during fetal life, so that IgM, IgG3, and IgA are transcribed and secreted into serum. However, no environmental antigen is present during this time and it is unknown whether this CSR involves germinal center formation. There is also low level somatic hypermutation (SHM) in rearranged VDJs resulting in <10 mutation per kilobase (Butler et al., 2011a). In heavy chain rearrangement these mutations accumulate in CDR regions. In lambda rearrangement mutations are equally distributed in CDR and FR regions, although the total mutation frequency is 10-fold lower than in heavy chain rearrangements (Vazquez et al., 2012). Tests for expression of AID during fetal life have not been undertaken.

THE PRE-IMMUNE ANTIBODY REPERTOIRE OF SWINE

We define the pre-immune repertoire as the one present in fetal and newborn piglets. Conventionally reared swine have been previously exposed to both environmental antigen and regulatory influences from maternal passive antibodies, but isolator piglets are free of such influences. In their circulation, newborns have ~ 30 μg/ml of IgG, 1 μg/ml of IgM, and 2 μg/ml of IgA (Butler et al., 2001, 2009b). If maintained for 5 weeks in germfree conditions in which dietary protein is the sole source of environmental antigen, IgM and IgA levels increase 3- to 5-fold to ~ 6 μg/ml, but there is only a 20% increase in IgG to 40–45 μg/ml. Since these animals are immuno-unresponsive (see below) we suspect this small increase is an intrinsic developmental effect much as is the CSR and SHM that occur during fetal life. We base this on the fact that isolator piglets that become immunoresponsive have a 20- to 35-fold increase in serum Ig across all major isotypes. Of the six subclasses of IgG, IgG3 accounts for >60% of the Cγ transcripts in mucosal tissues during the period prior to environmental exposure (Butler and Wertz, 2006).

A notable variation on the theme of repertoire development and diversification from what is presented in textbooks and reviews concerns VH gene usage. Swine use 7 VH genes to form nearly their entire VDJ repertoire starting first in YS and continuing throughout gestation and beyond into postnatal life (**Figure 4**; Butler et al., 2011a). With minor exceptions, proportional usage remains constant and the usage does not depend on the position of the VH gene in the genome (Eguchi-Ogawa et al., 2010; Butler et al., 2011a). VHG (IGHV2) which is the most 3″ functional gene is seldom used whereas VHN (IGHV15) can account for 13% of the repertoire in YS at 20 DG (Butler et al., 2011a; see Antibody Repertoire Development and the Origin of the Genomic Repertoire). Exceptions to the constancy of VH usage involves decreased usage of VHN in older fetuses and a reciprocal increase in usage of VHC. As will be discussed in more detail in the next section (see Development of Adaptive Immunity Depends on an Encounter with MAMPs) this constancy of VH usage continues after birth in antigenized animals including those reared conventionally and consequently exposed to a plethora of environmental antigens. There is no consistent change in the frequency of usage between the two DH segments and swine have only one functional JH (Butler et al., 1996; Eguchi-Ogawa et al., 2010). The small number of VH, DH, and JH segments used means that combinatorial diversity is very small, i.e., 14 possibilities compared to ~9000 in humans. Thus, we estimated that junctional diversity in CDR3 accounts for >95% of the swine pre-immune repertoire (Butler et al., 2000a). As indicated above, the frequency of SHM remains low during this period but the complexity of CDR3 is high and the Gaussian spectratype pattern of CDR3 lengths suggests an unselected repertoire (Navarro et al., 2000; Butler et al., 2007).

As indicated in Section "The Genomic Potential for the Antibody Repertoire in Swine," the overall genomic structure of the kappa and lambda loci of swine is similar to that in other well-studied mammals. Genomic gene annotation may not totally predict the expressed repertoire. In the case of kappa, 11 functional Vκ genes and 5 Jκ genes are present in the genome, yet 2 Vκ families and 1 Jκ segment account for most of the repertoire (Butler et al., 2004; Schwartz et al., 2012a). In the case of lambda, Vλ usage appears to closely agree with the genomic potential but only two of the four Jλ genes are used (Schwartz et al., 2012b; Vazquez et al., 2012).

Certain features of the pre-immune light chain repertoire differ substantially from those in the heavy chain but these features are not unique to swine. First, SHM is 10-fold lower in light chain rearrangement than in heavy chain rearrangement of piglets from the same population. Furthermore there is little junctional diversity in kappa or lambda rearrangement and CDR3 length is ~30 ± 2 (Butler et al., 2004; Vazquez et al., 2012). These observations are nearly identical to studies in humans (Victor et al., 1994; Bridges et al., 1995; Girschick and Lipsky, 2001; Richl et al., 2008). Of some notice is that in the pre-immune repertoire, SHM is concentrated in the CDR region of heavy chain rearrangements but both are lower and widely distributed in rearranged light chains (Butler et al., 2006b, 2011a; Vazquez et al., 2012). The significance of this difference is unclear. However, one might speculate that because the antibody binding site is primarily determined by the heavy chain and its CDR3 (Padlan, 1994) light chain may provide only a supporting role and their presence primarily affects the conformation of the heavy chain binding site. Their complete absence in the camelids partially supports this view (Nguyen et al., 2002).

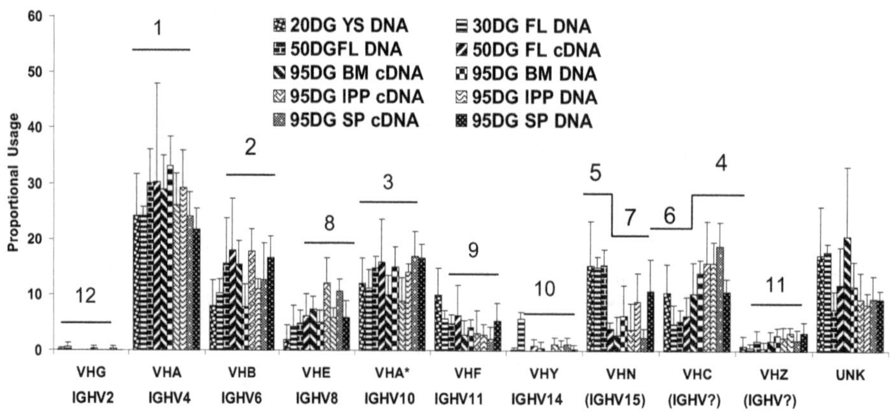

FIGURE 4 | The proportional usage of 11 porcine VH genes during fetal life. VHB and VHB* (IGHV6 and IGHV12) are considered as a group in this analysis. Both the familiar and IMGT nomenclature (if available) are given. Data are based on >5500 VDJ clones and were analyzed using a computer modeling program. The horizontal bars and numbers above each VH gene correspond to the frequency of usage; 1 = highest frequency. For VHN and VHC, the order changes during development. UNK includes VH genes other than those shown and mutated versions of those shown. From Butler et al. (2011a).

DEVELOPMENT OF ADAPTIVE IMMUNITY DEPENDS ON AN ENCOUNTER WITH MAMPs

COLONIZATION AND MAMPs

Piglets maintained germfree in isolators for 5–6 weeks show only minor changes in serum Ig levels until after colonized (Butler et al., 2000b, 2009b; see The Pre-Immune Antibody Repertoire of Swine), do not have antibodies to dietary proteins (J.E. Butler and Patrick Weber, unpublished observations) and are unable to respond to T cell dependent (TD) and T cell independent (TI-2) antigens. However, colonization with benign *Escherichia coli* or a probiotic cocktail, allows responses to both types of antigens (Butler et al., 2002). In lieu of living bacteria, purified MAMPs (bacterial DNA as CpG-ODN, muramyl dipeptide or LPS) have the same affect (Butler et al., 2005b). Thus, bacterial MAMPs provide the adjuvant necessary for innate immune receptors to stimulate the development of adaptive immunity. The impact of such exposure results in 100- to 1000-fold increase in serum Igs (Butler et al., 2009b), CSR to downstream Cγ genes, (Butler et al., 2012a) a 3- to 5-fold increase in the frequency of SHM and a 1–2 log increase in the RDI (Butler et al., 2011a). CpG-ODN and LPS are polyclonal B cell activators and can also expand the existing B cell populations to secrete IgM, IgA, and IgG3 antibodies. However, such expansion cannot be considered a "somatically adapted" repertoire.

REPERTOIRE DIVERSIFICATION FOLLOWING INFECTION WITH RNA VIRUSES

Viruses have a broad range of effects on adaptive immunity. Some are polyclonal activators while others suppress immune responses by interfering with antigen presentation by a variety of mechanisms (Coutelier et al., 1990; Ehrlich, 1995; Hahn et al., 1998; Acha-Orbea et al., 1999; Hunziker et al., 2003). However some, such as influenza (FLU), stimulate robust antibody responses, the apparent basis of generally high efficacy FLU vaccines. Such viruses generate dsRNA during replication, a known adjuvant (Cunnington and Naysmith, 1975). In piglets, we have studied three pandemic viruses including swine influenza (S-FLU) and another RNA virus called porcine respiratory and reproductive syndrome virus (PRRSV) which acts as a polyclonal activator of B cells in both germfree and colonized piglets and fetuses inoculated *in utero*. Polyclonal activation by PRRSV results in lymphoid adenopathy, hypergammaglobulinemia, the appearance of autoantibodies and the deposition of immune complexes in kidney (Lemke et al., 2004). Infection with PRRSV expands certain B cells clones that display hydrophobic CDR3s, a feature common to antibodies that comprise the pre-immune repertoire (Butler et al., 2007, 2008; Schelonka et al., 2007). In addition to polyclonal activation there is also diversification of the repertoire, not dissimilar from that seen in piglets infected with S-FLU or colonized with gut flora (**Figure 5**). However, the degree of repertoire diversification does not parallel the increase in serum Igs (Sun et al., 2012b). This results in only a very small proportion of virus-specific Igs (Lemke et al., 2004).

Infection of isolator piglets with S-FLU results in a robust IgG response to the virus but a much weaker response to irrelevant model TI-2 and TD antigen than does gut colonization (Butler et al., 2012a). Thus, S-FLU does not have the same robust adjuvant impact as does bacterial colonization. This may be due to the fact that S-FLU offers primarily one TLR ligand, double-stranded

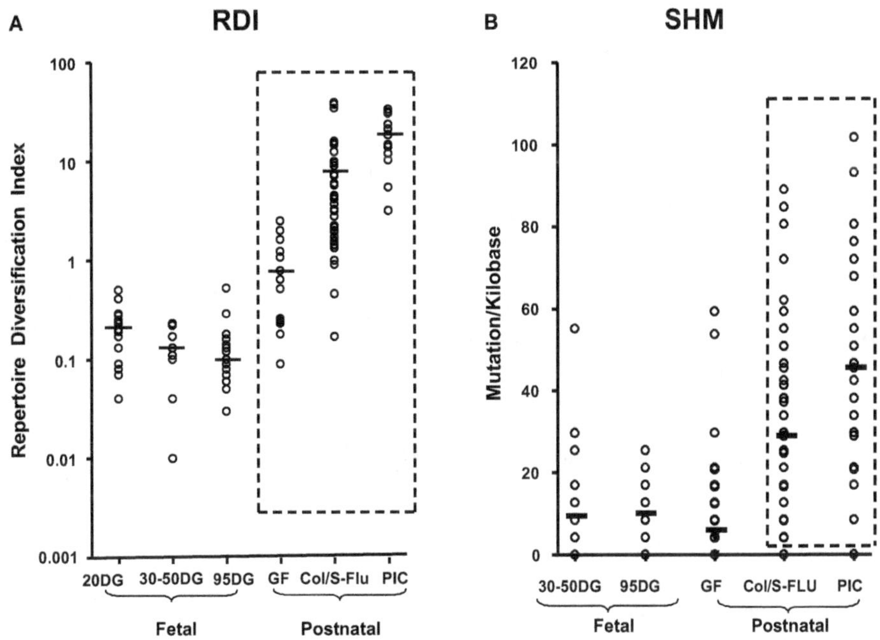

FIGURE 5 | Diversification of the porcine antibody repertoire during fetal and postnatal life expressed as a repertoire diversification index [RDI; (A)] or as the frequency of somatic hypermutation [SHM; (B)]. DG, days of gestation. Values for 95 DG are pooled from clone frequencies recovered from spleen, IPP, and MLN since there were no tissue differences. GF, germfree isolator piglets; Col S-FLU, colonized or S-FLU infected isolator piglets; PIC, parasite-infected young adults reared conventionally. From Butler et al. (2011a).

RNA or that the gut innate immune system is more responsive than that of the respiratory tract. In any case, the result of S-FLU infection supports the concept that MAMPs awakens the adaptive immune system.

A third pandemic disease of swine is porcine circo virus Type 2, a small DNA virus (PCV2; Allan and Ellis, 2000; Merial, 2004). In the piglet model, PCV2 has little or no adjuvant effect in terms of stimulating the production of antibodies to irrelevant model TI-2 and TD antigens. However infection with PCV2 nevertheless results in a generally robust response to a recombinant ORF2 antigen of the virus (Sun et al., 2012c). This IgG response in serum occurs in the context of elevated IgA levels in serum and bronchial-alveolar lavage (BAL). PCV2 infection does not result in polyclonal B cell activation, rather it targets IgA-producing cells. These findings further emphasize that the humoral immune response to any one particular viral infection, should not be projected to other viral infections.

DIVERSIFICATION OF THE HEAVY VARIABLE REGION REPERTOIRE IS BY SHM OF VH GENES THAT COMPRISE THE PRE-IMMUNE REPERTOIRE

The user friendly and simple VDJ system of swine combined with the other advantages of the piglet model (see The Piglet Model for Studies of Antibody Repertoire Development) make it possible to follow the developmental history of the seven major VH genes that comprise >90% of the pre-immune repertoire in postnatal animals under various environmental conditions. The surprising result is that exposure to environmental antigen does not result in the recruitment of other VH genes from the genomic repertoire that are not present in the pre-immune repertoire. Rather, somatic mutants of the "magnificent seven" VH genes that comprise the pre-immune repertoire comprise the adaptive repertoire (**Figure 6**). In piglets infected with S-FLU, colonized with bacteria or helminth parasites, the same VH genes comprise the repertoire but ∼90% of them are somatically mutated (Butler et al., 2011a; **Figure 6**). The use of somatic gene conversion, prominent in the rabbit (Knight, 1992; Schiaffella et al., 1999; Winstead et al., 1999) has not been observed in swine.

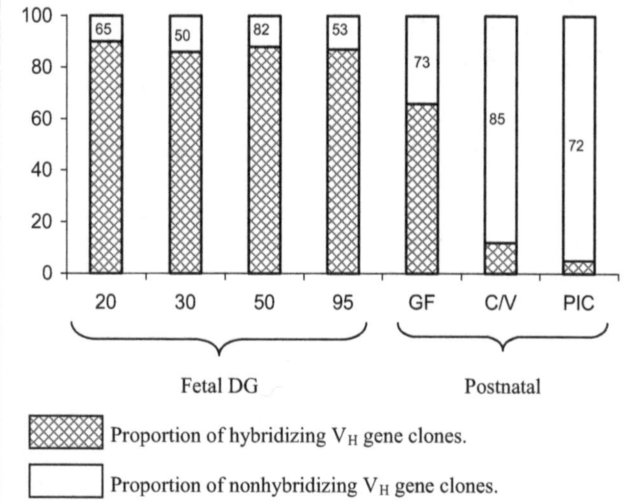

FIGURE 6 | The proportion of VDJ clones from fetal and postnatal piglets that hybridize with cocktails that contain probes for the CDR1 and CDR2 regions of the major seven VH genes used to form the pre-immune repertoire (see Figure 4). Legend for hybridization/non-hybridization is on the figure. Failure to hybridize means that either other VH genes are used or the major seven VH have been mutated to the extent that they no long hybridize with the CDR-specific probes. The number within the bar representing non-hybridizing VH genes indicates the proportion that are the major VH genes as determined by sequence analysis. This means, e.g., that in C/V piglets, 85% are a mutated version of the seven major genes. GF, germfree; C/V, colonized and/or virus infected; PIC, parasite-infected conventional pigs.

ENVIRONMENTAL EXPOSURE RESULTS IN CSR TO DOWNSTREAM Cγ GENES

We described above that in naïve newborns and fetal piglets, >60% of IgG transcripts encode IgG3. However, fetal infection or postnatal exposure to virus, normal gut flora or parasitic infection reduces IgG3 transcription to ∼5% (Butler et al., 2012a). The resultant IgG is now encoded by downstream Cγ genes of which IgG1 is a major player (Butler and Wertz, 2006). The switch to downstream Cγ genes (**Figure 7A**) parallels the diversification of their VH genes while the repertoire associated with IgM and IgG3 does not diversify (**Figure 7B**). These observations are further evidence that environmental exposure of fetal and newborn piglets turns on the machinery of the adaptive immune system. However, since IgA and IgG3 are already transcribed and secreted by the fetus, environmental exposure is not obligatory for CSR.

THE SWINE VERSUS ESTABLISHED PARADIGMS OF ANTIBODY REPERTOIRE DEVELOPMENT

The paradigms for development of the mammalian antibody repertoire decorate the pages of immunology textbooks and are embodied in a number of classic reviews (Rajewsky et al., 1987; Cohn and Langman, 1990). Discussed in this section is how well the swine system fits these paradigms. In the swine system, some level of CSR and SHM occurs in the absence of environmental exposure. This may also be the case in lab rodents and in human, but is ambiguous in these species because such changes could result from the regulatory effects of maternal antibodies (Wikler et al., 1980; Rodkey and Adler, 1983; Yamaguchi et al., 1983; Wang and Shlomchik, 1998) or may be the result of antigen trafficking across the maternal-fetal barrier (Tristram, 2005). In any case, newborn piglets enter the world with a "natural antibody repertoire" of IgM, IgA, and IgG3 antibodies; a phenomenon that is probably universal among all vertebrates (Ochsenbein and Zinkernagel, 2000).

In swine, the evolution of antibody repertoire development appears to have followed a somewhat different path than in mice and humans. However, we have been unable to identify vertical studies on VH usage in rodents or humans, equivalent to those done in swine to thoroughly confirm these differences (Sun et al., 1998; Butler et al., 2011a). In swine, proportional VH gene usage appears to be constant from the time of the initial B cell development in the YS to adulthood (Butler et al., 2011a). Adaptive diversification of the repertoire depends on SHM of the same major VH genes that comprise the pre-immune repertoire. In humans and mice, adaptive responses are often ascribed to the selective use of certain VH genes (Sheehan et al., 1993; Glas et al., 2000). Despite these differences between mice and swine,

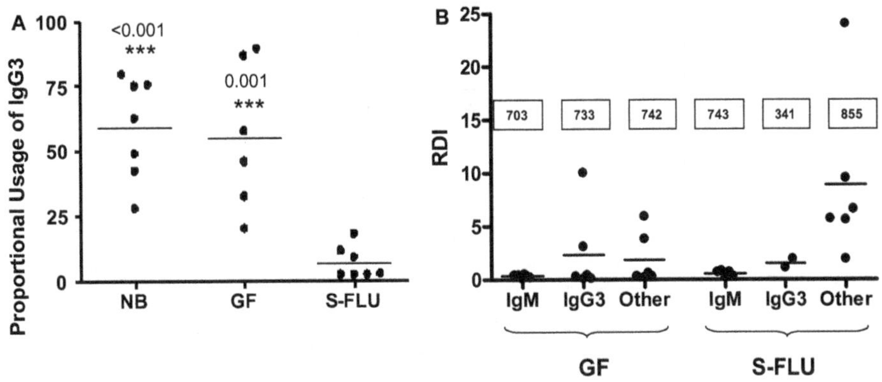

FIGURE 7 | Adaptive changes to the antibody repertoire as a result of postnatal infection with S-FLU. (A) Effect on IgG3 transcription in the tracheal-bronchial lymph node (TBLN). NB, newborn; GF, 5-week germfree isolator piglets; S-FLU, 5-week S-FLU infected isolator piglets. **(B)** The repertoire diversification index (RDI) for VH genes transcribed with IgM, IgG3 and downstream Cγ transcripts (called: "other") in GF and S-FLU infected piglets. The boxed values are the number of clones examined. Data indicate that the IgM and IgG3 repertoire does not diversify in S-FLU infection.

there are many similarities. For example, repertoire diversification is by SHM with mutations accumulating in the CDR regions (Berek and Milstein, 1987; Butler et al., 2006a, 2011a) with no evidence of somatic gene conversion as has been reported in the rabbit and chicken (Reynaud et al., 1987; Becker and Knight, 1990; Schiaffella et al., 1999; Winstead et al., 1999; Ratcliffe, 2006). Consistent with studies in humans, light chains provide limited diversity (see The Pre-Immune Antibody Repertoire of Swine). Also similar to mice and human is the duplication of the Cγ genes and the changes in their expression upon antigenic stimulation (Mossman and Coffman, 1989). This of course differs from lagomorphs that have a single Cγ gene but 13 genes for IgA that comprise their repertoire (Burnett et al., 1989; **Figure 1**). Like humans and rodents, there is no apparent equivalent to the specialized IgG1 of ruminant artiodactyls that is believed to be essential for passive immunity from mother to young, and which also appears to function as a mucosal antibody (Butler, 1983; Butler and Kehrle, 2005). In regard to mucosal immunity, swine have essentially the same IgA-dependent system as rodents and humans including a well-developed gut-mammary gland axis. Both swine and rodents lack the specialized long-hinged IgA1 of humans and primates, which is especially susceptible to bacterial proteases (Plaut et al., 1974) although *H. suis* produces an unrelated protease that cleaves both porcine IgA allotypic variants and may well cleave the IgA of most mammals (Mullens et al., 2011).

At this point, information on diversification of the light chain repertoire of swine may be inadequate. At this time there is little to suggest that only a small number of Vλ or Vκ genes comprise the diversified repertoire of the light chains in the manner we have described for the VH genes in this species. Rather, a much larger array of Vk and Vλ genes are used (Butler et al., 2004; Vazquez et al., 2012). However, like mice and humans, length junctional diversity in the light chain repertoire is restricted (Victor et al., 1994; Bridges et al., 1995; Girschick and Lipsky, 2001; Richl et al., 2008). But unlike the camelids, another Ungulate, light chains have not become obsolete (Hamers-Casterman et al., 1993; Nguyen et al., 2002). There is much to favor the idea that light chains help stabilize the heavy chain binding site and allow specificity modification and therefore the rescue of autoreactive B cells through receptor editing (Tiegs et al., 1993).

As regards the adjuvant effect of bacterial and viral MAMPs that act on innate immune receptors, this is most likely a universal phenomenon among higher vertebrates that go on to develop an effective adaptive immune system. In any case, this topic falls outside the main theme of this review.

ANTIBODY REPERTOIRE DEVELOPMENT AND THE ORIGIN OF THE GENOMIC REPERTOIRE

ORIGIN AND IMPORTANCE OF THE GENOMIC REPERTOIRE

Discussion of the expressed antibody repertoire should also consider its genomic origin. The presence of an annotated gene is not alone evidence for its function; the many breeds of dogs are a poignant example. Insight into why the genomic repertoire of Ig genes greatly exceeds the functional repertoire may help to explain their phylogeny. This can help to explain the redundancy that is a feature of the genomic repertoire which can assure an effective adaptive immune system among higher vertebrates.

DUPLICATION AND GENOMIC GENE CONVERSION EXPLAINS THE PORCINE VH AND Cγ GENOMIC REPERTOIRE

Figure 8 aligns the sequences of a number of porcine VH genes to show that with minor exceptions, they only differ in their CDR1 and CDR2 regions. Thus, the genomic repertoire is a "mix and match" CDR potpourri, with CDR regions shared among different VH genes. Certain VH genes like VHA and VHA* (IGHV4 and IGHV10) and VHB and VHB* (IGHV6 and IGHV12) are duplications with several mutation; one in the CDR1 region of VHB* and two in FR3 of VHA*. In fact there is evidence that the genes segments encoding these duplicated VH genes and several others were duplicated as a block (Eguchi-Ogawa et al., 2010) similar to the duplicons in the human heavy chain constant region and the JλCλ loci of all studied mammals (**Figure 1B**). These features of duplicated genes are also seen among the VH genes of bats (Bratsch et al., 2011; Butler et al., 2011d). These comparisons support the hypothesis that the germline VH repertoire in swine

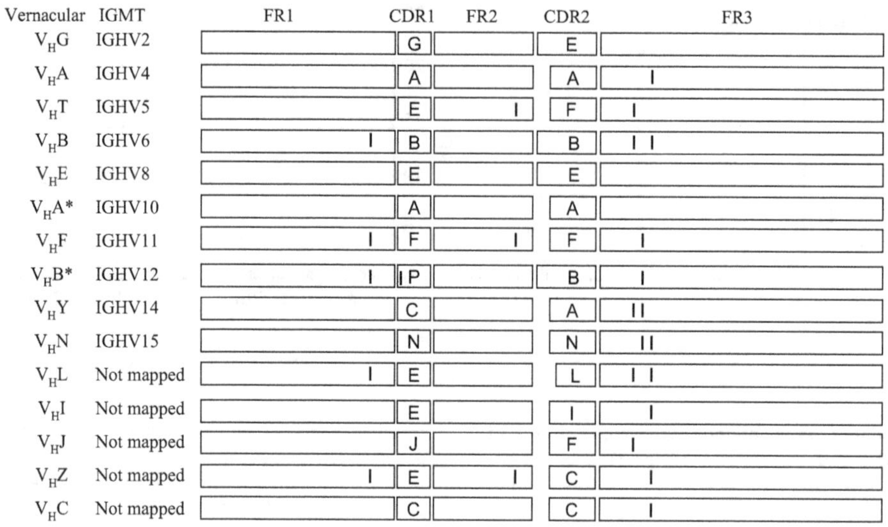

FIGURE 8 | Evidence in support of duplication of VH genes in swine. Diagrammatic comparison of 16 of 32 VH3 family genes described for swine. The sequences are drawn to approximate scale. CDR sequences are identified by capital letter. Only the first fifteen 3′ VH genes have been mapped; pseudogenes are not shown. Those VH genes with the same A,B, etc. CDR designations share the same CDR1 or CDR2 regions. In the case where small differences (genomic point mutations) in FR and CDR regions are involved, vertical lines are drawn.

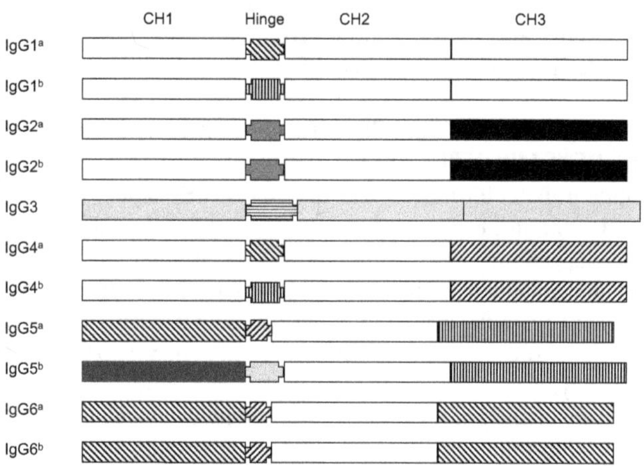

FIGURE 9 | The gene structure of 11 porcine Cγ genes representing the six expressed IgG subclasses and allotypes of swine. Different marking patterns are used to identify domain sequences. Domains with the same pattern indicate they are shared among Cγ genes. Note that no domains are shared with IgG3.

results from gene duplication that occurred simultaneously with genomic gene conversion. The same mechanism appears evident when the sequences of the six expressed porcine Cγ genes and their allotypic variants are compared (**Figure 9**). For example, the allotypic variants of IgG1 and IgG4 have the same hinge exons and the hinge of $IgG5^a$ is shared with the allelic variants of IgG6. With exception of $IgG5^b$ and IgG3, the Cγ1 domain of all Cγ subclass genes and their alleles are identical.

Dendogram analyses of sequence data that are often called phylogenetic studies, indicate that IgG3 is the ancestral IgG for swine. This and other evidence indicates that subclass diversification occurred after speciation (Kehoe and Capra, 1974; Nguyen, 2001; Butler et al., 2009c). We believe the other five Cγ genes then diversified from IgG3. Convincing evidence could be best obtained by studying the Cγ subclasses of other swine related species that are related to the ancestors of the domesticated pig. Consistent with studies on human Cγ (LeFranc et al., 1991), there is also evidence for deletion of some Cγ genes in some pigs (Butler and Wertz, 2006; Eguchi-Ogawa et al., 2012).

THE RESTRICTED USE OF VH GENES IN SWINE QUESTIONS THE IMPORTANCE OF COMBINATORIAL DIVERSITY

As shown in **Table 1**, lab rodents, rabbits, humans, and bats have and/or express large numbers of VH genes; the same is true for the more primitive Zebrafish (Weinstein et al., 2009). In swine and ruminant artiodactyls, the number is surprisingly low. In swine with ∼30 VH genes, only seven appear to be used/needed for a healthy adaptive immune system. Many of the others may represent only allelic variants, so the actual number of germline VH genes may be <20. This raises a question about the textbook paradigms of the importance of multiple VH genes and combinatorial diversity in generating a protective antibody repertoire. This was tested by Xu and Davis (2000) who used a mouse with a single functional VH gene, but with an intact DH and JH region. They showed this transgenic mouse could make antibodies to nearly all environmental antigens. This can be interpreted to mean that extensive duplication of VH genes is not required for the ability to make antibodies to many specificities. This may explain why ruminant artiodactyls and swine have a small genomic repertoire yet are among the most successful mammals on the planet (**Table 1**). However the Xu and Davis work also suggests that the critical feature is DH and JH polygeny, which invokes the next question of how swine generate diversity with only two functional diversity segments and a single JH. This brings the focus to junctional diversity in the formation of CDR3 and away from the emphasis on the number of functional VH, DH, and JH segments. CDR3 is considered most important for the specificity of antibodies (Padlan, 1994), whether generated from a genome with many available DH and JH segments, or from a genome with just one or several DH and JH segments. Perhaps this is compensated by light chain diversity, yet the camelids do it without the assistance of light chains (Hamers-Casterman et al., 1993; Nguyen et al., 2002).

IS THE DIVERSIFICATION OF THE IgG SUBCLASSES IN MAMMALS REALLY NECESSARY FOR SPECIES SURVIVAL?

Textbooks and reviews emphasize the importance of the division of labor among different antibody isotypes; each constant region permitting some special biological function, i.e., following the accepted concept of structure function relationship. While this is clear for IgM, IgE, IgA, and IgG, applying this to the subclasses of IgG is less convincing, especially in species like the horse, swine, and bats that have large numbers of Cγ variants while the highly successful rabbit lacks subclass variants. We also know that IgD knockout mice behave normally (Nitschke et al., 1993), rabbits lack IgD altogether (Lanning et al., 2003) and even mammals with a gene for IgD apparently do not express it. In humans, deficiencies of individual IgG subclasses are well known but these have not translated to an effect on human health, even in environmentally stress underdeveloped countries (LeFranc et al., 1983; Olsson et al., 1993; Rabbani et al., 1995). In mice, differential IgG subclass expression is related to the balance between inflammatory and regulatory cytokine (Mossman and Coffman, 1989) but there is little evidence that the resulting subclasses make a difference in protective immunity; i.e., does the absence either of IgG1 or IgG2b antibodies really affect protective immunity? Four decades of phenomenological studies in the veterinary world would suggest that the IgG1 subclass is indispensable for passive immunity in ruminant artiodactyls. However, an IgG1 knockout cow or ewe has not been produced to experimentally test this assumption. The same is true in horses in which antibodies of different IgG subclasses have long been described, seven IgG subclasses are known from gene sequences but evidence in support of a unique role for each of these subclass antibodies in the horse immune response is lacking. The study of the many IgG subclasses in swine is only in its infancy because until recently, the subclasses had not been defined (Butler et al., 2009c; Kloep et al., 2012). This lack of progress has been largely due to the lack of IgG subclass reagents for use in immunoassays and, of course, the lack of subclass knockout animals. A solution to the first problem is now underway (Butler et al., 2012a,b)

The point to be made is that with the possible exception of ruminant IgG1, evidence is not strong that subclass diversification of IgG is really necessary for survival of the host especially since rabbits accomplish this with one gene for IgG. Perhaps the IgA polygeny of rabbits compensates for this "deficiency," but there are no data that address this point and evidence for a unique role for each of the 13 different IgA subclasses in rabbits is missing.

THE ORIGIN OF VH AND Cγ POLYGENY

As early as 1932, gene duplication was discussed as an essential feature of the evolutionary process (Haldane, 1932; Bridges, 1936; Ohno, 1970). Various mechanisms are known or proposed including RNA/DNA transposition, non-homologous crossing over, and even entire gene duplication (Woody and McConkey, 2011). The first two are often referred to as genomic gene conversion, although this term seems most appropriate to explain non-homologous crossing over (Meselson and Radding, 1975; Szostak et al., 1983). In humans, mouse and rat genomes, ~15% of all genes represent tandemly arrayed genes (Shoja and Zhang, 2006). Tandem duplication also creates redundancy (Li et al., 2005) and this is what is seen among Ig genes, especially those encoding the variable heavy and light chain loci and in some species the Cγ genes. Tandem arrayed duplicons are quite often conserved among species (Zhang, 2003); a phenomenon that also appears true for the Ig variable region genes of swine (Eguchi-Ogawa et al., 2010). Since tandem duplicates are mainly attributed to non-homologous cross-overs, many or most emerge as functional genes (Woody and McConkey, 2011). During evolution these duplicons appear to be retained in the genome despite their apparent redundancy (Xue and Fu, 2009). Duplication reduced selective pressure on single genes since one or several of the duplicated "offspring" genes can more rapidly accumulate mutations and therefore assume new functions while not comprising the function of the parent gene (Ohno, 1970; Lynch and Conery, 2000; Kondrashov et al., 2002).

While the exact mechanism remains unknown, evidence points to non-homologous recombination (gene conversion), acting together with gene duplication, as the mechanism for VH and Cγ polygeny in mammals. This is consistent with studies that some proportion of these duplicated genes will be non-functional, i.e., pseudogenes (Wolfe and Shields, 1997). This is specifically seen among the tandem duplicons in the VH, Vκ, Vλ loci, and among especially the Cγ genes of the constant heavy chain sublocus in all higher vertebrates. Among the duplicated VH and Cγ gene in swine, the 5′ region that encodes FR1 or CH1 respectively, is most conserved among duplicons and among species. While this might suggest progressive 5′ to 3′ mutation of the duplicated genes during evolution, this does not seem to be the case for the for VH and Cγ genes of swine. For example, the hinge regions of Cγ genes are most variable in swine and other mammals (**Figure 9**; Butler et al., 2009c). While the FR regions of porcine VH genes are nearly identical, the CDR1 and CDR2 segments differ and are shared. Thus the CDR regions of VH genes and the hinge segment of Cγ genes are perhaps the best candidates for genomic gene conversion rather than point mutation during evolution.

SHM REDUCES THE VALUE OF VARIABLE REGION GENE POLYGENY

Most evolutionary genetic studies of protocaryotic and eucaryotic species focus on changes in the genome that are transmitted to the offspring in Mendelian fashion. Studies on adaptive immunity, a system most developed in mammals, introduced a new mechanism for variability, namely somatic generation of antibody specificity. This process involves somatic rearrangement of gene segments, additions/subtractions of nucleotide at the boundaries of rearranged segments plus SHM of these rearrangements. The rate of the latter is several logs greater than for the mutations that accumulate in the genome.

Well-developed adaptive immune systems that follow this pattern are primarily restricted to mammals and the chicken and are associated with the expression of AID (see below). Such somatic processes are difficult to identify in cartilaginous and bony fishes and are present at reduced frequency in amphibians (Du Pasquier et al., 1998, 2000). At least SHM and CSR in mammals are associated with the formation of germinal centers that involves the expression of a member of the APOBEC family called antigen-activated cytidine deaminase (AID; Honjo et al., 2002). In lieu of this feature, elasmobranches have ~200 cassettes of fused V-D-J-C genes in their genome although there are some variations on this theme (Dooley and Flajnik, 2006). The genome of *Xenopus tropicalis* contains 11 VH gene families and 37 Vλ genes encoded at three loci (Qin et al., 2008). Among eutherian mammals, some bats have >250 VH genes, lab rodents and human ~100, and rabbits ~200 (Bratsch et al., 2011; **Table 1**). Many of these VH genes are known to be pseudogenes, consistent with data on tandem gene duplication (Wolfe and Shields, 1997). In general, bats (Chiroptera) and rodents which are considered primitive eutherian mammals, have more VH genes whereas Ungulates, that emerged later, have few VH genes (**Table 1**). This is superficial support for the hypothesis that the generation of antibody diversity by SHM or somatic gene conversion has minimized the need for large numbers of variable region gene segments and the importance of combinatorial diversity in more recently evolved mammals.

We believe that vertebrates initially evolved the need for multiple VH genes to create a repertoire of specific antibodies but with the subsequent development of somatic rearrangement and especially SHM, the needs for such polygeny became increasingly redundant. Thus, tandemly duplicated VH genes remain in the genome as evolutionary relics.

LESSONS FROM STUDIES ON ANTIBODY REPERTOIRE DEVELOPMENT IN PIGLETS

The use of the piglet model to study antibody repertoire development has provided useful information on the B cell system of this species that often differs from the textbook models describing the process. Thus, the basis of the title of the review. It is also inconsistent with proposals that place hoofed mammals in the GALT category in which development of the B cell repertoire depends on hindgut lymphoid tissue (Lanning et al., 2004). Collectively considered, our studies indicate that:

(1) Diversity of the pre-immune repertoire in swine is almost exclusively dependent on junctional diversity in CDR3 of the heavy chain followed by SHM, since only seven VH genes with shared CDRs, two DH genes and one functional JH comprise the functional repertoire and such diversity is greatly restricted in light chain rearrangements.
(2) Repertoire diversification after antigen encounter is by SHM primarily in the CDR regions of the rearranged heavy chain variable regions. Evidence for somatic gene conversion, junctional diversity or SHM in light chains that might contribute to extensive antibody repertoire diversification is lacking.
(3) Light chain rearrangement occurs first in the lambda locus and there is no evidence of a special Vλ gene like λ5 that is used in the earliest phases of B cell lymphogenesis. This raises the question of whether the conventional pre-BCR is present in swine or any artiodactyls.
(4) The prominent hindgut lymphoid tissue of swine, the IPP, is not required for B cell lymphogenesis, maintenance of B cell levels or repertoire development. This opens the question regarding the true function of this lymphoid organ. Here we propose it represents "first responder" mucosal lymphoid tissue. A key factor in this scenario is that IgG3, which is encoded by the most 5′ Cγ gene, shares this same genomic feature with mice, cattle, and humans. Perhaps this primordial IgG provides the "natural antibodies" that target the polysaccharide antigens of intestinal bacteria.

REFERENCES

Acha-Orbea, H., Finke, D., Attinger, A., Schmid, S., Wehrli, N., Vacheron, S., Xenarios, I., Scarpellino, L., Toellner, K. M., MacLennan, I. C., and Lutter, S. A. (1999). Interplay between mouse mammary tumor virus and the cellular and humoral immune response. *Immunol. Rev.* 168, 287–303.

Allan, G. M., and Ellis, J. A. (2000). Porcine circoviruses: a review. *J. Vet. Diagn. Invest.* 12, 3–14.

Becker, R. S., and Knight, K. L. (1990). Somatic diversification of immunoglobulin heavy chain VDJ genes: evidence for somatic gene conversion in rabbit. *Cell* 63, 987–997.

Berek, C., and Milstein, C. (1987). Mutation drift and repertoire shift in the maturation of the immune response. *Immunol. Rev.* 96, 23–41.

Brambell, F. W. R. (1970). *The Transmission of Passive immunity from Mother to Young.* Amsterdam: North-Holland Publishing Company.

Bratsch, S., Wertz, N., Chaloner, K., Kunz, T. H., and Butler, J. E. (2011). The little brown bat displays a highly diverse VH, DH and JH repertoire but little evidence of somatic hypermutation. *Dev. Comp. Immunol.* 35, 421–430.

Bridges, C. B. (1936). The bar "gene" a duplication. *Science* 83, 210–211.

Bridges, S. L. Jr., Lee, S. K., Johnson, M. L., Lavelle, J. C., Fowler, P. G., Koopman, W. J., and Schroeder, H. W. Jr. (1995). Somatic mutation and CDR3 lengths of immunoglobulin kappa light chains expressed in patients with rheumatoid arthritis and in normal individuals. *J. Clin. Invest.* 96, 831–841.

Burnett, R. C., Hanly, W. C., Zhai, S. K., and Knight, K. L. (1989). The IgA heavy chain gene family in rabbits: cloning and sequence analysis of 13 Ca genes. *EMBO J.* 8, 40410–44047.

Butler, J. E. (1974). "Immunoglobulins of the mammary secretions" in Lactation, a Comprehensive Treatise, Vol. III, Chap. V, eds B. L. Larson and V. Smith (New York: Academic Press), 217–255.

Butler, J. E. (1983). Bovine immunoglobulins: an augmented review. *Vet. Immunol. Immunopathol.* 4, 43–152.

Butler, J. E. (1997). Immunoglobulin gene organization and the mechanism of repertoire development. *Scand. J. Immunol.* 45, 455–462.

Butler, J. E., and Kehrle, M. E. Jr. (2005). "Immunocytes and immunoglobulins in milk," in *Mucosal Immunology*, 3rd Edn, eds J. Mestecky, M. E. Lamm, W. Strober, J. R. McGhee, L. Mayer, and J. Bienenstock (New York: Academic Press), 1763–1793.

Butler, J. E., Lager, K. M., Splichal, I., Francis, D., Kacskovics, I., Sinkora, M., Wertz, N., Sun, J., Zhao, Y., Brown, W. R., DeWald, R., Dierks, S., Muyldermanns, S., Lunney, J. K., McCray, P. B., Rogers, C. S., Welsh, M. J., Navarro, P., Klobasa, F., Habe, F., and Ramsoondar, J. (2009a). The piglet as a model for B cell and immune system development. *Vet. Immunol. Immunopathol.*128, 147–170.

Butler, J. E., Sinkora, M., Wertz, N., and Kacskovics, I. (2009b). Immunoglobulins, B cells and repertoire development. *Dev. Comp. Immunol.* 33, 321–333.

Butler, J. E., Wertz, N., Deschacht, N., and Kacskovics, I. (2009c). Porcine IgG: structure, genetics and evolution. *Immunogenetics* 61, 209–230.

Butler, J. E., Lemke, C. D., Weber, P., Sinkora, M., and Lager, K. D. (2007). Antibody repertoire development in fetal and neonatal piglets. XIX. Undiversified B cells with hydrophobic HCDR3s preferentially proliferate in PRRS. *J. Immunol.* 178, 6320–6331.

Butler, J. E., Sun, J., and Navarro, P. (1996). The swine immunoglobulin heavy chain locus has a single JH and no identifiable IgD. *Int. Immunol.* 8, 1897–1904.

Butler, J. E., Sun, J., Weber, P., Ford, S. P., Rehakova, Z., Sinkora, J., and Lager, K. (2001). Antibody repertoire development in fetal and neonatal piglets. IV. Switch recombination, primarily in fetal thymus occurs independent of environmental antigen and is only weakly associated with repertoire diversification. *J. Immunol.* 167, 3239–3249.

Butler, J. E., Sun, X.-Z., Wertz, N., Lager, K. M., Urban, J. Jr., Nara, P., and Tobin, G. (2011a). Antibody repertoire development in fetal and neonatal piglets. XXI. VH usage remains constant in fetal piglets and postnatally development. *Mol. Immunol.* 49, 483–494.

Butler, J. E., Mateo, K., Sun, X.-Z., Wertz, N., Sinkora, M., Harvey, R., and Francis, D. L. (2011b). Antibody repertoire development in fetal and neonatal piglets XX: the ileal Peyers patches are not a site of B cell lymphogenesis and are not required for systemic B cell proliferation and Ig synthesis. *J. Immunol.* 187, 5141–5149.

Butler, J. E., Sun, X.-Z., and Wertz, N. (2011c). "Immunoglobulin polygeny: an evolutionary perspective" in *Gene Duplication*, ed. F. Friedberg (Rijeka: InTech), 113–140.

Butler, J. E., Wertz, N., Zhao, Y., Kunz, T. H., Bratsch, S., Whitaker, J., and Schountz, T. (2011d). Two suborders of bats have the canonical isotypes repertoire of other eutherian mammals. *Dev. Commun. Immunol.* 35, 272–284.

Butler, J. E., Sun, X.-Z., Wertz, N., Vincent, A. L., Zanella, E. L., and Lager, K. M. (2012a). Antibody repertoire development in fetal and neonatal piglets. XVI. Influenza stimulates adaptive immunity, class switch and diversification of the IgG repertoire encoded by downstream Cγ genes. *Immunology* (in press).

Butler, J. E., Wertz, N., Sun, X.-Z., Lunney, J. K., and Muyldermanns, J. (2012b). Resolution of an immunodiagnostic dilemma: heavy chain chimeric antibodies for species in which plasmocytomas are unknown. *Mol. Immunol.* (pending).

Butler, J. E., Weber, P., Sinkora, M., Baker, D., Schoenherr, A., Mayer, B., and Francis, D. (2002). Antibody repertoire development in fetal and neonatal piglets. VIII. Colonization is required for newborn piglets to make serum antibodies to T-dependent and type 2 T-independent antigens. *J. Immunol.* 169, 6822–6830.

Butler, J. E., Weber, P., Sinkora, M., Sun, J., Ford, S. J., and Christenson, R. (2000a). Antibody repertoire development in fetal and neonatal piglets. II. Characterization of heavy chain CDR3 diversity in the developing fetus. *J. Immunol.* 165, 6999–7011.

Butler, J. E., Sun, J. Weber, P., and Francis, D. (2000b). Antibody repertoire development in fetal and neonatal piglets. III. Colonization of the gastrointestinal tracts results in preferential diversification of the pre-immune mucosal B-cell repertoire. *Immunology* 100, 119–130.

Butler, J. E., Weber, P., and Wertz, N. (2006a). Antibody repertoire development in fetal and neonatal pigs. XIII. "Hybrid VH genes" and the pre-immune repertoire revisited. *J. Immunol.* 177, 5459–5470.

Butler, J. E., Sinkora, M., Wertz, N., Holtmeier, W., and Lemke, C. D. (2006b). Development of the neonatal B- and T-cell repertoire in swine: implications for comparative and veterinary immunology. *Vet. Res.* 37, 417–441.

Butler, J. E., Weber, P., Wertz, N., and Lager, K. M. (2008). Porcine reproductive and respiratory syndrome virus (PRRSV) subverts development of adaptive immunity by proliferation of germline-encoded B cells with hydrophobic HCDR3s. *J. Immunol.* 180, 2347–2356.

Butler, J. E., and Wertz, N. (2006). Antibody repertoire development in fetal and neonatal piglets. XVII. IgG subclass transcription revisited with emphasis on new IgG3. *J. Immunol.* 177, 5480–5489.

Butler, J. E., Wertz, N., Sun, J., Wang, H., Lemke, C., Chardon, P., Puimi, F., and Wells, K. (2005a). The pre-immune variable kappa repertoire of swine is selectively generated from certain subfamilies of Vκ2 and one Jκ gene. *Vet. Immunol. Immunopathol.* 108, 127–137.

Butler, J. E., Francis, D., Freeling, J., Weber, P., Sun, J., and Krieg, A. M. (2005b). Antibody repertoire development in fetal and neonatal piglets. IX. Three PAMPs act synergistically to allow germfree piglets to respond to TI-2 and TD antigens. *J. Immunol.* 175, 6772–6785.

Butler, J. E., Wertz, N., Wang, H., Sun, J., Chardon, P., Piumi, F., and Wells, K. (2004). Antibody repertoire in fetal and neonatal pigs. VII. Characterization of the pre-immune kappa light chain repertoire. *J. Immunol.* 173, 6794–6805.

Cohn, M., and Langman, R. E. (1990). The protecton: the unit of humoral immunity selected by evolution. *Immunol. Rev.* 115, 11–147.

Coutelier, J.-P., Coulie, G., Wauters, P., Heremans, H. and der Logt, J. T. (1990). In vivo polyclonal B-lymphocyte activation elicited by murine viruses. *J. Virol.* 64, 5383–5388.

Cunnington, P. G., and Naysmith, J. D. (1975). Naturally occurring double-stranded RNA and immune responses. III. Immunogenicity and antigenicity in animals. *Immunology* 29, 1001–1017.

Dooley, H., and Flajnik, M. F. (2006). Antibody repertoire development in cartilaginous fish. *Dev. Comp. Immunol.* 30, 43–56.

Du Pasquier, L., Robert, J., Courtet, M., and Mussmann, R. (2000). B cell development in the amphibian *Xenopus*. *Immunol. Rev.* 175, 201–213.

Du Pasquier, L., Wilson, M., Greenberg, A. S, and Flajnik, M. F. (1998). Somatic mutation in ectothermic vertebrates: musings on selection and origins. *Curr. Top. Microbiol. Immunol.* 229, 199–216.

Eguchi-Ogawa, T., Sun, X.-Z., Wertz, N., Uenishi, H., Puimi, F., Chardon, P., Wells, K., Tobin, G. J., and Butler, J. E. (2010). Antibody repertoire development in fetal and neonatal piglets. XI. The relationship of VDJ usage and the genomic organization of the variable heavy chain locus. *J. Immunol.* 184, 3734–3742.

Eguchi-Ogawa, T., Toki, D., Wertz, N., Butler, J. E., and Uenishchi, H. (2012). Complete structure of the genomic sequence encoding the constant region of the porcine immunoglobulin heavy chain. *Mol. Immunol.* (in press).

Ehrlich, R. (1995). Selective mechanisms utilized by persistent and oncogenic viruses to interfere with antigen producing and presentation. *Immunol. Res.* 14, 77–97.

Girschick, H. J., and Lipsky, P. E. (2001). The kappa repertoire of human neonatal B cells. *Mol. Immunol.* 38, 1113–1127.

Glas, A. M., van Monfort, E. H. N., and Milner, E. C. B. (2000). "The human antibody repertoire: old notions, current realities and VH gene-dependent biases," in *The Antibodies*, Vol. 6, eds M. Zanetti and J. D. Capra (Amsterdam: Harwood Academic Publishers), 63–79.

Hahn, G., Jores, R., and Mocarski, E. S. (1998). Cytomegalovirus remains latent in a common precursor of dendritic and myeloid cells. *Proc. Natl. Acad. Sci. U.S.A.* 95, 3937–3942.

Haldane, J. B. S. (1932). *The Causes of Evolution*. London: Longmans and Green.

Hamers-Casterman, C., Atarhouch, T., Muylermans, S., Robinson, G., Hamers, C., Bajyana Songa, E., Bendahman, N., and Hamers, R. (1993). Naturally occurring antibodies devoid of light chains. *Nature* 363, 446–448.

Herzenberg, L. A., Stall, A. M., Lalor, P. A., Sidman, C., Moore, W. A., Parks, D., and Herzenberg, L. A. (1986). The Ly-1 B cell lineage. *Immunol. Rev.* 93, 81–102.

Honjo, T., Kinoshita, K., and Muranmatsu, M. (2002). Molecular mechanisms of lass switch recombination: linkage with somatic hypermutation. *Annu. Rev. Immunol.* 20, 165–196.

Hood, L., Gray, W. R., Saunders, B. G. and Dreyer, W. J. (1967). Light chain evolution. *Cold Spring Harb. Symp. Quant. Biol.* 32, 133–146.

Hunziker, L., Recher, M., Macpherson, A. J., Ciurea, A., Freigang, S., Hengartner, H., and Zinkernagel, R. M. (2003). Hypergammaglobulinemia and autoantibody induction mechanisms in viral infection. *Nat. Immunol.* 4, 343–349.

Kehoe, J. M., and Capra, J.D. (1974). Nature and significance of immunoglobulin subclasses. *NY State J. Med.* 74, 489–491.

Kloep, A., Wertz, N., Mendicino, M., and Butler, J. E. (2012). Linkage haplotype for IgG and IgA subclass genes. *Immunogenetics* 64, 469–473.

Knight, K. L. (1992). Restrictive VH gene usage and generation of antibody diversity in rabbit. *Annu. Rev. Immunol.* 10, 593–616.

Kondrashov, F. A., Rogozin, I. B., Wolf, Y. I., and Koonin, E. V. (2002). Selection in the evolution of gene duplications. *Genome Biol.* 3, RESEARCH0008.

Lanning, D., Osbourne, B. A., and Knight, K. L. (2004). "Immunoglobulin genes and generation of antibody repertoires in higher vertebrates: a key role for GALT," in *Molecular Biology of B Cells*, eds F. W. Alt, T. Honjo, and M. S. Neuberger (London: Elsevier Science Ltd.), 433–448.

Lanning, D. K., Zhao, S. K., and Knight, K. L. (2003). Analysis of the 3′ Cmu region of the rabbit Ig heavy chain locus. *Gene* 309, 135–144.

LeFranc, G., Chaabani, H., Van Loghem, E., Lefranc, M. P., De Lange, G., and Helal, A. N. (1983). Simultaneous absence of the human IgG1, IgG2, IgG4 and IgA1 subclasses:

immunological and immunogenetic considerations. *Eur. J. Immunol.* 13, 240–244.

LeFranc, M. P., Hammarstrom, L., Smith, C. I., and Lefranc, G. (1991). Gene deletion in the human immunogolubulin heavy chain constant region locus: molecular and immunological analysis. *Immunol. Rev.* 2, 265–281.

Lemke, C. D., Haynes, J. S., Spaete, R., Adolphson, D., Vorwald, A., Lager, K., and Butler, J. E. (2004). Lymphoid hyperplasia resulting in immune dysregulation is caused by PRRSV infection in pigs. *J. Immunol.* 172, 1916–1925.

Li, W. H., Yang, J., and Guo, X. (2005). Expression divergence between duplicate genes. *Trends Genet.* 21, 602–607.

Lynch, M., and Conery, J. S. (2000). The evolutionary fate and consequences of duplicate genes. *Science* 290, 1151–1155.

Mage, R. G., Lanning, D., and Knight, K. L. (2006). B cell and antibody repertoire development in rabbits: the requirement of gut-associated lymphoid tissues. *Dev. Comp. Immunol.* 30, 137–153.

Merial, Inc. (2004). PCV2 diseases: from research back to the field again, Vol. 5. Kansas City, MO: Corporate Publication by Merial Inc.

Meselson, M. S., and Radding, C. M. (1975). A general model for genetic recombination. *Proc. Natl. Acad. Sci. U.S.A.* 72, 358–361.

Mossman, T. R., and Coffman, R. L. (1989). TH1 and TH2 cells: different patterns of lymphokine secretion lead to different functional properties. *Annu. Rev. Immunol.* 7, 143–173.

Mullens, M. A., Register, K. B., Bayles, D. O., and Butler, J. E. (2011). *Haemophilus parasuis* exhibits IgA protease activity but lacks homologs of the IgA protease genes of *Haemophilus influenzae. Vet. Microbiol.* 153, 407–412.

Navarro, P., Christenson, R., Weber, P., Rothschild, M., Ekhard, G., Lemky, J., and Butler, J. E. (2000). Porcine IgA allotypes are not equally transcribed or expressed in heterozygous swine. *Mol. Immunol.* 37, 653–664.

Nguyen, V. K. (2001). *Generation of Heavy Chain Antibodies in Camelids.* Ph.D. thesis, Free University of Brussels, Brussels, 109–111.

Nguyen, V. K., Su, C., Muyldermans, S., and van der Loo, W. (2002). Heavy chain antibodies in Camelids; a case of evolutionary innovation. *Immunogenetics* 54, 39–47.

Nitschke, L., Kosco, M. L., Kohler, G., and Lamers, M. C. (1993). Immunoglobulin D deficient mice can mount normal immune responses to thymus-independent and -dependent antigens. *Proc. Natl. Acad. Sci. U.S.A.* 90, 1887–1891.

Ochsenbein, A. F., and Zinkernagel, R. (2000). Natural antibodies and complement link innate and acquired immunity. *Immunol. Today* 1, 624–630.

Ohno, S. (1970). *Evolution by Gene Duplication.* New York: Springer-Verlag.

Olsson, P. G., Rabbani, H., Hammarstrom, L., and Smith, C. I. (1993). Novel human immunoglobulin heavy chain constant region gene deletion haplotypes characterized by pulsed-field electrophoresis. *Clin. Exp. Immunol.* 94, 84–90.

Padlan, E. A. (1994). Anatomy of the antibody molecule. *Mol. Immunol.* 31, 169–217.

Plaut, A. G., Wustar, R. Jr., and Capra, J. D. (1974). Differential susceptibility of human IgA immunoglobulins to streptocococcal IgA proteases. *J. Clin. Invest.* 54, 1295–1300.

Qin, T., Ren, L., Hu, X., Guo, Y., Fei, J., Pan-Hammarstrom, Q., Butler, J. E., Wu, C., Li, L., Hammarstrom, L., and Zhao, Y. (2008). Genomic organization of the immunoglobulin gene loci in *Xenopus tropcalis*: evolutionary implications. *Dev. Comp. Immunol.* 32, 156–165.

Rabbani, H., Kondo, N. Smith, C. I., and Hammarstrom, L. (1995). The influence of gene deletion and duplication within the IGHC locus on serum immunoglobulin subclass levels. *Clin. Immunol. Immunopathol.* 76, 214–218.

Rajewsky, K., Forster, I., and Cumano, A. (1987). Evolutionary and somatic selection of the antibody repertoire in the mouse. *Science* 238, 1088–1094.

Ratcliffe, M. J. H. (2006). Antibodies, immunoglobulin genes and the bursa of Fabricius in chicken. B cell development. *Dev. Comp. Immunol.* 30, 101–118.

Reynaud, C. A., Anquez, V., Daher, A., and Weill, J.-C. (1987). A hyperconversion mechanism generates the chicken pre-immune light chain repertoire. *Cell* 48, 379–388.

Richl, P., Stern, U., Lipsky, P. E., and Girschick, H. J. (2008). The lambda gene immunoglobulin repertoire of human neonatal B cells. *Mol. Immunol.* 45, 320–327.

Rodkey, L. S., and Adler, F. L. (1983). Regulation of natural anti-allotypic antibody responses by network induced auto-anti-idiotypic responsiveness of their offspring. *J. Exp. Med.* 152, 1024–1035.

Schelonka, R. L., Tanner, J., Zhang, Y., Gartland, G. L., Zemlin, M., and Schroeder, H. W. Jr. (2007). Categorized selection of the antibody repertoire in splenic B cells. *Eur. J. Immunol.* 4, 1010–1021.

Schiaffella, E., D. Sehgal, A.O., Anderson, and Mage, R. G. (1999). Gene conversion and hypermutation during diversification of VH sequences in developing germinal centers of immunized rabbits. *J. Immunol.* 162, 3984–3995.

Schwartz, J. C., Lefranc, M., and Murtaugh, M. P. (2012a). Evolution of the porcine kappa locus through germline gene conversion. *Immunogenetics* 64, 303–311.

Schwartz, J. C., Lefranc, M., and Murtaugh, M. P. (2012b). Organization, complexity and allelic diversity of the porcine immunoglobulin lambda locus. *Immunogenetics* 64, 399–407.

Sheehan, K. M., Mainville, C. V. A., Willert, S., and Brodeur, P. H. (1993). The utilization of individual VH exons in the primary repertoire of adult BALB/c mice. *J. Immunol.* 151, 5363–5375.

Shoja, V., and Zhang, L. (2006). A roadmap of tandemly arrayed genes in the genomes of human, mouse and rat. *Mol. Biol. Evol.* 23, 2134–2141.

Sinkora, M., Sun, J., Sinkorova, J., Christenson, R. K., Ford, S. P., and Butler, J. E. (2003). Antibody repertoire development in fetal and neonatal piglets. VI. B cell lymphogenesis occurs in multiple sites with differences in the frequency of in-frame rearrangements. *J. Immunol.* 170, 1781–1788.

Sinkora, M., Zelena, K., Butler, J. E., Francis, D., Santiago-Mateo, K., Potockova, H., and Sinkorova, J. (2011). Ileal Peyers patches (IPP) are not necessary for B cell development and maintenance and do not contribute significantly to the overall B cell pool in swine. *J. Immunol.* 187, 5150–5161.

Skvaril, F., Baranden, S., Kuffer, F., and Probst, M. (1976). Changes of kappa/lambda ratio of human serum immunoglobulins in the course of development. *Blut* 33, 281–284.

Sun, J., and Butler, J. E. (1997). Sequence analysis of swine switch μ, Cμ and Cμm. *Immunogenetics* 46, 452–460.

Sun, J., Hayward, C., Shinde, R., Christenson, R., Ford, S. P., and Butler, J. E. (1998). Antibody repertoire development in fetal and neonatal piglets. I. Four VH genes account for 80% of VH usage during 84 days of fetal life. *J. Immunol.* 161, 5070–5078.

Sun, J., Kacskovics, I., Brown, W. R, and Butler, J. E. (1994). Expressed swine VH genes belong to a small VH gene family homologous to human VH III. *J. Immunol.* 153, 5618–5627.

Sun, X.-Z., Wertz, N., Lager, K., Sinkora, M., Stepanova, K., Tobin, G., and Butler, J. E. (2012a). Antibody repertoire development in fetal and neonatal piglets. XXII. Lambda rearrangement precedes kappa rearrangement during B cell lymphogenesis in swine. *Immunol. (British)* (in press).

Sun, X.-Z., Wertz, N., Lager, K. L., Tobin, G., and Butler, J. E. (2012b). Antibody repertoire development in fetal and neonatal piglets XXIII: fetal piglets infected with a vaccine strain of PRRS Virus display the same immune dysregulation seen in isolator piglets. *Vaccine* 30, 3646–3652.

Sun, X.-Z., Wertz, N., Lager, K. L., and Butler, J. E. (2012c). Antibody repertoire development in fetal and neonatal piglets. XV. Porcine circovirus type 2 infection results in serum IgG antibodies to ORF 2, elevated IgA levels but little evidence for immune suppression. *Vaccine* (pending).

Szostak, J. W., Orr-Weaver, T. L., and Rothstein, R. J. (1983). The double-strand break repair model for recombination. *Cell* 33, 25–35.

Tiegs, S. L., Russell, D. M., and Nemazee, D. (1993). Receptor editing in self-reactive bone marrow B cells. *J. Exp. Med.* 177, 1009–1020.

Tristram, D. A. (2005). "Maternal genital tract infection and the neonates," in *Mucosal Immunology*, 3rd Edn, Vol II, eds J. Mestecky, M. E. Lamm, W. Strober, J. Bienestock, J. R. McGhee, and L. Mayer (Elsevier/Academic Press), 1721–1731.

Vazquez, J., Wertz, N., Sun, J., Wells, K., Sun, X.-Z., and Butler, J. E. (2012). Antibody repertoire development in fetal and neonatal piglets. XI. Characterization of the expressed lambda repertoire. *Mol. Immunol.* (pending).

Victor, K. D., Vu, K., and Feeney, A. J. (1994). Limited junctional diversity in kappa light chains. Junctional sequences from CD431B2201 early B cell progenitors resemble those from peripheral B cells. *J. Immunol.* 152, 3467–3475.

Wang, H., and Shlomchik, M. J. (1998). Maternal Ig mediates neonatal tolerance in rheumatoid factor transgenic mice but tolerance breaks down in adult mice. *J. Immunol.* 160, 2263–2271.

Weinstein, J. A., Jiang, N., White R. A. III, Fisher, D. S., and Quake, S. R. (2009). High throughput sequencing of the Zebrafish antibody repertoire. *Science* 324, 807–810.

Wikler, M., Demeur, C., Dewasne, G. and Urbain, J. (1980). Immunoregulatory role of maternal idiotypes. Ontogeny of immune networks. *J. Exp. Med.* 152, 1024–1035.

Winstead, C. R, Zhai, S. K., Sethupathi, P., and Knight, K. L. (1999). Antigen-induced somatic diversification of rabbit IgA genes: gene conversion and point mutation. *J. Immunol.* 162, 6602–6612.

Wolfe, K. H., and Shields, D. C. (1997). Molecular evidence for an ancient duplication of the entire yeast genome. *Nature* 387, 708–713.

Woody, O. Z., and McConkey, B. J. (2011). "Detection and analysis of functional specialization in duplicated genes," in *Gene Duplication*, ed. F. Friedberg (Croatia: InTeck Rijeka), 37–58.

Xu, J. L., and Davis, M. M. (2000). Diversity in the CDR3 region of VH is sufficient for most antibody specificities. *Immunity* 13, 37–45.

Xue, C., and Fu, Y. (2009). Preservation of duplicate genes by originalization. *Genetica* 136, 69–78.

Yamaguchi, N., Shimizu, S., Hara, A., and Saito, T. (1983). The effector maternal antigenic stimulation upon the active immune responsiveness of their offspring. *Immunology* 50, 229–238.

Zhang, J. (2003). Evolution by gene duplication: an update. *Trends Ecol. Evol.* 18, 292–298.

Zhao, Y., Pan-Hammarstrom, Q., Kacskovics, I., and Hammarstrom, L. (2003). The porcine Ig delta gene: unique chimeric splicing of the fist constant region domain in its heavy chain transcripts. *J. Immunol.* 171, 1312–1318.

7

Multi step selection in IgH chains is initially focused on CDR3 and then on other CDR regions

Gilad Liberman[1†], Jennifer Benichou[2†], Lea Tsaban[2], Jacob Glanville[3] and Yoram Louzoun[1,2]*

[1] *Gonda Multidisciplinary Brain Research Center, Bar-Ilan University, Ramat Gan, Israel*
[2] *Department of Mathematics, Bar-Ilan University, Ramat Gan, Israel*
[3] *Protein Engineering and Applied Quantitative Genotherapeutics, Rinat-Pfizer Inc., South San Francisco, CA, USA*

Edited by:
Michal Or-Guil, Humboldt University Berlin, Germany

Reviewed by:
Sho Yamasaki, Kyushu University, Japan
Nikolai Petrovsky, Flinders Medical Centre, Australia

****Correspondence:***
Yoram Louzoun, Department of Mathematics, Gonda Multidisciplinary Brain Research Center, Bar-Ilan University, Ramat Gan 52900, Israel e-mail: louzouy@math.biu.ac.il

[†] *Gilad Liberman and Jennifer Benichou have contributed equally to this work.*

Affinity maturation occurs through two selection processes: the choice of appropriate clones (clonal selection), and the internal evolution within clones, induced by somatic hyper-mutations, where high affinity mutants are selected for. When a final population of immunoglobulin sequences is observed, the genetic composition of this population is affected by a combination of these two processes. Different immune induced diseases can result from the failure of regulation of clonal selection or of the regulation of the within clone affinity maturation. In order to understand each of these processes separately, we propose a mixed lineage tree/sequence based method to detect within clone selection as defined by the effect of mutations on the average number of offspring. Specifically, we measure the imbalance in the number of leaves in lineage trees branches following synonymous and non-synonymous (NS) mutations. If a mutation is positively selected, we expect the number of leaves in the sub-tree below this mutation to be larger than in the parallel sub-tree without the mutation. The ratio between the number of leaves in such branches following NS mutations can be used to measure selection within a clone. We apply this method to the sampled Ig repertoire from multiple healthy volunteers and show that within clone selection is positive in the CDR2 region and either positive or negative in the CDR3 and FWR3 regions. Selection occurs already at the IgM isotype level mainly in the DH gene region, with a strong negative selection in the join region. This is followed in the later memory stages in the CDR2 region. We have not studied here the FWR1 and CDR1 regions. An important advantage of this method is that it is very weakly affected by the baseline mutation model or by sampling biases, as are most synonymous to NS mutations ratio based methods.

Keywords: adaptive evolution, phylogenetic tree, immune system, micro-evolution, tree shapes

INTRODUCTION

The humoral adaptive immune response is based on the production of high affinity antibodies against pathogenic antigens. These antibodies are produced through an affinity maturation process, where high affinity antibodies are produced from a large number of cells with different B Cell Receptors (BCRs). The affinity maturation process involves two stages. The first one is clonal selection, where a set of cells with initially mid-high affinity of their BCR to the antigen are expanded. Following this stage, each clone passes a within clone increase in affinity, through somatic hypermutation (SHM) (1) that alter the properties of the BCR, mainly in the complementarity determining region (CDR)3 region (2). The end product of this affinity maturation process is a large population of B cells, with varying BCR that often contain at least one high affinity clone (3).

While the choice of a clone is equivalent to the selection of one specie among many, the dynamics of specific clones in the B cell response against pathogens (4, 5) is a classical example of a process involving rapid asexual reproduction, where constant diversification and adaptation occurs following a high mutation rate. While many tools to study the evolution of species have been developed, tools for the analysis of within population evolution are lacking. We here propose a new method to analyze the within clone affinity maturation process and use it to analyze the healthy B cell repertoire in a large cohort of healthy volunteers.

Multiple methods have been proposed for the measures of selection in populations or between populations, in the sense of evolving toward a higher fitness phenotype (**Table 1**). A now classical measure is the synonymous (S) to non-synonymous (NS) mutations. Specifically, a comparison of the observed and expected NS/(NS + S) ratios is often used as a measure for selection. The expected ratio is calculated based on an underlying mutation probability model [e.g., Ref. (6–8)], or based on genetic regions where no selection is assumed to occur (9). An increased frequency of NS mutations is treated as an indication for positive selection and a decreased one indicates negative selection. Important drawbacks of such methods are: (a) their strong sensitivity to the baseline mutation model (i.e., the expected probability of each mutation type), especially when the mutations rate is position dependent, as happens for example in immunoglobulin sequences (10), and (b) the effect of sampling biases. However, the main problem lies in

Table 1 | List of existing methods based on their reference (first column), the method they use (second column), whether they can detect the direction of selection (third column) and the baseline to which they compare in order to define if selection took place (last column).

Reference	Method	Directional	Baseline reference
Nei and Gojobori (6)	S vs. NS ratio	Yes	Mutation probability model
Yang (7)	S vs. NS ratio	Yes	Mutation probability model
Yang and Nielsen (8)	S vs. NS ratio	Yes	Mutation probability model
Shlomchik et al. (9)	S vs. NS ratio	Yes	Genetic region with no selection pressure
Hershberg et al. (10)	S vs. NS ratio	Yes	Position dependent mutation probability model
Sackin (11)	Tree morphology	No	Yule model
Colless (12)	Tree morphology	No	Yule model
Tajima (16), others	Mutation statistic	No	Naive evolution

the fact that they were developed for an analysis of the comparison between species (clones in this case), and not within a specie.

A different approach for detecting selection is to use properties of lineage trees. Two of the most powerful such methods are Sackin's and Colless's statistics (11–14). Sackin's index is the average root'-leaf distance (over all leaves). Colless's index is the sum of imbalance over all nodes, where a node's imbalance is taken to be the difference in number of leaves between the bigger and smaller sub-trees. These measures are tested vs. a neutral model, which is usually the Yule model, where a tree is constructed by giving each branch the same probability to split (15). Other statistics do not use trees but are based on properties of the full sequences, most notably Tajima's D (16). Such methods have two well-known limitations. They do not distinguish between S and NS mutations and statistical power is lost. However, perhaps the most significant limitation is that in most cases, these methods cannot differ between different types of selection, e.g., positive and negative ones.

We here offer a more direct approach to measure selection within a clone, as well as a better definition of its meaning. This new method overcomes limitations of the S to NS mutation ratio and of the tree shape based selection detection methods, by accounting for the completing information found in each of the two, that is, the classification into mutation types, and the imbalance between different sub-trees.

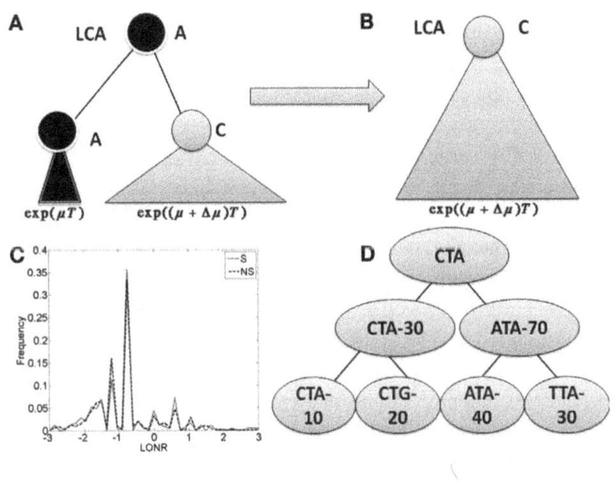

FIGURE 1 | The branch imbalance framework and examples. **(A)** Schematic view of a branch corresponding to a mutation event. Following a mutation, the population can be expanded (or reduced), the advantage will lead to an exponentially growing difference in the number of offspring in parallel branches descending from the same internal origin. T is the time from the mutation to the sampling time. **(B)** After some time, one branch will take over the entire sample, and the information carried in the ratio between the branches will be lost. **(C)** LONR values histogram for one simulated sequence pool, simulated under naive multiplication from unique ancestral sequence. While the average is not 0, there is no difference between branches following S and NS mutations. **(D)** Example of tree. In the left branch, a mutation occurred from CTA to CTG, and the ratio between the mutated and un-mutated branches number of offspring is 20/10. In the right branch, a mutation from ATA to TTA occurred, with a ratio of 30/40. In the root, a mutation from CTA to ATA occurred with a ratio of 70/30.

MATERIALS AND METHODS

SELECTION SCORE

Given a tree, each mutation event is assigned: (a) a NS or S mutation flag by its effect on the amino-acid translation of the containing codon; (b) the location of the mutation (related gene where applicable, and number of nucleotides from the beginning of the sequence, otherwise); and (c) the log of the ratio between the number of leaves (sequences) in the sub-tree following the mutation branch and the number of leaves in the sub-tree following the non-mutated branch (see **Figure 1**; **Figure A1** in Appendix). This ratio is denoted the Log Offspring Number Ratio (LONR). This log-ratio is thus positive if the number of final sequences marked by the tree construction algorithm as descendants of the mutated sequence is larger than the number of final sequences marked as descendants of the non-mutated sequence. This suggests some better fitness of the mutated sequence, or positive selection for such mutation, and negative in the opposite case. For each area of the sequence, a t-test is performed (unpaired, unequal variances) between the NS and S mutations (see **Figure A4** in Appendix for flow chart).

SIMULATION

A sequence pool simulating neutral reproduction was generated from a random original sequence of 348 nt, with a constant multiplication rate of two offspring per organism. Two regions were defined with uniform mutation probabilities with average mutation rate of 1/2 and 1 mutation per generation. The population was sampled in different sample sizes and along different generations.

In each sampling, one of the first eight siblings (the third generation) was chosen randomly, and its descendants had a twice higher probability of being sampled, effectively simulating sampling bias for a specific clone. The process was repeated 1000 times, and selection was computed in the described process. NS and S mutations were defined relative to their direct ancestor, resulting in unequal NS and S probabilities. All mutations had similar probabilities (i.e., we did not differentiate between Purines and Pyrimidines).

STATISTICAL ANALYSIS

For the immunoglobulin data, the receptors where clustered by isotype (IgA and IgG). Lineage trees were constructed and the sequences were divided into CDR and FWR regions. Mean LONR NS-S difference was computed per clone and per region along with two sample t-test p-values.

IMMUNOGLOBULIN SEQUENCES

Over 500,000 BCRs were sampled from each donor in 12 donors (17), using 454 sequencing, and a RACE protocol. The details of the sequencing and the validity checks are beyond the scope of this manuscript. For each sequence, the most fitting VH, JH, and V-J distance was found by maximizing the relative number of non-mutations for both VH and JH segments. Only sequences that matched higher than 0.5 in both segments were kept for further analysis. The sequences were then clustered according to the most fitting VH and JH as well as the distance between VH and JH, and were truncated to 159 nt from the end of the germline VH and 20 nt from the beginning of the germline JH. Only trees with a sufficient number of mutations were analyzed, which automatically removed sequences defined with ORF and pseudo VH genes (**Figure A3** in Appendix).

CLONE DEFINITION

Sequences were grouped into clones using a two-step approach. First, the germline VH and JH of each sequence were determined by aligning all possible germline VH and JH (based on the IMGT germline library) (18) against the sequence using the Basic Local Alignment Search Tool (BLAST) (19).

Next, in order to count the clones, we grouped all sequences according to their VH and JH usage as well as the distance between VH and JH, since SHMs usually do not produce additions or deletions of nucleotides. Thus, every clone emerging from the same founder cell should have the same distance between VH and JH. We then took all of the sequences with the same VH, JH, and distance between VH and JH and grouped them using a phylogenic approach. The distance between VH and JH was computed by positioning the IMGT germline VH and JH genes on the observed sequence and determining the distance between the last nucleotide of VH and the first nucleotide of JH.

All the sequences with equal VH, JH, and distance were aligned together with an artificial sequence composed of the germline and gaps between them. Within each group, the sequences were aligned (using MUSCLE 3.6) (20), and a phylogenetic tree was built using maximum parsimony (21) and/or neighbor joining (22) methods (from the PHYLIP 3.69 program package). We then parsed this tree with a cutoff distance of four mutations into clones. Thus, a clone was defined as a set of sequences that are similar one to each other, up to a distance of four mutations.

RESULTS

SELECTION

Before discussing B cells specifically, let us discuss how selection can be estimated in a rapidly mutating population. Assume a population originating from a single founder through asexual division. In the case of B cells, this would be a clone seeded by an ancestral B cell with a given H chain rearrangement. We ignore the L chain at this stage. The genetic sequence of the founder can be changed by mutations that can affect the population dynamics. In such a case we would define positive selection in the population as an increased average division/birth rate or a decreased average death rate following mutations. Note that these are not precisely the same, especially in the context of B cell dynamics (23), but this is beyond the scope of the current analysis. A decrease in the division rate would be defined as negative selection. Note that each mutation by itself can have a positive, null, or negative effect, but the definition of selection is based on the average population dynamics and not with the dynamics following a single mutation.

Let us follow a mutation that occurs within a population. If this mutation increases the average number of offspring per generation from μ to $\mu + \Delta\mu$, then by a time proportional to log of the total population size, the advantageous mutation will take over the population. When we compare the population to its latest common ancestor (LCA), we will have no evidence that such a mutation has occurred (**Figures 1A,B**). If the original sequence cannot be known (as often occurs in the CDR3 region), we will not be able to detect the presence of such a mutation. If the original sequence is known (as typically occurs in mutations within the germline VH gene), the genetic composition of the population would be equivalent to the one expected in a neutral model (model with no selection). The only difference would be the addition of a single NS mutation to a gene in the entire population. This information can be used to infer that selection has taken place. This is basically the logic behind S to NS mutation ratio tests for selection.

During the intermediate period when the two sub-clones still exist (the mutated and the un-mutated one), one can compare the population size of the two sub-clones. We expect the ratio between the two population sizes to be proportional to $e^{\Delta\mu T}$, where T is the time from the mutation to the sampling time (**Figure 1A**).

For a single mutation, it will be hard to differentiate between the effect of selection and a non-uniform sampling where one branch is sampled more deeply. However, if many mutations occur in the genetic region of interest, and if on average mutations in this region increase the average number of offspring, we expect more offspring in branches that follow a mutation in this region than in branches emerging from the same direct ancestor with no mutations, and inversely in the case of negative selection.

We thus propose to detect selection using this imbalance in cases where the total mutation rate (mutation rate per organism multiplied by population sample size) is significantly higher than one, as typically occur in within clone B cell evolution.

LOG OFFSPRING NUMBER RATIO

We define a measure of selection in a gene as the ratio of the number of leaves (measured descendants) under the branch where a mutation occurred and the number of decedents in its direct sibling where no such mutation occurred. We compare the distribution of these ratios (more precisely the log of the ratios) in S and NS mutations to estimate whether the distribution deviates from the one induced by neutral drift (**Figure 1D**).

Specifically, for each mutation occurring in one son of an internal node and not in the other, we compute the sub-tree size under the son with a mutation and the sub-tree under the son without a mutation. The log of the ratio between these two sizes is defined as the LONR of this mutation. We then compute the LONR value for all S and NS mutations in the tree, and compare the S and NS LONR distributions (**Figure 1C; Figures A1** and **A2** in Appendix).

Note that this analysis is not sensitive to the details of the baseline model for the probability of either silent or replacement mutations, since their absolute number is never used in the analysis. The only case where such a model would affect the current measurement is in the extreme case that the probability for S would differ by orders of magnitude from the probability of NS mutations.

In order to check that the LONR does not detect selection in its absence, we simulated mutating clones, sampled the resulting sequences (see Materials and Methods for details), produced lineage trees, and compared the LONR distribution following S and NS mutations. When the number of mutations is very small, or the number of samples is small, the False Positive (FP) rate (the cases where the LONR average is significantly different following S and NS mutations with a *p*-value of 0.05) is higher than the expected 5%. However, in the regime of over 10–20 mutations per sequence and at least 300 sequences per tree, the FP rates are near the expected 5% (data not shown). We have repeated the analysis with non-uniform mutation rates (position dependent mutation rates) and with sampling biases, and obtained similar results, as long as the S and NS mutation rates are of the same order of magnitude. A detailed methodological analysis of the LONR will be given in a separate analysis.

SELECTION ALONG HUMAN Ig CLONES

We have used the LONR score to analyze the healthy repertoire from 12 donors. In such a repertoire two opposite forces operate: (a) mutations can ruin the functionality of the receptor and decrease its survival probability, (b) mutations can on the other hand increase the affinity to the antigen and thus lead to a higher division rate. The CDRs of the BCR determine its interaction with the antigen, and mutations there were reported to have a higher probability to increase the affinity than mutations in the framework (FWR) region (5, 24). However, the net selection effect in each of these regions still remains unclear. Beyond the effect of SHM, B cells are affected by isotype switches from naïve IgM to memory IgM, and from there to memory IgG and IgA. The memory (IgM, IgG, and IgA) isotypes occur at the advanced stages of the immune response and thus lineage trees based on such receptors are expected to represent the full evolution following selection.

We have used high-throughput sequencing to sequence over 500,000 BCR samples from each donor, in 12 donors. We built lineage trees from the sequences [see (17) for details of sequences, and production of lineage trees]. We measured the LONR distribution in all naïve and memory, IgM as well as IgA and IgG sequences trees (over 50,000 lineage trees) and compared the LONR distribution in NS and S mutations. The results are actually quite striking. We analyzed separately CDR2, FWR3, and CDR3, using the standard IMGT definition (18).

We did not analyze the CDR1 and FWR1 and FWR2 regions, since we did not have enough samples with reliable sequences in these regions. Thus, our results only apply to the comparison of the more 3′ regions (CD2,3 and FWR3). Also, we here include the JH region within the CDR3 analysis. This was done in order to avoid artifacts of the DH gene length. In this specific point, our notation slightly deviates from the standard IMGT analysis that ends the CDR3 region at the beginning of the JH gene region.

As expected in both IgG and IgA memory cells, the positive selection is much stronger for the CDR regions than for the FWR (**Figure 2**). However, in the memory IgM, even the FWR region passes a positive selection during the immune response. Thus, one cannot conclude as a generic conclusion that FWR regions are under negative selection, while CDR regions are under a positive selection. Within different CDR regions, CDR2 is under a much more stringent positive selection than the CDR3 region. Highlighting the fact that while the CDR3 is selected at clone level, where clones with an appropriate CDR3 sequence are selected for expansion, mutations in the CDR2 region may induce a much stronger positive selection than mutations in the CDR3 that can induce a more balanced effect. When analyzing only trees where there is a significant difference between the LONR score ($p < 0.01$) of S and NS mutations, the results are qualitatively similar to the analysis of all trees (**Figure 2**, inset).

In order to ensure that the LONR is not an artifact of the sampling depth or the number of mutations, we computed a correlation between the average S vs. NS mutations LONR difference in each sample (a sample being defined as a single donor, a given isotype, and a given VH gene) and the sample size, or the average number of mutations in each region separately or in all regions in this sample. In all cases there was practically no correlation (the

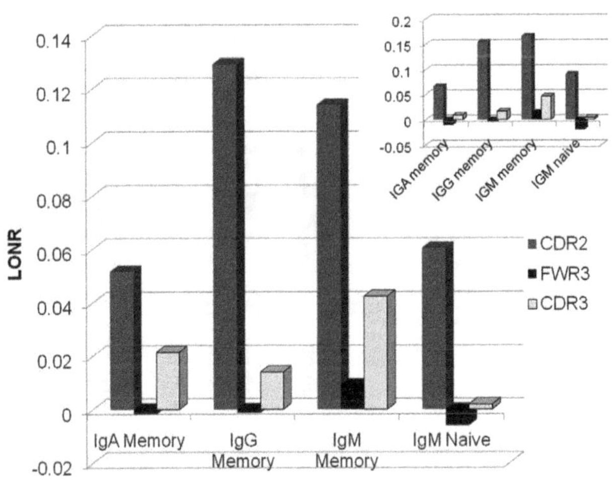

FIGURE 2 | Average LONR score per region and per isotype for all lineage trees (main figure) and for trees with a significant difference (*t*-test, $p < 0.01$; inset). The main positive selection occurs in CDR2, followed by CDR3. FWR3 has a limited if any negative selection. Selection occurs mainly in the memory isotype, but some systematic selection is already observed in the IgM naïve isotype.

highest Spearman correlation was $R = 0.05$). The same occurs if S or NS mutations are used separately. Thus, the observed selection effect is not a sampling or a mutation rate effect.

COMPARISON OF ISOTYPES

Selection and mutations are accompanied by an isotype switch process. It is not clear from the current literature whether isotype switch precedes mutations and selection or if it occurs in parallel. If selection occurs only following isotype switch, we expect no selection to be observed in lineage trees composed of purely IgM sequences. However, the selection level in IgM memory trees is as high as the one observed in IgG lineage trees, and higher than the one observed in IgA lineage trees. Moreover, even in trees composed only of naïve (CD27−) sequences (25, 26), a clear advantage in the division rate following mutations in the CDR2 region is observed. One can thus conclude that even before they become memory cells, B cells pass an antigen induced selection. Note that the CD27− cells can be activated cells, and are not of a pure naïve type (27, 28).Thus, the observed mutations and selection may actually represent an activated phenotype which is a part of the CD27− sub population.

COMPARISON BETWEEN DONORS AND BETWEEN VH GENES

The results presented in **Figure 2** are the average of the selection score over many donors. Some variability exists between donors, and the average selection score can represent a combination of positive selection in some donors and negative selection in others. We have thus separated the analysis into different donors (**Figure 3**). A clear difference emerges between the different regions. While in the CDR2 region practically all donors show a positive selection in all isotypes, in FWR3 and CDR3, the results are highly variables in all isotypes, with some donors showing a marked positive selection and some a negative selection. The main difference between FWR3 and CDR3 is not in the sign of the selection but in its variance. In CDR3 the variance among donors is much larger than in FWR3.

POSITION EFFECT

A more complex picture emerges when each position is analyzed by itself, instead of merging all positions belonging to the same region. At the naïve IgM level, positive selection is mainly focused on the DH region within the CDR3 region, while negative selection takes place in the junction regions (**Figure 4**). When moving to the IgM memory isotype the selection in the CDR3 becomes much weaker, and the selection in the CDR2 starts to rise. Finally, when moving to the IgA and IgG isotype selection is fully focused on CDR2. Note that we here plot the net selection per nucleotide, without considering the total number of mutations per nucleotide. Thus some nucleotide may contribute significantly more than other nucleotides to the average. This different weighting induces some quantitative differences between **Figures 3** and **4**. Note also that while the total number of mutations per sequences is much larger in IgG and IgA than in the naïve IgM serotype, the selection is actually maximal at the naïve level.

These results are highly consistent among the different independent donors, with selection patterns practically overlapping in 10 donors out of 12 (**Figure 4**). In two donors the observed

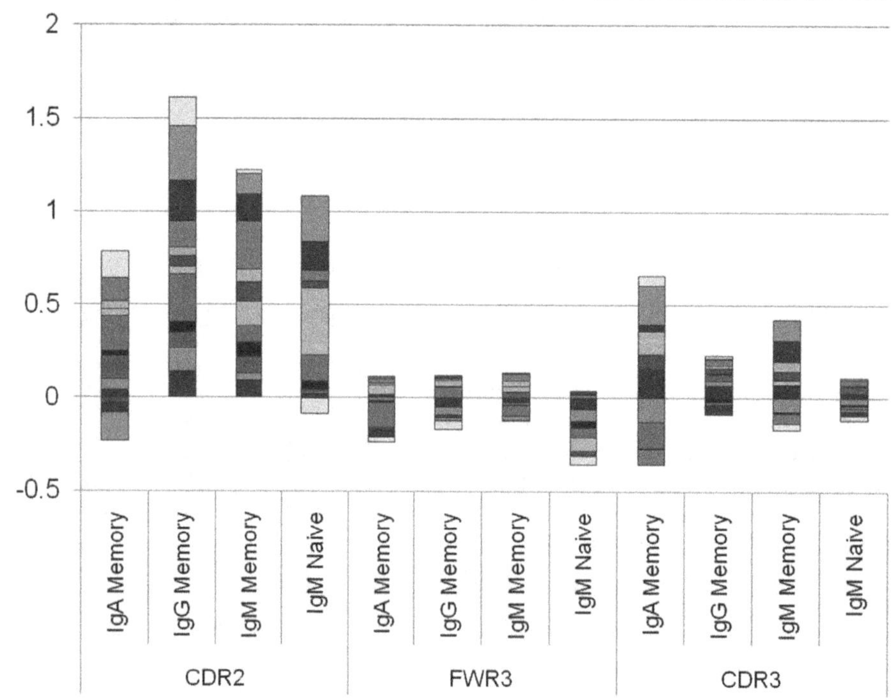

FIGURE 3 | Log offspring number ratio per donor and per isotype. Each column is an isotype in a different region, and each color is a different donor. Each column represents the aggregate over many donors, where negative and positive values are drawn separately. While in the CDR2 there are practically no donors where the average selection is negative (with the exception of two IgA samples and one naïve IgM sample), in the CDR3 there are approximately the same number of donors with negative selection and with positive selection. This shows that the selection in CDR2 is a universal feature, while in CDR3 it may depend on the random junction initially produced or in the different exposures to antigens.

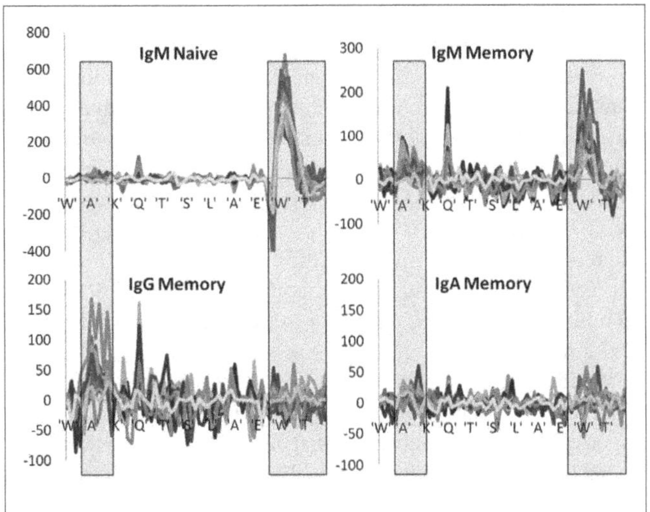

FIGURE 4 | Position specific effects. Total LONR score per amino acid (averaged over the 3-nt composing the amino acid). The LONR is drawn for the four isotypes discussed in previous figures: naïve IgM, memory IgM, IgG, and IgA. Each line represents a different donor. The highlighted regions represent the CDR2 (to the left) and CDR3 (to the right). The sequence at the bottom is a typical sequence. The zone of very strong negative selection at the beginning of the CDR3 is the junction region. One can observe a switch from a very strong positive selection in the naïve IgM isotype focused on the CDR3 to a much weaker selection in the IgG and IgA focused on the CDR2. Note that the scales of the y axes are different between the plots.

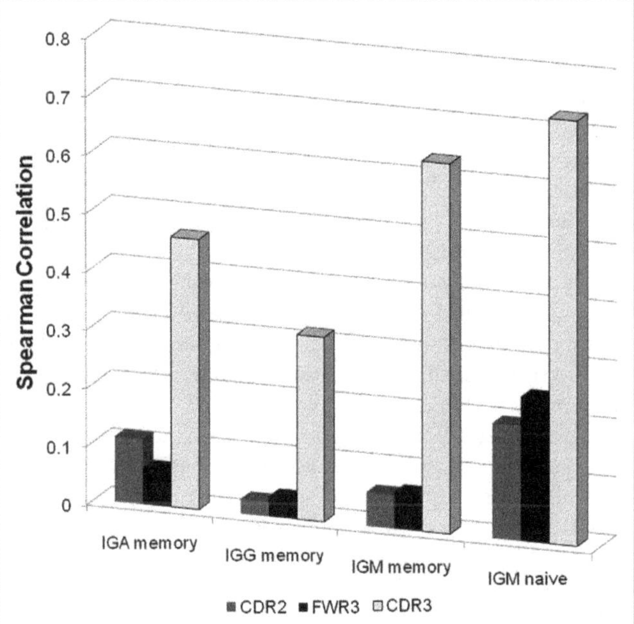

FIGURE 5 | Spearman correlation between the NS/(S + NS) fraction and the total number of B cells for different isotype and different regions. For each sample we produced a vector of 46 values (all functional VH genes with enough samples) representing the total number of B cells in this sample with such a V gene. When all samples are taken together, this leads to a 12*2*46 values (12 donors, 2 technical repeats per donor). We computed the correlation of these values with the NS/(S + NS) values in the same categories. As one can clearly see the highest correlation is with the CDR3 regions of naïve IgM samples.

selection was weak and noisy, but these donors had much smaller sample sizes (data not shown).

These results suggest the following two stage selection process occurring in Ig lineage trees. The first stage of selection occurs early in the CDR3 and is generic and uniform. This would be equivalent to the "key mutation" concept (29, 30). Following these key mutations, selection becomes much weaker and focused on the CDR2 regions in the IgG isotype. The memory IgM shows a translational mutation distribution from the key-mutation selection event, to the weaker mutation in the CDR2, which may alters the affinity in a limited way.

In order to check that there is indeed a correlation between mutations in the CDR3 regions of naïve cells, we compared the correlation between the NS/(S + NS) ratio and the total number of B cells for different regions, VH genes, and isotypes (**Figure 5**). The total clone size was defined as the number of sequences with a give VH in a give sample. The NS and S mutations were defined as the average number of mutations in the leaves compared with the ancestral sequence of each clone (a similar analysis with the number of unique mutations led to similar results). The total number of B cells is the total number of B cells sequenced in a given sample with the same VH gene. As expected the highest correlation was with the NS/(S + NS) ratio in the CDR3 region of naïve IgM cells. Note that a trivial correlation is expected between the number of B cells and the total number of mutations, since large clones may be older clones and as such accumulate a large number of mutations. However, here we have compares the NS fraction, which is not expected to be correlated with the population size, unless selection is involved.

DISCUSSION

While multiple sequence based methods have been proposed to detect selection (10, 31–36), most of them are sensitive to the baseline mutation model, or to sampling effects. Moreover, many existing methods conclude the existence of positive or negative selection from highly frequent or rare mutations. Such an under or over expression of a sequence can simply represent the random expansion of a population, a bottleneck effect, or the random association of this mutation with another mutation which is selected. Indeed even in models of neutral evolution, alleles carrying some sequences are expected to be much more frequent than others, since alleles, and sequence distributions have a fat tail. Instead, positive selection should be defined by the systematic increase of the population size following replacement mutations in a given region.

We have here used this precise definition to define the LONR score as the increase/decrease in the relative branch size following a mutation. A comparison between the LONR score following synonymous and NS mutations. A detailed methodological analysis is left to a different framework; we here describe an application of the LONR score to immunoglobulin clones in healthy volunteers.

The LONR differs in two basic aspects from most other S to NS mutation frequencies methods. First this method does not count the absolute number of sequences; instead it measures for each mutation the effect it has on its number of offspring. The second difference is the definition of mutations and their classification as

S/NS in respect to their direct ancestor, and not to a consensus or ancestral sequence.

Since each mutation is counted once, independent of the total number of sequences that end up containing this mutation, it is practically not affected by sampling biases or by the expansion of specific sub-populations. Moreover the LONR does not require a baseline mutation model, since it does not compare the number of synonymous or NS mutations. Instead, it measures the effect of each mutation on the total number of offsprings.

Tree shape based methods were developed (11–14). However, these methods often cannot detect the direction of selection, and cannot detect which region in the sequence is selected. Moreover, many of these tree shapes are sensitive to sampling effects making them impractical to use in realistic situations (37).

The observed selection in Ig clones has a well conserved pattern among donors. It is consistently positive in the CDR2 region, and positive in average in the CDR3 region. The mutation pattern in the CDR3 region is composed of strong positive selection in the DH region, and strong negative selection in the junctions between the VH and DH genes and between DH and JH genes. We currently have no clear explanation for the negative selection in the junction. However, one can hypothesize that only B cells with appropriate junctions are selected to pass affinity maturation, and that following within clone selection must maintain these junctions. Such a behavior has been clearly observed in H chain transgenic models of selection in mice (23). At later stages, selection is focused on the CDR2 region and is much lower in the CDR3 regions. This can represent a fine tuning of the affinity, where the main limiting step is the accumulation of key mutations in the CDR3, which is then followed by the expression of more specific mutations in the CDR2 region.

We did not analyze the CDR1 and FWR1 and FWR2 regions, since we did not have enough samples with reliable sequences in these regions. We can only guess that CDR1 should behave approximately like CDR2. FWR1 and FWR2 may be quite different than FWR3 as previously proposed (38). Advances in B cell sequencing technologies (39) will hopefully provide longer reads allowing us to study these regions as well.

REFERENCES

1. Nossal G. The molecular and cellular basis of affinity maturation in the antibody response. *Cell* (1992) **68**:1. doi:10.1016/0092-8674(92)90198-L
2. Kocks C, Rajewsky K. Stepwise intraclonal maturation of antibody affinity through somatic hypermutation. *Proc Natl Acad Sci U S A* (1988) **85**:8206–10. doi:10.1073/pnas.85.21.8206
3. Berek C, Milstein C. Mutation drift and repertoire shift in the maturation of the immune response. *Immunol Rev* (1987) **96**:23–41. doi:10.1111/j.1600-065X.1987.tb00507.x
4. Liu Y, Joshua D, Williams G, Smith C, Gordon J, Maclennan I. Mechanism of antigen-driven selection in germinal centres. *Nature* (1989) **342**(6252):929–31. doi:10.1038/342929a0
5. Berek C, Berger A, Apel M. Maturation of the immune response in germinal centers. *Cell* (1991) **67**:1121–9. doi:10.1016/0092-8674(91)90289-B
6. Nei M, Gojobori T. Simple methods for estimating the numbers of synonymous and nonsynonymous nucleotide substitutions. *Mol Biol Evol* (1986) **3**:418–26.
7. Yang Z. Likelihood ratio tests for detecting positive selection and application to primate lysozyme evolution. *Mol Biol Evol* (1998) **15**:568–73. doi:10.1093/oxfordjournals.molbev.a025957
8. Yang Z, Nielsen R. Estimating synonymous and nonsynonymous substitution rates under realistic evolutionary models. *Mol Biol Evol* (2000) **17**:32–43. doi:10.1093/oxfordjournals.molbev.a026236
9. Shlomchik MJ, Aucoin AH, Pisetsky DS, Weigert MG. Structure and function of anti-DNA autoantibodies derived from a single autoimmune mouse. *Proc Natl Acad Sci U S A* (1987) **84**:9150–4. doi:10.1073/pnas.84.24.9150
10. Hershberg U, Uduman M, Shlomchik MJ, Kleinstein SH. Improved methods for detecting selection by mutation analysis of Ig V region sequences. *Int Immunol* (2008) **20**:683–94. doi:10.1093/intimm/dxn026
11. Sackin M. "Good" and "bad" phenograms. *Syst Biol* (1972) **21**:225–6. doi:10.1093/sysbio/21.2.225
12. Colless D. Phylogenetics: the theory and practice of phylogenetic systematics. *Syst Zool* (1982) **31**:100–4. doi:10.2307/2413420
13. Kirkpatrick M, Slatkin M. Searching for evolutionary patterns in the shape of a phylogenetic tree. *Evolution* (1993) **47**:1171–81. doi:10.2307/2409983
14. Blum MGB, François O. On statistical tests of phylogenetic tree imbalance: the Sackin and other indices revisited. *Math Biosci* (2005) **195**:141–53. doi:10.1016/j.mbs.2005.03.003
15. Yule GU. A mathematical theory of evolution, based on the conclusions of Dr. JC Willis, FRS. *Phil Trans R Soc Lond B* (1925) **213**:21–87.
16. Tajima F. Statistical method for testing the neutral mutation hypothesis by DNA polymorphism. *Genetics* (1989) **123**:585–95.
17. Benichou J, Glanville J, Prak ETL, Azran R, Kuo TC, Pons J, et al. The restricted DH gene reading frame usage in the expressed human antibody repertoire is selected based upon its amino acid content. *J Immunol* (2013) **190**:5567–77. doi:10.4049/jimmunol.1201929
18. Lefranc M-P, Giudicelli V, Ginestoux C, Bodmer J, Müller W, Bontrop R, et al. IMGT, the international ImMunoGeneTics database. *Nucleic Acids Res* (1999) **27**:209–12. doi:10.1093/nar/27.1.209
19. Altschul SF, Gish W, Miller W, Myers EW, Lipman DJ. Basic local alignment search tool. *J Mol Biol* (1990) **215**:403–10. doi:10.1016/S0022-2836(05)80360-2
20. Edgar RC. MUSCLE: multiple sequence alignment with high accuracy and high throughput. *Nucleic Acids Res* (2004) **32**:1792–7. doi:10.1093/nar/gkh340
21. Kolaczkowski B, Thornton JW. Performance of maximum parsimony and likelihood phylogenetics when evolution is heterogeneous. *Nature* (2004) **431**:980–4. doi:10.1038/nature02917
22. Saitou N, Nei M. The neighbor-joining method: a new method for reconstructing phylogenetic trees. *Mol Biol Evol* (1987) **4**:406–25.
23. Anderson SM, Khalil A, Uduman M, Hershberg U, Louzoun Y, Haberman AM, et al. Taking advantage: high-affinity B cells in the germinal center have lower death rates, but similar rates of division, compared to low-affinity cells. *J Immunol* (2009) **183**:7314–25. doi:10.4049/jimmunol.0902452
24. Cowell LG, Kim HJ, Humaljoki T, Berek C, Kepler TB. Enhanced evolvability in immunoglobulin V genes under somatic hypermutation. *J Mol Evol* (1999) **49**:23–6. doi:10.1007/PL00006530
25. Klein U, Rajewsky K, Küppers R. Human immunoglobulin (Ig) M+ IgD+ peripheral blood B cells expressing the CD27 cell surface antigen carry somatically mutated variable region genes: CD27 as a general marker for somatically mutated (memory) B cells. *J Exp Med* (1998) **188**:1679–89. doi:10.1084/jem.188.9.1679
26. Agematsu K, Hokibara S, Nagumo H, Komiyama A. CD27: a memory B-cell marker. *Immunol Today* (2000) **21**:204–6. doi:10.1016/S0167-5699(00)01605-4
27. Fecteau JF, Côté G, Néron S. A new memory CD27-IgG+ B cell population in peripheral blood expressing VH genes with low frequency of somatic mutation. *J Immunol* (2006) **177**:3728–36.
28. Cagigi A, Du L, Dang LVP, Grutzmeier S, Atlas A, Chiodi F, et al. CD27(-) B-cells produce class switched and somatically hypermutated antibodies during chronic HIV-1 infection. *PLoS One* (2009) **4**:e5427. doi:10.1371/journal.pone.0005427
29. Radmacher MD, Kelsoe G, Kepler TB. Predicted and inferred waiting times for key mutations in the germinal centre reaction: evidence for stochasticity in selection. *Immunol Cell Biol* (1998) **76**:373–81. doi:10.1046/j.1440-1711.1998.00753.x
30. Kleinstein SH, Singh JP. Toward quantitative simulation of germinal center dynamics: biological and modeling insights from experimental validation. *J Theor Biol* (2001) **211**:253–75. doi:10.1006/jtbi.2001.2344

31. Yang Z, Bielawski JP. Statistical methods for detecting molecular adaptation. *Trends Ecol Evol* (2000) **15**:496–503.
32. Plotkin JB, Dushoff J, Fraser HB. Detecting selection using a single genome sequence of *M. tuberculosis* and *P. falciparum*. *Nature* (2004) **428**:942–5. doi:10.1038/nature02458
33. Wong WSW, Nielsen R. Detecting selection in non-coding regions of nucleotide sequences. *Genetics* (2004) **167**:949–58. doi:10.1534/genetics.102.010959
34. Massingham T, Goldman N. Detecting amino acid sites under positive selection and purifying selection. *Genetics* (2005) **169**:1753–62. doi:10.1534/genetics.104.032144
35. Pond SLK, Frost SDW. A genetic algorithm approach to detecting lineage-specific variation in selection pressure. *Mol Biol Evol* (2005) **22**:478–85. doi:10.1093/molbev/msi031
36. Zhang J, Nielsen R, Yang Z. Evaluation of an improved branch-site likelihood method for detecting positive selection at the molecular level. *Mol Biol Evol* (2005) **22**:2472–9. doi:10.1093/molbev/msi237
37. Stam E. Does imbalance in phylogenies reflect only bias? *Evolution* (2002) **56**:1292–5. doi:10.1554/0014-3820(2002)056[1292:DIIPRO]2.0.CO;2
38. Shapiro GS, Aviszus K, Ikle D, Wysocki LJ. Predicting regional mutability in antibody V genes based solely on di- and trinucleotide sequence composition. *J Immunol* (1999) **163**:259–68.
39. Benichou J, Ben-Hamo R, Louzoun Y, Efroni S. Rep-Seq: uncovering the immunological repertoire through next-generation sequencing. *Immunology* (2012) **135**(3):183–91. doi:10.1111/j.1365-2567.2011.03527.x

APPENDIX

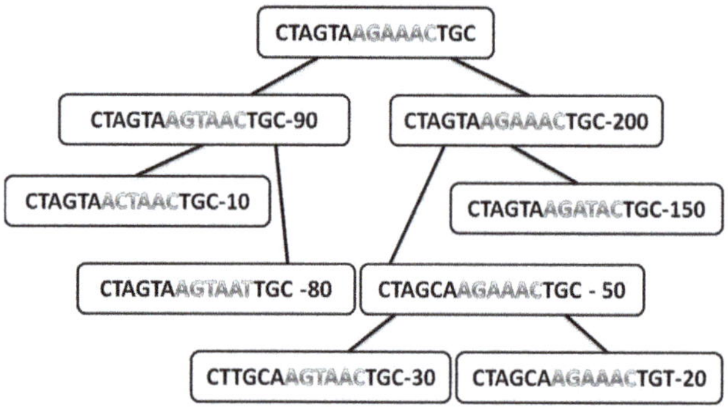

FIGURE A1 | Typical tree with the sequences in each node and the total number of offspring of each node. Only internal nodes are drawn here (leaves are not used for the analysis, since they have no mutations under them). The sequences are divided into two regions (different colors). The number in each node is the total number of offspring.

Position	Mutation	Translation	Type	Zone	LONR
9	AGA->AGT	R->S	NS	2	Log(90/200)
8	AGT->ACT	S->T	NS	2	Log(10/80)
12	AAC->AAT	N->N	S	2	Log(80/10)
10	AAC->TAC	N->Y	NS	2	Log(150/50)
3	CTA->CTT	L->L	S	1	Log(30/20)
15	TGC->TGT	C->C	S	1	Log(20/30)
5	GTA->GCA	V->A	NS	1	Log(50/150)

FIGURE A2 | Log offspring number ratio values for S and NS mutations as given in Figure A1. For each mutation its region is give (1 or 2), its type (S or NS), its position along the gene in nucleotides, the mutation itself in nucleotides, and amino acids, as well as the LONR score. The distribution of LONR scores is used to assess selection.

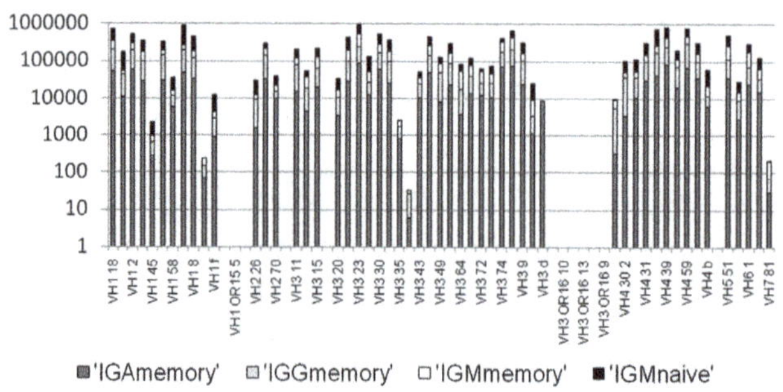

FIGURE A3 | Number of mutation events per VH gene per isotype. There are practically no mutations assigned to pseudogenes, since practically none of the sequenced in-frame lineage trees are based on pseudogenes (<0.05%). However, there are also some functional VH genes with practically no lineage trees. We removed those from the current analysis.

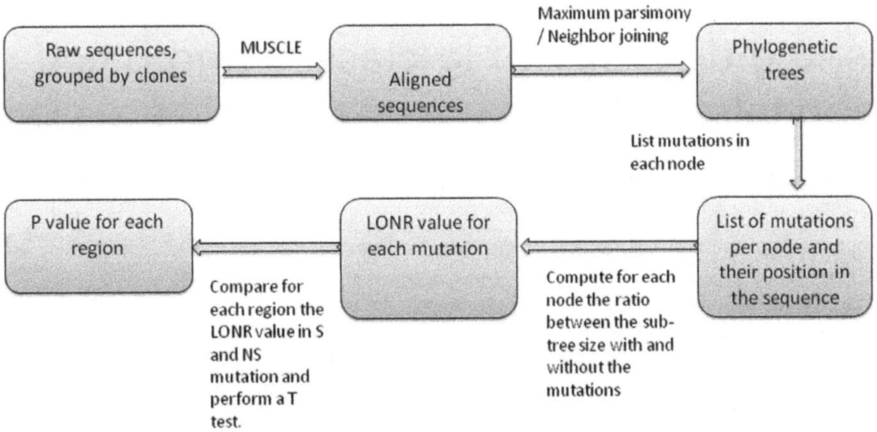

FIGURE A4 | Flow chart of LONR score production. First sequences are aligned, then phylogenetic trees are produced. For each internal node in the trees, a list of mutations is produced (between the internal node and one of its direct descendents). For each such mutation the LONR score is computed resulting in a list of LONR score for each mutation. For genetic region, the LONR score of the mutations in this regions are analyzed and the resulting *p*-value is the result of a *t*-test between S and NS mutations.

8

The astonishing diversity of Ig classes and B cell repertoires in teleost fish

Simon Fillatreau[1], Adrien Six[2,3], Susanna Magadan[4], Rosario Castro[4], J. Oriol Sunyer[5] and Pierre Boudinot[4]*

[1] *Deutsches Rheuma-Forschungszentrum, Leibniz Institute, Berlin, Germany*
[2] *UPMC Univ Paris 06, UMR 7211, "Immunology, Immunopathology, Immunotherapy," F-75013 Paris, France*
[3] *UMR 7211, "Immunology, Immunopathology, Immunotherapy," CNRS, Paris, France*
[4] *Virologie et Immunologie Moléculaires, Institut National de la Recherche Agronomique, Jouy-en-Josas, France*
[5] *Department of Pathobiology, School of Veterinary Medicine, University of Pennsylvania, Philadelphia, PA, USA*

Edited by:
Harry W. Schroeder, University of Alabama at Birmingham, USA

Reviewed by:
Michael Zemlin, Philipps University Marburg, Germany
Peter D. Burrows, University of Alabama at Birmingham, USA

****Correspondence:***
Pierre Boudinot, Virologie et Immunologie Moléculaires, Institut National de la Recherche Agronomique, Domaine de Vilvert, 78352 Jouy-en-Josas, France.
e-mail: pierre.boudinot@jouy.inra.fr

With lymphoid tissue anatomy different than mammals, and diverse adaptations to all aquatic environments, fish constitute a fascinating group of vertebrate to study the biology of B cell repertoires in a comparative perspective. Fish B lymphocytes express immunoglobulin (Ig) on their surface and secrete antigen-specific antibodies in response to immune challenges. Three antibody classes have been identified in fish, namely IgM, IgD, and IgT, while IgG, IgA, and IgE are absent. IgM and IgD have been found in all fish species analyzed, and thus seem to be primordial antibody classes. IgM and IgD are normally co-expressed from the same mRNA through alternative splicing, as in mammals. Tetrameric IgM is the main antibody class found in serum. Some species of fish also have IgT, which seems to exist only in fish and is specialized in mucosal immunity. IgM/IgD and IgT are expressed by two different sub-populations of B cells. The tools available to investigate B cell responses at the cellular level in fish are limited, but the progress of fish genomics has started to unravel a rich diversity of IgH and immunoglobulin light chain locus organization, which might be related to the succession of genome remodelings that occurred during fish evolution. Moreover, the development of deep sequencing techniques has allowed the investigation of the global features of the expressed fish B cell repertoires in zebrafish and rainbow trout, in steady state or after infection. This review provides a description of the organization of fish Ig loci, with a particular emphasis on their heterogeneity between species, and presents recent data on the structure of the expressed Ig repertoire in healthy and infected fish.

Keywords: fish, antibody, repertoire, evolution, B cells

INTRODUCTION

Teleost fish form a large zoological group with about 40,000 identified species, in comparison to 10,000 species for birds, and only around 5700 species for mammals. Fish are heterogeneous with regards to size, morphology, physiology, and behavior. They are ubiquitous throughout almost all aquatic environments, which have diverse oxygen concentrations, water pressures, temperatures, and salinities. Related representatives from the same group can be found in different ecosystems. For instance, Perciformes are adapted to both freshwater and marine habitats, including Antarctic. These diverse milieus certainly host a broad variety of pathogens. Fish can be infected by viruses (rhabdoviruses, bornaviruses, reoviruses, nodaviruses, iridoviruses, herpesviruses, etc.), bacteria (*Vibrio, Aeromonas, Flavobacterium, Yersinia, Lactococcus, Mycobacterium*, etc.), and many parasites. Thus, it is expected that a considerable diversity of host/pathogen interactions characterize fish immune defense mechanisms.

Most of our current knowledge on the immune systems and pathogens of fish comes from aquaculture species. In this context, pathogen diagnostic and vaccination are of considerable economic importance. As an illustration of this, the vaccination program established in Norway to protect Atlantic salmon against vibriosis and furunculosis during the last decades has dramatically reduced the impact of these pathogens, yielding a sharp increase in salmon production that now allows an export value of more than 35 billions Norwegian Kroner (close to 5 billions €) per year. The main aquaculture species of interest for immunology are rainbow trout and Atlantic salmon (*Salmo salar*, Salmoniformes), common, and crucian carp (*Cyprinus carpio* and *Carassius auratus*, Cypriniformes), channel catfish (*Ictalurus punctatus*, Siluriformes), tilapia, sea bass, and sea bream (*Oreochromis niloticus, Dicentrarchus labrax*, and *Sparus aurata*, Perciformes), Japanese flounder (*Paralichthys olivaceus*, Pleuronectiformes), as well as cod (*Gadus morhua*, Gadiformes). The immune systems of several additional species of economical importance in Asia like Grass carp (*Ctenopharyngodon idella*, Cypriniformes), and mandarin fish (*Siniperca chuatsi*, Perciformes) have been increasingly studied during the last years. In addition, a few freshwater fish species originally studied in developmental biology for their capacity to provide eggs, or for their ecological/morphological characteristics, later became experimental models in Immunology. These include zebrafish (*Danio rerio*, Cypriniformes), medaka (*Oryzias latipes*, Beloniformes/Cyprinodontiformes), and stickleback (*Gasterosteus aculeatus*, Gasterosteiformes). In sum, it stands out that our knowledge of fish immunology relates only to a minor fraction of the 40,000 known fish species. It is therefore important not to generalize observations made in individual groups, especially since our knowledge on the model species listed above already illustrates that the organization of the immune system differs among distinct fish species.

Besides its direct relevance for aquaculture, the study of the immune system of fish is also of interest to understand the evolution of the adaptive immune system in Vertebrates. The primordial adaptive immune system of extinct vertebrates is not accessible, but it can be inferred through comparative analyses of the B and T cell systems from distant living groups like fish and mammals. Although fish lack bone marrow and lymph nodes, fish infections by bacterial or viral pathogens can lead to the production of specific antibodies, which in some cases correlates perfectly with protection against re-infection by these pathogens. Such a protection may persist for more than 1 year. It is therefore possible to compare how the humoral immune system functions in fish and in mammals.

Research on the immune system of fish has generally been limited by the lack of reagents suitable for classical cellular immunology research, but it has greatly benefited from the sequencing of their genomes (**Table 1**), which have particular structural features directly relevant for their immune system. In particular, a cycle of tetraploidization and re-diploidization occurred during the early evolution of fish genomes, which was followed by further cycles of whole-genome duplications, and differential loss of various genome parts during the subsequent evolution of many fish families (**Figure 1**). As a result, fish genomes are especially heterogeneous. Some genes involved in the immune system have been affected by these re-modelings; in fact, the great number of gene duplicates has probably played an important role in the diversification of the immune genes through sub-functionalization and specific adaptations. This might also account for the fact that the immunoglobulin (Ig) loci of some fish species are among the largest and most complex described yet. Salmonids have two IgH loci per haplotype with several hundreds of V genes, while mammals have only one IgH loci per haplotype and fewer VH genes.

The availability of genomic resources has been particularly useful to investigate B cell repertoires in fish, both for the description of the genomic organization of Ig loci, which defines the potential repertoire, and for the characterization of the primary repertoire expressed by B cells in healthy and infected fish (Jerne, 1971). When considering the importance of efficient adaptive immune responses for the control of infectious diseases, and for successful vaccination, one realizes the relevance of understanding how lymphocyte repertoires are selected during B cell development and modified upon antigenic challenge. In this review, we will first examine fish Ig classes, the structure of the loci, and the IgH splicing patterns. We will then study the B cell system and the features of the available (expressed) repertoires of antibodies in healthy or infected fish.

DIVERSIFICATION OF IG GENES IN FISH: POTENTIAL REPERTOIRES AND DIVERSIFICATION MECHANISMS

Ig LOCI IN FISH

Fish have three Ig classes

Three classes of Ig have been identified in teleost fish. These are IgM, which is found in all vertebrate species (reviewed in Flajnik and Kasahara, 2009), IgD, which also has a wide distribution among vertebrates, and IgT/Z (for Teleost/Zebrafish), which is specific to fish. Hereafter, fish IgM, D, and T/Z classes refer to the protein products of the isotypes μ, δ, and τ/ζ, respectively, which correspond to their associated constant genes.

IgM was the first Ig class identified in fish. It can be expressed at the surface of B cells or secreted. Secreted tetrameric IgM represents the main serum Ig in fish.

IgD was initially thought to be expressed only in rodents and primates, and to be of recent evolutionary origin. However, the first fish IgD was identified in Wilson et al. (1997) in the channel catfish.

Table 1 | Status of genome sequencing of the main model species for fish immunology.

AQUACULTURE SPECIES	
Rainbow trout (*Oncorhynchus mykiss*)	Genome in progress
Atlantic salmon (*Salmo salar*)	Genome in progress
Atlantic cod (*Gadus morhua*)	Genome published (Star et al., 2011)
Common carp (*Cyprinus carpio*)	Genome published (Henkel et al., 2012)
Crucian carp (*Carassius carassius*)	
Channel catfish (*Ictalurus punctatus*)	Genome in progress
Tilapia (*Oreochromis niloticus*)	Genome available at http://www.ensembl.org/Oreochromis_niloticus/Info/Index
Sea bass (*Dicentrarchus labrax*)	Genome in progress
Sea bream (*Sparus aurata*)	
Japanese flounder (*Paralichthys olivaceus*)	
MODEL SPECIES	
Zebrafish (*Danio rerio*)	Genome available at http://www.ensembl.org/Danio_rerio/Info/Index
Medaka (*Oryzias latipes*)	Genome published (Kasahara et al., 2007)
Three-spined stickleback (*Gasterosteus aculeatus*)	Genome published (Jones et al., 2012)

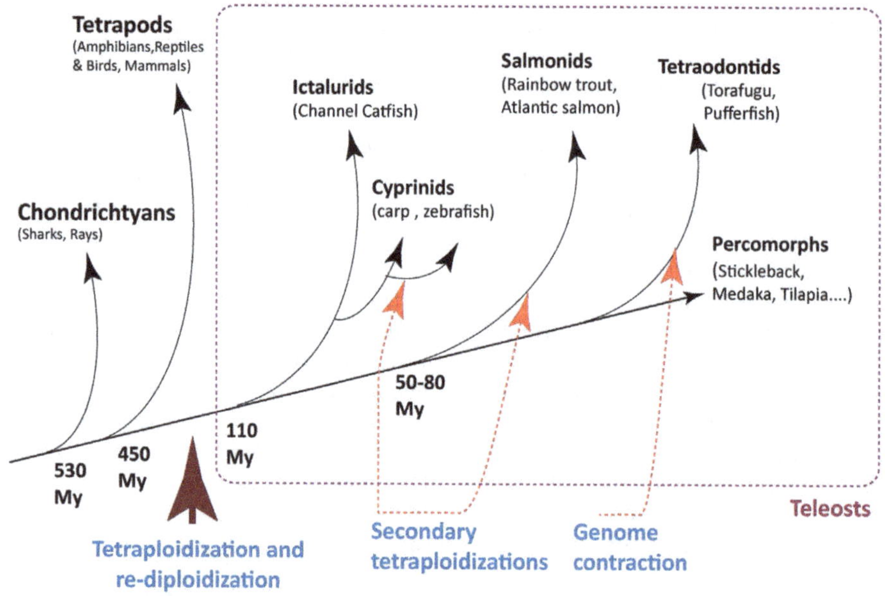

FIGURE 1 | Milestones of genome evolution within the fish lineage. A few key events of tetraploidization/re-diploidization and contraction are represented. Note that red arrows indicate a segment on the tree where an event is assumed, not a precise time point. The time arrow is not on scale.

It differs from mammalian IgD because it is a chimeric protein containing a Cμ1 domain followed by a number of Cδ. This chimeric structure was also found in Atlantic salmon (Hordvik et al., 1999), and other fish species (Stenvik and Jørgensen, 2000; Aparicio et al., 2002; Hordvik, 2002; Srisapoome et al., 2004; Xiao et al., 2010). To date, no complete fish IgD heavy chain without Cμ1 has been described. Intriguingly, a similar Cμ1–Cδ structure has been discovered in some non-fish species of the order of the Artiodactyls (Zhao et al., 2002, 2003). Fish IgD also differs from eutherian IgD by the large number (7–17) of Cδ domains it can contain, and by the absence of a hinge. Secreted IgD have been found in catfish (Edholm et al., 2010), and in rainbow trout (Ramirez-Gomez et al., 2012), but with some differences because it did not contain V domain in the former, while it did in rainbow trout. Of note, IgD has been found in most vertebrates, and it has orthologs even in Chondrichthyans (known as IgW), suggesting that it represents a primordial Ig class, like IgM (Ohta and Flajnik, 2006). To date, IgD seems to be missing only in birds, and in few mammalian species. No IgD sequence was found in the chicken *IgH* locus (Zhao et al., 2000) and seems to be absent from the chicken genome. *IgD* could not be found from available sequences from duck and ostrich either (Lundqvist et al., 2001; Huang et al., 2012). In the same line, *IgD* is apparently absent from the elephant and opossum IgH loci (Wang et al., 2009; Guo et al., 2011).

IgT/IgZ was discovered in Hansen et al. (2005) in rainbow trout (IgT) and zebrafish (IgZ; Danilova et al., 2005). It does not exist in other vertebrates but fish. IgHτ/ζ may contain different numbers of C domains: four C domains are found in most species (Salinas et al., 2011), whereas stickleback (*G. aculeatus*) has three and fugu (*Takifugu rubripes*) has two. In carp (*C. carpio*) IgT is a chimeric protein containing a Cμ1 domain and a Cτ/ζ domain (Savan et al., 2005). No Igτ/ζ locus could be found in the Medaka genome or in the Channel catfish, but it might be identified in catfish when the full genome sequence will be available. Recent studies performed in trout demonstrate that IgT is especially critical for the protection of mucosal territories in this species (Zhang et al., 2010), as suggested by the fact that the local ratio of IgT to IgM is >60-fold higher in the gut mucus than in serum. Furthermore, fish surviving an infection by the gut parasite *Ceratomyxa shasta* had elevated titers of parasite-specific IgT only in the gut mucus but not in the serum, while high titers of parasite-specific IgM were measured in the serum but generally not in the mucus. Additionally, as for IgA in human, an important property of IgT in the gut of rainbow trout seems to be its ability to recognize and coat a large percentage of luminal bacteria at steady state. Secreted IgT is found in trout serum as a monomer, and in mucus as a tetramer (Zhang et al., 2010).

Remarkably, neither IgG nor IgE are present in fish, even though long-lasting protection against secondary infection exists, and many parasites can infect fish.

Fish IgH loci: structure and number across fish species

The archetypal structure of the IgH loci follows a pattern of translocon organization with a region containing VH genes in 5′, followed by units comprising several D, J, and then C region genes in 3′. The Dτ-Jτ-Cτ cluster(s) encoding IgT specific genes are generally located between the region containing the VH genes and the Dμ/δ-Jμ/δ-Cμ-Cδ locus. This structure is found for example in the zebrafish, grass carp, and fugu (**Figure 2A**). In this case, the configuration of IgH loci imposes the alternative production of either IgT or IgM/D rearrangements at a given locus since the recombination of VH to Dμ deletes the Dτ-Jτ-Cτ region(s). Since most VH genes are located upstream of both DHτ and Dμ/δ, they can probably be used by IgT, IgM, and IgD

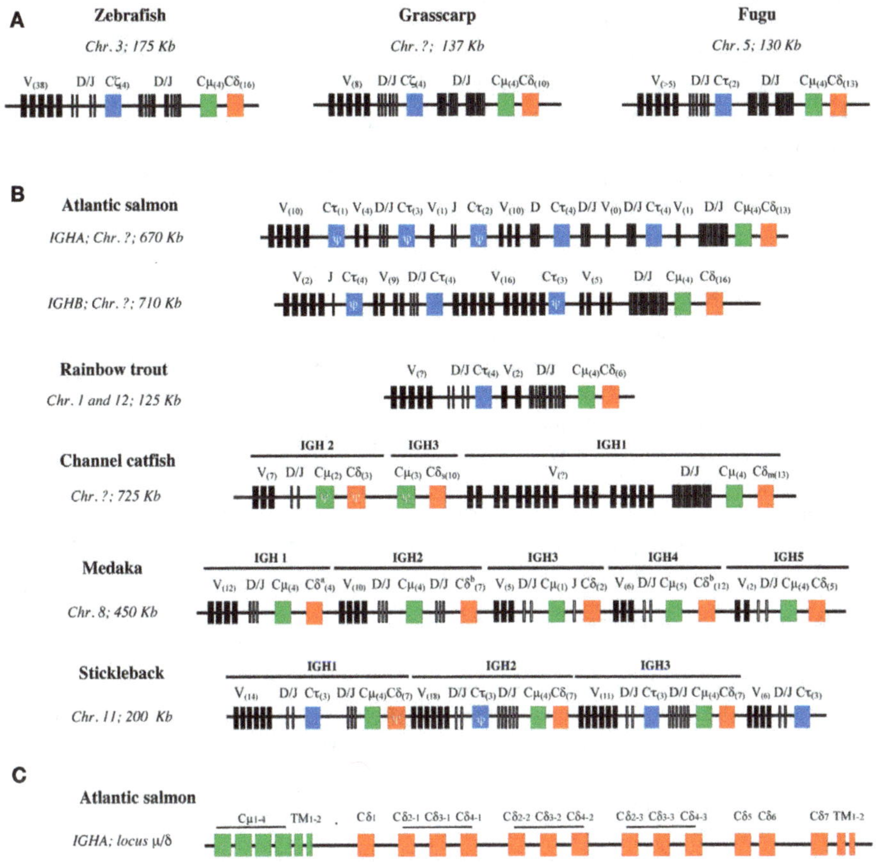

FIGURE 2 | Schematic structure of IgH loci in different teleost species. **(A)** IgH loci with archetypic structure in zebrafish, grass carp, and fugu. **(B)** Variants of IgH structure found in other species with partial or complete duplications present in different chromosomes (Chr.) (Atlantic salmon, rainbow trout) or in the same chromosome (channel catfish, three-spined stickleback, and Japanese medaka) (Chr.). The schemes are not in scale and depict the genomic configuration of V sets (black boxes), D and J sets (narrow gray boxes), and CH gene sets. $C\mu$ are represented as green boxes, $C\delta$ as red boxes, and $C\tau/\zeta$ as blue boxes. The number of in frame V genes and CH exons are indicated in brackets within boxes. CH sequences with frameshift mutations are considered as pseudogenes (Ψ). Catfish IgH: $C\delta_s$ and $C\delta_m$ correspond to the secreted and membrane IgD coding genes, respectively. Medaka IgH: in the $C\delta^a$, the genomic sequence presents a gap and the actual number of $C\delta$ domains is unknown; $C\delta^b$ indicates the presence of $C\mu$ domains inserted between $C\delta$ exons. The "?" symbol indicates a lack of data. **(C)** Detailed exon structure of the IgHA μ-δ region in Atlantic salmon.

(Danilova et al., 2005; Hansen et al., 2005). A large number of VH genes are either pseudogenes, or their sequence is not complete in the genome assembly. Therefore, the diversity of functional VH genes is difficult to estimate. Beyond these general features, the structure of the loci coding for the isotypes corresponding to IgM, IgD, and IgT is surprisingly diverse among teleost fish species, due to successive episodes of genome duplications and gene loss.

Various number of IgH loci can be found in teleost species. The number of IgH loci varies among teleosts, and in some cases isoloci can even be found on different chromosomes (**Figure 2B**).

Salmonids such as Atlantic Salmon and rainbow trout possess two IgH isoloci (IgHA and IgHB) due to the tetraploidization of Salmonidae (Yasuike et al., 2010). The two corresponding IgM subtypes seem to be expressed at the mRNA level in Atlantic salmon and brown trout, but only one is found in rainbow trout and arctic char, suggesting that one of the two isoloci may be non-functional in these last two species. In Atlantic salmon, considering both IgHA and IgHB isoloci, there are eight $C\tau$ loci with variable numbers of $D\tau$ and $J\tau$ genes likely due to tandem duplications, but only three out of these eight loci seem to be functional (two for IgHA and one for IgHB). In contrast, there is only one $D\mu/\delta$-$J\mu/\delta$-$C\mu$-$C\delta$ region per isolocus.

Cyprinids can also have different types of IgH loci. Zebrafish has only one IgH locus with the archetypic structure, as mentioned above (Danilova et al., 2005). The common carp has two subclasses of IgT/Z: IgZ1 is similar to the zebrafish IgZ while the IgZ2 contains a $C\mu1$ domain (Ryo et al., 2010). It seems that the two carp IgZ are expressed from two distinct loci, but it is not clear at present whether these loci are located on the same chromosome. The common carp genome has been recently sequenced, and may provide novel information when fully annotated (Henkel et al., 2012).

In other species like channel catfish, medaka, and three-spined stickleback, tandem duplications of the IgH locus have been found (**Figure 2B**). The channel catfish IgH region contains three μ/δ loci, yet only 1 μ is functional and τ/ζ has not been found so far. The absence of IgT, which still has to be confirmed by full genome sequencing, might be due to a gene loss in the early evolution of Ictalurids. Intriguingly, in catfish the membrane IgD and the (V-less) secreted IgD are always produced from the two different functional Cδ (Bengtén et al., 2006). It remains to be determined whether they could be expressed from the same haplotype. In the medaka genome, five regions encoding constant domains of IgM and IgD have been identified in one large locus (Magadán-Mompó et al., 2011). The analysis of Expressed Sequence Tags (ESTs) suggests that the IGH3 region is disorganized and might be non-functional (**Figure 2B**). No IgT gene has been found so far in this species. In the stickleback genome, three sets of τ/ζ-μ-δ loci separated by VH-containing regions have been described, evoking recombination units as found in mouse λ light chains or shark IgH loci (Bao et al., 2010; Gambón-Deza et al., 2010).

The structure of the IgHδ locus differs between fish species. A precise examination of fish IgH shows that the structure of IGHδ is remarkably heterogeneous among fish species with frequent C-domain duplications, while IgHμ and likely IgHτ appear to be more conserved. For example, Cδ2–Cδ3–Cδ4 domains are repeated three times in Atlantic salmon IgHA (**Figure 2C**) and catfish, and four times in zebrafish and Atlantic salmon IgHB. In puffer fish, the IgD gene comprises a longer tandem Cδ1 → Cδ6 duplication (Saha et al., 2004). The rainbow trout IgD gene is also particular as it carries a Cδ1–Cδ2a–Cδ3a–Cδ4a–Cδ2b–Cδ7 configuration, which seems to be the result of a first duplication of Cδ2–Cδ4 present in Cδ1–Cδ2–Cδ3–Cδ4–Cδ5–Cδ6–Cδ7, leading to Cδ1–Cδ2a–Cδ3a–Cδ4a–Cδ2b–Cδ3b–Cδ4b–Cδ5–Cδ6–Cδ7, followed by deletion of the Cδ3b–Cδ6 domains (Hansen et al., 2005). In the Japanese flounder and stickleback there is no Cδ domain duplication (Hirono et al., 2003; Hansen et al., 2005; Bao et al., 2010; Gambón-Deza et al., 2010). Of note, fish IgM and IgD are co-produced through alternative splicing of a long pre-mRNA containing the VDJ region, the Cμ exons, and the Cδ exons, as in mammals (**Figure 3A**). Precisely, fish IgHδ mature transcripts are produced by splicing of the donor site at the end of the Cμ1 exon to the acceptor site of the first Cδ exon (Wilson et al., 1997), which results in a chimeric Cμ1/Cδ molecules.

Different Ig splicing patterns are used by distinct fish species to generate membrane IgM

In mice and humans, membrane, and secreted IgM H chains are produced from the same pre-mRNA through alternative splicing. A membrane Igμ transcript is made if a cryptic splice site located within Cμ4 is spliced to the acceptor site of the transmembrane (TM)1 exon, and a secreted Igμ transcript is produced when the mRNA is polyadenylated between the last constant (C) region domain Cμ4 and the TM exons. In fish, membrane Igμ transcripts have the TM exons spliced to the donor site located at the 3′end of the Cμ3 exon, hence they lack the last Cμ domain (Cμ4) that is present in the secreted Igμ transcripts (**Figure 3B**; Bengtén et al., 1991; Lee et al., 1993; van Ginkel et al., 1994). Exceptions to this rule have been found in different species. The medaka membrane Igμ lacks both Cμ3 and Cμ4 domains because the TM exons are spliced directly to the 3′end of the Cμ2 domain (Magadán-Mompó et al., 2011). In the Antarctic Notothenioids fish, membrane Igμ transcripts also lack these domains (Coscia et al., 2010) but two exons consisting of 39-nt (RA and RB) are present between the Cμ2 and TM1 exons (Coscia et al., 2010). This splicing pattern, which is found in most of the Antarctic Notothenioids, may represent an adaptive selection of IgM during Notothenioid evolution (Coscia and Oreste, 2003). In the zebrafish, in addition to the classical VDJ–Cμ1–Cμ2–Cμ3–TM1–TM2 mRNA, an alternative VDJ–Cμ1–TM1–TM2 membrane Igμ transcript has been reported, which encodes only one CH domain (Hu et al., 2011). This implies that B cells can express two different forms of membrane IgM in this species, which increases the number of expressed Ig isotypes. Noteworthy, the functional implication of these various splicing patterns for B cell functions is unknown.

In ancient lineages of fish such as holosteans, the bowfin (*Amia calva*), and the long-nose gar (*Lepisosteus osseus*) a remarkable diversity of splicing patterns of the membrane Igμ transcripts was also observed (Wilson et al., 1995a,b). In chondrosteans, another ancient fish lineage, the diversity of membrane Igμ transcripts is even higher: in Siberian sturgeon (*Acipenser baerii*) the TM1 exon is alternatively spliced to three possible donor sites: a cryptic site at the end of Cμ4, a cryptic site at the end of Cμ3, and the

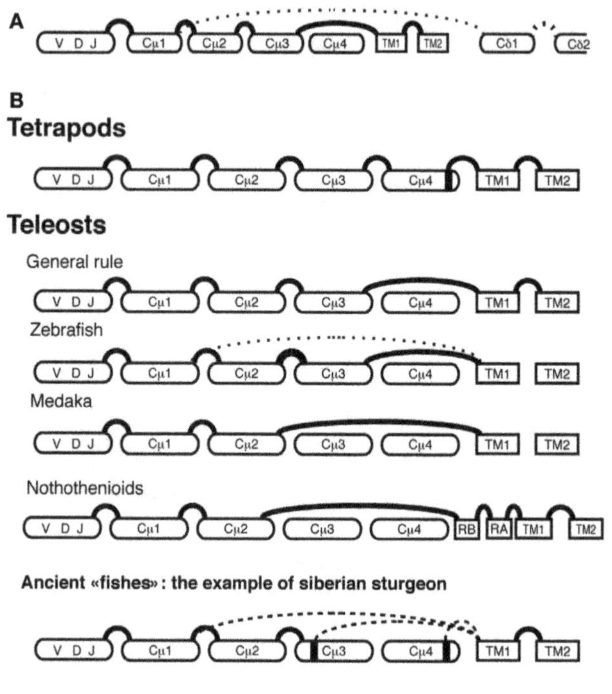

FIGURE 3 | Representation of IgH splicing alternative pathways in fish and tetrapods. The alternative splicing leading to IgHμ (plain line) and to IgHδ (dotted line) mature mRNAs **(A)**. IgHμ RNA splicing pathways in different fish groups and in Tetrapods **(B)**: plain and dotted lines represent general and alternative splicing pathways, respectively.

donor splice site at the 3′end of Cμ1, leading to IgM H chains with four, two, or only one complete Cμ domain(s) (Lundqvist et al., 2009; **Figure 3B**). The shortest membrane Igμ splice variant might have specialized functions because it was retrieved only in transcripts expressing VH2 (Lundqvist et al., 2009). This diversification of splicing pathways to produce membrane IgM in the "ancient fish" lineages evokes a highly diverse situation after whole-genome duplication in the early fish evolution, followed by standardization to the Cμ3 → TM1 splicing pattern in teleosts before their great radiation. However, the particular situations found in ice fish (Notothenioids) or even in zebrafish or medaka indicate that this standardization is not universal.

IgL loci in teleost fish

Four immunoglobulin light chain (IgL) isotypes have been described in teleosts: L1, L2, L3, and λ (Edholm et al., 2009; Bao et al., 2010). A recent comprehensive phylogenetic analysis of vertebrate VL and CL sequences suggested that fish L1 and L3 chains are κ orthologous (Criscitiello and Flajnik, 2007), and fish L2 are orthologs of Xenopus σ (Partula et al., 1996). The current general classification of IgL from all vertebrates distinguishes four clans based on phylogenetic relationships: κ (mammalian κ, elasmobranch Type III, Teleost L1, and L3, Xenopus ρ), λ (mammalian λ, elasmobranch type II), σ (Xenopus σ, teleost L2, elasmobranch type IV), and σ cart (σ-cart, that is restricted to elasmobranch).

Light chain genes in fish genomes are found as multiple VL–JL–CL units. The genomic organization of VL–JL–CL unit is conserved in teleosts. For the L1 and L3 loci, the V genes are in opposite transcriptional orientation with respect to the J and C segments. In contrast, in L2 and λ clusters V, J, and C genes are in same orientation (Daggfeldt et al., 1993; Ghaffari and Lobb, 1993, 1997; Timmusk et al., 2000), with the exception of stickleback L2 (Bao et al., 2010). In a genome wide study in zebrafish, such clusters have been found in five different chromosomes (Zimmerman et al., 2008). Interestingly, VL–JL rearrangements between distinct units were reported in this species, which might be a means of increasing the potential combinatorial diversity.

It is intriguing that to date no pseudo light chain corresponding to eutherian mammal VpreB or λ5 has been reported in fish. In mammals, these chains play a crucial role in the stepwise process of Ig chains rearrangements that take place during B cell development. A deficiency in VpreB or λ5 results in a block of B cell development at the pre-B cell stage in mice (Kitamura et al., 1992). In fish, it is still unknown if an alternative pre-B cell receptor that lacks the VpreB/λ5 surrogate light chain forms during B cell development. In fact, it is not known if Ig gene rearrangements in fish follow the ordered model described in mouse and human; moreover, no pre-Tα receptor has been found in fish, while it was recently discovered in sauropsids (Smelty et al., 2010). Similarly, the mechanisms ensuring allelic exclusion in fish are unknown.

PATHWAYS AND ENZYMATIC MACHINERY OF Ig REARRANGEMENT AND DIVERSIFICATION

The enzymatic machinery of Ig gene rearrangement: similarities between fish and mammals

The rearrangement of VDJ genes is mediated in mammals by a complex enzymatic machinery that includes recombination activating genes (RAG)-1 and 2, proteins from the non-homologous end joining (NHEJ) pathway of repair of DNA double strand breaks, and DNA polymerases of the X family polymerase λ, polymerase μ, and terminal deoxynucleotidyl transferase (TdT). RAG are lymphocyte-specific enzymes that mediate the first steps of VDJ recombination including recognition of the Recognition Sequence Signal (RSS) situated on the sides of the Ig gene segments recruited in the rearrangement, cleavage of DNA at these RSS sites, and hairpin formation as well as resolution. The NHEJ components (Ku70, Ku80, DNAPK, XRCC4, ligase IV, and ARTEMIS) constitute the major pathway involved in the repair of the double strand DNA breaks introduced by the RAG enzymes. The resolution of the DNA breaks is preceded by the action of polymerases λ and μ, which mediate DNA deletional trimming at the junction site, and TdT, which adds "N" nucleotides in a template-independent manner in VDJ junctions. The enzymes implicated in the molecular machinery of Ig rearrangements are remarkably conserved between mammals and fish (**Table 2**).

RAG1 and RAG2 from fish were first cloned in rainbow trout (Hansen and Kaattari, 1996; Hansen, 1997) and zebrafish (Greenhalgh and Steiner, 1995; Willett et al., 1997). They are expressed in tissues where rearrangement activity is expected, and a zebrafish with a truncated RAG1, identified by screening of *N*-ethyl-*N*-nitrosourea mutants, is unable to make VDJ rearrangements, indicating that this enzyme is required for this process in zebrafish as in mammals (Wienholds et al., 2002). In line with this, V, D, and J segments of fish IgH and IgL are flanked by typical RSS (Ghaffari and Lobb, 1997; Hayman and Lobb, 2000). Of note, RSS-like heptamers and nonamers were found within some JL–CL introns (Ghaffari and Lobb, 1997) as well as in 3' region of the majority of the zebrafish CL genes (Zimmerman et al., 2011), evoking the isolated RSS heptamer recombination element located in mouse Jκ–Cκ intron, which can recombine with the κ-deleting element located downstream of Cκ exon to delete the Cκ exon and silence the Igκ locus (Vela et al., 2008). Such process of locus inactivation might provide a mechanism to achieve allelic exclusion for fish IgL (Vela et al., 2008).

The genes coding for the main enzymes of the NHEJ machinery appear to be present in fish genomes, with (recent) duplications for some of them in zebrafish (**Table 2**). An ortholog of Ku70 was identified in zebrafish that was critical for protection from radiation-induced DNA damage because embryos in which this gene was knocked-down were highly sensitive to ionizing radiation (Bladen et al., 2007).

Orthologs of the X family of DNA polymerases involved in diversification of VDJ junctions have also been identified in fish. The gene coding for TdT was found in rainbow trout and zebrafish genomes (Hansen, 1997; Beetz et al., 2007). It is expressed in lymphoid tissues where rearrangements occur (thymus, pronephros, mesonephros, spleen, and gut). Both TCR and Ig junctions contain N diversity, suggesting that fish TdT has similar functions as in mammals. In zebrafish polymerase μ is expressed also in primary lymphoid tissues, as well as in ovary and testis (Beetz et al., 2007). Thus, the mechanisms of Ig rearrangement might be similar in teleosts and mammals.

Table 2 | Genes of the key participants of the rearrangement machinery in fish.

	Reference	Zebrafish	Stickleback
Rag1	Hansen and Kaattari (1995), Hansen and Kaattari (1996), Greenhalgh and Steiner (1995), Willett et al. (1997)	ENSDARG00000052122	ENSGACG00000011465
Rag2		ENSDAzRG00000052121	ENSGACG00000011461
NHEJ			
Ku70	Bladen et al. (2007)	ENSDARG00000090718 ENSDARG00000071551	ENSGACG00000004868
Ku80		ENSDARG00000068862 ENSDARG00000015599	ENSGACG00000006130
XRCC4		ENSDARG00000010732	? (But present in a number of other fish)
DNAPK		ENSDARG00000075083	ENSGACG00000001974
Artemis/DCLRE1C		ENSDARG00000045704	ENSGACG00000020073
Ligase IV		ENSDARG00000060620	ENSGACG00000014135
POLYMERASES X			
Polymerases λ		ENSDARG00000039613	ENSGACG00000018272
Polymerases μ	Beetz et al. (2007)	ENSDARG00000042507	ENSGACG00000001887
TdT	Hansen (1997), Beetz et al. (2007)	ENSDARG00000038540	ENSGACG00000002880

It is interesting to note that the genes coding for some of these enzymes are present in the genomes of ancient fish such as cartilaginous elasmobranch (which include shark, ray, and skates). TdT from elasmobranch has structural similarities with the mouse TdT, in agreement with the fact that both enzymes have template-independent mode of DNA elongation without strong nucleotide bias (Bartl et al., 2003). These data suggest that TdT and other polymerases from the ancient family of polymerases X were used by the rearrangement machinery even before the divergence of fish and mammals (Beetz et al., 2007).

Mechanisms of hypermutation: presence and limits

The affinity maturation of antibody responses is less efficient in cold blood vertebrates compared to mammals (Wilson et al., 1992). For example after immunization of rainbow trout with the hapten-carrier antigen TNP-KLH (trinitrophenyl-linked to keyhole limpet hemocyanin), the affinity of the antigen-specific antibody response progressively increased over 27 weeks, with initial production of low affinity antibodies, which were replaced within 5 weeks by antibodies of intermediate affinity, and after 15 weeks by antibodies that had the highest affinity for antigen (Ye et al., 2011). It is assumed that the low efficiency of the affinity maturation of the antigen-specific antibody response in fish is due to the absence of typical germinal centers (GC), which are the specialized anatomical structures supporting the selection of B cells expressing high affinity B cell receptor (BCR) for antigen in mammals (Wilson et al., 1992). However, clusters of cells containing melano-macrophages were found in spleen and kidney of channel catfish, which might represent primordial GC because activation-induced deaminase (AID) was expressed in these structures (Saunders et al., 2010). AID is a critical enzyme for somatic hypermutation and class switch recombination of Ig genes in mammals. Fish AID differ from their mammalian counterparts at the level of the catalytic sites, but puffer fish and zebrafish AID could nonetheless mediate Ig class switch recombination in mouse B cells (Barreto et al., 2005). In catfish hypermutated IgH sites show an accumulation of G → A and C → T substitutions consistent with AID activity. However, the pattern of Ig somatic hypermutation has particular characteristics in fish, with sequence motifs containing hypermutation hotspots different from those known in mammals (Yang et al., 2006). Interestingly, there was no difference in the ratio of replacement-to-silent mutations in the complementarity determining regions (CDR), which correspond to the Ig parts involved in antigen binding, and in the framework regions, which are normally not involved in antigen binding. Thus, the mechanism of Ig somatic mutation did not coevolve in fish with the pathways mediating selection of B cells with non-synonymous substitutions specifically within CDR-encoded regions. Fish Ig structure suggests that as in mammals CDR are most important for antigen binding, and that they form the main part of the antigen binding surface. A possible explanation for this finding is that mutated Ig sequences do not undergo positive selection for affinity maturation efficiently due to the lack of an appropriate micro-environment. In this context, the primary role of the process of somatic hypermutation might have been to diversify the available repertoire by targeting hotspot motifs preferentially located within CDR-encoded regions. Whether part of this diversity might have deleterious specificity and require particular negative selection remains unknown. In zebrafish, a comprehensive analysis of IgHμ transcripts via deep sequencing indicated that the frequency of Ig sequences with high numbers of somatic mutations increased with age (up through 1 year), in agreement with the notion that hypermutation brings a significant contribution to the diversification of the Ig repertoire (Jiang et al., 2011). Fish Ig light chains can also be subjected to hypermutation (Marianes and Zimmerman, 2011), as previously observed in shark (Lee et al., 2002). It is so far unknown whether fish AID, like mammalian ones, can specifically target additional genes with frequent translocations in tumors, repetitive sequences, and histone H3K4 trimethylation (Kato et al., 2011). The gene *aid* is found in the genome of the main fish model species within conserved synteny groups, indicating they represent true orthologs of the mammalian gene (see zebrafish ENSDARG00000015734, stickleback ENSGACG00000010521, fugu ENSTRUG00000007079 in the Ensembl website).

THE CENTRAL B CELL SYSTEM IN FISH

Three modes of early hematopoiesis have been described in fish (Zapata et al., 2006): hematopoiesis can start in the yolk sac blood islands like in the angelfish, or in intraembryonic intermediate cell mass (ICM) as in zebrafish; alternatively it may initiate for a short time in the yolk sac before continuing in the ICM as in rainbow trout. In zebrafish, the hematopoietic activity appears at 4 days post-fertilization (dpf), but gives rise first to erythroblasts and myeloid cells. Fish B cell lymphopoiesis appears and occurs mainly in the kidney. The expression of zebrafish RAG2 was observed at 8 dpf in the pronephros of *Rag2-Gfp* transgenic fish, which was the earliest extrathymic site of RAG expression (Trede et al., 2004). AID mRNA was even detected at 2 dpf in this species by analysis of gene expression on the whole embryo (Trede et al., 2004). The first VHDHJH rearrangements were detected around 4 dpf (Danilova and Steiner, 2002), but cells expressing IgM (Lam et al., 2004) appeared in the kidney only at 3 weeks post-fertilization, suggesting a slow process of B cell maturation. In the rainbow trout, RAG expression occurred earlier, from 10 dpf onward, and membrane IgM-expressing cells became detectable at hatching (Razquin et al., 1990), around 3 wpf (Hansen, 1997). The spleen seems to have much less importance for B cell lymphopoiesis than the kidney tissue, if any.

In adult fish, B cells reside in the anterior and posterior kidney, spleen, gut lamina propria, and blood (Rombout et al., 1993; Abelli et al., 1997). Several B cell subsets can be distinguished according to their expression of distinct Ig class combinations. In some fish species two subsets of B cells can be identified by their expression of both IgM and D, or IgT only. The development of IgM^+IgD^+ B cells and IgT^+ B cells involves two different pathways because in zebrafish with a deficiency in *Ikaros* gene IgT^+ B cells are totally lacking, while IgM^+ B cells are present, even though their appearance shows a delayed kinetic (Schorpp et al., 2006). Moreover, these two types of B cells are differently localized in the organism. IgM^+ B cells are the main B cell population (75–80%) in spleen, kidney, and blood, while IgT^+ B cells represent the main B cell subset (55%) in gut-associated lymphoid tissues (Zhang et al., 2010). The existence and importance of $IgM^-IgD^+IgT^-$ B cells in fish is a matter of debate. While in most fish species it is considered that IgD is always co-expressed with IgM, a distinct population of IgM^-IgD^+ B cells has recently been identified in the channel catfish, which preferentially expresses σ IgL (Edholm et al., 2010). The frequency of this population is highly variable between individuals, ranging from a few percent to more than 70% of B cells within peripheral blood leukocytes. The participation of these cells to immune responses is not known.

Fish B cells show different homing patterns depending on their development and activation stages. B cell progenitors and plasma cells are dominant in the anterior kidney, while mature B cells and plasma blasts are primarily found in posterior kidney (Zwollo et al., 2005; Zwollo, 2011). Spleen leukocytes also contain B cells that can differentiate into plasma cells. Based on these data, it can be envisioned that B cell development occurs in the anterior kidney, from where mature B cells enter the blood/lymph to reach the spleen and posterior kidney, where they can become activated and differentiate into plasma blasts and then plasma cells, which migrate back to the anterior kidney where they might subsist as long-lived cells in particular niches. Such model suggests that B cells use the same tissue for their development as plasma cells for their residence, as previously observed in mammals.

The B cell repertoire in the healthy fish

The modalities of B cell selection to produce a naïve repertoire remain unknown in fish. The development of high-throughput sequencing methods now makes possible a comprehensive description of expressed immune repertoires. The first exhaustive sequencing of a B cell expressed diversity in a vertebrate was performed in zebrafish by Weinstein et al. (2009) using 454 GS FLX pyrosequencing. In this study, whole-fish mRNA was prepared from 14 individuals belonging to 4 families, and the variable domain (VDJ region) of IgHμ sequenced. The expressed IgM repertoire was studied in quiescent state, from healthy fish that had been raised in classical aquarium environment and possessed a normal gut microbial flora. It was estimated that a large proportion of the possible V/J combinations (50–86%) were expressed. Interestingly, the distribution of VDJ diversity was similar between individuals, and identical μ heavy chains were found in distinct fish more often than expected. This study established that the expressed IgM repertoire of different fish belonging to distinct families shared some patterns, a property which was called stereotypy. The same laboratory also followed the evolution of the expressed IgM repertoire during zebrafish development (Jiang et al., 2011). In 2-weeks-old fish, the repertoire of VDJ combinations showed a high level of stereotypy, suggesting that the primary repertoire was strongly constrained. In such young fish, which have few (if any) antibody-secreting cells, the abundance, and the junctional sequence diversity of VDJ combinations correlated. In contrast, this correlation was lost in 3-month-old fish. This was likely due to the higher frequency of antibody-secreting cells in these older animals. Nevertheless, the frequencies of VDJ combinations correlated between individuals, substantiating further the notion that deterministic forces regulate the structure of the primary repertoire. The apparent contradiction between a deterministic view of the expression of VDJ combinations and the loss of correlation between VDJ frequency and diversity in adult fish may be explained by the accumulation of different numbers of plasma cells in distinct adult fish.

In a different study, a combination of CDR3 length spectratyping and pyrosequencing was used to describe the expressed IgM, IgD, and IgT repertoires in rainbow trout (Castro et al., 2013). The VDJ domains expression was studied in the spleen of naïve individuals. Clonal isogenic animals were analyzed to avoid fish-to-fish variation due to genetic heterogeneity. As in zebrafish, it was found that not all V/J combinations were expressed. In fact, only 7 out of 13 VH families were retrieved. CDR3 length spectratyping and pyrosequencing showed that spleen Ig repertoires were very diverse for all three isotypes in healthy fish. IgM and IgD repertoires were rather similar for most VH, while being significantly different from the IgT repertoire. This observation suggested that IgM and IgD repertoires were not subjected to drastic differential selection. The strong difference between IgT and IgM/IgD CDR3 length profiles was consistent with the usage of a different set of rearrangements with specific D and J segments in B cells expressing either IgM/IgD or IgT. A more detailed analysis focused on the VDJ junctions. To compare the distributions of junctional sequences between individuals, sequence reads encoding a CDR3 region were annotated using IMGT/highV-QUEST for VH, JH, and C genes, and aggregated into "junction sequence types" (JST). The abundance distribution of JST computed from pyrosequencing datasets indicated that 90–99% of junction sequences were found less than five times, likely corresponding to naive non-expanded B cells. Only few JST were found more than 20 times, possibly reflecting the presence of few antibody-secreting cells in the spleen of these fish, in good accordance with previous studies about spleen B cell subsets in rainbow trout (Bromage et al., 2004).

Taken together, these observations indicate that all VDJ combinations are not equally expressed, and suggest that, at least in zebrafish, the expressed repertoire exhibits a significant level of stereotypy.

THE MODIFICATIONS OF FISH EXPRESSED Ab REPERTOIRES BY INFECTIONS AND VACCINES

In fish, B cell responses occur against a variety of pathogens, and must occur in microenvironments different from those described in mammals, due to the lack of GC and lymph nodes. In this context, the clonal complexity of trout B cell responses is largely unknown. The development of high-throughput sequencing approaches of Ig transcripts combined with CDR3 length spectratyping can provide comprehensive analyses of B cell responses, which are required to understand the dynamics of their clonal complexity (Ademokun et al., 2011).

Such an approach was used to characterize the B cell response of rainbow trout against a rhabdovirus, the Viral Hemorrhagic Septicemia Virus (VHSV). Clonal fish were vaccinated using an attenuated virus, then challenged 3 weeks later with the same virus, and finally analyzed after three more weeks. At this stage, all fish had neutralizing antibodies against VHSV, and increased levels of total IgM as well as IgT in serum. The titer of IgM remained more than 10 times higher than of IgT after infection, and the ratio of $IgM^{+}IgT^{-}/IgM^{-}IgT^{+}$ B cells was similar between infected and control fish. CDR3 length spectratyping showed that the VHSV infection triggered a strong IgM response. Indeed, VHCμ spectratypes were extensively and significantly skewed in infected fish for all the analyzed VH, as shown by a comparison of each peak in each spectratype profile using the ISEApeaks software (Collette and Six, 2002). Interestingly, the VH5.1-Cμ profile showed a great amplification of the same peak in all infected individuals, suggesting a public response. In contrast, VHCδ profiles showed only weak and sporadic alterations, which were not statistically validated. The low contribution of IgD to the response might reflect a down regulation of its expression in activated B cells, as in human and mice. This analysis also revealed a significant IgT response in spleen of infected fish. After VHSV infection, most splenic IgT spectratyping profiles were affected, although to a lesser extent compared to IgM. No peak expansion common to all infected fish was observed for IgT, suggesting the absence of a public response. Hence, the spleen might be a site of activation for VHSV-specific IgT^{+} B cells. This is intriguing because IgT is a specialized mucosal Ig.

The molecular diversity of IgM and IgT responses was further characterized by pyrosequencing of VHC junctions for different VH groups. Since a JST corresponds to a CDR3 protein sequence associated with a (VH, JH) pair, the distribution of the relative abundance of JST in different fish provides a description of the importance of antibody clonal responses. IgM JST distributions showed that the virus induced a major shift of the IgM expressed repertoire, with appearance of a significant number of highly represented JST (**Figure 4**).

Further analysis indicated that these large JST sets corresponded essentially to transcripts encoding secreted IgH, hence to antibody-secreting cells. When comparing the JST expanded in different infected fish, similar VH5.1-J5 rearrangements with CDR3 of 10 amino acids were present in all individuals. The CDR3 with the amino acid sequence ARYNNNAFDY was the most frequent, but a number of other related JST were found repeated in several individuals, with exchange of small or polar amino acids: ARYNN**D**AFDY, ARY**D**NNAFDY, ARYN**S**NAFDY, ARYNN**V**AFDY, ARY**DD**NAFDY, ARYN**T**NAFDY, ARYN**GD**AFDY, ARY**SGD**AFDY, and ARYN**GR**AFDY. Such expansion of a number

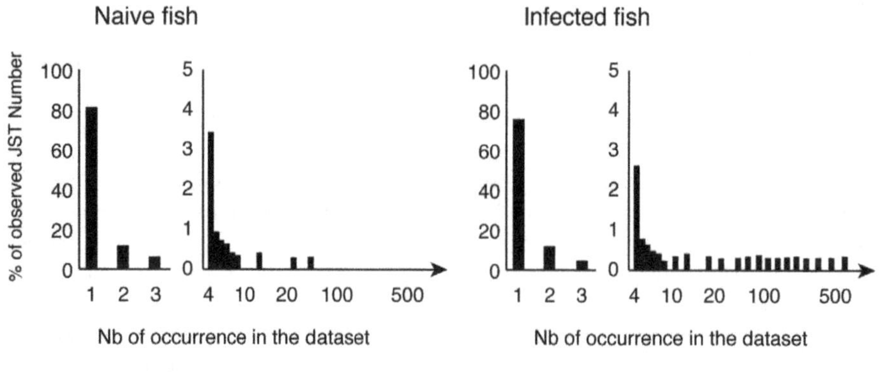

FIGURE 4 | Typical normalized distributions of JST in the pyrosequencing datasets. JST observed n times from control and virus infected fish for a given VH/C combination are represented as percentages of the total number of JST. Large clonal expansions are indicated by high number of occurrences of expressed JST in infected animals.

of similar junctions found in several fish, and differing from the most frequent one by only one (or a few) conservative substitution(s) is typical of "public" responses in mammals (Bousso et al., 1998; Lin and Welsh, 1998). Importantly, this observation suggests that rainbow trout possess a common pool of pre-existing spleen VH5.1^{+} B cells among which the public IgM response to VHSV is recruited.

This pyrosequencing study also revealed the great importance and diversity of private clonal expansions in infected fish. It is at present unclear whether these expansions represent only VHSV-specific responses or include bystander-activated cells. It will be important to clarify this point, and whether bystander effects could be beneficial or detrimental to the host. In this regard, it is intriguing that fish injected with oil-adjuvanted vaccines developed an autoimmune syndrome with autoantibodies and liver lesions (Koppang et al., 2008).

PERSPECTIVES

The aim of this review was to provide a concise description of our current knowledge of fish Ig repertoire. It is clear that a lot of important unknowns remain in fish B cell biology. As perspectives, we have listed five topics below, which might provide interesting areas for future investigation.

B CELL RECEPTOR ALLELIC EXCLUSION IN FISH

Many aspects of Ig gene rearrangement and B cell biology remain mysterious in fish. In particular, the absence of the pseudo light chains VpreB and λ5, which are required for the formation of pre-BCR in mammals, suggests that allelic exclusion is achieved by different mechanisms in fish and mammals. In fact, the regulation of VDJ recombination to ensure allelic and isotypic exclusion in fish is far from being understood. This question evokes the situation in sharks where the IgH locus organization consists of many (up to 200) independently rearranging miniloci: in these species, the rearrangement takes place within a minilocus, and only one or few H chain genes are fully rearranged in each B cell, whereas the other loci retain their germline configuration (Malecek et al., 2008). The mechanisms by which sharks and bony fishes regulate the progression of VDJ rearrangements might reveal pathways of general interest.

MATURATION OF B CELL RESPONSE WITHOUT GC

The process of hypermutation of Ig genes observed in fish in absence of typical GC is reminiscent of the affinity maturation that can occur in mammals in extra follicular foci in the spleen red pulp (Matsumoto et al., 1996). Its potential role in the diversification of the fish Ig repertoire also bears some similarities with the fact that at least a part of human marginal zone B cell pool expresses a BCR repertoire diversified through somatic hypermutation independently of GC, even though antigen stimulation via BCR does not seem to be involved in the latter case (Weill et al., 2009). Collectively, these examples highlight the diverse utilizations made during evolution of this remarkable process of somatic hypermutation of Ig genes, for the diversification of antibody repertoires. In fish, the existence of long-term protection and antigen-specific B cell memory raises the question of differentiation of memory B cells in absence of classical GC. In fact, memory B cells expressing high affinity, hypermutated IgG1 were found in lymphotoxin-alpha deficient mice, which lack GC (Matsumoto et al., 1996). The alternative site of memory B cells differentiation has not been identified. The modalities of memory B cell formation outside GC represent both a practical issue for vaccination and a fundamental question in B cell biology.

DIVERSITY OF B CELL REPERTOIRES

The comprehensive description of fish B cell repertoires and in-depth statistical analyses have opened the way to comparative studies of the population dynamics of B cells in different fish species. The seminal work of Quake's group suggests that zebrafish antibody repertoires may harbor a higher level of stereotypy than expected. It will be interesting to understand if the total number of B cells present at a given time has a strong influence on such patterns: a zebrafish may contain a few millions of B cells, while a trout has around 100–1000 times more, and a large tuna probably 1000–10,000 times more. It appears likely that the constraints exerted on B cell diversity to express at once a complete repertoire able to cope properly with the diversity of relevant pathogens will be different in these species. Also, some fish species like Atlantic cod show very poor antibody responses (Espelid et al., 1991; Pilström and Petersson, 1991; Schrøder et al., 1992; Magnadottir et al., 2001), when having high level of serum antibodies and a repertoire strongly skewed toward the VHIII family (Stenvik et al., 2001), possibly reflecting a particular importance of natural antibodies. These particularities must be put in the context of the absence of CD4, LI, and MHC class II molecules (hence, lack of the equivalent of a CD4^{+} T cell help activity) recently revealed by the analysis of the complete sequence of the cod genome (Star et al., 2011). As a group, teleost fish represent a rich diversity of species with a wide range of size and a complex history of whole-genome duplications. Future studies on B cell repertoires from different fish species will provide insightful information about the general rules of adaptation of this system, in fish and more generally in vertebrates.

METHODOLOGIES FOR B CELL REPERTOIRE ANALYSIS

CDR3 length spectratyping, also called Immunoscope, has been the standard technique for large-scale analysis of antigen receptors repertoire diversity for about 15 years (Pannetier et al., 1993, 1995). Systematic sequencing of "all" Ig transcripts expressed in a lymphocyte population of interest represents a step forward, and is made possible by the "next generation" sequencing technologies. A benefit of these approaches is clearly that several angles of analysis can be taken to focus on different aspects of the repertoire such as clonotypes frequency, Ig V-C or V-J CDR3 diversity, CDR3 sequence analysis, V allele identification, etc. The ability to process the complexity of the information provided in such amounts of data remains limited, and specific software developments for automatic annotation of Ig sequences, and statistical modeling of repertoire diversity can still be improved. New strategies will have to be developed, possibly from existing scoring systems. The most common is the Shannon entropy, introduced by Claude Shannon in 1948 for the information theory. Then, in 1961, Alfred Rényi has generalized the utilization of an entropy index to several functions, including Species Richness, Simpson, Quadratic, and Berger–Parker indexes to quantify the diversity, uncertainty, or randomness of a system, respectively. Among these,

Simpson's diversity and Shannon's entropy indices have already been applied to analyze TCR sequence data. A comparative review of such scoring strategies was published by Miqueu et al. (2007). Deep sequencing repertoire analysis calls for advanced statistical analysis and graphical representations, such as multivariate analysis (e.g., hierarchical clustering, principal component analysis, multidimensional scaling, etc.) and probabilistic or network modeling of sequence distributions (Mora et al., 2010; Ben-Hamo and Efroni, 2011; Murugan et al., 2012). In this perspective, different parameters can be computed to quantify the differences between repertoires at distinct levels. An important feature is the total diversity of the repertoire, which can be estimated from a dataset following approaches (Fisher et al., 1943; Efron and Thisted, 1976). At another level, a deep sequencing dataset can be summarized in various groups of sequences sharing common features (e.g., V or J gene segment, CDR3 length, sample origin, frequency), which allows comparisons between different conditions. For example, a perturbation score can be computed from the Hamming distance (Gorochov et al., 1998) to compare antibody repertoires between infected fish and a reference from control animals.

EFFECT OF TEMPERATURE ON FISH B CELL RESPONSES

While fish have colonized aquatic environments across a wide temperature range, only a few species control their internal temperature. The adaptation of fish immune system to various temperature is not fully understood, but the magnitude of the primary response to T dependent antigens is suppressed at lower temperatures for example in the channel catfish (Bly and Clem, 1991) and carp (Le Morvan et al., 1996). More recently, it was also observed that the highest magnitude of rainbow trout specific IgM – but not IgT – response against *Yersinia ruckeri* was obtained at high temperature (25°C; Raida and Buchmann, 2007). Differential sensitivity of lymphocyte responses to temperature variations may affect immune repertoires – perhaps especially regarding natural antibodies and mucosal locations – since different pathogens may be adapted to distinct temperature ranges.

With a large number of species and a wide diversity of anatomy, physiological, and ecological adaptations to the aquatic environments and their pathogens, fish offer interesting perspectives for comparative analysis of B cell repertoire biology. New sequencing technologies have already made it possible.

ACKNOWLEDGMENTS

This work was supported by Institut National de la Recherche Agronomique and the European Community's Seventh Framework Program (FP7/2007-2013) under Grant Agreement 222719 LIFECYCLE and by the European Commission under the Work Programme 2012 of the seventh Framework Programme for Research and Technological Development of the European Union (Grant Agreement 311993 TARGETFISH). We acknowledge Dr. Oystein Evensen for helpful discussions and Dr. Vicky Lampropoulou for critical reading of the manuscript.

REFERENCES

Abelli, L., Picchietti, S., Romano, N., Mastrolia, L., and Scapigliati, G. (1997). Immunohistochemistry of gut-associated lymphoid tissue of the sea bass Dicentrarchus labrax (L.). *Fish Shellfish Immunol.* 7, 235.

Ademokun, A., Wu, Y., Martin, V., Mitra, R., Sack, U., Baxendale, H., et al. (2011). Vaccination-induced changes in human B-cell repertoire and pneumococcal IgM and IgA antibody at different ages. *Aging Cell* 10, 922–930.

Aparicio, S., Chapman, J., Stupka, E., Putnam, N., Chia, J.-M., Dehal, P., et al. (2002). Whole-genome shotgun assembly and analysis of the genome of Fugu rubripes. *Science* 297, 1301–1310.

Bao, Y., Wang, T., Guo, Y., Zhao, Z., Li, N., and Zhao, Y. (2010). The immunoglobulin gene loci in the teleost Gasterosteus aculeatus. *Fish Shellfish Immunol.* 28, 40–48.

Barreto, V. M., Pan-Hammarstrom, Q., Zhao, Y., Hammarstrom, L., Misulovin, Z., and Nussenzweig, M. C. (2005). AID from bony fish catalyses call switch recombination. *J. Exp. Med.* 202, 733.

Bartl, S., Miracle, A. L., Rumfelt, L. L., Kepler, T. B., Mochon, E., Litman, G. W., et al. (2003). Terminal deoxynucleotidyl transferases from elasmobranchs reveal structural conservation within vertebrates. *Immunogenetics* 55, 594–604.

Beetz, S., Diekhoff, D., and Steiner, L. A. (2007). Characterization of terminal deoxynucleotidyl transferase and polymerase mu in zebrafish. *Immunogenetics* 59, 735–744.

Bengtén, E., Leanderson, T., and Pilström, L. (1991). Immunoglobulin heavy chain cDNA from the teleost Atlantic cod (Gadus morhua L.): nucleotide sequences of secretory and membrane form show an unusual splicing pattern. *Eur. J. Immunol.* 21, 3027–3033.

Bengtén, E., Quiniou, S., Hikima, J., and Waldbieser, G. (2006). Structure of the catfish IGH locus: analysis of the region including the single functional IGHM gene. *Immunogenetics* 58, 831–844.

Ben-Hamo, R., and Efroni, S. (2011). The whole-organism heavy chain B cell repertoire from Zebrafish self-organizes into distinct network features. *BMC Syst. Biol.* 5:27. doi:10.1186/1752-0509-5-27

Bladen, C. L., Navarre, S., Dynan, W. S., and Kozlowski, D. J. (2007). Expression of the Ku70 subunit (XRCC6) and protection from low dose ionizing radiation during zebrafish embryogenesis. *Neurosci. Lett.* 422, 97–102.

Bly, J. E., and Clem, L. W. (1991). Temperature-mediated processes in teleost immunity: in vitro immunosuppression induced by in vivo low temperature in channel catfish. *Vet. Immunol. Immunopathol.* 28, 365–377.

Bousso, P., Casrouge, A., Altman, J., Haury, M., Kanellopoulos, J., Abastado, J.-P., et al. (1998). Individual variations in the murine T cell response to a specific peptide reflect variability in naive repertoires. *Immunity* 9, 169–178.

Bromage, E. S., Kaattari, I. M., Zwollo, P., and Kaattari, S. L. (2004). Plasmablast and plasma cell production and distribution in trout immune tissues. *J. Immunol.* 173, 7317–7323.

Castro, R., Jouneau, L., Pham, H.-P., Bouchez, O., Giudicelli, V., Lefranc, M.-P., et al. (2013). Teleost fish mount complex clonal IgM and IgT responses in spleen upon systemic viral infection. *PLoS Pathog.* 9:e1003098. doi: 10.1371/journal.ppat.1003098

Collette, A., and Six, A. (2002). ISEApeaks: an Excel platform for GeneScan and Immunoscope data retrieval, management and analysis. *Bioinformatics* 18, 329–330.

Coscia, M. R., and Oreste, U. (2003). Limited diversity of the immunoglobulin heavy chain variable domain of the emerald rockcod Trematomus bernacchii. *Fish Shellfish Immunol.* 14, 71–92.

Coscia, M. R., Varriale, S., De Santi, C., Giacomelli, S., and Oreste, U. (2010). Evolution of the Antarctic teleost immunoglobulin heavy chain gene. *Mol. Phylogenet. Evol.* 55, 226–233.

Criscitiello, M. F., and Flajnik, M. F. (2007). Four primordial immunoglobulin light chain isotypes, including lambda and kappa, identified in the most primitive living jawed vertebrates. *Eur. J. Immunol.* 37, 2683–2694.

Daggfeldt, A., Bengtén, E., and Pilström, L. (1993). A cluster type organization of the loci of the immunoglobulin light chain in Atlantic cod (Gadus morhua L.) and rainbow trout (Oncorhynchus mykiss Walbaum) indicated by nucleotide sequences of cDNAs and hybridization analysis. *Immunogenetics* 38, 199–209.

Danilova, N., Bussmann, J., Jekosch, K., and Steiner, L. A. (2005). The immunoglobulin heavy-chain locus in zebrafish: identification and expression of a previously unknown isotype, immunoglobulin Z. *Nat. Immunol.* 6, 295–302.

Danilova, N., and Steiner, L. A. (2002). B cells develop in the zebrafish pancreas. *Proc. Natl. Acad. Sci. U.S.A.* 99, 13711–13716.

Edholm, E.-S., Bengtén, E., Stafford, J. L., Sahoo, M., Taylor, E. B., Miller, N. W., et al. (2010). Identification of two IgD+ B cell populations in channel catfish, Ictalurus punctatus. *J. Immunol.* 185, 4082–4094.

Edholm, E.-S., Wilson, M., Sahoo, M., Miller, N. W., Pilström, L., Wermenstam, N. E., et al. (2009). Identification of Igsigma and Iglambda in channel catfish, Ictalurus punctatus, and Iglambda in Atlantic cod, Gadus morhua. *Immunogenetics* 61, 353–370.

Efron, B., and Thisted, R. (1976). Estimating the number of unseen species: how many words did Shakespeare know? *Biometrika* 63, 435–447.

Espelid, S., Rødseth, O., and Jørgensen, T. (1991). Vaccination experiments and studies of the humoral immune responses in cod, Gadus morhua L., to four strains of monoclonal defined Vibrio anguillarum. *J. Fish Dis.* 14, 185–198.

Fisher, R. A., Steven-Corbet, A., and Williams, C. B. (1943). The relation between the number of species and the number of individuals in a random sample of an animal population. *J. Anim. Ecol.* 12, 42–58.

Flajnik, M. F., and Kasahara, M. (2009). Origin and evolution of the adaptive immune system: genetic events and selective pressures. *Nat. Rev. Genet.* 11, 47–59.

Gambón-Deza, F., Sánchez-Espinel, C., and Magadán-Mompó, S. (2010). Presence of an unique IgT on the IGH locus in three-spined stickleback fish (Gasterosteus aculeatus) and the very recent generation of a repertoire of VH genes. *Dev. Comp. Immunol.* 34, 114–122.

Ghaffari, S. H., and Lobb, C. J. (1993). Structure and genomic organization of immunoglobulin light chain in the channel catfish. An unusual genomic organizational pattern of segmental genes. *J. Immunol.* 151, 6900–6912.

Ghaffari, S. H., and Lobb, C. J. (1997). Structure and genomic organization of a second class of immunoglobulin light chain genes in the channel catfish. *J. Immunol.* 159, 250–258.

Gorochov, G., Neumann, A. U., Kereveur, A., Parizot, C., Li, T., Katlama, C., et al. (1998). Perturbation of CD4+ and CD8+ T-cell repertoires during progression to AIDS and regulation of the CD4+ repertoire during antiviral therapy. *Nat. Med.* 4, 215–221.

Greenhalgh, P., and Steiner, L. A. (1995). Recombination activating gene 1 (Rag1) in zebrafish and shark. *Immunogenetics* 41, 54–55.

Guo, Y., Bao, Y., Wang, H., Hu, X., Zhao, Z., Li, N., et al. (2011). A Preliminary analysis of the immunoglobulin genes in the African elephant (Loxodonta africana). *PLoS ONE* 6:e16889. doi:10.1371/journal.pone.0016889

Hansen, J., Landis, E., and Phillips, R. (2005). Discovery of a unique Ig heavy-chain isotype (IgT) in rainbow trout: implications for a distinctive B cell developmental pathway in teleost fish. *Proc. Natl. Acad. Sci. U.S.A.* 102, 6919–6924.

Hansen, J. D. (1997). Characterization of rainbow trout terminal deoxynucleotidyl transferase structure and expression. TdT and RAG1 co-expression define the trout primary lymphoid tissues. *Immunogenetics* 46, 367–375.

Hansen, J. D., and Kaattari, S. L. (1995). The recombination activation gene 1 (RAG1) of rainbow trout (Oncorhynchus mykiss): cloning, expression, and phylogenetic analysis. *Immunogenetics* 42, 188–195.

Hansen, J. D., and Kaattari, S. L. (1996). The recombination activating gene 2 (RAG2) of the rainbow trout Oncorhynchus mykiss. *Immunogenetics* 44, 203–211.

Hayman, J. R., and Lobb, C. J. (2000). Heavy chain diversity region segments of the channel catfish: structure, organization, expression and phylogenetic implications. *J. Immunol.* 164, 1916–1924.

Henkel, C. V., Dirks, R. P., Jansen, H. J., Forlenza, M., Wiegertjes, G. F., Howe, K., et al. (2012). Comparison of the exomes of common carp (Cyprinus carpio) and zebrafish (Danio rerio). *Zebrafish* 9, 59–67.

Hirono, I., Nam, B.-H., Enomoto, J., Uchino, K., and Aoki, T. (2003). Cloning and characterisation of a cDNA encoding Japanese flounder Paralichthys olivaceus IgD. *Fish Shellfish Immunol.* 15, 63–70.

Hordvik, I. (2002). Identification of a novel immunoglobulin delta transcript and comparative analysis of the genes encoding IgD in Atlantic salmon and Atlantic halibut. *Mol. Immunol.* 39, 85–91.

Hordvik, I., Thevarajan, J., Samdal, I., Bastani, N., and Krossøy, B. (1999). Molecular cloning and phylogenetic analysis of the Atlantic salmon immunoglobulin D gene. *Scand. J. Immunol.* 50, 202–210.

Hu, Y.-L., Zhu, L.-Y., Xiang, L.-X., and Shao, J.-Z. (2011). Discovery of an unusual alternative splicing pathway of the immunoglobulin heavy chain in a teleost fish, Danio rerio. *Dev. Comp. Immunol.* 35, 253–257.

Huang, T., Zhang, M., Wei, Z., Wang, P., Sun, Y., Hu, X., et al. (2012). Analysis of immunoglobulin transcripts in the ostrich Struthio camelus, a primitive avian species. *PLoS ONE* 7:e34346. doi:10.1371/journal.pone.0034346

Jerne, N. K. (1972). "What precedes clonal selection? Ontogeny of acquired immunity," in *Proceedings of the A CIBA Foundation Symposium 1971*, Amsterdam, 1–15.

Jiang, N., Weinstein, J. A., Penland, L., White, R. A., and Fisher, D. S. (2011). Determinism and stochasticity during maturation of the zebrafish antibody repertoire. *Proc. Natl. Acad. Sci. U.S.A.* 108, 5348–5353.

Jones, F. C., Grabherr, M. G., Chan, Y. F., Russell, P., Mauceli, E., Johnson, J., et al. (2012). The genomic basis of adaptive evolution in threespine sticklebacks. *Nature* 484, 55–61.

Kasahara, M., Naruse, K., Sasaki, S., Nakatani, Y., Qu, W., Ahsan, B., et al. (2007). The medaka draft genome and insights into vertebrate genome evolution. *Nature* 447, 714–719.

Kato, L., Begum, N. A., Maxwell Burroughs, A., Doi, T., Kawaib, J., Daubb, C. O., et al. (2011). Nonimmunoglobulin target loci of activation-induced cytidine deaminase (AID) share unique features with immunoglobulin genes. *Proc. Natl. Acad. Sci. U.S.A.* 109, 2479.

Kitamura, D., Kudo, A., Schaal, S., Müller, W., Melchers, F., and Rajewsky, K. (1992). A critical role of lambda 5 protein in B cell development. *Cell* 69, 823–831.

Koppang, E. O., Bjerkås, I., Haugarvoll, E., Chan, E. K. L., Szabo, N. J., Ono, N., et al. (2008). Vaccination-induced systemic autoimmunity in farmed Atlantic salmon. *J. Immunol.* 181, 4807–4814.

Lam, S. H., Chua, H. L., Gong, Z., Lam, T. J., and Sin, Y. M. (2004). Development and maturation of the immune system in zebrafish, Danio rerio: a gene expression profiling, in situ hybridization and immunological study. *Dev. Comp. Immunol.* 28, 9–28.

Le Morvan, C., Deschaux, P., and Troutaud, D. (1996). Effects and mechanisms of environmental temperature on carp (Cyprinus carpio) anti-DNP antibody response and non-specific cytotoxic cell activity: a kinetic study. *Dev. Comp. Immunol.* 20, 331–340.

Lee, M. A., Bengtén, E., Daggfeldt, A., Rytting, A. S., and Pilström, L. (1993). Characterisation of rainbow trout cDNAs encoding a secreted and membrane-bound Ig heavy chain and the genomic intron upstream of the first constant exon. *Mol. Immunol.* 30, 641–648.

Lee, S. S., Tranchina, D., Ohta, 3Y., Flajnik, M. F., and Hsu, E. (2002). Hypermutation in shark immunoglobulin light chain genes results in contiguous substitutions. *Immunity* 16, 571.

Lin, M. Y., and Welsh, R. M. (1998). Stability and diversity of T cell receptor repertoire usage during lymphocytic choriomeningitis virus infection of mice. *J. Exp. Med.* 188, 1993–2005.

Lundqvist, M., Strömberg, S., Bouchenot, C., Pilström, L., and Boudinot, P. (2009). Diverse splicing pathways of the membrane IgHM pre-mRNA in a Chondrostean, the Siberian sturgeon. *Dev. Comp. Immunol.* 33, 507–515.

Lundqvist, M. L., Middleton, D. L., Hazard, S., and Warr, G. W. (2001). The immunoglobulin heavy chain locus of the duck. Genomic organization and expression of D, J, and C region genes. *J. Biol. Chem.* 276, 46729–46736.

Magadán-Mompó, S., Sánchez-Espinel, C., and Gambón-Deza, F. (2011). Immunoglobulin heavy chains in medaka (Oryzias latipes). *BMC Evol. Biol.* 11:165. doi:10.1186/1471-2148-11-165

Magnadottir, B., Jonsdottir, H., Helgason, S., Bjoörnson, B., Solem, S., and Pilström, L. (2001). Immune parameters of immunised cod. *Fish Shellfish Immunol.* 10, 75–89.

Malecek, K., Lee, V., Feng, W., Huang, J. L., Flajnik, M. F., Ohta, Y., et al. (2008). Immunoglobulin heavy chain exclusion in the shark. *PLoS Biol.* 6:e157. doi:10.1371/journal.pbio.0060157

Marianes, A. E., and Zimmerman, A. M. (2011). Targets of somatic hypermutation within immunoglobulin light chain genes in zebrafish. *Immunology* 132, 240–255.

Matsumoto, M., Lo, S. F., Carruthers, C. J., Min, J., Mariathasan, S., Huang, G., et al. (1996). Affinity maturation without germinal centres in lymphotoxin-alpha-deficient mice. *Nature* 382, 462–466.

Miqueu, P., Guillet, M., Degauque, N., and Dor, J. (2007). Statistical analysis of CDR3 length distributions for the assessment of T and B cell repertoire biases. *Mol. Immunol.* 44, 1057–1064.

Mora, T., Walczak, A. M., Bialek, W., and Callan, C. G. (2010). Maximum entropy models for antibody diversity. *Proc. Natl. Acad. Sci. U.S.A.* 107, 5405–5410.

Murugan, A., Mora, T., Walczak, A. M., and Callan, C. G. (2012). Statistical inference of the generation probability of T-cell receptors from sequence repertoires. *Proc. Natl. Acad. Sci. U.S.A.* 109, 16161–16166.

Ohta, Y., and Flajnik, M. (2006). IgD, like IgM, is a primordial immunoglobulin class perpetuated in most jawed vertebrates. *Proc. Natl. Acad. Sci. U.S.A.* 103, 10723–10728.

Pannetier, C., Cochet, M., Darche, S., Casrouge, A., Zöller, M., and Kourilsky, P. (1993). The sizes of the CDR3 hypervariable regions of the murine T-cell receptor beta chains vary as a function of the recombined germline segments. *Proc. Natl. Acad. Sci. U.S.A.* 90, 4319–4323.

Pannetier, C., Even, J., and Kourilsky, P. (1995). T-cell repertoire diversity and clonal expansions in normal and clinical samples. *Immunol. Today* 16, 176–181.

Partula, S., Schwager, J., Timmusk, S., Pilström, L., and Charlemagne, J. (1996). A second immunoglobulin light chain isotype in the rainbow trout. *Immunogenetics* 45, 44–51.

Pilström, L., and Petersson, A. (1991). Isolation and partial characterization of immunoglobulin from cod (Gadus morhua L.). *Dev. Comp. Immunol.* 15, 143–152.

Raida, M. K., and Buchmann, K. (2007). Temperature-dependent expression of immune-relevant genes in rainbow trout following Yersinia ruckeri vaccination. *Dis. Aquat. Org.* 77, 41–52.

Ramirez-Gomez, F., Greene, W., Rego, K., Hansen, J. D., Costa, G., Kataria, P., et al. (2012). Discovery and characterization of secretory IgD in rainbow trout: secretory IgD is produced through a novel splicing mechanism. *J. Immunol.* 188, 1341–1349.

Razquin, B., Castillo, A., Lopez-Fierro, P., Alvarez, F., Zapata, A., and Villena, A. (1990). Ontogeny of IgM-producing cells in the lymphoid organs of rainbow trout, Salmo gairdneri Richardson: an immunological and enzyme-histochemical study. *J. Fish Biol.* 36, 159.

Rombout, J. H., Taverne-Thiele, A. J., and Villena, M. I. (1993). The gut-associated lymphoid tissue (GALT) of carp (Cyprinus carpio L.): an immunocytochemical analysis. *Dev. Comp. Immunol.* 17, 55–66.

Ryo, S., Wijdeven, R. H. M., Tyagi, A., Hermsen, T., Kono, T., Karunasagar, I., et al. (2010). Common carp have two subclasses of bonyfish specific antibody IgZ showing differential expression in response to infection. *Dev. Comp. Immunol.* 34, 1183–1190.

Saha, N. R., Suetake, H., Kikuchi, K., and Suzuki, Y. (2004). Fugu immunoglobulin D: a highly unusual gene with unprecedented duplications in its constant region. *Immunogenetics* 56, 438–447.

Salinas, I., Zhang, Y.-A., and Sunyer, J. O. (2011). Mucosal immunoglobulins and B cells of teleost fish. *Dev. Comp. Immunol.* 35, 1346–1365.

Saunders, H. L., Oko, A. L., Scott, A. N., Fan, C. W., and Magor, B. G. (2010). The cellular context of AID expressing cells in fish lymphoid tissues. *Dev. Comp. Immunol.* 34, 669.

Savan, R., Aman, A., Nakao, M., Watanuki, H., and Sakai, M. (2005). Discovery of a novel immunoglobulin heavy chain gene chimera from common carp (Cyprinus carpio L.). *Immunogenetics* 57, 458–463.

Schorpp, M., Bialecki, M., Diekhoff, D., Walderich, B., Odenthal, J., Maischein, H.-M., et al. (2006). Conserved functions of Ikaros in vertebrate lymphocyte development: genetic evidence for distinct larval and adult phases of T cell development and two lineages of B cells in zebrafish. *J. Immunol.* 177, 2463–2476.

Schrøder, M., Espelid, S., and Jørgensen, T. (1992). Two serotypes of Vibrio salmonicida isolated from diseased cod (Gadus morhua L.); virulence immunological studies and vaccination experiments. *Fish Shellfish Immunol.* 2, 211–221.

Smelty, P., Marchal, C., Renard, R., Sinzelle, L., Pollet, N., Dunon, D., et al. (2010). Identification of the pre-T-cell receptor alpha chain in non-mammalian vertebrates challenges the structure-function of the molecule. *Proc. Natl. Acad. Sci. U.S.A.* 107, 19991–19996.

Srisapoome, P., Ohira, T., Hirono, I., and Aoki, T. (2004). Genes of the constant regions of functional immunoglobulin heavy chain of Japanese flounder, Paralichthys olivaceus. *Immunogenetics* 56, 292–300.

Star, B., Nederbragt, A. J., Jentoft, S., Grimholt, U., Malmstrøm, M., Gregers, T. F., et al. (2011). The genome sequence of Atlantic cod reveals a unique immune system. *Nature* 477, 207–210.

Stenvik, J., and Jørgensen, T. Ø. (2000). Immunoglobulin D (IgD) of Atlantic cod has a unique structure. 51, 452–461.

Stenvik, J., Schrøder, M., Olsen, K., Zapata, A., and Jørgensen, T. (2001). Expression of immunoglobulin heavy chain transcripts (VH-families, IgM, and IgD) in head kidney and spleen of the Atlantic cod (Gadus morhua L.). *Dev. Comp. Immunol.* 25, 291–302.

Timmusk, S., Partula, S., and Pilström, L. (2000). Different genomic organization and expression of immunoglobulin light-chain isotypes in the rainbow trout. *Immunogenetics* 51, 905–914.

Trede, N. S., Langenau, D. M., Traver, D., Look, A. T., and Zon, L. I. (2004). The use of zebrafish to understand immunity. *Immunity* 20, 367–379.

van Ginkel, F. W., Miller, N. W., Cuchens, M. A., and Clem, L. W. (1994). Activation of channel catfish B cells by membrane immunoglobulin cross-linking. *Dev. Comp. Immunol.* 18, 97–107.

Vela, J. L., Aït-Azzouzene, D., Duong, B. H., Ota, T., and Nemazee, D. (2008). Rearrangement of mouse immunoglobulin kappa deleting element recombining sequence promotes immune tolerance and lambda B cell production. *Immunity* 28, 161–170.

Wang, X., Olp, J. J., and Miller, R. D. (2009). On the genomics of immunoglobulins in the gray, short-tailed opossum Monodelphis domestica. *Immunogenetics* 61, 581–596.

Weill, J.-C., Weller, S., and Reynaud, C.-A. (2009). Human marginal zone B cells. *Annu. Rev. Immunol.* 27, 267–285.

Weinstein, J. a, Jiang, N., White, R. a, Fisher, D. S., and Quake, S. R. (2009). High-throughput sequencing of the zebrafish antibody repertoire. *Science* 324, 807–810.

Wienholds, E., Schulte-Merker, S., Walderich, B., and Plasterk, R. H. A. (2002). Target-selected inactivation of the zebrafish ragl gene. *Science* 297, 99–102.

Willett, C. E., Cherry, J. J., and Steiner, L. A. (1997). Characterization and expression of the recombination activating genes (ragl and rag2) of zebrafish. *Immunogenetics* 45, 394–404.

Wilson, M., Bengtén, E., Miller, N. W., Clem, L. W., Du Pasquier, L., and Warr, G. W. (1997). A novel chimeric Ig heavy chain from a teleost fish shares similarities to IgD. *Proc. Natl. Acad. Sci. U.S.A.* 94, 4593–4597.

Wilson, M., Hsu, E., Marcuz, A., Courtet, M., Du Pasquier, L., and Steinberg, C. (1992). What limits affinity maturation of antibodies in Xenopus-the rate of somatic mutation or the ability to select mutants? *EMBO J.* 11, 4337–4347.

Wilson, M. R., van Ravenstein, E., Miller, N. W., Clem, L. W., Middleton, D. L., and Warr, G. W. (1995a). cDNA sequences and organization of IgM heavy chain genes in two holostean fish. *Dev. Comp. Immunol.* 19, 153–164.

Wilson, M., Ross, D., Miller, N., Clem, L., Middleton, D., and Warr, G. (1995b). Alternate pre-mRNA processing pathways in the production of membrane IgM heavy chains in holostean fish. *Dev. Comp. Immunol.* 19, 165–177.

Xiao, F. S., Wang, Y. P., Yan, W., Chang, M. X., Yao, W. J., Xu, Q. Q., et al. (2010). Ig heavy chain genes and their locus in grass carp Ctenopharyngodon idella. *Fish Shellfish Immunol.* 29, 594–599.

Yang, F., Waldbieser, G. C., and Lobb, C. J. (2006). The nucleotide targets of somatic mutation and the role of selection in immunoglobulin heavy chains of a teleost fish. *J. Immunol.* 176, 1655.

Yasuike, M., Boer, J. D., Schalburg, K. R. V., Cooper, G. A., McKinnel, L., Messmer, A., et al. (2010). Evolution of duplicated IgH loci in Atlantic salmon, Salmo salar. *BMC Genomics* 11:486. doi:10.1186/1471-2164-11-486

Ye, J., Kaattari, I. M., and Kaattari, S. L. (2011). The differential dynamics of antibody subpopulation expression during affinity maturation in a teleost. *Fish Shellfish Immunol.* 30, 372–377.

Zapata, A., Diez, B., Cejalvo, T., Gutiérrez-de Frías, C., and Cortés, A. (2006). Ontogeny of the immune system of fish. *Fish Shellfish Immunol.* 20, 126–136.

Zhang, Y., Salinas, I., Li, J., Parra, D., Bjork, S., Xu, Z., et al. (2010). IgT, a primitive immunoglobulin class specialized in mucosal immunity. *Nat. Immunol.* 11, 827–835.

Zhao, Y., Kacskovics, I., Pan, Q., Liberles, D. A., Geli, J., Davis, S. K., et al. (2002). Artiodactyl IgD: the missing link. *J. Immunol.* 169, 4408–4416.

Zhao, Y., Pan-Hammarström, Q., Kacskovics, I., and Hammarström, L. (2003). The porcine Ig delta gene: unique chimeric splicing of the first constant region domain in its heavy chain transcripts. *J. Immunol.* 171, 1312–1318.

Zhao, Y., Rabbani, H., Shimizu, A., and Hammarström, L. (2000). Mapping of the chicken immunoglobulin heavy-chain constant region gene locus reveals an inverted alpha gene upstream of a condensed upsilon gene. *Immunology* 101, 348–353.

Zimmerman, A. M., Romanowski, K. E., and Maddox, B. J. (2011). Targeted annotation of immunoglobulin light chain (IgL) genes in zebrafish from BAC clones reveals kappa-like recombining/deleting elements within IgL constant regions. *Fish Shellfish Immunol.* 31, 697–703.

Zimmerman, A. M., Yeo, G., Howe, K., Maddox, B. J., and Steiner, L. A. (2008). Immunoglobulin light chain (IgL) genes in zebrafish: genomic configurations and inversional rearrangements between (V(L)-J(L)-C(L)) gene clusters. *Dev. Comp. Immunol.* 32, 421–434.

Zwollo, P. (2011). Dissecting teleost B cell differentiation using transcription factors. *Dev. Comp. Immunol.* 35, 898–905.

Zwollo, P., Cole, S., Bromage, E., and Kaattari, S. (2005). B cell heterogeneity in the teleost kidney: evidence for a maturation gradient from anterior to posterior kidney. *Immunol.* 174, 6608–6616.

9

The structural basis of antibody-antigen recognition

Inbal Sela-Culang[†], Vered Kunik[†] and Yanay Ofran[*]

The Goodman Faculty of Life Sciences, Bar Ilan University, Ramat Gan, Israel

Edited by:
Michal Or-Guil, Humboldt University Berlin, Germany

Reviewed by:
Gur Yaari, Yale University, USA
Chaim Putterman, Albert Einstein College of Medicine, USA

***Correspondence:**
Yanay Ofran, The Goodman Faculty of Life Sciences, Bar Ilan University, Ramat-Gan 52900, Israel
e-mail: yanay@ofranlab.org

[†]Inbal Sela-Culang and Vered Kunik have contributed equally to this work.

The function of antibodies (Abs) involves specific binding to antigens (Ags) and activation of other components of the immune system to fight pathogens. The six hypervariable loops within the variable domains of Abs, commonly termed complementarity determining regions (CDRs), are widely assumed to be responsible for Ag recognition, while the constant domains are believed to mediate effector activation. Recent studies and analyses of the growing number of available Ab structures, indicate that this clear functional separation between the two regions may be an oversimplification. Some positions within the CDRs have been shown to never participate in Ag binding and some off-CDRs residues often contribute critically to the interaction with the Ag. Moreover, there is now growing evidence for non-local and even allosteric effects in Ab-Ag interaction in which Ag binding affects the constant region and vice versa. This review summarizes and discusses the structural basis of Ag recognition, elaborating on the contribution of different structural determinants of the Ab to Ag binding and recognition. We discuss the CDRs, the different approaches for their identification and their relationship to the Ag interface. We also review what is currently known about the contribution of non-CDRs regions to Ag recognition, namely the framework regions (FRs) and the constant domains. The suggested mechanisms by which these regions contribute to Ag binding are discussed. On the Ag side of the interaction, we discuss attempts to predict B-cell epitopes and the suggested idea to incorporate Ab information into B-cell epitope prediction schemes. Beyond improving the understanding of immunity, characterization of the functional role of different parts of the Ab molecule may help in Ab engineering, design of CDR-derived peptides, and epitope prediction.

Keywords: antibody, CDRs, antigen, paratope, epitope, framework, constant domain

INTRODUCTION

Antibodies (Abs) have two distinct functions: one is to bind specifically to their target antigens (Ags); the other is to elicit an immune response against the bound Ag by recruiting other cells and molecules. The association between an Ab and an Ag involves myriad of non-covalent interactions between the epitope – the binding site on the Ag, and the paratopes – the binding site on the Ab. The ability of Abs to bind virtually any non-self surface with exquisite specificity and high affinity is not only the key to immunity but has also made Abs an enormously valuable tool in experimental biology, biomedical research, diagnostics and therapy. The diversity of their binding capabilities is particularly striking given the high structural similarity between all Abs. The availability of increasing amounts of structural data in recent years now allows for a much better understanding of the structural basis of Ab function in general, and of Ag recognition in particular. This review surveys the recent developments and the current gaps and challenges in this field. We focus specifically on the current understanding of the determinants within the Ab structure that contribute to Ag binding. We first discuss the motivations for, and applications of, the study of the structural basis of Ag recognition. Then we describe and discuss the Ab-Ag interface, with specific focus on the paratopes and the complementarity determining regions (CDRs), and their role in Ag binding. The last part focuses on the contribution of the non-CDRs parts of the Ab [i.e., framework regions (FRs) and the constant domains] to Ag binding and on the recent suggestions regarding non-local and allosteric effects in Ab function. Over the last few years numerous reviews have addressed issues that are related or tangential to the topics we review here. This includes reviews of the engineering of Abs (1), their stability (2), affinity maturation (3), and isotype selection (4). While these important topics are relevant to the findings and ideas we review here, they are beyond the scope of this review.

THE MOTIVATIONS FOR, AND APPLICATIONS OF, THE STUDY OF Ab-Ag RECOGNITION

UNDERSTANDING IMMUNITY AND AUTOIMMUNITY

The adaptive immune response involves two types of lymphocytes: T cells, which recognizes Ags that have been processed and their fragments are presented by MHC molecules, and B cells which produce soluble Abs that can identify also the intact Ag in its native form. While the way in which T cells recognize their epitopes has been extensively studied to a level that enables the successful prediction of T-cell epitopes (5, 6), the rules that govern Ab-Ag recognition, including which parts of the Ab structure underlie Ag recognition and how and why certain determinants on the Ag are selected as epitopes, are not as well characterized. Understanding the mechanisms that underlie Ab-Ag recognition, therefore, is crucial for understanding immunity.

The immune system enables Abs to distinguish between foreign and self molecules (7). Autoimmune diseases are characterized by the inappropriate response to self-Ags. It is not always clear what role is played by Abs and what role is played by other components of the immune system in autoimmunity. A variety of molecular mechanisms have been proposed, including sequestered Ags, molecular mimicry, and polyclonal B-cell activation (8). Better understanding of the underpinnings of Ab-Ag recognition may also shed light on these questions.

A MODEL FOR STUDYING BIO-MOLECULAR RECOGNITION

A fundamental characteristic of the immune system is its ability to continuously generate novel protein recognition sites. Ab-Ag interfaces, therefore, are often considered a model system for elucidating the principles governing biomolecular recognition (9–13). For example, Keskin (14) and McCoy et al. (15) used X-ray crystallographic structures of Ab-Ag complexes to elucidate principles of the molecular architecture of protein–protein interfaces. Other studies, however, view Ab-Ag interfaces as a specific case that may not allow for generalization to all types of protein–protein interfaces (16). Thus, large scale studies of protein–protein interactions often exclude Ab-Ag complexes from the dataset analyzed (16–19). It is, therefore, important to determine to what extent Ab-Ag complexes could serve as a general model for protein–protein interactions.

ANTIBODY ENGINEERING

The specificity of the Ab molecule to its cognate Ag has been exploited for the development of a variety of immunoassays, vaccinations, and therapeutics. Ab engineering may offer to expand the application of Abs by permitting improvements of affinity (20, 21) and specificity (22, 23). Understanding of the role each structural element in the Ab plays in Ag recognition is essential for successful engineering of better binders. The engineering of Abs is also important for the clinical use of Abs from non-human sources. Early studies on the use of rodent Abs in humans determined that they can be immunogenic (24). Humanization by grafting of the CDRs from a mouse Ab to a human FR is a commonly used engineering strategy for reducing immunogenicity (25, 26). In most cases, the successful design of high-affinity, CDR-grafted, Abs requires that key residues in the human acceptor FRs that are crucial for preserving the functional conformation of the CDRs will be back-mutated to the amino acids of the original murine Ab (26, 27). Several groups (28–30) used the experimentally determined 3-D structures of Ab-Ag complexes in the Protein Data Bank (PDB) (31) to determine which residues participate in Ag recognition and binding. Such knowledge can be exploited to identify residues that are important for the function of the Ab in general and for Ag recognition in particular and may guide Ab engineering (32, 33). Residues that help maintain the functional conformation of the CDRs, for example, can be used to improve Ab humanization efforts by CDR-grafting.

Ab EPITOPE PREDICTION

Antibody epitopes (sometimes referred to as B-cell epitopes) are the molecular structures within an Ag that make specific contacts with the Ab paratope. B-cell epitopes are used in the development of vaccines and in immunodiagnostics. Correct identification of B-cell epitopes within an antigenic protein, may open the door for the design of molecules (biologic or synthetic) that mimic potentially protective epitopes and could be used to raise specific Abs or be used as a prophylactic or therapeutic vaccines. Identification of B-cell epitopes could promote protective immunity in the context of emerging and re-emerging infectious diseases and potential bioterrorist threats. This may be achieved by choosing from among the putative epitopes those that may provide immunity (e.g., by eliciting Abs that hamper the molecular function of pathogenic Ags). The choice of such epitopes is believed to be relevant for understanding and controlling protective immunity. In the case of the vaccinia virus, for example, which was used as smallpox vaccine and is the only vaccine that has led to the complete eradication of an infectious disease from the human population, individuals possessing a high frequency of memory B-cells specific for major neutralizing Ags of the vaccinia virus are better protected from smallpox than individuals with a memory B-cell pool dominated by specificities for non-protective Ags (34). Thus, understanding the way in which an Ab recognizes its cognate epitope is of particular interest for vaccine design and disease prevention (35). Existing tools for identification of Ab epitopes (such as X-ray crystallography, pepscan, phage display, expressed fragments, partial proteolysis, mass spectrometry, and mutagenesis analysis) are not only expensive, laborious, and time consuming but also fail to identify many epitopes (36). When talking about protein Ags, most of these methods typically identify linear stretches as epitopes, while, arguably, most of the epitopes on protein Ags are conformational and even discontinuous. As for computational approaches, despite more than 30 years of efforts (37), existing B-cell epitope prediction methods are not accurate enough (38, 39) and are, therefore, not widely used. This is exemplified in **Figure 1**, in which the structure of hen egg lysozyme (HEL) Ag and three Abs that bind it are shown (**Figures 1A,B**), as well as the epitopes predicted by three different methods (**Figure 1C**).

In general, current methods are trying to identify epitopic residues based on the presence of features associated with residues that bind the Ab (40–50). One possible explanation for the failure of these methods is that the differences between epitopes and other residues are not substantial. Indeed, several analyses (51–53) have shown that the amino-acid composition of epitopes is essentially indistinguishable from that of other surface-exposed non-epitopic residues.

This lack of intrinsic properties that clearly differentiate between epitopic and non-epitopic residues and the fact (demonstrated in **Figure 1**) that most of the Ag surface may become a part of an epitope under some circumstances (54–57) suggest that epitopes depend, to a great extent, on the Abs that recognize them. This is exemplified in **Figure 1**: most of the HEL surface residues are part of an epitope of at least one Ab (**Figures 1A,B**), even though this figure shows only three Abs (out of dozens known to bind HEL). Almost all the residues predicted to be epitopic may be considered as correct predictions as they bind some Ab (**Figure 1C**) but also as false predictions as they don't bind the others. Similarly, predicting that a residue is not in an epitope may be either a true negative or a false negative, depending on the Ab considered. It has recently been suggested by us (Sela-Culang et al., submitted)

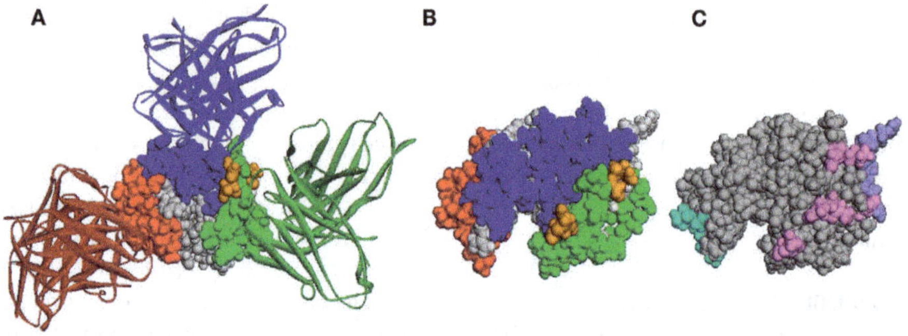

FIGURE 1 | Predicted epitopes vs. the actual epitopes of HEL. **(A)** The 3-D structure of HEL (CPK representation) together with three Abs (ribbon representation). PDB IDs 1JHL, 3D9A, and 1MLC were superimposed according to HEL structure. Epitope residues are colored blue, green, and red according to the corresponding Ab. Residues that are common to two epitopes are colored orange. **(B)** The structure of HEL colored according to the same three epitopes as in **(A)**, presented in a different orientation. **(C)** The structure of HEL colored according to the epitopes predicted by Discotope (light blue), ellipro (purple), and seppa (pink). Note, not all predicted residues of Discotope and ellipro are observable in the presented orientation.

and by others (58–60) that predicting epitopes should be done for a certain Ab. A similar concept was successfully applied in the case of T-cell epitope prediction methods: these methods do not examine the Ag for general features. Rather, different predictions are made, dependent on the specific MHC molecule binding and presenting the epitope to T cells.

THE ROLE OF CDRs AND THEIR DEFINITION

As shown in **Figure 2**, Abs are all-beta proteins consisting of four polypeptide chains: two identical heavy (H) chains and two identical light (L) chains (61). The light and heavy chains are linked by disulfide bonds to form the arms of a Y-shaped structure, each arm is known as a Fab (61). The Fab is composed of two variable domains (VH in the heavy chain and VL in the light chain) and two constant domains (CH1 and CL) (62). In the pairing of light and heavy chains, the two variable domains dimerize to form the Fv fragment which contains the Ag binding site. Within each variable domain lie six hypervariable loops (63), three in the light chain (L1, L2, and L3) and three in the heavy chain (H1, H2, and H3), supported by a conserved FR of β-sheets. The light and heavy variable domains fold in a manner that brings the hypervariable loops together to create the Ag binding site or paratope. Two additional domains of the heavy chain, CH2, and CH3, compose the Fc region which is responsible for mediating the biological activity of the Ab molecule.

CDRs IDENTIFICATION

As indicated by their names, CDRs are believed to account for the recognition of the Ag. Therefore, a major focus in analyzing the structural basis for Ag recognition has been in identifying the exact boundaries of the CDRs in a given Ab. It is a common practice to identify paratopes through the identification of CDRs. Kabat and co-authors (63, 64) were the first to introduce a systematic approach to identify CDRs in newly sequenced Abs. It was based on the assumption that CDRs are the most variable regions between Abs. Therefore, they aligned the (fairly limited) set of Ab sequences available at that time and identified the most variable positions. Based on the alignment, they introduced a numbering scheme for the residues in the hypervariable regions and determined which positions mark the beginning and the end of each CDR. As structural data became available, Chothia and Lesk (65, 66) manually analyzed a small number of experimentally solved 3-D structures and determined the structural location of the loop regions. The boundaries of the FRs and CDRs were determined and the latter have been shown to adopt a restricted set of conformations, based on the presence of certain residues at key positions in the CDRs and the flanking FRs. Their finding that Kabat's definitions of L1 and H1 are structurally incorrect led to the introduction of the Chothia numbering scheme. With the increase of available structural data, they ran their analysis anew and introduced a new definition of L1 (66) in 1989. In 1997 (67), however, they concluded that this correction was erroneous, and reverted to their original 1987 numbering scheme. While the Kabat and Chothia schemes treated separately the different families of immunoglobulin domains, Lefranc and colleagues (68, 69) proposed a unified numbering scheme (referred to as IMGT numbering scheme) for immunoglobulin variable domain genomic sequences, including Ab light and heavy variable domains, as well as T-cell receptor variable domains. To correlate between the sequence, structure, and domain folding behavior of all immunoglobulin variable domains, the Aho numbering scheme spatially aligned known 3-D structures of immunoglobulins and unified their numbering (70).

A drawback of the Kabat, Chothia, and IMGT numbering schemes is that CDRs length variability takes into account only the most common loop lengths; While both Kabat and Chothia schemes accommodate insertions with insertion letters (e.g., 27A), the IMGT scheme avoids the use of insertion codes for all but the least common very long loops, and the Aho numbering scheme places insertions and deletions symmetrically around a key position. However, Abs with unusually long insertions may be hard to annotate using these methods and, as a result, their CDRs may not be identified correctly. For instance, the recently determined 3-D crystal structure of two bovine Abs (71) reveal exceptionally long H3 CDRs (>60 residues), with long insertions which these methods cannot accommodate and thus cannot identify the CDRs of these Abs.

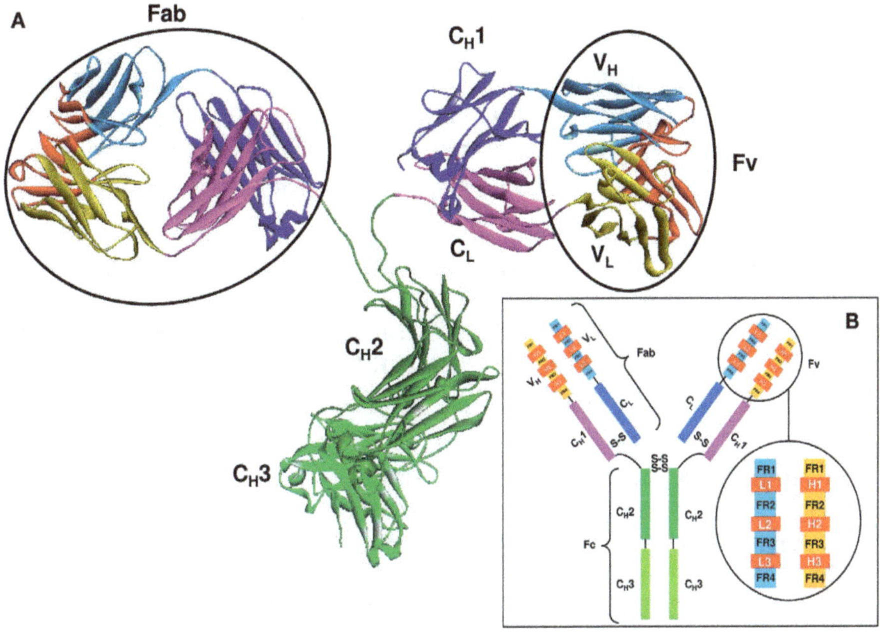

FIGURE 2 | The structure of an Ab molecule. (A) The 3-D structure of an Ab molecule (PDB ID: 1IGT). **(B)** A schematic representation of the Ab scaffold.

ARE CDRs GOOD PROXIES FOR THE PARATOPE?

While identification of paratopes is often done through identification of CDRs, not all the residues within the CDRs bind the Ag. In fact, an early analysis of the 3-D structures of Abs suggested that only 20–33% of the residues within the CDRs participate in Ag binding (72). In 1996, MacCallum and colleagues (73) performed a detailed residue-level analysis of Ag contacts. They suggested that contacting residues are more common at CDRs residues which are located at the center of the Ag combining site, and that non-contacting residues within the CDRs correspond with residues that are important for maintaining the structural conformations of the hypervariable loops and not necessarily for recognition of the Ag. Thus, they introduced a mapping of Ag-contacting propensities for each Ab position and proposed a new definition for CDRs based on these propensities. Padlan and co-workers (28) utilized Abs sequence and structure data to perform a by-position summary of Ag contacts. They found that the residues that are directly involved in the interaction with the Ag are also, in general, the most variable ones. They suggested that the residues that interact with the Ag should be called Specificity Determining Residues (SDRs).

The number of publicly available structures of Ab-Ag complexes increased in recent years to a level that enabled large-scale analyses. In a recent analysis (29) we utilized all available protein-Ab complexes in the PDB to identify the structural regions in which Ag binding actually occurs. This approach was implemented into a method dubbed Paratome (30, 74) that is based on a multiple structure alignment (MSTA) of all available Ab-Ag complexes in the PDB. The MSTA revealed regions of structural consensus where the pattern of structural positions that bind the Ag is highly similar among all Abs. These regions of structural binding consensus were termed antigen binding regions (ABRs). While CDRs, as identified by methods such as Kabat (63), Chothia (65), and IMGT (69), may miss ~20% of the Ag binding residues, ABRs cover ~96% of the residues that actually bind the Ag (30). To avoid confusions and cumbersome nomenclature, herein we generically refer to CDRs, SDRs, and ABRs as "CDRs" unless otherwise specified. **Figure 3** shows an example of CDRs as identified by Kabat, Chothia, IMGT, and Paratome for one Ab (anti-IL-15, PDB ID: 2XQB), compared to the actual Ag binding residues. It can be seen that in this example, some of the CDRs (e.g., L3, H3) identified by the four methods are almost identical, while in other CDRs (e.g., L2, H1, and H2) there are substantial differences between the methods. The MSTA of Abs with known 3-D structure also confirmed previous observations that there are structural positions within the CDRs in which none, or only a small percentage of the Abs contact the Ag. This is shown in **Figure 4** where an example of such a position is marked by a green arrow.

INTEGRALITY VS. MODULARITY

Designed systems are often characterized as either modular or integral. In a modular system different components, or modules, function independent of the function of other modules. The generation of Abs in the immune system is based on combining different elements, in a way that may be considered modular where each component is capable of binding the Ag regardless of the others. However, some analyses suggest that Ag binding warrants a more integrative view of the relationships between the different components of the Ab.

The binding-sites of interacting proteins are usually composed of surface patches that have good shape and electrostatic complementary (15, 75, 76). It has been shown that CDRs

```
A                              L1
Contacts TQPPSASGTPGQRVTISCSGSTSNLKRNYVYWYQQLPGTAPK
Kabat    TQPPSASGTPGQRVTISCSGSTSNLKRNYVYWYQQLPGTAPK
Chothia  TQPPSASGTPGQRVTISCSGSTSNLKRNYVYWYQQLPGTAPK
IMGT     TQPPSASGTPGQRVTISCSGSTSNLKRNYVYWYQQLPGTAPK
Paratome TQPPSASGTPGQRVTISCSGSTSNLKRNYVYWYQQLPGTAPK

            L2
Contacts LLIYRDRRRPSGVPDRFSGSKSGTSASLAISGLRSEDEADYY
Kabat    LLIYRDRRRPSGVPDRFSGSKSGTSASLAISGLRSEDEADYY
Chothia  LLIYRDRRRPSGVPDRFSGSKSGTSASLAISGLRSEDEADYY
IMGT     LLIYRDRRRPSGVPDRFSGSKSGTSASLAISGLRSEDEADYY
Paratome LLIYRDRRRPSGVPDRFSGSKSGTSASLAISGLRSEDEADYY

            L3
Contacts CAWYDRELSEWVFGGGTKLTVLQPKAAPSVTLFPPSSEELQ
Kabat    CAWYDRELSEWVFGGGTKLTVLQPKAAPSVTLFPPSSEELQ
Chothia  CAWYDRELSEWVFGGGTKLTVLQPKAAPSVTLFPPSSEELQ
IMGT     CAWYDRELSEWVFGGGTKLTVLQPKAAPSVTLFPPSSEELQ
Paratome CAWYDRELSEWVFGGGTKLTVLQPKAAPSVTLFPPSSEELQ

B                                   H1
Contacts VQLVQSGAEVKKPGASVKVSCKASGYSFSSFGISWVRQAPGQG
Kabat    VQLVQSGAEVKKPGASVKVSCKASGYSFSSFGISWVRQAPGQG
Chothia  VQLVQSGAEVKKPGASVKVSCKASGYSFSSFGISWVRQAPGQG
IMGT     VQLVQSGAEVKKPGASVKVSCKASGYSFSSFGISWVRQAPGQG
Paratome VQLVQSGAEVKKPGASVKVSCKASGYSFSSFGISWVRQAPGQG

                     H2
Contacts LEWLGWISAFNGYTKYAQKFQDRVTMTTDTSTSTAYMELRSLR
Kabat    LEWLGWISAFNGYTKYAQKFQDRVTMTTDTSTSTAYMELRSLR
Chothia  LEWLGWISAFNGYTKYAQKFQDRVTMTTDTSTSTAYMELRSLR
IMGT     LEWLGWISAFNGYTKYAQKFQDRVTMTTDTSTSTAYMELRSLR
Paratome LEWLGWISAFNGYTKYAQKFQDRVTMTTDTSTSTAYMELRSLR

                          H3
Contacts SDDTAVYYCARDPAAWPLQQSLAWFDPWGQGTMVTVSSASTKG
Kabat    SDDTAVYYCARDPAAWPLQQSLAWFDPWGQGTMVTVSSASTKG
Chothia  SDDTAVYYCARDPAAWPLQQSLAWFDPWGQGTMVTVSSASTKG
IMGT     SDDTAVYYCARDPAAWPLQQSLAWFDPWGQGTMVTVSSASTKG
Paratome SDDTAVYYCARDPAAWPLQQSLAWFDPWGQGTMVTVSSASTKG
```

FIGURE 3 | Comparison of different CDR identification methods. The light **(A)** and heavy **(B)** chains of PDB ID 2XQB were numbered according to Kabat (colored green) and Chothia (colored red) using the Abnum tool (www.bioinf.org.uk/abs/abnum) and CDRs were extracted according to the CDR definitions table (www.bioinf.org.uk/abs/#cdrs). CDRs according to IMGT (colored orange) were identified using the IMGT-gap tool (www.imgt.org/3Dstructure-DB/cgi/DomainGapAlign.cgi). ABRs according to Paratome (colored blue) were identified using the Paratome server (www.ofranlab.org/paratome). Contacts (colored purple) between the Ab and IL-15 were defined using a 6-Å cutoff value.

are characterized by an amino-acid composition that is different from that of other protein loops (77) and also from other types of protein–protein interfaces (58). Thus, one would expect that epitopes, just like paratopes, should have a distinct amino-acid composition. However, several recent analyses (51, 53) have shown that this is not the case: while epitopes differ from other types of interfaces (10, 29, 60), their amino-acid composition is virtually the same as that of non-epitopic surface residues.

Several studies have shown that each CDR has its own unique amino-acid composition, different from the composition of the other CDRs (52, 58, 78). Additionally, we have shown that each CDR has a unique set of contact preferences, therefore, favoring

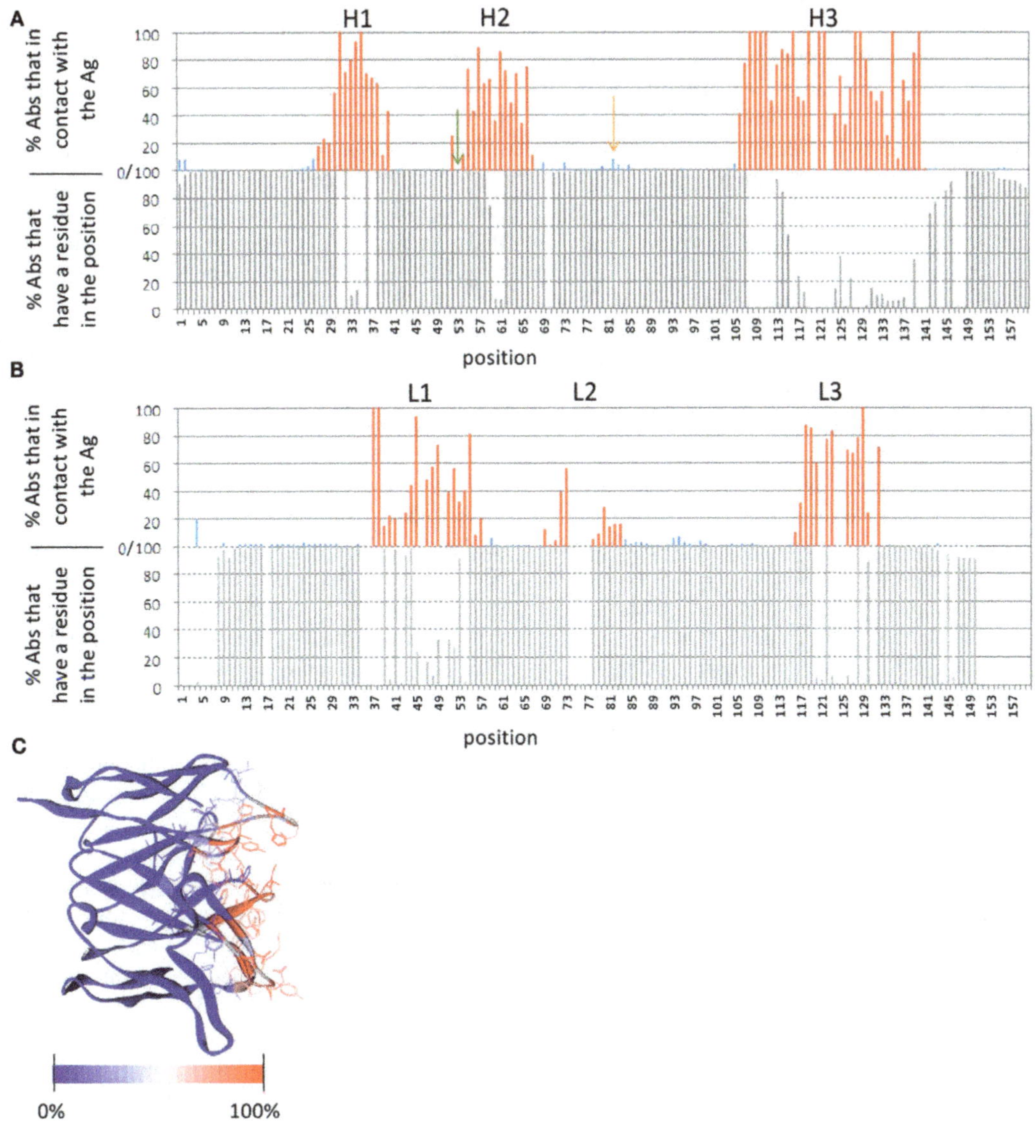

FIGURE 4 | Ab positions that contact the Ag. **(A,B)** The lower graphs show the percentage of Abs with known 3-D structure that have a residue in a given position (i.e., in other Abs there is a gap in the MSTA in that position). The upper graphs show the percentage of Abs that contact the Ag out of those Abs that have a residue in that position. **(A)** Depicts the heavy chain and **(B)** depicts the light chain. In the upper graphs, the ABRs are colored red and the FRs are colored blue. An example of a position within an ABR that is not in contact with the Ag in any of the Abs, is marked by a green arrow. An example of a position in the FRs that is in contact with the Ag in many (8%) of the Abs is marked by an orange arrow. **(C)** The Ab Fv domain (PDB ID: 1QFU) is colored according to the percentage of all Abs with known 3-D structure in which the residue in that position is in contact with the Ag: from red (100% of the Abs) to blue (0%). ABR residues are presented as lines. The definition of the ABRs is according to the Paratome server. A 6-Å cutoff value was used to define residues in contact. Percentages of contacts were calculated based on an MSTA of all protein Ab-Ag complexes in the PDB (30).

certain amino-acids over others (52). Dividing epitope residues into six subsets according to the CDR they bind, we found that each of the subsets has a distinct amino-acid composition, distinguishable from non-epitope surface (52). In other words, when the six subsets of epitope residues are considered together the unique composition of each subset disappears so that the overall amino-acid composition of the entire epitope is indistinguishable from the rest of the surface. Pathogenic epitopes may have evolved to resemble Ag surface to escape recognition. On the other hand, the integration of the six CDRs together, each with its own unique amino-acid composition and contact preferences, could be the evolutionary response of the immune system that enables Abs to recognize virtually any surface patch on the Ag.

Despite this integrated effect of the CDRs, Abs can be also considered as a modular system, composed of different elements (such as the Fab, VH and VL, or the six CDRs), which may bind the Ag on their own. Such smaller Ab fragments that retain Ag binding affinity and specificity, hold a great potential for drug design (79–81) as they have improved pharmacokinetics, tissue and tumor penetration, and can be produced more economically (80, 81).

They may also be combined with other fragments to yield better binders. Although such smaller fragments cannot induce effector function such as complement activation (due to the lack of the constant domains), they may neutralize the targeted Ag. Fab and single-chain variable (scFv) fragments usually maintain specific binding to the Ag (82). VH and VL fragments usually show sticky behavior, low solubility, and reduced Ag binding affinity (83–85), although, they sometime retain specificity to the Ag (83, 85–87).

The CDRs may provide additional level of modularity. According to the commonly accepted hotspot hypothesis, the binding energy of two proteins is largely determined by a very small number of critical interface residues (12, 88–90). Thus, one may wonder whether an individual CDR could bind the Ag on its own provided that it harbors hotspots. Several linear peptides containing one or more of the CDRs that retained Ag specificity have been reported (91–98). Although their affinity was usually in the micromolar range, it could be significantly improved by introducing relatively minor modifications (91, 99). However, many attempts to isolate and design such CDR derived peptides failed (100, 101). One possible reason is that a CDR, on its own, may not fold to the same conformation as in the context of the entire Fab, which may be crucial for binding. Cyclizing the CDR by adding Cys residues at its edges was suggested as a solution for this problem (96, 102–104). Another reason might lie in the fact that many attempts for the design of CDR-derived peptides are made based on CDR-H3, as it is considered to be the most important CDR for Ag binding (67, 105–107). However, the median length of ABR-H2 is substantially longer than that of H3, and both typically form the same number of interactions with the Ag (52). In addition, while ABR-H3 was shown to have the highest contribution to Ag binding energy on average (52), there are individual cases in which other CDRs are the dominant ones (52, 102). It is also possible that in some cases the binding depends on specific contacts from residues in different CDRs, which may preclude the design of CDR-derived peptides that maintain specificity. We have shown (102) that CDRs that are able to bind the Ag on their own have unique characteristics and, thus, can be computationally identified given the Ab-Ag complex structure. This may enhance the design of CDR-derived peptides that are not necessarily based on CDR-H3.

NON-CDR DETERMINANTS THAT HAVE A ROLE IN Ag BINDING

FR RESIDUES

Within the variable domain, the CDRs are believed to be responsible for Ag recognition, while the FR residues are considered a scaffold for the CDRs. However, it is now well established that some of the FR residues may play an important role in Ag binding (32, 108). As mentioned above, many such FR residues were identified during the process of Ab humanization by CDR grafting. While grafting only the CDRs usually results in a significant drop or a complete loss of binding, the binding affinity can be retained by back mutating some of the FR residues to the original murine sequence, emphasizing their role in Ag binding (26, 109–115).

Framework region residues that affect Ag binding can be divided into two categories. The first are FR residues that contact the Ag, thus are part of the binding-site (108, 109, 111, 116–123). Some of these residues are close in sequence to the CDRs (in fact they may be within the boundaries of CDRs according to some CDR identification methods, but not according to others, as shown in **Figure 3**). Other residues are those that are far from the CDRs in sequence, but are in close proximity to it in the 3-D structure. In particular, a loop in the heavy chain FR-3, sometimes referred to as CDR-H4, accounts for 1.3% of human Ab-Ag contacts (78, 124). This CDR-H4 is also enriched (in human Abs) in somatic hypermutations (Burkovitz et al., submitted). **Figure 4** shows positions that are not in the CDRs but are in contact with the Ag in many Abs [e.g., the one marked by an orange arrow (4A), which corresponds to CDR-H4].

In the second category of FR residues that affect Ag binding, are residues that are not in contact with the Ag, but affect Ag binding indirectly (108, 109, 120, 121). These residues can be further divided to those that are in spatial proximity to the CDRs, and those that are not. The former are assumed to affect binding by providing a structural support to the CDRs, enabling them to adopt the right conformation and orientation, shaping the binding-site required for Ag binding (32). For example, it has been suggested that a certain position in heavy chain FR-3, close in structure but not in sequence to CDR-H1 and CDR-H2, affects the orientation of CDR-H2 relative to CDR-H1 in such a way that a large side-chain packs between them and separates them while a small side-chain allows them to be closer to each other (109, 120). Nevertheless, this is not always true, as was shown in the case of the anti-lysozyme D1.3 Ab: while mutating Lys in this position to either Val, Ala, or Arg resulted in affinity difference, no structural change was observed (121).

Framework region residues that are more distant from the paratope are suggested to play a role in maintaining the overall structure of the Fv domains (32). However, these FR residues may also affect the Ag binding-site itself, by directing the relative orientation of the VH vs. the VL, and thus the orientation of the CDRs relative to each other (125–128). In particular, FR-2 residues were shown to play an important role in VH-VL interaction (129). Moreover, Masuda et al. (130) pointed to a specific position in the FR-2 loop, which controls the strength of the VH-VL interaction as well as its dependence on Ag binding. We have shown that the conformation of this loop changes upon Ag binding more than other residues in the FRs, and that the binding related conformational changes in this loop are similar in their magnitude to those of the CDRs (107). The potential role of the VH-VL interface in Ag binding is further supported by the observation that residues that are in the VH-VL interface (and are not a part of the Ab-Ag interface), are more likely to be mutated during the somatic hypermutation process, than residues that are not in either of these interfaces (Burkovitz et al., submitted).

Understanding the role of FR residues in Ag binding is crucial for efficient Ab design in general and for humanization in particular. Specifically, knowing in advance which FR residues may affect Ag binding, one may consider back-mutating these residues into their murine sequence, to improve affinity during CDR grafting. To this end, attempts were made to identify positions that contribute to Ag binding in multiple cases (32, 113, 119). For example, Haidar et al. (32) used a non-redundant dataset of Ab-Ag complex structures to identify positions that frequently contact the CDRs, and combined these positions with those that were back-mutated frequently in the humanization literature. The 17 FR positions they identified were successfully used to design a combinatorial library for Ab humanization. Additional Abs, for which structures of both wild-type and a mutant(s) are available, may reveal the structural mechanisms by which each FR position affects Ag binding.

CONSTANT REGION

Until recently, Ab constant domains were considered responsible for the isotype and for effector function, such as complement activation, Fc receptor binding, avidity, and serum half-life (131). However, many studies now provide a strong evidence for a role for the constant region in Ag binding (131–147). There are many examples of Abs with identical variable domains but different isotypes that bind the same Ag with a different affinity or specificity (134–146). For instance, two Abs sharing identical variable domains but expressing different isotypes were shown to bind tubulin with significantly different affinities (135). Consistent with these studies, it has been shown that the complex of HEL and the Fv version of the HyHEL-10 Ab has an order of magnitude lower dissociation constant than the complex of HEL with the Fab version of this Ab (147). A probable explanation for this phenomenon would be an allosteric influence of the constant domains on the structure of the variable domains. Indeed, several structural studies provided some evidence for such structural effects (133, 146, 147). For example, Janda et al. (133) analyzed by Circular Dichroism (CD) spectra four different Ab isotypes of the 3E5 family that share identical variable domains, and showed that the different isotypes undergo different structural changes upon binding a common Ag. Similar results were obtained for anti-nuclear Abs as well: Xia et al. (146) compared four different isotypes of the PL9–11 anti-nuclear Ab sharing the same variable region, and found that the changes in secondary structure content (as revealed by CD analysis) as well as the wave length shifts of tryptophan fluorescence emission, upon Ag binding, are both isotype dependent. Recently, Tudor et al. (144) showed that this allosteric effect may control not only Ag binding affinity and specificity, but also the epitope recognized. They showed that two anti-HIV-1 IgG1 and IgA2 Abs with identical variable regions, recognize only partially overlapping epitopes.

Differences in affinity and specificity of Abs with the same variable region but different isotypes may play a role in autoimmunity if they occur in a self-reactive Ag. For example, different isotypes have been shown to be associated with different clinical outcomes for lupus erythematosus: a set of anti-PL9–11 Abs sharing the same variable domain but different isotypes were shown to bind DNA and chromatin, as well as the renal Ags, with different affinities that were associated with significant differences in renal pathogenicity *in vivo* and survival (148).

Several studies have suggested that allosteric effects in Abs may occur on the other direction as well: structural changes in the variable region caused by Ag binding may be transferred into the constant domains, potentially influencing effector activation and cellular response (131, 149–151). For example, Oda et al. (149) showed that the binding of staphylococcal protein A (SPA) or streptococcal protein G (SPG) to the constant region was inhibited by hapten binding in several Abs. A different example was provided by Horgan et al. (151) who observed differences in complement activation of two Abs which differ only in their VH domain.

An allosteric effect in Abs is further supported by a systematic computational analysis we have performed on all available free and Ag-bound pairs of structures (107). Many of the Ag-binding-related structural changes occur distant from the Ag binding-site, including changes in the relative orientation of the heavy and light chains in both the variable and constant domains as well as a change in the elbow angle between the variable and the constant domains. Moreover, the most consistent and substantial conformational change outside of the binding site was found in a loop in the heavy chain constant domain, which is a part of the CH1-CL interface, and is involved in complement binding (152).

What could be the mechanism for these allosteric effects? Changes in the constant domains sequence (different isotypes of the same Ab) or in its conformation (e.g., by effector binding) may lead to a rearrangement of the constant domains relative to each other and relative to the variable domains, which may result in a change to the VH-VL relative orientation (72), thus re-shaping the Ag binding-site (153–155).

The potential influence of the constant region on Ag affinity or specificity suggests that the process of class-switch may be considered, in combination with somatic hypermutations, as a mechanism for Ab diversity (131, 132). Engineering of an Ab of interest is usually associated with the optimization of its affinity to the Ag. Since the constant region may affect this affinity, the isotype selected should be carefully considered. Moreover, the constant region should be taken into account in vaccine design as well since different isotypes may bind the pathogenic Ag with different affinities, thus affecting the response to infection. For example, the anti HIV-1 IgG1 and IgA2 Abs mentioned above share the same variable region, nevertheless, they have been shown to block HIV-1 infection differently (144). While IgA2 blocked HIV-1 transcytosis and $CD4^+$ cell infection more efficiently, IgG1 and IgA2 act synergistically to block HIV-1 transfer from Langerhans cells to T cells. Thus, it has been suggested that a mucosal IgA-based vaccine response should complement an IgG-based vaccine response in blocking HIV-1 transmission.

CONCLUDING REMARKS

As Abs are one of the most versatile naturally occurring biosensors, it is of high importance to decipher the structural and molecular mechanisms by which they recognize and bind their Ags. Such knowledge is crucial for understanding immunity, may enable better prediction of Ab epitopes, and assist in Ab engineering.

While the commonly accepted view has been that CDRs hold the key for Ab-Ag recognition, recent findings indicate that not all the positions in the traditionally defined CDRs are important for binding. Furthermore, it has been shown that many positions that contribute critically to the binding energy reside outside of the transitional CDRs. Moreover, different CDR identification methods may often identify radically different stretches as "CDRs," indicating that CDRs are not well defined and thus are not necessarily a good proxy for the binding site. The hypervariable loops that accommodate the CDRs differ significantly from each other on various aspects. Understanding the way in which their binding preferences are integrated to yield the overall specificity of the Ab is an intriguing structural and biophysical challenge.

Accumulation of recent data suggests that elements that may be spatially distant from the Ag binding site also play a crucial role in Ag recognition. The unorthodox suggestion that non-local and even allosteric effects influence epitope recognition warrants additional analysis and research.

Addressing the open questions regarding the structural basis of Ag recognition requires additional structural data in the form of crystal structures of Abs bound to Ags of different types (proteins, peptides, nucleic acids, and haptens). Large-scale analysis of such structures will allow for the generation and testing of new hypotheses regarding the way in which Abs find and bind their epitopes.

ACKNOWLEDGMENTS

The authors are supported in part by NIAID contract N01-AI-90048C (http://www.niaid.nih.gov/).

REFERENCES

1. Vincent KJ, Zurini M. Current strategies in antibody engineering: Fc engineering and pH-dependent antigen binding, bispecific antibodies and antibody drug conjugates. *Biotechnol J* (2012) **7**:1444–50. doi:10.1002/biot.201200250
2. Wang W, Singh S, Zeng DL, King K, Nema S. Antibody structure, instability, and formulation. *J Pharm Sci* (2007) **96**:1–26. doi:10.1002/jps.20727
3. Sheedy C, MacKenzie CR, Hall JC. Isolation and affinity maturation of hapten-specific antibodies. *Biotechnol Adv* (2007) **25**:333–52. doi:10.1016/j.biotechadv.2007.02.003
4. Salfeld JG. Isotype selection in antibody engineering. *Nat Biotechnol* (2007) **25**:1369–72. doi:10.1038/nbt1207-1369
5. Brusic V, Bajic VB, Petrovsky N. Computational methods for prediction of T-cell epitopes – a framework for modelling, testing, and applications. *Methods* (2004) **34**:436–43. doi:10.1016/j.ymeth.2004.06.006
6. Kim Y, Sette A, Peters B. Applications for T-cell epitope queries and tools in the Immune Epitope Database and Analysis Resource. *J Immunol Methods* (2011) **374**:62–9. doi:10.1016/j.jim.2010.10.010
7. Frank SA. Specificity and cross-reactivity (Chapter 4). In: *Immunology and Evolution of Infectious Disease*. Princeton, NJ: Princeton University Press (2002). p. 33–54.
8. Rose NR, MacKay IR, editors. T-cells and autoimmunity. In: *The Autoimmune Diseases*, 4th ed. San Diego: Elsevier Academic Press (2006). 1160 p.
9. Jones S, Thornton JM. Principles of protein-protein interactions. *Proc Natl Acad Sci U S A* (1996) **93**:13–20. doi:10.1073/pnas.93.1.13
10. Jones S, Thornton JM. Analysis of protein-protein interaction sites using surface patches. *J Mol Biol* (1997) **272**:121–32. doi:10.1006/jmbi.1997.1234
11. Lo Conte L, Chothia C, Janin J. The atomic structure of protein-protein recognition sites. *J Mol Biol* (1999) **285**:2177–98. doi:10.1006/jmbi.1998.2439
12. Bogan AA, Thorn KS. Anatomy of hot spots in protein interfaces. *J Mol Biol* (1998) **280**:1–9. doi:10.1006/jmbi.1998.1843
13. Chakrabarti P, Janin J. Dissecting protein-protein recognition sites. *Proteins* (2002) **47**:334–43. doi:10.1002/prot.10085
14. Keskin O. Binding induced conformational changes of proteins correlate with their intrinsic fluctuations: a case study of antibodies. *BMC Struct Biol* (2007) **7**:31. doi:10.1186/1472-6807-7-31
15. McCoy AJ, Chandana Epa V, Colman PM. Electrostatic complementarity at protein/protein interfaces. *J Mol Biol* (1997) **268**:570–84. doi:10.1006/jmbi.1997.0987
16. Neuvirth H, Raz R, Schreiber G. ProMate: a structure based prediction program to identify the location of protein-protein binding sites. *J Mol Biol* (2004) **338**:181–99. doi:10.1016/j.jmb.2004.02.040
17. Ma B, Elkayam T, Wolfson H, Nussinov R. Protein–protein interactions: structurally conserved residues distinguish between binding sites and exposed protein surfaces. *Proc Natl Acad Sci U S A* (2003) **100**:5772–7. doi:10.1073/pnas.1030237100
18. Bordner AJ, Abagyan R. Statistical analysis and prediction of protein-protein interfaces. *Proteins* (2005) **60**:353–66. doi:10.1002/prot.20433
19. Ofran Y, Rost B. Analysing six types of protein-protein interfaces. *J Mol Biol* (2003) **325**:377–87. doi:10.1016/S0022-2836(02)01223-8
20. Marks JD, Griffiths AD, Malmqvist M, Clackson TP, Bye JM, Winter G. By-passing immunization: building high affinity human antibodies by chain shuffling. *Biotechnology (N Y)* (1992) **10**:779–83. doi:10.1038/nbt0792-779
21. Soderlind E, Ohlin M, Carlsson R. Complementarity-determining region (CDR) implantation: a theme of recombination. *Immunotechnology* (1999) **4**:279–85.
22. Hemminki A, Niemi S, Hautoniemi L, Soderlund H, Takkinen K. Fine tuning of an anti-testosterone antibody binding site by stepwise optimisation of the CDRs. *Immunotechnology* (1998) **4**:59–69. doi:10.1016/S1380-2933(98)00002-5
23. Ohlin M, Owman H, Mach M, Borrebaeck CA. Light chain shuffling of a high affinity antibody results in a drift in epitope recognition. *Mol Immunol* (1996) **33**:47–56. doi:10.1016/0161-5890(95)00123-9
24. Mirick GR, Bradt BM, Denardo SJ, Denardo GL. A review of human anti-globulin antibody (HAGA, HAMA, HACA, HAHA) responses to monoclonal antibodies. Not four letter words. *Q J Nucl Med Mol Imaging* (2004) **48**:251–7.
25. Jones PT, Dear PH, Foote J, Neuberger MS, Winter G. Replacing the complementarity-determining regions in a human antibody with those from a mouse. *Nature* (1986) **321**:522–5. doi:10.1038/321522a0
26. Queen C, Schneider WP, Selick HE, Payne PW, Landolfi NF, Duncan JF, et al. A humanized antibody that binds to the interleukin 2 receptor. *Proc Natl Acad Sci U S A* (1989) **86**:10029–33. doi:10.1073/pnas.86.24.10029
27. Co MS, Queen C. Humanized antibodies for therapy. *Nature* (1991) **351**:501–2. doi:10.1038/351501a0
28. Padlan EA, Abergel C, Tipper JP. Identification of specificity-determining residues in antibodies. *FASEB J* (1995) **9**:133–9.
29. Ofran Y, Schlessinger A, Rost B. Automated identification of complementarity determining regions (CDRs) reveals peculiar characteristics of CDRs and B cell epitopes. *J Immunol* (2008) **181**:6230–5.
30. Kunik V, Peters B, Ofran Y. Structural consensus among antibodies defines the antigen binding site. *PLoS Comput Biol* (2012) **8**:e1002388. doi:10.1371/journal.pcbi.1002388
31. Berman HM, Westbrook J, Feng Z, Gilliland G, Bhat TN, Weissig H, et al. The Protein Data Bank. *Nucleic Acids Res* (2000) **28**:235–42. doi:10.1093/nar/28.1.235
32. Haidar JN, Yuan QA, Zeng L, Snavely M, Luna X, Zhang H, et al. A universal combinatorial design of antibody framework to graft distinct CDR sequences: a bioinformatics approach. *Proteins* (2012) **80**:896–912. doi:10.1002/prot.23246
33. Hanf KJ, Arndt JW, Chen LL, Jarpe M, Boriack-Sjodin PA, Li Y, et al. Antibody humanization by redesign of complementarity-determining region residues proximate to the acceptor framework. *Methods* (2013). doi:10.1016/j.ymeth.2013.06.024
34. Amanna IJ, Slifka MK, Crotty S. Immunity and immunological memory following smallpox vaccination. *Immunol Rev* (2006) **211**:320–37. doi:10.1111/j.0105-2896.2006.00392.x
35. Yang XD, Yu XL. An introduction to epitope prediction methods and software. *Rev Med Virol* (2009) **19**:77–96. doi:10.1002/rmv.602
36. Xu XL, Sun J, Liu Q, Wang XJ, Xu TL, Zhu RX, et al. Evaluation of spatial epitope computational tools based on experimentally-confirmed dataset for protein antigens. *Chin Sci Bull* (2010) **55**:2169–74. doi:10.1007/s11434-010-3199-z
37. Hopp TP, Woods KR. Prediction of protein antigenic determinants from amino acid sequences. *Proc Natl Acad Sci U S A* (1981) **78**:3824–8. doi:10.1073/pnas.78.6.3824
38. Ponomarenko JV, Bourne PE. Antibody-protein interactions: benchmark datasets and prediction tools evaluation. *BMC Struct Biol* (2007) **7**:64. doi:10.1186/1472-6807-7-64
39. Blythe MJ, Flower DR. Benchmarking B cell epitope prediction: underperformance of existing methods. *Protein Sci* (2005) **14**:246–8. doi:10.1110/ps.041059505

40. Ansari HR, Raghava GP. Identification of conformational B-cell epitopes in an antigen from its primary sequence. *Immunome Res* (2010) **6**:6. doi:10.1186/1745-7580-6-6
41. Kulkarni-Kale U, Bhosle S, Kolaskar AS. CEP: a conformational epitope prediction server. *Nucleic Acids Res* (2005) **33**:W168–71. doi:10.1093/nar/gki460
42. Liang SD, Zheng DD, Zhang C, Zacharias M. Prediction of antigenic epitopes on protein surfaces by consensus scoring. *BMC Bioinformatics* (2009) **10**:302. doi:10.1186/1471-2105-10-302
43. Ponomarenko J, Bui HH, Li W, Fusseder N, Bourne PE, Sette A, et al. ElliPro: a new structure-based tool for the prediction of antibody epitopes. *BMC Bioinformatics* (2008) **9**:514. doi:10.1186/1471-2105-9-514
44. Rubinstein ND, Mayrose I, Pupko T. A machine-learning approach for predicting B-cell epitopes. *Mol Immunol* (2009) **46**:840–7. doi:10.1016/j.molimm.2008.09.009
45. Rubinstein ND, Mayrose I, Martz E, Pupko T. Epitopia: a web-server for predicting B-cell epitopes. *BMC Bioinformatics* (2009) **10**:287. doi:10.1186/1471-2105-10-287
46. Sun J, Wu D, Xu T, Wang X, Xu X, Tao L, et al. SEPPA: a computational server for spatial epitope prediction of protein antigens. *Nucleic Acids Res* (2009) **37**:W612–6. doi:10.1093/nar/gkp417
47. Sweredoski MJ, Baldi P. PEPITO: improved discontinuous B-cell epitope prediction using multiple distance thresholds and half sphere exposure. *Bioinformatics* (2008) **24**:1459–60. doi:10.1093/bioinformatics/btn199
48. Ambroise J, Giard J, Gala JL, Macq B. Identification of relevant properties for epitopes detection using a regression model. *IEEE/ACM Trans Comput Biol Bioinform* (2011) **8**:1700–7. doi:10.1109/TCBB.2011.77
49. Liang S, Zheng D, Standley DM, Yao B, Zacharias M, Zhang C. EPSVR and EPMeta: prediction of antigenic epitopes using support vector regression and multiple server results. *BMC Bioinformatics* (2010) **11**:381. doi:10.1186/1471-2105-11-381
50. Zhang W, Xiong Y, Zhao M, Zou H, Ye X, Liu J. Prediction of conformational B-cell epitopes from 3D structures by random forests with a distance-based feature. *BMC Bioinformatics* (2011) **12**:10. doi:10.1186/1471-2105-12-341
51. Janin J, Chothia C. The structure of protein-protein recognition sites. *J Biol Chem* (1990) **265**:16027–30.
52. Kunik V, Ofran Y. The indistinguishability of epitopes from protein surface is explained by the distinct binding preferences of each of the six antigen-binding loops. *Protein Eng Des Sel* (2013). doi:10.1093/protein/gzt027
53. Kringelum JV, Nielsen M, Padkjær SB, Lund O. Structural analysis of B-cell epitopes in antibody:protein complexes. *Mol Immunol* (2013) **53**:24–34. doi:10.1016/j.molimm.2012.06.001
54. Benjamin DC, Berzofsky JA, East IJ, Gurd FR, Hannum C, Leach SJ, et al. The antigenic structure of proteins: a reappraisal. *Annu Rev Immunol* (1984) **2**:67–101. doi:10.1146/annurev.iy.02.040184.000435
55. Greenbaum JA, Andersen PH, Blythe M, Bui HH, Cachau RE, Crowe J, et al. Towards a consensus on datasets and evaluation metrics for developing B-cell epitope prediction tools. *J Mol Recognit* (2007) **20**:75–82. doi:10.1002/jmr.815
56. Novotný J, Handschumacher M, Haber E, Bruccoleri RE, Carlson WB, Fanning DW, et al. Antigenic determinants in proteins coincide with surface regions accessible to large probes (antibody domains). *Proc Natl Acad Sci U S A* (1986) **83**:226–30. doi:10.1073/pnas.83.2.226
57. Thornton JM, Edwards MS, Taylor WR, Barlow DJ. Location of "continuous" antigenic determinants in the protruding regions of proteins. *EMBO J* (1986) **5**:409–13.
58. Zhao L, Li JY. Mining for the antibody-antigen interacting associations that predict the B cell epitopes. *BMC Struct Biol* (2010) **10**(Suppl 1):S6. doi:10.1186/1472-6807-10-S1-S6
59. Zhao L, Wong L, Li JY. Antibody-specified b-cell epitope prediction in line with the principle of context-awareness. *IEEE/ACM Trans Comput Biol Bioinform* (2011) **8**:1483–94. doi:10.1109/TCBB.2011.49
60. Soga S, Kuroda D, Shirai H, Kobori M, Hirayama N. Use of amino acid composition to predict epitope residues of individual antibodies. *Protein Eng Des Sel* (2010) **23**:441–8. doi:10.1093/protein/gzq014
61. Edelman GM, Benacerraf B. On structural and functional relations between antibodies and proteins of the gamma-system. *Proc Natl Acad Sci U S A* (1962) **48**:1035–42. doi:10.1073/pnas.48.6.1035
62. Putnam FW, Liu YS, Low TL. Primary structure of a human IgA1 immunoglobulin. IV. Streptococcal IgA1 protease, digestion, Fab and Fc fragments, and the complete amino acid sequence of the alpha 1 heavy chain. *J Biol Chem* (1979) **254**:2865–74.
63. Wu TT, Kabat EA. An analysis of the sequences of the variable regions of Bence Jones proteins and myeloma light chains and their implications for antibody complementarity. *J Exp Med* (1970) **132**:211–50. doi:10.1084/jem.132.2.211
64. Kabat EA, Wu TT, Bilofsky H, Reid-Miller M, Perry H. *Sequence of Proteins of Immunological Interest*. Bethesda: National Institute of Health (1983).
65. Chothia C, Lesk AM. Canonical structures for the hypervariable regions of immunoglobulins. *J Mol Biol* (1987) **196**:901–17. doi:10.1016/0022-2836(87)90412-8
66. Chothia C, Lesk AM, Tramontano A, Levitt M, Smith-Gill SJ, Air G, et al. Conformations of immunoglobulin hypervariable regions. *Nature* (1989) **342**:877–83. doi:10.1038/342877a0
67. Al-Lazikani B, Lesk AM, Chothia C. Standard conformations for the canonical structures of immunoglobulins. *J Mol Biol* (1997) **273**:927–48. doi:10.1006/jmbi.1997.1354
68. Giudicelli V, Chaume D, Bodmer J, Muller W, Busin C, Marsh S, et al. IMGT, the international ImMunoGeneTics database. *Nucleic Acids Res* (1997) **25**:206–11. doi:10.1093/nar/25.1.206
69. Lefranc MP, Pommié C, Ruiz M, Giudicelli V, Foulquier E, Truong L, et al. IMGT unique numbering for immunoglobulin and T cell receptor variable domains and Ig superfamily V-like domains. *Dev Comp Immunol* (2003) **27**:55–77. doi:10.1016/S0145-305X(02)00039-3
70. Honegger A, Pluckthun A. Yet another numbering scheme for immunoglobulin variable domains: an automatic modeling and analysis tool. *J Mol Biol* (2001) **309**:657–70. doi:10.1006/jmbi.2001.4662
71. Wang F, Ekiert DC, Ahmad I, Yu W, Zhang Y, Bazirgan O, et al. Reshaping antibody diversity. *Cell* (2013) **153**:1379–93. doi:10.1016/j.cell.2013.04.049
72. Padlan EA. Anatomy of the antibody molecule. *Mol Immunol* (1994) **31**:169–217. doi:10.1016/0161-5890(94)90001-9
73. MacCallum RM, Martin AC, Thornton JM. Antibody-antigen interactions: contact analysis and binding site topography. *J Mol Biol* (1996) **262**:732–45. doi:10.1006/jmbi.1996.0548
74. Kunik V, Ashkenazi S, Ofran Y. Paratome: an online tool for systematic identification of antigen binding regions in antibodies based on sequence or structure. *Nucleic Acids Res* (2012) **40**(Web Server issue):W521–4. doi:10.1093/nar/gks480
75. Jones S, Thornton JM. Prediction of protein-protein interaction sites using patch analysis. *J Mol Biol* (1997) **272**:133–43. doi:10.1006/jmbi.1997.1234
76. Cohen GH, Silverton EW, Padlan EA, Dyda F, Wibbenmeyer JA, Willson RC, et al. Water molecules in the antibody-antigen interface of the structure of the Fab HyHEL-5-lysozyme complex at 1.7 A resolution: comparison with results from isothermal titration calorimetry. *Acta Crystallogr D Biol Crystallogr* (2005) **61**:628–33. doi:10.1107/S0907444905007870
77. Collis AV, Brouwer AP, Martin AC. Analysis of the antigen combining site: correlations between length and sequence composition of the hypervariable loops and the nature of the antigen. *J Mol Biol* (2003) **325**:337–54. doi:10.1016/S0022-2836(02)01222-6
78. Raghunathan G, Smart J, Williams J, Almagro J. Antigen-binding site anatomy and somatic mutations in antibodies that recognize different types of antigens. *J Mol Recognit* (2012) **25**:103–13. doi:10.1002/jmr.2158
79. Nelson AL, Reichert JM. Development trends for therapeutic antibody fragments. *Nat Biotechnol* (2009) **27**:331–7. doi:10.1038/nbt0409-331
80. Holliger P, Hudson PJ. Engineered antibody fragments and the rise of single domains. *Nat Biotechnol* (2005) **23**:1126–36. doi:10.1038/nbt1142

81. Hudson PJ, Souriau C. Engineered antibodies. *Nat Med* (2003) **9**:129–34. doi:10.1038/nm0103-129
82. Jain M, Kamal N, Batra SK. Engineering antibodies for clinical applications. *Trends Biotechnol* (2007) **25**:307–16. doi:10.1016/j.tibtech.2007.05.001
83. Ward ES, Güssow D, Griffiths AD, Jones PT, Winter G. Binding activities of a repertoire of single immunoglobulin variable domains secreted from *Escherichia coli. Nature* (1989) **341**:544–6. doi:10.1038/341544a0
84. Rinfret A, Horne C, Dorrington KJ, Klein M. Noncovalent association of heavy and light chains of human immunoglobulins. IV. The roles of the CH1 and CL domains in idiotypic expression. *J Immunol* (1985) **135**:2574–81.
85. Berry MJ, Davies J. Use of antibody fragments in immunoaffinity chromatography. Comparison of FV fragments, VH fragments and paralog peptides. *J Chromatogr* (1992) **597**:239–45. doi:10.1016/0021-9673(92)80116-C
86. Pereira B, Benedict CR, Le A, Shapiro SS, Thiagarajan P. Cardiolipin binding a light chain from lupus-prone mice. *Biochemistry* (1998) **37**:1430–7. doi:10.1021/bi972277q
87. Dubnovitsky AP, Kravchuk ZI, Chumanevich AA, Cozzi A, Arosio P, Martsev SP. Expression, refolding, and ferritin-binding activity of the isolated VL-domain of monoclonal antibody F11. *Biochemistry (Mosc)* (2000) **65**:1011–8.
88. Clackson T, Wells JA. A hot spot of binding energy in a hormone-receptor interface. *Science* (1995) **267**:383–6. doi:10.1126/science.7529940
89. Sheinerman FB, Norel R, Honig B. Electrostatic aspects of protein-protein interactions. *Curr Opin Struct Biol* (2000) **10**:153–9. doi:10.1016/S0959-440X(00)00065-8
90. Ofran Y. *Prediction of Protein Interaction Sites. Computational Protein-Protein Interactions R Nussinov and G Schreiber.* Boca Raton: CRC Press (2009). p. 167–84.
91. Park BW, Zhang HT, Wu C, Berezov A, Zhang X, Dua R, et al. Rationally designed anti-HER2/neu peptide mimetic disables P185HER2/neu tyrosine kinases in vitro and in vivo. *Nat Biotechnol* (2000) **18**:194–8. doi:10.1038/72651
92. Polonelli L, Pontón J, Elguezabal N, Moragues MD, Casoli C, Pilotti E, et al. Antibody complementarity-determining regions (CDRs) can display differential antimicrobial, antiviral and antitumor activities. *PLoS One* (2008) **3**(6):e2371. doi:10.1371/journal.pone.0002371
93. Kang CY, Brunck TK, Kieber-Emmons T, Blalock JE, Kohler H. Inhibition of self-binding antibodies (autobodies) by a VH-derived peptide. *Science* (1988) **240**:1034–6. doi:10.1126/science.3368787
94. Taub R, Hsu JC, Garsky VM, Hill BL, Erlanger BF, Kohn LD. Peptide sequences from the hypervariable regions of two monoclonal anti-idiotypic antibodies against the thyrotropin (TSH) receptor are similar to TSH and inhibit TSH-increased cAMP production in FRTL-5 thyroid cells. *J Biol Chem* (1992) **267**:5977–84.
95. Saragovi HU, Fitzpatrick D, Raktabutr A, Nakanishi H, Kahn M, Greene MI. Design and synthesis of a mimetic from an antibody complementarity-determining region. *Science* (1991) **253**:792–5. doi:10.1126/science.1876837
96. Levi M, Sällberg M, Rudén U, Herlyn D, Maruyama H, Wigzell H, et al. A complementarity-determining region synthetic peptide acts as a miniantibody and neutralizes human immunodeficiency virus type 1 in vitro. *Proc Natl Acad Sci U S A* (1993) **90**:4374–8. doi:10.1073/pnas.90.10.4374
97. Tsumoto K, Misawa S, Ohba Y, Ueno T, Hayashi H, Kasai N, et al. Inhibition of hepatitis C virus NS3 protease by peptides derived from complementarity-determining regions (CDRs) of the monoclonal antibody 8D4: tolerance of a CDR peptide to conformational changes of a target. *FEBS Lett* (2002) **525**:77–82. doi:10.1016/S0014-5793(02)03090-9
98. Feng Y, Chung D, Garrard L, McEnroe G, Lim D, Scardina J, et al. Peptides derived from the complementarity-determining regions of anti-Mac-1 antibodies block intercellular adhesion molecule-1 interaction with Mac-1. *J Biol Chem* (1998) **273**:5625–30. doi:10.1074/jbc.273.10.5625
99. Feng J, Li Y, Zhang W, Shen B. Rational design of potent mimic peptide derived from monoclonal antibody: antibody mimic design. *Immunol Lett* (2005) **98**:311–6. doi:10.1016/j.imlet.2004.12.006
100. Lasonder E, Bloemhoff W, Welling GW. Interaction of lysozyme with synthetic anti-lysozyme D1.3 antibody fragments studied by affinity chromatography and surface plasmon resonance. *J Chromatogr A* (1994) **676**:91–8. doi:10.1016/0021-9673(94)00125-1
101. Schellekens GA. *Molecular Aspects of Antibody-Antigen Interactions: Size Reduction of a Herpes Simplex Virus Neutralizing Antibody and its Antigen.* Groningen: University of Groningen (1996).
102. Burkovitz A, Leiderman O, Sela-Culang I, Byk G, Ofran Y. Computational identification of antigen-binding antibody fragments. *J Immunol* (2013) **190**:2327–34. doi:10.4049/jimmunol.1200757
103. Bourgeois C, Bour JB, Aho LS, Pothier P. Prophylactic administration of a complementarity-determining region derived from a neutralizing monoclonal antibody is effective against respiratory syncytial virus infection in BALB/c mice. *J Virol* (1998) **72**:807–10.
104. Williams WV, Kieber-Emmons T, VonFeldt J, Greene MI, Weiner DB. Design of bioactive peptides based on antibody hypervariable region structures. Development of conformationally constrained and dimeric peptides with enhanced affinity. *J Biol Chem* (1991) **266**:5182–90.
105. Barrios Y, Jirholt P, Ohlin M. Length of the antibody heavy chain complementarity determining region 3 as a specificity-determining factor. *J Mol Recognit* (2004) **17**:332–8. doi:10.1002/jmr.679
106. Kuroda D, Shirai H, Kobori M, Nakamura H. Structural classification of CDR-H3 revisited: a lesson in antibody modeling. *Proteins* (2008) **73**:608–20. doi:10.1002/prot.22087
107. Sela-Culang I, Alon S, Ofran Y. A systematic comparison of free and bound antibodies reveals binding-related conformational changes. *J Immunol* (2012) **189**:4890–9. doi:10.4049/jimmunol.1201493
108. Sedrak P, Hsu K, Mohan C. Molecular signatures of anti-nuclear antibodies – contribution of heavy chain framework residues. *Mol Immunol* (2003) **40**:491–9. doi:10.1016/S0161-5890(03)00223-2
109. Xiang J, Sha Y, Jia Z, Prasad L, Delbaere L. Framework residue-71 and residue-93 of the chimeric B72.3 antibody are major determinants of the conformation of heavy-chain hypervariable loops. *J Mol Biol* (1995) **253**:385–90. doi:10.1006/jmbi.1995.0560
110. Verhoeyen M, Milstein C, Winter G. Reshaping human antibodies: grafting an antilysozyme activity. *Science* (1988) **239**:1534–6. doi:10.1126/science.2451287
111. Kettleborough CA, Saldanha J, Heath VJ, Morrison CJ, Bendig MM. Humanization of a mouse monoclonal antibody by CDR-grafting: the importance of framework residues on loop conformation. *Protein Eng* (1991) **4**:773–83. doi:10.1093/protein/4.7.773
112. Carter P, Presta L, Gorman CM, Ridgway JB, Henner D, Wong WL, et al. Humanization of an anti-p185HER2 antibody for human cancer therapy. *Proc Natl Acad Sci U S A* (1992) **89**:4285–9. doi:10.1073/pnas.89.10.4285
113. Baca M, Presta L, O'Connor S, Wells J. Antibody humanization using monovalent phage display. *J Biol Chem* (1997) **272**:10678–84. doi:10.1074/jbc.272.16.10678
114. Rodríguez-Rodríguez ER, Ledezma-Candanoza LM, Contreras-Ferrat LG, Olamendi-Portugal T, Possani LD, Becerril B, et al. A single mutation in framework 2 of the heavy variable domain improves the properties of a diabody and a related single-chain antibody. *J Mol Biol* (2012) **423**:337–50. doi:10.1016/j.jmb.2012.07.007
115. Chiu WC, Lai YP, Chou MY. Humanization and characterization of an anti-human TNF-alpha murine monoclonal antibody. *PLoS One* (2011) **6**:e16373. doi:10.1371/journal.pone.0016373
116. Davies DR, Chacko S. Antibody structure. *Acc Chem Res* (1993) **26**:421–7. doi:10.1021/ar00032a005
117. Schroeder H, Hillson J, Perlmutter R. Structure and evolution of mammalian VH families. *Int Immunol* (1990) **2**:41–50. doi:10.1093/intimm/2.1.41
118. Amit A, Mariuzza R, Phillips S, Poljak R. 3-Dimensional structure of an antigen-antibody complex at 2.8 a resolution. *Science* (1986) **233**:747–53. doi:10.1126/science.2426778
119. Foote J, Winter G. Antibody framework residues affecting the

conformation of the hypervariable loops. *J Mol Biol* (1992) **224**:487–99. doi:10.1016/0022-2836(92)91010-M

120. Tramontano A, Chothia C, Lesk A. Framework residue-71 is a major determinant of the position and conformation of the 2nd hypervariable region in the VH domains of immunoglobulins. *J Mol Biol* (1990) **215**:175–82. doi:10.1016/S0022-2836(05)80102-0
121. Holmes M, Buss T, Foote J. Structural effects of framework mutations on a humanized anti-lysozyme antibody. *J Immunol* (2001) **167**:296–301.
122. Potter K, Hobby P, Klijn S, Stevenson F, Sutton B. Evidence for involvement of a hydrophobic patch in framework region 1 of human v4-34-encoded igs in recognition of the red blood cell I antigen. *J Immunol* (2002) **169**:3777–82.
123. Pospisil R, Youngcooper G, Mage R. Preferential expansion and survival of B-lymphocytes based on VH framework-1 and framework-3 expression: "positive" selection in appendix of normal and VH-mutant rabbits. *Proc Natl Acad Sci USA* (1995) **92**:6961–5. doi:10.1073/pnas.92.15.6961
124. Capra J, Kehoe J. Variable region sequences of 5 human immunoglobulin heavy chains of VH3 subgroup: definitive identification of four heavy chain hypervariable regions. *Proc Natl Acad Sci USA* (1974) **71**:845–8. doi:10.1073/pnas.71.3.845
125. Banfield M, King D, Mountain A, Brady R. V-L:V-H domain rotations in engineered antibodies: crystal structures of the Fab fragments from two murine antitumor antibodies and their engineered human constructs. *Proteins* (1997) **29**:161–71. doi:10.1002/(SICI)1097-0134(199710)29:2<161::AID-PROT4>3.0.CO;2-G
126. Nakanishi T, Tsumoto K, Yokota A, Kondo H, Kumagai I. Critical contribution of VH-VL interaction to reshaping of an antibody: the case of humanization of anti-lysozyme antibody, HyHEL-10. *Protein Sci* (2008) **17**:261–70. doi:10.1110/ps.073156708
127. Stanfield R, Takimotokamimura M, Rini J, Profy A, Wilson I. Major antigen-induced domain rearrangements in an antibody. *Structure* (1993) **1**:83–93. doi:10.1016/0969-2126(93)90024-B
128. Tan P, Sandmaier B, Stayton P. Contributions of a highly conserved VHNL hydrogen bonding interaction to scFv folding stability and refolding efficiency. *Biophys J* (1998) **75**:1473–82. doi:10.1016/S0006-3495(98)74066-4
129. Essen L, Skerra A. The de-novo design of an antibody combining site – crystallographic analysis of the V-L domain confirms the structural model. *J Mol Biol* (1994) **238**:226–44. doi:10.1006/jmbi.1994.1284
130. Masuda K, Sakamoto K, Kojima M, Aburatani T, Ueda T, Ueda H. The role of interface framework residues in determining antibody V-H/V-L interaction strength and antigen-binding affinity. *Febs J* (2006) **273**:2184–94. doi:10.1111/j.1742-4658.2006.05232.x
131. Torres M, Casadevall A. The immunoglobulin constant region contributes to affinity and specificity. *Trends Immunol* (2008) **29**:91–7. doi:10.1016/j.it.2007.11.004
132. Casadevall A, Janda A. Immunoglobulin isotype influences affinity and specificity. *Proc Natl Acad Sci U S A* (2012) **109**:12272–3. doi:10.1073/pnas.1209750109
133. Janda A, Casadevall A. Circular dichroism reveals evidence of coupling between immunoglobulin constant and variable region secondary structure. *Mol Immunol* (2010) **47**:1421–5. doi:10.1016/j.molimm.2010.02.018
134. Dam TK, Torres M, Brewer CF, Casadevall A. Isothermal titration calorimetry reveals differential binding thermodynamics of variable region-identical antibodies differing in constant region for a univalent ligand. *J Biol Chem* (2008) **283**:31366–70. doi:10.1074/jbc.M806473200
135. Pritsch O, Hudry-Clergeon G, Buckle M, Petillot Y, Bouvet JP, Gagnon J, et al. Can immunoglobulin C(H)1 constant region domain modulate antigen binding affinity of antibodies? *J Clin Invest* (1996) **98**:2235–43. doi:10.1172/JCI119033
136. Pritsch O, Magnac C, Dumas G, Bouvet JP, Alzari P, Dighiero G. Can isotype switch modulate antigen-binding affinity and influence clonal selection? *Eur J Immunol* (2000) **30**(12):3387–95. doi:10.1002/1521-4141(200012)30:12<3387::AID-IMMU3387>3.0.CO;2-K
137. Torres M, May R, Scharff MD, Casadevall A. Variable-region-identical antibodies differing in isotype demonstrate differences in fine specificity and idiotype. *J Immunol* (2005) **174**:2132–42.
138. Torres M, Fernández-Fuentes N, Fiser A, Casadevall A. The immunoglobulin heavy chain constant region affects kinetic and thermodynamic parameters of antibody variable region interactions with antigen. *J Biol Chem* (2007) **282**:13917–27. doi:10.1074/jbc.M700661200
139. McLean GR, Torres M, Elguezabal N, Nakouzi A, Casadevall A. Isotype can affect the fine specificity of an antibody for a polysaccharide antigen. *J Immunol* (2002) **169**:1379–86.
140. Cooper LJ, Shikhman AR, Glass DD, Kangisser D, Cunningham MW, Greenspan NS. Role of heavy chain constant domains in antibody-antigen interaction. Apparent specificity differences among streptococcal IgG antibodies expressing identical variable domains. *J Immunol* (1993) **150**:2231–42.
141. McCloskey N, Turner MW, Steffner P, Owens R, Goldblatt D. Human constant regions influence the antibody binding characteristics of mouse-human chimeric IgG subclasses. *Immunology* (1996) **88**:169–73. doi:10.1111/j.1365-2567.1996.tb00001.x
142. Michaelsen TE, Ihle Ø, Beckstrøm KJ, Herstad TK, Sandin RH, Kolberg J, et al. Binding properties and anti-bacterial activities of V-region identical, human IgG and IgM antibodies, against group B *Neisseria meningitidis*. *Biochem Soc Trans* (2003) **31**:1032–5. doi:10.1042/BST0311032
143. Liu F, Bergami PL, Duval M, Kuhrt D, Posner M, Cavacini L. Expression and functional activity of isotype and subclass switched human monoclonal antibody reactive with the base of the V3 loop of HIV-1 gp120. *AIDS Res Hum Retroviruses* (2003) **19**:597–607. doi:10.1089/088922203322230969
144. Tudor D, Yu H, Maupetit J, Drillet AS, Bouceba T, Schwartz-Cornil I, et al. Isotype modulates epitope specificity, affinity, and antiviral activities of anti-HIV-1 human broadly neutralizing 2F5 antibody. *Proc Natl Acad Sci U S A* (2012) **109**:12680–5. doi:10.1073/pnas.1200024109
145. Torosantucci A, Chiani P, Bromuro C, De Bernardis F, Palma AS, Liu Y, et al. Protection by anti-beta-glucan antibodies is associated with restricted beta-1,3 glucan binding specificity and inhibition of fungal growth and adherence. *PLoS One* (2009) **4**:e5392. doi:10.1371/journal.pone.0005392
146. Xia Y, Janda A, Eryilmaz E, Casadevall A, Putterman C. The constant region affects antigen binding of antibodies to DNA by altering secondary structure. *Mol Immunol* (2013) **56**:28–37. doi:10.1016/j.molimm.2013.04.004
147. Adachi M, Kurihara Y, Nojima H, Takeda-Shitaka M, Kamiya K, Umeyama H. Interaction between the antigen and antibody is controlled by the constant domains: normal mode dynamics of the HEL-HyHEL-10 complex. *Protein Sci* (2003) **12**:2125–31. doi:10.1110/ps.03100803
148. Xia Y, Pawar RD, Nakouzi AS, Herlitz L, Broder A, Liu K, et al. The constant region contributes to the antigenic specificity and renal pathogenicity of murine anti-DNA antibodies. *J Autoimmun* (2012) **39**:398–411. doi:10.1016/j.jaut.2012.06.005
149. Oda M, Kozono H, Morii H, Azuma T. Evidence of allosteric conformational changes in the antibody constant region upon antigen binding. *Int Immunol* (2003) **15**:417–26. doi:10.1093/intimm/dxg036
150. Piekarska B, Drozd A, Konieczny L, Król M, Jurkowski W, Roterman I, et al. The indirect generation of long-distance structural changes in antibodies upon their binding to antigen. *Chem Biol Drug Des* (2006) **68**:276–83. doi:10.1111/j.1747-0285.2006.00448.x
151. Horgan C, Brown K, Pincus SH. Effect of H-chain V-region on complement activation by immobilized immune-complexes. *J Immunol* (1992) **149**:127–35.
152. Vidarte L, Pastor C, Mas S, Blazquez AB, de los Rios V, Guerrero R, et al. Serine 132 is the C3 covalent attachment point on the CH1 domain of human IgG1. *J Biol Chem* (2001) **276**(41):38217–23.
153. Braden BC, Poljak RJ. Structural features of the reactions – between antibodies and protein antigens. *FASEB J* (1995) **9**:9–16.

10

Fundamental roles of the innate-like repertoire of natural antibodies in immune homeostasis

Jaya Vas*[1], *Caroline Grönwall*[1] and *Gregg J. Silverman*[1,2]

[1] *Laboratory of B Cell Immunobiology, Department of Medicine, New York University School of Medicine, New York, NY, USA*
[2] *Laboratory of B Cell Immunobiology, Department of Pathology, New York University School of Medicine, New York, NY, USA*

Edited by:
Harry W. Schroeder, University of Alabama at Birmingham, USA

Reviewed by:
Harry W. Schroeder, University of Alabama at Birmingham, USA
David Nemazee, The Scripps Research Institute, USA

****Correspondence:***
Gregg J. Silverman, Laboratory of B Cell Immunobiology, Department of Medicine, New York University School of Medicine, Alexandria Center for Life Science, 450 East 29th Street, Room 804, New York, NY 10016, USA.
e-mail: gregg.silverman@nyumc.org

The composition of the early immune repertoire is biased with prominent expression of spontaneously arising B cell clones that produce IgM with recurrent and often autoreactive binding specificities. Amongst these naturally arising antibodies (NAbs) are IgM antibodies that specifically recognized amaged and senescent cells, often via oxidation-associated neo-determinants. These NAbs are present from birth and can be further boosted by apoptotic cell challenge. Recent studies have shown that IgM NAb to apoptotic cells can enhance phagocytic clearance, as well as suppress proinflammatory responses induced via Toll-like receptors, and block pathogenic IgG-immune complex (IC)-mediated inflammatory responses. Specific antibody effector functions appear to be involved, as these anti-inflammatory properties are dependent on IgM-mediated recruitment of the early recognition factors of complement. Clinical surveys have suggested that anti-apoptotic cell (AC) IgM NAbs may modulate disease activity in some patients with autoimmune disease. In mechanistic studies, anti-AC NAbs were shown to act in dendritic cells by inhibition of the mitogen-activated protein kinase (MAPK) pathway, a primary signal transduction pathway that controls inflammatory responses. This immunomodulatory pathway has an absolute requirement for the induction of MAPK phosphatase-1. Taken together, recent studies have elucidated the novel properties of a class of protective NAbs, which may directly blunt inflammatory responses through a primitive pathway for regulation of the innate immune system.

Keywords: immunoregulation, innate-like, natural antibody

INTRODUCTION

The evolutionary emergence of the combinatorial antigen receptor system of variable region (V) gene rearrangements in lymphocytes has provided a greatly enhanced capacity for specific recognition of an immense range of ligands. In humans, the antibody system can generate B cell antigen receptors (BCR) encoded by more than 10^{20} genetically distinct variable region rearrangements. Considering that each individual has only about 10^{11} lymphocytes, if the primary B cell repertoire was indeed generated randomly, there would belittle or no recurrence in the antibody gene sequences in the somatically generated repertoires of the billions of humans on the planet. In the following sections, we review evidence the B cell compartment arises during development with a restricted and biased repertoire, and that the antibody products of these B cell clones may serve to protect the host from both external threats and for the maintenance of internal homeostasis.

RESTRICTION IN THE EARLY REPERTOIRE

In the mouse, there is a remarkable restriction in the usage patterns of the heavy chain V region (V_H) genes during early repertoire development (Perlmutter et al., 1985). Surveys of murine antibody sequences have provided extensive evidence of recurrent lymphocyte clones with the same V gene rearrangements in different individuals (Seidl et al., 1997), and emerging data suggests there may be similar patterns in the human B cell repertoire (Jackson et al., 2012). In fact, these biases in the expression of V_H rearrangements are first detectable at a time point at which representation cannot be affected by antigenic selection of these IgM-associated clones (Schroeder et al., 1987; Schroeder and Wang, 1990). Moreover, a recent report suggested that the perinatal V_H repertoire expressed in human IgA may be even more restricted than the IgM pool (Rogosch et al., 2012). Recurrent biases in the V_H expression in the early B cell repertoire have also been reported in other species, such as swine (Sun et al., 1998) and sheep (Jenne et al., 2006), as well as more primitive species, such as the amphibian *Xenopus laevis* (Flajnik and Rumfelt, 2000), and zebrafish (Du Pasquier et al., 2000).

Both humans and mice have circulating IgM antibodies that arise early life without immunogenic challenge and have therefore been termed natural antibodies (NAbs). In fact, neonatal B cells produce IgM antibodies that are readily detectable in the bloodstream at birth, and studies in mice have shown that more than 80% of circulating IgM are produced by a phenotypically distinct mature B cell subset, termed the B-1a cell subset, and characterized by membrane-associated CD5. In general, while some B-1 cells express antigen-receptors for recognition of common bacterial Ags, some B-1 cell clones can also recognize self-antigens, including the phospholipidphosphatidylcholine (PtC), the phospholipid-associated phosphorylcholine (PC) head group, as well as DNA and certain cell membrane proteins (Kantor and Herzenberg, 1993).

B-1 cells are believed to represent a developmentally distinct lineage from their adult counterpart, the bone marrow-derived B-2 subset (reviewed in Hardy, 2006; Baumgarth, 2011). Murine B-1 clones are self-replenishing, which ensures the maintenance of this repertoire, as later in life the capacity for *de novo* generation of mature lymphocytes with the B-1 cell phenotype is limited. Studies by Notkins and colleagues have shown that CD5-bearing human B cells also have a bias toward the production of certain types of autoantibodies (Casali and Notkins, 1989). However, CD5 molecules can represent an activation marker on human B cells, and hence by itself CD5 may not be a rigorous phenotypic marker for this B cell subset in humans (Cong et al., 1991). To address this long standing issue, Rothstein and coworkers have reported a detailed phenotyping scheme, in addition to CD5, for identifying human B cells with the diagnostic features of B-1 cells. The repertoire of these human B-1 cells also appeared to include prominent expression of self-specificities for native DNA and PC-containing antigens (Griffin et al., 2011).

AUTOREACTIVITY OF B LYMPHOCYTE SUBSETS

In mice, mature B-1 and B-2 lymphocyte subsets can play discrete but complementary functional roles in host defenses (reviewed in Baumgarth, 2011). There are also subpopulations within B-1 cells in addition to $CD5^+$ B-1a cells, as B-1b cells (that do not express CD5) make essential contributions to T cell-independent defenses for certain types of infections (Alugupalli and Abraham, 2009). The clonal selection of these distinct B cell subsets may in part reflect differences in their cellular thresholds for negative selection (i.e., BCR-induced cell death) and in their activation requirements for second signals after BCR stimulation. By one estimate, over 70% of BCR-expressing immature B cells in the bone marrow display some level of autoreactivity while the level is much less in recirculating naïve mature B-2 cells (Wardemann et al., 2003). Hence, the immune tolerance checkpoints for B-2 cells that arise from precursors in the bone marrow appear to be generally more stringent in the removal of self-reactivity (i.e., negative selection). In contrast, conserved B-1 cell clonotypes may be positively selected (i.e., enhanced survival and clonal proliferation) by certain types of non-protein self-antigens (Hayakawa et al., 1999), which may include specific types of intracellular antigens (Ferry et al., 2007). As B-1 cells are a major source of circulating IgM in neonates, this may explain why neonatal IgM–NAbs from umbilical cord commonly display features of self-reactivity (Chou et al., 2009).

In the human immune system there is a remarkably strong association between the immune recognition of cell surface *N*-acetyllactosamine/polylactosamine determinants in glycoconjugates and the usage of the V_H4-34 gene segment (originally termed V_H4-21; Silberstein et al., 1991). *N*-acetyllactosamine/polylactosamine moieties are common on cell surfaces throughout the body, as these are structural components of the I/i blood group antigens and also constitute the antigenic target of pathogenic autoantibodies in cold-agglutinin disease (Silverman et al., 1990; Silberstein et al., 1991; Grillot-Courvalin et al., 1992; Pascual and Capra, 1992).

The immune recognition of I/i related non-protein antigens may be involved in very different types of immune responses. Using a lectin microarray system, exosomes released by human tumor cell lines were shown to express a shared polylactosamine glycan signature (Batista et al., 2011). These findings extend earlier evidence that I/i related determinants can be preferentially expressed on cells during early development and on their malignant counterparts (i.e., onco-fetal antigens; Feizi, 1988). In addition, V_H4-34 encoded autoantibodies were found to commonly bind to HIV-1 envelope determinants (Kobie et al., 2012). Batista et al. (2011) have suggested that these glycans reflect a recurrent type of glycan epitope profile on stressed and apoptotic cells (ACs). Taken together, these findings highlight the intertwined nature of immunodominant determinants on microparticles, exosomes, and HIV-1 virions that arise by budding through the membranes of stressed host cells.

B cell receptor encoded by V_H4-34 rearrangements recognize I/i determinants via contact sites associated with a V_H germline framework subdomain sequences – there is little apparent contribution from the somatically generated heavy chain CDR3 or by the paired light chain (Pascual et al., 1991). Using the 9G4 anti-idiotype antibody, B cells that bear non-mutated V_H4-34 products have been shown to be highly represented, and whereas in healthy individuals these autoreactive germline B cells were shown to be excluded from T cell-dependent germinal center reactions (Pugh-Bernard et al., 2001), these V_H defined clones can be actively recruited into the germinal center reactions in patients with systemic lupus erythematosus (SLE; Cappione et al., 2005). These findings have been interpreted as evidence of immune defects in SLE patients related to the regulation of autoreactive B cells, although this topic remains controversial.

NATURAL ANTIBODIES AND IMMUNE RECOGNITION OF DAMAGED AND APOPTOTIC CELLS

During the process of AC death, different cell membrane-associated phospholipids can undergo selective enzyme-mediated and oxidation associated modifications, and these cell membrane neo-determinants become available for recognition by the immune system. Among these, phosphatidylserine (PS) becomes oxidized and rapidly translocates from the inner to the outer leaflet of the cell membrane upon the initiation of apoptosis, where it can serve as a recognition signal for ingestion by professional phagocytes (i.e., "eat me" signal). Apoptosis can also be associated with other lipid neo-determinants, such as malondialdehyde (MDA), which is formed from interactions of unsaturated lipids with reactive oxidation species. Oxidative modifications of the abundantly distributed neutral phospholipid, PtC, also affect the distribution and/or conformation of the PC head group (Friedman et al., 2002), which renders it accessible for antibody recognition. These PC-antigens, as well as MDA-containing antigens, are immunodominant within murine B cell clonal responses that are boosted by intravenous infusions of ACs (Chen et al., 2009b).

The dominant natural antibody-producing anti-PC B cell clone, termed T15 (also TEPC15), has recurrently been isolated in anti-PC responses. The high representation of this clone in the early repertoire in part reflects a bias for increased representation of the specific V_HS107.1 gene rearrangements used by the

T15 clone (Feeney, 1991). In fact both of the V_H and V_L rearrangements in the T15 clone are formed by primary sequence direct rearrangements, and are without somatic mutations. The invariance of the T15 clonotypic NAb therefore is reminiscent of germline encoded receptors of the innate immune system (discussed in Shaw et al., 2000). In fact, T15 clonotypic antibodies are highly specific for PC determinants (Kearney et al., 1981) and in microarray analysis demonstrated little or no cross-reactivity to a large number of structurally distinct antigens (Chen et al., 2009b). Throughout life, T15-related B-1 cells are a major source of NAbs to a range of PC-containing antigens (Masmoudi et al., 1990), including those present on AC membranes, oxidized low-density lipoprotein (LDL), as well as in pneumococcal bacterial cell wall polysaccharide (Shaw et al., 2003; Chou et al., 2009). Many other B-1 cell clones have been demonstrated to be polyreactive and relatively low-affinity (Kantor and Herzenberg, 1993). However, crystallographic analysis of a V_HS107.1 encoded (i.e., T15-related) Fab revealed a deep antigen-binding cleft with substantial binding affinity for the small PC moiety (reviewed in Davies et al., 1975). As a consequence of the dependence of the *in vivo* anti-PC response on T15 clonotypic B cells, otherwise immunocompetent mice which were made deficient only for the S107.1 V_H gene segment, have highly impaired responses to immune challenge with PC determinants on either ACs or bacteria, and also display impaired immune defenses for *S. pneumoniae* infection (Mi et al., 2000; Chen et al., 2009b). Taken together, these studies suggest that the antigen binding sites of T15-related antibodies have innate-like properties for recognition of PC-containing antigens are highly represented in the pre-immune repertoire (Kearney, 2005), in part because of their preferentially formation by biases in the somatic diversification mechanisms (Feeney, 1992).

Within the NAb pool there are also other antibodies that recognize distinct sets of neo-determinants that arise following cellular injury. There are at least two self-antigen specificities that have been reported to be associated with post-ischemic injury of endothelial cells (Zhang et al., 2008; Kulik et al., 2009). In addition, there are IgM–NAbs that specifically recognize erythrocytes with cell membrane-associated changes due to senescence or from damage by experimental treatment with the protease, bromalein (Cox and Hardy, 1985; Mercolino et al., 1986; Hardy and Hayakawa, 2005). These antibodies are reported to recognize a determinant involving PtC, although it is unclear whether the accessibility of this PtC-associated red cell epitope results from oxidative modification, or due to loss of erythrocyte membrane proteins. Red cell membrane intrinsic proteins have also been implicated as antigenic targets for IgG–NAbs (Lutz, 2012). Notably, as red cells have neither mitochondria nor nuclei, these cells do not undergo the same apoptosis-associated metabolic changes seen in conventional mitochondria-containing cells. This may explain why PC-related antigens are not prominently displayed on erythrocytes as a consequence of aging. Taken together, the cumulative data suggest that the IgM repertoire may include a range of distinct subsets of autoreactive NAbs, which recognize different cell types affected by apoptosis, injury and senescence, and these NAbs may help to regulate the clearance of different cell types and tissue remodeling as well as modulate innate immune responses.

EFFECTS OF PC-SPECIFIC NATURAL IgM ON TOLL-LIKE RECEPTOR-INDUCED INFLAMMATION

Earlier studies have shown that C1q can directly binding to AC membranes and then serve as an "eat-me" signal for the phagocytic clearance of these dying cells (Korb and Ahearn, 1997; Navratil et al., 2001; Ogden et al., 2001). In explanation, C1q may directly interact with externalized PS on these damaged cells (Paidassi et al., 2008). In some settings, the deposition of C1q onto ACs can subsequently have an immunomodulatory effect and inhibit the secretion of proinflammatory cytokines, although by itself these effects are limited (Fraser et al., 2009). Similar properties have also been associated with the mannose-binding lectin (MBL), which triggers the lectin pathway of complement activation. MBL is structurally related to C1q and these two recognition molecules share a common ancestral genetic origin (Matsushita et al., 2004). Furthermore, MBL can also bind directly to ACs. This may suggest that initiation of apoptosis is associated with a change in the distribution of high-mannose glycoconjugates on the cell membrane (Stuart et al., 2005). These findings are consistent with reports that phagocytes of C1q-deficient mice, as well as MBL-deficient mice, display defects in AC clearance (Quartier et al., 2005; Stuart et al., 2005).

The potential roles of T15 IgM–NAb have been investigated in the innate immune responses of professional phagocytes. As mentioned above, while this IgM natural antibody does not bind healthy cells it can specifically recognize exposed PC determinants on ACs and form complexes (Chen et al., 2009a,b). In turn, these AC–IgM complexes have greatly enhanced capacity to recruit the early complement factors, C1q and the structurally related MBL, at levels several-fold higher than in the absence of bound IgM. Notably the recruitment of C1q or MBL by IgM–NAb complexes greatly amplifies the capacity for AC phagocytic clearance (Chen et al., 2009a,b; illustrated in **Figure 1**). These properties are explained by reports that some polymeric IgM, when bound to their cognate antigen, are highly efficient at recruitment of C1q, while other studies have shown that polymeric IgM themselves can contain high mannose glycoconjugates (Arnold et al., 2006). Hence, AC-reactive polymeric IgM may serve to integrate these complement associated innate immune functions (Quartier et al., 2005; Chen et al., 2009a,b).

The formation of IgM–NAb complexes with ACs can also result in strong suppression of *in vivo* and *in vitro* inflammatory responses, including those induced by ligands for both membrane-associated and endosomal Toll-like receptors (TLRs), which include TLR3, TLR4, TLR7, and TLR9 (Chen et al., 2009b). These activities are also dependent on the recruitment of C1q and MBL, which are postulated to serve as bridging molecules that trigger phagocyte functions in a way that does not require activation of the complement cascade (Chen et al., 2009a,b). Hence, both the enhancement of apoptotic clearance and the down-modulation of inflammatory responses are therefore pathways by which some NAbs may augment and amplify housekeeping functions that serve to protect the host.

EFFECTS OF THE APOPTOTIC CELL-SPECIFIC NAb–IgM ON IMMUNE COMPLEX DRIVEN PATHOGENESIS

During autoimmune pathogenesis high-affinity IgG autoantibodies can make direct contributions by multiple mechanisms

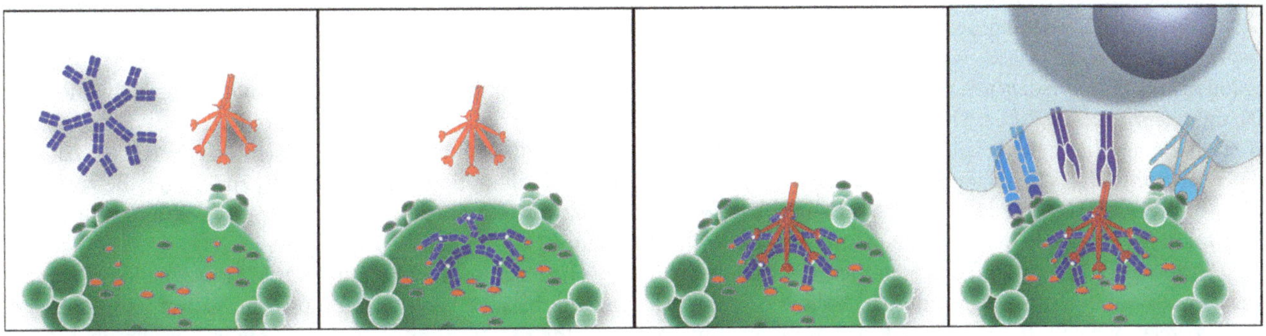

FIGURE 1 | Model of an IgM–NAb complex that enhances interactions between an apoptotic cell and professional phagocytes. In this idealized model, apoptotic death results in membrane alterations that expose a range of neo-determinants. PC-associated membrane determinants are recognized by antigen-binding sites of a pentameric IgM. Binding of PC determinants results in conformational changes in the mu constant regions, which expose a conformational site responsible for recruitment of the globular heads of C1q (Czajkowsky and Shao, 2009). Alternatively, MBL binds to nearby high mannose N-linked glycoconjugates on mu-associated sites (not shown). This polymeric IgM–C1q complex is involved in generating or stabilizing interactions with receptors on professional phagocytes, which enhance apoptotic phagocytosis and blocks inflammatory responses.

(reviewed in Elkon and Casali, 2008; Lleo et al., 2010). Central to these pathways, many IgG autoantibodies implicated in systemic autoimmune diseases form immune complexes (ICs) with their target antigen, which alter their potential interactions with the host immune system. In sera of patients with conditions such as SLE and Sjogren's syndrome, nucleic acid-recognizing autoantibodies can form ICs with their antigens, ribonucleoproteins, or deoxyribonucleoproteins. These ICs can deposit in tissues such as the kidney, skin, and joints and drive local inflammation and tissue injury by triggering complement cascades (reviewed in Bagavant and Fu, 2009). IgG-ICs might additionally serve as a delivery system to transport self-antigens to endosomal pattern-recognition receptors (PRRs) via uptake by activating Fc receptors. Studies by Marshak-Rothstein, Rifkin, and Rönnblom have demonstrated that DNA or RNA-containing ICs consisting of IgG autoantibodies bound to nuclear debris from dying cells can activate mouse B cells (Leadbetter et al., 2002), conventional dendritic cells (DCs; Boulé et al., 2004), and plasmacytoid DCs (Yasuda et al., 2007) as well as human peripheral blood mononuclear cells (Lövgren et al., 2004). These IgG-nucleic acid ICs can interact with rheumatoid factor autoantibody-bearing B cells (Leadbetter et al., 2002) or with DCs bearing activating FcγR, which enables the delivery to otherwise inaccessible intracellular compartments. The outcome of this targeted DNA/RNA internalization is the activation of PRRs of the innate immune system, such as the nucleic acid-recognizing TLRs; TLR7 (activated by ssRNA) and TLR8 and TLR9 (activated by DNA). IgG antibodies to the citrullinated self-protein, fibrinogen, which are prevalent in rheumatoid arthritis patients, have also been shown *in vitro* to activate macrophages through a co-stimulatory pathway involving both FcγR and TLR4 (Sokolove et al., 2011).

The pathogenic influence of IgG autoantibody-ICs can be opposed by IgM natural antibodies to ACs. *In vivo* studies have shown that administration of anti-PC natural IgM greatly attenuated disease severity in a murine model of collagen-induced arthritis (CIA; Chen et al., 2009a). In this model, immunization with xenogenic collagen II emulsified in complete Freund's adjuvant induces a pathogenic autoimmune response to type II collagen (Terato et al., 1992; Nandakumar et al., 2003), with tissue injury in part mediated through the activating Fc-γ receptors (Kleinau et al., 2000). Infusions of IgM–NAbs to ACs also blocked the disease process induced by passive transfer of anti-type II collagen autoantibodies (Chen et al., 2009a), in which inflammatory arthritis is mediated by FcγR and innate immune cells, while lymphocytes do not play central roles (Terato et al., 1992; Nandakumar et al., 2003).

In vitro studies have shown that anti-AC IgM antibodies can directly block the activating effects of lupus-associated IgG autoantibodies on bone marrow-derived DCs (Vas et al., 2012). In fact, the inflammatory effects of both anti-DNA and -RNA IgG-nucleic acid ICs in myeloid DCs were inhibited with suppression of the secretion of inflammatory cytokines IL-6 and TNF-α (Vas et al., 2012). This IgM–NAb also suppressed IC-mediated induction of cell surface expression of CD80 and CD86, as well as CD40 and other co-stimulatory molecules.

NATURAL ANTIBODY REGULATORY PATHWAYS THAT MODULATE INFLAMMATORY AND AUTOIMMUNE DISEASES

Serologic surveys of a large cohort of well-characterized SLE patients have further evaluated the potential clinical relevance of IgM autoantibodies to defined oxidation-associated antigenic-specificities, including the apoptosis-associated neo-antigens, PC and MDA. In the lupus cohort, levels of both of these types of IgM autoantibodies were significantly higher compared to healthy adult controls (Grönwall et al., 2012a). Importantly, higher levels of IgM anti-PC correlated with less long-term organ damage, as defined by the SLICC/ACR damage index score, as well as lower disease activity as assessed by the SELENA revision of the SLE disease activity index (SLEDAI) at the time of visit. IgM anti-PC levels also correlated with an absence of cardiovascular events, while there were no associations with renal disease (Grönwall et al., 2012a). These results are consistent with a previous report from a smaller cohort of Swedish patients (Su et al., 2008) and with studies showing that lower IgM anti-PC levels are associated with more frequent cardiovascular events in non-autoimmune patients (de Faire et al., 2010; Fiskesund et al., 2010). These findings were in fact predicted by earlier studies in atherosclerosis-prone mice (Shaw et al., 2000). Indeed, pneumococcal vaccination, which induces PC-specific antibody responses, was shown to arrest plaque progression in LDL receptor-deficient mice with cholesterol levels over 1000 mg/dl (Binder et al., 2003). These findings have therefore further strengthened the hypothesis that some anti-AC IgM–NAbs can play protective roles in inflammatory disease.

Yet not every IgM–NAb that recognizes ACs may have equivalent clinical implications. In fact, levels of antibodies to PC and to MDA showed significant differences in their associations with lupus clinical manifestations. IgM anti-MDA showed only weak inverse correlations with the SLICC/ACR damage index but not the SELENA-SLEDAI score and there were also no significant associations with renal disease or cardiovascular events (Grönwall et al., 2012a). These studies also showed that higher levels of the IgM antibody to β2-GPI correlated with less organ damage by SLICC/ACR damage index. Furthermore, patients without renal disease had higher levels of IgM anti-CL, and IgM anti-dsDNA (Grönwall et al., 2012a). This may indicate that higher levels of some IgM antibodies may protect some patients from kidney disease, as suggested in an earlier and more focused report (Mehrani and Petri, 2011). Taken together, these studies refute the notion that circulating IgM autoantibodies are inherently polyreactive. Instead, these data strongly argue that the antigenic fine binding specificity of the IgM determines whether there is an association with protection from certain lupus disease features (Grönwall et al., 2012a). In a recent clinical study, Ajeganova et al. (2011) examined RA patients treated with TNF-α blockers. They observed that levels of PC-specific natural IgM levels were increased in patients treated with TNF-α blockade, while lower anti-PC IgM levels correlated with inferior response to therapeutic intervention for RA disease. Further investigations will be needed to better understand how anti-AC NAbs may modulate the pathogenesis of different autoimmune rheumatic diseases.

MAPK PHOSPHATASE-1 IS REQUIRED FOR NATURAL ANTIBODY SUPPRESSION OF TLR RESPONSES

Investigations of signal transduction pathways have shown that IgM–NAbs to ACs can affect responses induced by agonists for a broad range of TLRs, by inhibition of the mitogen-activated protein kinase (MAPK) signal transduction system, which plays central roles in the induction and resolution of inflammatory responses (Grönwall et al., 2012b). Inflammatory responses can result from the induction of phosphorylation of one or more of the primary MAPKs; ERK1/2, JNK, and particularly p38, which then translocate to the nucleus where it can affect transcriptional regulation. In rheumatoid arthritis, activated (phosphorylated) p38 is increased in the RA synovium. However, despite evidence that small molecule p38 inhibitors have been effective in mouse models of inflammatory arthritis, efficacy in humans has been limited, which has suggested that an alternate approach to MAPK inhibition may provide greater clinical benefits (reviewed in Hammaker and Firestein, 2010).

To assess the potential relevance of this type of immunomodulatory NAb to clinical autoimmune diseases, the activity of the PC-specific IgM–NAb was also tested in a system in which inflammatory responses are induced by lupus IgG autoantibodies (Vas et al., 2012). These studies demonstrated that this natural IgM inhibited p38 phosphorylation induced in DCs by nucleic acid-containing IgG autoantibody ICs (Vas et al., 2012). Notably, this inhibitory pathway also blocked the nuclear accumulation of the activated primary MAPKs in myeloid DCs (Vas et al., 2012). *In vitro* studies of murine bone marrow-derived DCs confirmed that this inhibition was entirely dependent on the recruitment of either C1q or MBL (Grönwall et al., 2012b; illustrated in **Figure 1**).

The magnitude and duration of MAPK signaling is dependent on the balance between the upstream activators of the system and the deactivation of these kinases by specific phosphatases. Based on evidence that this NAb could affect the activation of each of the three primary MAPKs (Grönwall et al., 2012b), studies were therefore performed that assessed the potential involvement of the regulatory MAPK phosphatases (MKPs), also known as dual-specificity phosphatases (DUSPs). These studies highlighted the role of MKP-1, the archetype for the family, which can serve as the counter-regulatory factor for all three of the primary MAPKs (reviewed in Liu et al., 2007). In fact, the anti-AC IgM-mediated blockade of TLR-mediated MAPK signaling had an absolute requirement for the expression of MKP-1 (Grönwall et al., 2012b). In DCs activated by TLR agonists, the addition of the anti-AC IgM, in the presence of C1q or MBL in serum-free media, resulted in induction within minutes of MKP-1 at a transcript and a protein level, and it rapidly became localized within the nucleus (Grönwall et al., 2012b). Using deconvolutional immunofluorescence microscopy, NAb-mediated MKP-1 accumulation correlated with a reciprocal impairment in the phosphorylation and nuclear translocation of the activated primary MAPK protein molecules. To investigate the relative contribution of MKP-1 to NAb-mediated suppression, responses were compared in DCs from wild-type or MKP-1-deficient mice (Grönwall et al., 2012b). Such MKP-1-deficient mice are reported to exhibit overexuberant inflammatory responses, but no other immune developmental abnormalities (Dorfman et al., 1996; Salojin et al., 2006). These studies confirmed the absolute requirement for MKP-1 for IgM–NAb-mediated inhibition of TLR responses from DCs (Grönwall et al., 2012b).

CONCLUDING REMARKS

One of the most fundamental challenges faced by the immune system is the efficient recognition and clearance of the body's own cells, which because of senescence or injury enter programmed cell death pathways. While cells dying of apoptotic death pathways do not pose an immediate risk to the host, if these cell corpses are not efficiently removed there is the risk of progression to secondary necrosis. This can lead to the loss of integrity of cell membranes with release of cytoplasmic and nuclear components that can serve as ligands for proinflammatory cellular receptors, and the triggering of autoimmune responses. Hence, throughout the lifespan of multicellular organisms, there is an absolute need for the clearance of the immense number of cell corpses that are generated each day, even in health. As a direct consequence, the immune system has developed a redundant layering of superimposed mechanisms. Hence, the control of apoptotic clearance is intertwined with the regulation and resolution of inflammatory responses.

At birth, humans already have substantial levels of circulating IgM antibodies, which reflect a functional B cell compartment poised and ready to contribute to neonatal host defenses. These IgM antibodies arise in the womb from neonatal B lymphocytes that express clonally distributed BCRs. However, evidence of recurrent clones suggests that this early B cell repertoire may be affected by *in vivo* clonal selection that may be a response to evolutionary pressure to provide important housekeeping functions related to apoptotic clearance and avoidance of excessive and damaging inflammatory responses.

IgM-mediated protection from autoimmune disease was first demonstrated in mice deficient in the capacity to secrete IgM antibodies, as these mice were found to develop pathologic autoimmunity with the production of lupus IgG autoantibodies (Boes et al., 2000; Ehrenstein et al., 2000). Furthermore, in mice predisposed to the development of lupus-like disease, a bias toward secretion of monomeric IgM and lower levels of polymeric IgM can result in accelerated development of lupus-like disease (Youd et al., 2004). It may therefore be relevant that 8% of a cohort of 300 SLE patients were recently reported to have selective deficiency in serum IgM (Perrazio et al., 2012).

Our studies demonstrated that anti-AC IgM–NAbs, present from early in life, can suppress inflammatory responses mediated by phagocytic cells by induction of MKP-1, which in other settings have been shown to have potent regulatory roles for the MAPK system. MKP-1 is well known for its many counter-regulatory roles, which include the late negative feedback of responses to LPS stimulation, the blunting of responses after rapid re-exposure to a TLR agonist such as LPS tolerance, as well as contributing to the anti-inflammatory properties of glucocorticoids (reviewed in Liu et al., 2007). These studies also documented an additive effect of anti-AC IgM–NAb and dexamethasone for early MKP-1 induction and inhibition of LPS-induced p38 MAPK activation that, when combined, exceeded the maximum effects of either agent alone (Grönwall et al., 2012b). In part, this is likely explained by the additive integration of separate signals received via distinct cell membrane-associated receptors triggered by dexamethasone (i.e., glucocorticoid receptor) or by anti-AC IgM complexes (discussed below). As glucocorticoids are amongst the most widely prescribed treatments for inflammatory and autoimmune diseases, it is indeed intriguing that there is an overlap in the inhibitory signal transduction pathways of glucocorticoids and by the formation of regulatory ICs with early complement recognition factors that are coordinated in their organization by IgM autoantibodies to oxidation-associated neo-determinants on ACs.

Fundamental to the inhibitory effects of regulatory NAbs, polymeric IgMs that bind ACs can express constant regions with multiple sites for recruitment of C1q, and the Fcμ of some IgM–NAbs also have high mannose glycoconjugates on that bind MBL (Chen et al., 2009a,b). The potential properties of such complexes suggested by studies with targeted deficiencies in C1q, MBL, or secreted IgM, which each have impaired control of inflammatory responses, and in some cases are predisposed to the development of autoimmune disease (Botto et al., 1998; Boes et al., 2000; Ehrenstein et al., 2000; Stuart et al., 2005). Furthermore, we have previously shown that the complement-dependent immunomodulatory properties of anti-AC IgM, while the recruitment of C1q or MBL was essential, there was no absolute requirement for downstream activation of the complement cascade (Chen et al., 2009a).

These IgM–NAbs to AC-associated determinants can regulate responses mediated by diverse TLRs, an ancient type of innate immune receptor that was first characterized in insects (Lemaitre et al., 1996). Furthermore, mechanistic investigations have shown these effects are linked to modulation of the MAPK signaling system, which is one of the earliest evolutionarily conserved pathways of immunity, being present in plants and mammals (Asai et al., 2002). Likewise, MKP-1 orthologs have also been described in protozoans (Moncho-Amor et al., 2011), and as mentioned above, mice with MKP-1 deficiency have severe defects in the control of innate responses (Salojin et al., 2006). These regulatory properties are expressed by a class of naturally occurring autoreactive antibodies that are postulated to come from the most primitive tier of B cells in the adaptive immune system (Kantor and Herzenberg, 1993).

As ACs are ubiquitous, we wonder whether the high frequency of these innate-like NAb-producing clones in the "preimmune" repertoire in part reflects positive selection of the B-1 cell clones that are reactive with membrane-associated neo-determinants on cells wasted during development. The protective properties of anti-AC NAbs may be mediated by a previously unknown regulatory signaling pathway, which integrates and coordinates the influence of select innate immune factors on myeloid cell function.

ACKNOWLEDGMENTS

Work in our lab was supported by grants from the NIH; R01AI090118, R01 AI068063 and ARRA supplement, R01AI090118, and from the ACR REF Within Our Reach campaign, the Alliance for Lupus Research, the Arthritis Foundation, and the P. Robert Majumder Charitable Trust.

REFERENCES

Ajeganova, S., Fiskesund, R., de Faire, U., Hafström, I., and Frostegård, J. (2011). Effect of biological therapy on levels of atheroprotective antibodies against phosphorylcholine and apolipoproteins in rheumatoid arthritis – a one year study. *Clin. Exp. Rheumatol.* 29, 942–950.

Alugupalli, K. R., and Abraham, D. (2009). B cell multitasking is required to control nematode infection. *Immunity* 230, 317–319.

Arnold, J. N., Dwek, R. A., Rudd, P. M., and Sim, R. B. (2006). Mannan binding lectin and its interaction with immunoglobulins in health and in disease. *Immunol. Lett.* 106, 103–110.

Asai, T, Tena, G., Plotnikova, J., Willmann, M. R., Chiu, W. L., Gomez-Gomez, L., et al. (2002). MAP kinase signalling cascade in *Arabidopsis* innate immunity. *Nature* 415, 977–983.

Bagavant, H., and Fu, S. M. (2009). Pathogenesis of kidney disease in systemic lupus erythematosus. *Curr. Opin. Rheumatol.* 21, 489–494.

Batista, B. S., Eng, W. S., Pilobello, K. T., Hendricks-Muñoz, K. D., and Mahal, L. K. (2011). Identification of a conserved glycan signature for microvesicles. *J. Proteome Res.* 10, 4624–4633.

Baumgarth, N. (2011). The double life of a B-1 cell: self-reactivity selects for protective effector functions. *Nat. Rev. Immunol.* 11, 34–46.

Binder, C. J., Horkko, S., Dewan, A., Chang, M.-K., Kieu, E. P., Goodyear, C. S., et al. (2003). Pneumococcal vaccination decreases atherosclerotic lesion formation: molecular mimicry between *Streptococcus pneumoniae* and oxidized LDL. *Nat. Med.* 9, 736–743.

Boes, M., Schmidt, T., Linkemann, K., Beaudette, B. C., Marshak-Rothstein,

A., and Chen, J. (2000). Accelerated development of IgG autoantibodies and autoimmune disease in the absence of secreted IgM. *Proc. Natl. Acad. Sci. U.S.A.* 97, 1184–1189.

Botto, M., Dell'Agnola, C., Bygrave, A. E., Thompson, E. M., Cook, H. T., Petry, F., et al. (1998). Homozygous C1q deficiency causes glomerulonephritis associated with multiple apoptotic bodies. *Nat. Genet.* 19, 56–59.

Boulé, M. W., Broughton, C., Mackay, F., Akira, S., Marshak-Rothstein, A., and Rifkin, I. R. (2004). Toll-like receptor 9-dependent and -independent dendritic cell activation by chromatin–immunoglobulin G complexes. *J. Exp. Med.* 199, 1631–1640.

Cappione, A. III, Anolik, J. H., Pugh-Bernard, A., Barnard, J., Dutcher, P., Silverman, G, J., et al. (2005). Germinal center exclusion of autoreactive B cells is defective in human systemic lupus erythematosus. *J. Clin. Invest.* 115, 3205–3216.

Casali, P., and Notkins, A. L. (1989). Probing the human B-cell prertoire with EBV: polyreactive antibodies and CD5$^+$ lymphocytes. *Annu. Rev. Immunol.* 7, 513–535.

Chen, Y., Khanna, S., Goodyear, C. S., Park, Y. B., Raz, E., Thiel, S., et al. (2009a). Regulation of dendritic cells and macrophages by an anti-apoptotic cell natural antibody that suppresses TLR responses and inhibits inflammatory arthritis. *J. Immunol.* 183, 1346–1359.

Chen, Y., Park, Y. B., Patel, E., and Silverman, G. J. (2009b). IgM antibodies to apoptosis-associated determinants recruit C1q and enhance dendritic cell phagocytosis of apoptotic cells. *J. Immunol.* 182, 6031–6043.

Chou, M. Y., Fogelstrand, L., Hartvigsen, K., Hansen, L. F., Woelkers, D., Shaw, P. X., et al. (2009). Oxidation-specific epitopes are dominant targets of innate natural antibodies in mice and humans. *J. Clin. Invest.* 119, 1335–1349.

Cong, Y. Z., Rabin, E., and Wortis, H. H. (1991). Treatment of murine CD5$^-$ B cells with anti-Ig, but not LPS, induces surface CD5: two activation pathways. *Int. Immunol.* 3, 467–476.

Cox, K. O., and Hardy, S. J. (1985). Autoantibodies against mouse bromelain-modified RBC are specifically inhibited by a common membrane phospholipid, phosphatidylcholine. *Immunology* 55, 263–269.

Czajkowsky, D. M., and Shao, Z. (2009).The human IgM pentamer is a mushroom-shaped molecule with a flexural bias. *Proc. Natl. Acad. Sci. U.S.A.* 106, 14960–14965.

Davies, D. R., Padlan, E. A., and Segal, D. M. (1975). Three-dimensional structure of immunoglobulins. *Annu. Rev. Biochem.* 44, 639–667.

de Faire, U., Su, J., Hua, X., Frostegård, A., Halldin, M., Hellenius, M.-L., et al. (2010). Low levels of IgM antibodies to phosphorylcholine predict cardiovascular disease in 60-year old men: effects on uptake of oxidized LDL in macrophages as a potential mechanism. *J. Autoimmun.* 34, 73–79.

Dorfman, K., Carrasco, D., Gruda, M., Ryan, C., Lira, S. A., and Bravo, R. (1996). Disruption of the erp/mkp-1 gene does not affect mouse development: normal MAP kinase activity in ERP/MKP-1-deficient fibroblasts. *Oncogene* 13, 925–931.

Du Pasquier, L., Robert, J., Courtet, M., and Mußmann, R. (2000). B-cell development in the amphibian *Xenopus. Immunol. Rev.* 175, 201–213.

Ehrenstein, M. R., Cook, H. T., and Neuberger, M. S. (2000) Deficiency in serum immunoglobulin (Ig)M predisposes to development of IgG autoantibodies. *J. Exp. Med.* 19, 1253–1258.

Elkon, K., and Casali, P. (2008). Nature and functions of autoantibodies. *Nat. Clin. Pract. Rheumatol.* 4, 491–498.

Feeney, A. J. (1991). Predominance of the T15 anti-phosphorylcholine junctional sequence in neonatal pre-B cell. *J. Immunol.* 147, 4343–4350.

Feeney, A. J. (1992). Predominance of VH-D-JH junctions occurring at sites of short sequence homology results in limited junctional diversity in neonatal antibodies. *J. Immunol.* 149, 222–229.

Feizi, T. (1988). Carbohydrate structures as onco-developmental antigens and components of receptor systems. *Adv. Exp. Med. Biol.* 228, 317–329.

Ferry, H., Potter, P. K., Crockford, T. L., Nijnik, A., Ehrenstein, M. R., Walport, M. J., et al. (2007). Increased positive selection of B1 cells and reduced B cell tolerance to intracellular antigens in c1q-deficient mice. *J. Immunol.* 178, 2916–2922.

Fiskesund, R., Stegmayr, B., Hallmans, G., Vikström, M., Weinehall, L., de Faire, U., et al. (2010). Low levels of antibodies against phosphorylcholine predict development of stroke in a population-based study from Northern Sweden. *Stroke* 41, 607–612.

Flajnik, M., and Rumfelt, L. (2000). Early and natural antibodies in non-mammalian vertebrates. *Curr. Top. Microbiol. Immunol.* 252, 233–240.

Fraser, D. A., Laust, A. K., Nelson, E. L., and Tenner, A. J. (2009). C1q differentially modulates phagocytosis and cytokine responses during ingestion of apoptotic cells by human monocytes, macrophages, and dendritic cells. *J. Immunol.* 183, 6175–6185.

Friedman, P., Horkko, S., Steinberg, D., Witztum, J. L., and Dennis, E. A. (2002). Correlation of antiphospholipid antibody recognition with the structure of synthetic oxidized phospholipids. Importance of Schiff base formation and aldol condensation. *J. Biol. Chem.* 277, 7010–7020.

Griffin, D. O., Holodick, N. E., and Rothstein, T. L. (2011). Human B1 cells in umbilical cord and adult peripheral blood express the novel phenotype CD20$^+$CD27$^+$ CD43$^+$CD70$^-$. *J. Exp. Med.* 208, 67–80.

Grillot-Courvalin, C., Brouet, J.-C., Labaume, S., Piller, F., Rassenti, L. Z., Silverman, G. J., et al. (1992). An anti-B cell autoantibody from Wiskott-Aldrich syndrome which recognizes i blood group specificity on normal human B cells. *Eur. J. Immunol.* 22, 1781–1788.

Grönwall, C., Akhter, E., Oh, C., Burlingame, R. W., Petri, M., and Silverman, G. J. (2012a). IgM autoantibodies to distinct apoptosis-associated antigens correlate with protection from cardiovascular events and renal disease in patients with SLE. *Clin. Immunol.* 142, 390–398.

Grönwall, C., Chen, Y., Vas, J., Khanna, S., Thiel, S., Corr, M., et al. (2012b). MAPK phosphatase-1 is required for regulatory natural autoantibody-mediated inhibition of TLR responses. *Proc. Natl. Acad. Sci. U.S.A.* 109, 19745–19750.

Hammaker, D., and Firestein, G. S. (2010). "Go upstream, young man": lessons learned from the p38 saga. *Ann. Rheum. Dis.* 69, i77–i82.

Hardy, R. R. (2006). B-1 B cell development. *J. Immunol.* 177, 2749–2754.

Hardy, R. R., and Hayakawa, K. (2005). Development of B cells producing natural autoantibodies to thymocytes and senescent erythrocytes. *Springer Semin. Immunopathol.* 26, 363–375.

Hayakawa, K., Asano, M., Shinton, S. A., Gui, M., Allman, D., Stewart, C. L., et al. (1999). Positive selection of natural autoreactive B cells. *Science* 285, 113–116.

Jackson, K. J., Wang, Y., Gaeta, B. A., Pomat, W., Siba, P., Rimmer, J., et al. (2012). Divergent human populations show extensive shared IGK rearrangements in peripheral blood B cells. *Immunogenetics* 64, 3–14.

Jenne, C. N., Kennedy, L. J., and Reynolds, J. D. (2006). Antibody repertoire development in the sheep. *Dev. Comp. Immunol.* 30, 165–174.

Kantor, A. B., and Herzenberg, L. A. (1993). Origin of murine B lineages. *Annu. Rev. Immunol.* 11, 501–538.

Kearney, J. F. (2005). Innate-like B cells. *Springer Semin. Immunopathol.* 26, 377–383.

Kearney, J. F., Barletta, R., Quan, Z. S., and Quintáns, J. (1981). Monoclonal vs. heterogeneous anti-H-8 antibodies in the analysis of the anti- phosphorylcholine response in BALB/c mice. *Eur. J. Immunol.* 11, 877–883.

Kleinau, S., Martinsson, P., and Heyman, B. (2000). Induction and suppression of collagen-induced arthritis is dependent on distinct fcgamma receptors. *J. Exp. Med.* 191, 1611–1616.

Kobie, J. J., Alcena, D. C., Zheng, B., Bryk, P., Mattiacio, J. L., Brewer, M., et al. (2012). 9G4 autoreactivity is increased in HIV-infected patients and correlates with HIV broadly neutralizing serum activity. *PLoS ONE* 7:e35356. doi: 10.1371/journal.pone.0035356

Korb, L. C., and Ahearn, J. M. (1997). C1q binds directly and specifically to surface blebs of apoptotic human keratinocytes: complement deficiency and systemic lupus erythematosus revisited. *J. Immunol.* 158, 4525–4528.

Kulik, L., Fleming, S. D., Moratz, C., Reuter, J. W., Novikov, A., Chen, K., et al. (2009). Pathogenic natural antibodies recognizing annexin IV are required to develop intestinal ischemia-reperfusion injury. *J. Immunol.* 182, 5363–5373.

Leadbetter, E. A., Rifkin, I. R., Hohlbaum, A. M., Beaudette, B. C., Shlomchik, M. J., and Marshak-Rothstein, A. (2002). Chromatin–IgG complexes activate B cells by dual engagement of IgM and Toll-like receptors. *Nature* 416, 603–607.

Lemaitre, B., Nicolas, E., Michaut, L., Reichhart, J. M., and Hoffmann, J. A. (1996). The dorsoventral regulatory gene cassette spätzle/Toll/cactus controls the potent antifungal response in *Drosophila* adults. *Cell* 86, 973–983.

Liu, Y., Shepherd, E. G., and Nelin, L. D. (2007). MAPK phosphatases: regulating the immune response. *Nat. Rev. Immunol.* 7, 202–212.

Lleo, A., Invernizzi, P., Gao, B., Podda, M., and Gershwin, M. E. (2010). Definition of human autoimmunity – autoantibodies versus autoimmune disease. *Autoimmun. Rev.* 9, A259–A266.

Lövgren, T., Eloranta, M.-L., Båve, U., Alm, G. V., and Rönnblom, L. (2004). Induction of interferon-α production in plasmacytoid dendritic cells by immune complexes containing nucleic acid released by necrotic or late apoptotic cells and lupus IgG. *Arthritis Rheum.* 50, 1861–1872.

Lutz, H. U. (ed.) (2012). *Naturally Occurring Antibodies (NAbs).* Austin, TX: Lands Bioscience.

Masmoudi, H., Mota-Santos, T., Huetz, F., Coutinho, A., and Cazenave, P. A. (1990). All T15 Id-positive antibodies (but not of VHT15$^+$ antibodies) are produced by peritoneal CD5$^+$ B lymphocytes. *Int. Immunol.* 2, 515–520.

Matsushita, M., Matsushita, A., Endo, Y., Nakata, M., Kojima, N., Mizuochi, T., et al. (2004). Origin of the classical complement pathway: lamprey orthologue of mammalian C1q acts as a lectin. *Proc. Natl. Acad. Sci. U.S.A.* 101, 10127–10131.

Mehrani, T., and Petri, M. (2011). IgM anti-ß2 glycoprotein I is protective against lupus nephritis and renal damage in systemic lupus erythematosus. *J. Rheumatol.* 38, 450–453.

Mercolino, T. J., Arnold, L. W., and Haughton, G. (1986). Phosphatidyl choline is recognized by a series of Ly-1$^+$ murine B cell lymphomas specific for erythrocyte membranes. *J. Exp. Med.* 163, 155–165.

Mi, Q. S., Zhou, L., Schulze, D. H., Fischer, R. T., Lustig, A., Rezanka, L. J., et al. (2000). Highly reduced protection against *Streptococcus pneumoniae* after deletion of a single heavy chain gene in mouse. *Proc. Natl. Acad. Sci. U.S.A.* 97, 6031–6036.

Moncho-Amor, V., Galardi-Castilla, M., Perona, R., and Sastre, L. (2011). The dual-specificity protein phosphatase MkpB, homologous to mammalian MKP phosphatases, is required for *D. discoideum* post-aggregative development and cisplatin response. *Differentiation* 81, 199–207.

Nandakumar, K. S., Svensson, L., and Holmdahl, R. (2003). Collagen type II-specific monoclonal antibody-induced arthritis in mice: description of the disease and the influence of age, sex, and genes. *Am. J. Pathol.* 163, 1827–1837.

Navratil, J. S., Watkins, S. C., Wisnieski, J. J., and Ahearn, J. M. (2001). The globular heads of C1q specifically recognize surface blebs of apoptotic vascular endothelial cells. *J. Immunol.* 166, 3231–3239.

Ogden, C. A., Decathelineau, A., Hoffmann, P. R., Bratton, D., Ghebrehiwet, B., Fadok, V. A., et al. (2001). C1q and mannose binding lectin engagement of cell surface calreticulin and CD91 initiates macropinocytosis and uptake of apoptotic cells. *J. Exp. Med.* 194, 781–795.

Paidassi, H., Tacnet-Delorme, P., Garlatti, V., Darnault, C., Ghebrehiwet, B., Gaboriaud, C., et al. (2008). C1q binds phosphatidylserine and likely acts as a multiligand-bridging molecule in apoptotic cell recognition. *J. Immunol.* 180, 2329–2338.

Pascual, V., and Capra, J. D. (1992). VH4-21, a human VH gene segment overrepresented in the autoimmune repertoire. *Arthritis Rheum.* 35, 11–18.

Pascual, V., Victor, K., Lelsz, D., Spellerberg, M., Hamblin, T., Thompson, K., et al. (1991). Nucleotide sequence analysis of the V regions of two IgM cold agglutinins. Evidence that the VH4-21 gene segment is responsible for the major cross-reactive idiotype. *J. Immunol.* 146, 4385–4391.

Perlmutter, R., Kearney, J., Chang, S., and Hood, L. (1985). Developmentally controlled expression of immunoglobulin VH genes. *Science* 227, 1597–1601.

Perrazio, S. F., Salomao, R., Silva, N. P., Carneiro-Sampaio, M., and Andrade, L. E. C. (2012). Serial screening shows that 28% of systemic lupus erythematosus adult patients carry an underlying primary immunodeficiency. *Arthritis Rheum.* 64, S284.

Pugh-Bernard, A. E., Silverman, G. J., Cappione, A. J., Villano, M. E., Ryan, D. H., Insel, R. A., et al. (2001). Regulation of inherently autoreactive VH4-34 B cells in the maintenance of human B cell tolerance. *J. Clin. Invest.* 108, 1061–1070.

Quartier, P., Potter, P. K., Ehrenstein, M. R., Walport, M. J., and Botto, M. (2005). Predominant role of IgM-dependent activation of the classical pathway in the clearance of dying cells by murine bone marrow-derived macrophages *in vitro*. *Eur. J. Immunol.* 35, 252–260.

Rogosch, T., Kerzel, S., Hoß, K., Hoersch, G., Zemlin, C., Heckmann, M., et al. (2012). IgA response in preterm neonates shows little evidence of antigen-driven selection. *J. Immunol.* 189, 5449–5456.

Salojin, K. V., Owusu, I. B., Millerchip, K. A., Potter, M., Platt, K. A., and Oravecz, T. (2006). Essential role of MAPK phosphatase-1 in the negative control of innate immune responses. *J. Immunol.* 176, 1899–1907.

Schroeder, H., Hillson, J., and Perlmutter, R. (1987). Early restriction of the human antibody repertoire. *Science* 238, 791–793.

Schroeder, H. W., and Wang, J. Y. (1990). Preferential utilization of conserved immunoglobulin heavy chain variable gene segments during human fetal life. *Proc. Natl. Acad. Sci. U.S.A.* 87, 6146–6150.

Seidl, K. J., MacKenzie, J. D., Wang, D., Kantor, A. B., Kabat, E. A., Herzenberg L. A., et al. (1997). Frequent occurrence of dentical heavy, and light chain Ig rearrangements. *Int. Immunol.* 9, 689–670.

Shaw, P. X., Hörkkö, S., Chang, M.-K., Curtiss, L. K., Palinski, W., Silverman, G. J., et al. (2000). Natural antibodies with the T15 idiotype may act in atherosclerosis, apoptotic clearance, and protective immunity. *J. Clin. Invest.* 105,1731–1740.

Shaw, P. X., Goodyear, C. S., Chang, M. K., Witztum, J. L., and Silverman, G. J. (2003). The autoreactivity of anti-phosphorylcholine antibodies for atherosclerosis-associated neo-antigens and apoptotic cells. *J. Immunol.* 170, 6151–6157.

Silberstein, L., Jefferies, L., Goldman, J., Friedman, D., Moore, J., Nowell, P., et al. (1991). Variable region gene analysis of pathologic human autoantibodies to the related i and I red blood cell antigens. *Blood* 78, 2372–2386.

Silverman, G. J., Chen, P., and Carson, D. (1990). Cold agglutinins: specificity, idiotypy and structural analysis. *Chem. Immunol.* 48, 109–125.

Sokolove, J., Zhao, X., Chandra, P. E., and Robinson, W. H. (2011). Immune complexes containing citrullinated fibrinogen costimulate macrophages via Toll-like receptor 4 and Fcg receptor. *Arthritis Rheum.* 63, 53–62.

Stuart, L. M., Takahashi, K., Shi, L., Savill, J., and Ezekowitz, R. A. (2005). Mannose-binding lectin-deficient mice display defective apoptotic cell clearance but no autoimmune phenotype. *J. Immunol.* 174, 3220–3226.

Su, J., Hua, X., Concha, H., Svenungsson, E., Cederholm, A., and Frostegård, J. (2008). Natural antibodies against phosphorylcholine as potential protective factors in SLE. *Rheumatology* 47, 1144–1150.

Sun, J., Hayward, C., Shinde, R., Christenson, R., Ford, S. P., and Butler, J. E. (1998). Antibody repertoire development in fetal and neonatal piglets. I. Four VH genes account for 80 percent of VH usage during 84 days of fetal life. *J. Immunol.* 161, 5070–5078.

Terato, K., Hasty, K., Reife, R., Cremer, M., Kang, A., and Stuart, J. (1992). Induction of arthritis with monoclonal antibodies to collagen. *J. Immunol.* 148, 2103–2108.

Vas, J., Grönwall, C., Marshak-Rothsein, A., and Silverman, G. J. (2012). Natural antibody to apoptotic cell membranes inhibits the proinflammatory properties of lupus autoantibody immune complexes. *Arthritis Rheum.* 64, 3388–3398.

Wardemann, H., Yurasov, S., Schaefer, A., Young, J. W., Meffre, E., and Nussenzweig, M. C. (2003). Predominant autoantibody production by early human B cell precursors. *Science* 301, 1374–1377.

Yasuda, K., Richez, C., Maciaszek, J. W., Agrawal, N., Akira, S., Marshak-Rothstein, A., et al. (2007). Murine dendritic cell type I IFN production induced by human IgG-RNA immune complexes is IFN regulatory factor (IRF)5 and IRF7 dependent and is required for IL-6 production. *J. Immunol.* 178, 6876–6885.

Youd, M. E., Luus, L., and Corley, R. B. (2004). IgM monomers accelerate disease manifestations in autoimmune-prone Fas-deficient mice. *J. Autoimmun.* 23, 333–343.

Zhang, M., Alicot, E. M., and Carroll, M. C. (2008). Human natural IgM can induce ischemia/reperfusion injury in a murine intestinal model. *Mol. Immunol.* 245, 1036–1039.

11

A temporal model of human IgE and IgG antibody function

Andrew M. Collins* and Katherine J. L. Jackson

School of Biotechnology and Biomolecular Sciences, University of New South Wales, Sydney, NSW, Australia

Edited by:
Ramit Mehr, Bar-Ilan University, Israel

Reviewed by:
Tim L. Manser, Thomas Jefferson University, USA
Ramit Mehr, Bar-Ilan University, Israel
Michal Or-Guil, Humboldt University Berlin, Germany

****Correspondence:***
Andrew M. Collins, School of Biotechnology and Biomolecular Sciences, University of New South Wales, Sydney, NSW 2052, Australia
e-mail: a.collins@unsw.edu.au

The diversity of the human antibody repertoire that is generated by V(D)J gene rearrangement is extended by nine constant region genes that give antibodies their complex array of effector functions. The application of high throughput sequencing to the study of V(D)J gene rearrangements has led to significant recent advances in our understanding of the antigen-binding repertoire. In contrast, our understanding of antibody function has changed little, and mystery still surrounds the existence of four distinctive IgG subclasses. Recent observations from murine models and from human studies of VDJ somatic point mutations suggest that the timing of emergence of cells from the germinal center may vary as a consequence of class switching. This should lead to predictable differences in affinity between isotypes. These differences, and varying abilities of the isotypes to fix complement and bind FcRs, could help coordinate the humoral defenses over the time course of a response. We therefore propose a Temporal Model of human IgE and IgG function in which early emergence of IgE sensitizes sentinel mast cells while switching to IgG3 recruits FcγR-mediated functions to the early response. IgG1 then emerges as the major effector of antigen clearance, and subsequently IgG2 competes with IgG1 to produce immune complexes that slow the inflammatory drive. Persisting antigen may finally stimulate high affinity IgG4 that outcompetes other isotypes and can terminate IgG1/FcγR-mediated activation via the inhibitory FcγRIIB. In this way, IgG antibodies of different subclasses, at different concentrations and with sometimes opposing functions deliver cohesive, protective immune function.

Keywords: IgG subclasses, humoral immunity, class switching, affinity maturation, IgE, antibody function, B cell differentiation

It is almost 50 years since the complete set of human antibody isotypes was first described (1). For over 30 years, associations have been explored between antibody classes and subclasses and the response to particular pathogens (2). And for almost 30 years, the relationships between cytokine production and antibody class switching have been reported (3). Other rich sources of data that have guided thinking about antibody isotype function have been studies of immunodeficiencies, and the disease susceptibilities with which they are associated (2, 4). Yet despite literally thousands of such studies, and despite significant insights into the particularities of humoral immunity, no proposal has emerged that describes how IgG antibody subclasses and other antibody isotypes *work together* to provide protective immune functions. Here we propose a Temporal Model of human IgE and IgG antibody function, in which there is a programed order to the emergence of the different IgG isotypes that reflects their genomic organization, with switching and emergence being promoted or delayed at different critical points through the action of cytokines. We suggest that early in the germinal center reaction, IgM$^+$ B cells switch to both IgE and IgG3. Subsequently, IgG1 cells switch and emerge, followed by IgG2-committed cells and finally, if antigen persists, by IgG4-producing cells.

The Temporal Model has its genesis in recent observations of IgE-switched cells in the mouse. These studies suggest that the IgE response is not usually a late development arising from an expanded clone of IgG-committed cells that develops through the germinal center reaction. Rather, it has been shown that IgE class-switched murine cells usually develop and exit the germinal center reaction in the early phase of an immune response, and that they rapidly differentiate into plasmablasts and plasma cells (5, 6). The IgE-secreting plasma cells carry fewer somatic point mutations in their rearranged V(D)J genes than IgG-secreting plasma cells (6), and as a consequence their secreted antibodies are likely to be of lower affinity.

There can be no doubt that IgE antibodies can also be produced late in a response. Recent studies have confirmed the existence of high affinity IgE, and of sequential switching to IgE within the germinal centers of mice (7, 8). No attempt has been made here to incorporate such late IgE into the model. The functions of secretory IgA in mucosal secretions and of serum IgA are also not considered, but the temporal model provides a coherent view of the separate and joint activities of early IgE and the IgG subclasses.

Reports of early IgE in murine models provide a new perspective from which to consider some unusual features of human IgE antibody gene sequences. We have shown that IgE-associated VDJ genes from non-allergic individuals carry very few somatic point mutations, and some IgE sequences carry no mutations at all (9). In individuals with atopic dermatitis, unmutated sequences have also been seen at relatively high frequency (10). In parasitized individuals, we have seen more highly mutated IgE sequences (11), but these sequences did not carry the pattern of mutations that is considered the mutational signature of antigen selection within the germinal center reaction (12). In some, though not all allergic conditions, IgE sequences also lack this pattern of mutation (9, 10).

These studies can be understood if IgE class switching in humans, as in the mouse, can occur early in the germinal center reaction, and if such switching is rapidly followed by the differentiation of IgE-switched cells into plasmablasts that leave the germinal centers. Some continuing accumulation of somatic point mutations might then take place, outside the germinal centers (13). This would give the mutations in those IgE sequences a distinctly different pattern to that which is seen in IgG sequences that emerge after multiple rounds of selection within the germinal centers. Such selection typically leads to an accumulation of non-synonymous (replacement) mutations in the complementarity determining regions of the antibody genes (12).

In the context of invasion by pathogens, the production of early IgE antibodies could allow widely dispersed mast cells to function as sentinel cells (14), alerting the immune system to further incursions or spread of the pathogens. Early IgE could function in this way, despite its low affinity, because low affinity IgE has been shown to function well on the surface of mast cells and basophils, if it is directed against multiple epitopes on multivalent antigen (15, 16).

If class switching to IgE is rapidly followed by departure of cells from the germinal center, the possibility that switching to other isotypes may lead cells to follow other distinct developmental pathways cannot be ignored. We have therefore reconsidered the functions of human IgG subclasses, and this has been done in the light of our observations of somatic point mutations in antibodies of different IgG subclasses. These observations provide the broadest possible overview of humoral immunity. In an analysis of almost 1,000 VDJ genes isolated from people living in an area of endemic parasitism, a surprising and statistically significant relationship was seen (11). IgG3-associated VDJ genes were the least mutated VDJ gene sequences, and the mean number of mutations seen in sequences associated with the other subclasses corresponded to the position of each constant region gene within the IGH gene locus. That is, IgG3 < IgG1 < IgG2 < IgG4.

We hypothesize that differences in mean levels of mutation arise because human B cells tend to follow a programed sequence of class switching and departure from the germinal center reaction. We propose that cells first switch from IgM to IgG3, then to IgG1 and to IgG2 and finally to IgG4 following the genomic ordering of the constant region genes (**Figure 1**). This is not to deny the reality of alternative switch pathways under the influence of particular cytokines (17). We propose that class switching is driven by underlying probabilities, and switching is linked to emergence from the germinal centers, leading to the generalizable sequence of the Temporal Model. Through changes in probabilities associated with the expression of adhesion molecules and chemokine receptors, switching could be closely followed by emergence, or emergence could follow variable periods of proliferation, mutation, and selection within the germinal centers. The model does not attempt to resolve the timing of these events for each isotype.

The Temporal Model has parallels with models of division-linked phenotypic change, including class switching, which suggest that predictable order can emerge from stochastic processes

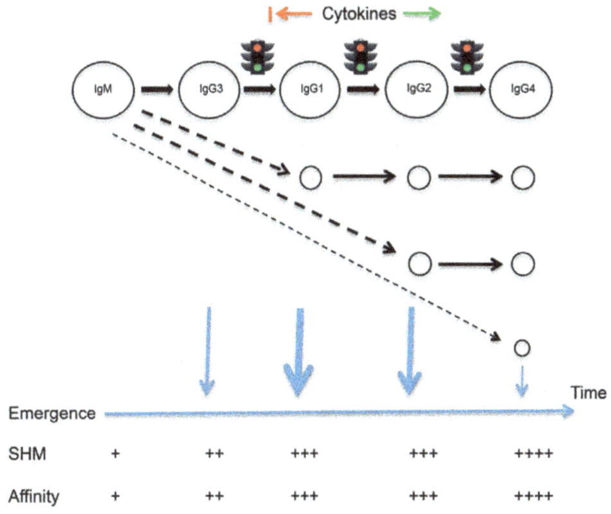

FIGURE 1 | The Temporal Model of IgE/IgG class switching and departure from the germinal center reaction. A programed sequence of sequential switching is highlighted, though alternative switch pathways are also indicated. The timing of switching events and the emergence of different cell types from the germinal center reaction is suggested by the extent of somatic point mutations carried by the cells. Many cytokines may act to promote or delay class switching, as indicated.

because of differences in the underlying probabilities of different outcomes (18, 19). It also is in line with modeling of the dynamics of murine division-linked isotype switching that suggested that the outcome of isotype switching, under the indirect influence of cytokines, is biased toward switching to the immediate downstream neighboring constant region gene (20).

Though a simple relationship between mutation numbers and affinity in any sequence cannot be assumed, accumulating mutations are generally considered to give rise to higher affinity antibodies through selection within the germinal centers (21). Sequential departure of cells from the germinal centers should therefore ensure that antibodies of different isotypes have predictable differences in affinity. This in turn should ensure that despite the different isotypes having some opposing actions, and despite the changing relative concentrations of the different isotypes over time (22), all antibodies at the time of their production should be able to play their assigned roles. It should also ensure that inflammatory processes are tightly controlled, through the temporal coordination of antibodies that have striking differences in their abilities to bind FcγR and to fix complement.

There is good evidence that the IgG3 response occurs early, is relatively transient and is of relatively low affinity (22, 23). This is supported by our sequencing study, for IgG3-associated VDJ genes had the fewest mutations of the IgG subclasses (mean 17.7 mutations), 31% of the sequences had less than 10 mutations and 7% of the sequences had no mutations at all (11). We propose that class switching to IgG3, the first IgG subclass gene in the human IGHC locus, first brings beneficial FcγR-mediated defenses into play. The accumulation of some somatic point mutations during the differentiation of IgG3-committed cells should ensure that most IgG3 antibodies have experienced some affinity maturation, and the specific physicochemical properties of IgG3 should mean that the switch from IgM to IgG3 does not lead to a crippling loss of binding avidity.

The principal "early" antibody, IgM, is able to provide useful protection despite its low affinity, because of the multivalent nature of secreted IgM, and because of its flexibility (24). The long hinge region of IgG3 makes it the most flexible human IgG antibody (25). This should facilitate bivalent binding of high avidity to repeated determinants on the surface of an invading pathogen. As part of the early response, IgG3 antibodies would have to work with IgM antibodies to efficiently trigger complement fixation and engagement with FcγR-bearing cells. In fact, IgG3 has the highest affinity of the IgG subclasses for C1q, the first component of the classical complement cascade (26). It also has the highest affinity for the FcγRIIIA and FcγRIIIB receptors, and its affinity for FcγRIIA is second only to IgG1 (27).

The elongated hinge region makes IgG3 vulnerable to catabolism. IgG3 has a half-life of just 7 days (28) and shares a short half-life with IgM (∼5 days) (29) and IgE (∼3 days) (30). This rapid turnover of all three kinds of "early antibody" should facilitate the ever-increasing dominance, as a response progresses, of higher affinity antibodies of other isotypes.

In our study of VDJ rearrangements, IgG1-associated sequences were significantly more mutated than IgG3 sequences. The mean mutation of VDJ utilizing the IgG1 gene, positioned immediately downstream from IgG3, was 21.0 somatic point mutations, and only 13% of sequences had fewer than 10 mutations (11). We therefore suggest that IgG1-committed cells are the next cell type to differentiate and depart the germinal centers. Although having on average just three more mutations than IgG3 sequences, we suggest that a number of days are likely to separate the average time of departure of IgG3-committed cells and IgG1-committed cells. It is generally accepted that mutations accumulate at the rate of about one mutation per cell division (31), and centroblast division time is thought to be around 7 h (32). It is likely, however, that as increasing numbers of mutations accumulate, the probability that further random mutations are beneficial is low (33). The speed with which selected sequences accumulate mutations is therefore likely to slow over the course of a response.

Class switching to IgG1 leads to the secretion of more highly mutated, complement-fixing, FcγR-binding IgG antibodies that often dominate the response to bacterial and viral invaders (34, 35). Certainly, IgG1 antibodies are the most abundant serum antibodies (36). With their shorter hinge regions, IgG1 molecules lack flexibility but with their higher affinity for antigen, even monovalent binding should be stable and effective. And with their high affinity for C1q (26) and FcγRI, FcγRII, and FcγRIII (27), such IgG1 antibodies would continue driving inflammatory processes and antigen clearance.

Many studies report that IgG1 antibodies appear relatively early in the immune response, and in fact IgG1 and IgG3 are often the only IgG subclasses detected in a response (37, 38). This could result from early antigen clearance preventing the appearance of IgG2 and IgG4 antibodies. It could also reflect delays in downstream class switching as a result of the prevailing cytokine milieu. T cell cytokines are often said to drive class switching to IgG1 and IgG3 (39). Alternatively, they could be said to delay class switching to IgG2 and IgG4, by their promotion of the IgG1 response.

IgG2 antibodies are the second most abundant serum antibodies and the IgG2 gene is positioned immediately downstream of IgG1. IgG2 antibodies are seen at concentrations that are comparable to IgG1 antibodies, and that are much higher than the typical serum concentrations of IgG3 and IgG4. In contrast to IgG1 antibodies, IgG2 antibodies fix complement very poorly (40, 41) and interact very weakly with FcγR (27). In our sequence study, IgG2 antibodies carried a higher mean number of mutations (22.0) than IgG1 antibodies (21.0) (11). It is difficult to believe that this higher level of mean mutations would lead to biologically significant differences in mean antibody affinity, but certainly IgG2 antibodies must share high affinity with IgG1 antibodies. All these features of the humoral response require explanation. In particular, any model of IgG subclass function must explain how IgG1 and IgG2 antibodies, the two most abundant antibody isotypes, work together to deliver protective immunity despite their diametrically opposed properties.

We hypothesize that IgG2-committed cells emerge from the germinal center reaction, on average, shortly after the development of the IgG1 response. We further hypothesize that IgG2 functions as an anti-inflammatory "partner" to more inflammatory IgG1 antibodies, "dampening down" the inflammatory response by its competition with the IgG1 isotype (**Figure 2**). Working together, IgG1 and IgG2 antibodies could provide a spectrum of activity, from the highly inflammatory "pure IgG1 response," to the "pure IgG2 response" that results in immune complexes that cannot interact with FcγR-bearing cells or with molecules of the complement system.

Mutation data suggests that IgG1 and IgG2 antibodies have similar affinities. If this is the case, they will compete on a level playing field, where antibody concentrations prevail. We propose that the relative concentrations of IgG1 and IgG2 are the result of the balance of cytokines that either promote or delay switching to IgG2. These proportions will be seen in the immune complexes that form during the response, and the outcome of varying proportions of IgG1 and IgG2 antibodies will be immune complexes having varying avidity for complement and for FcγR. IgG2 can therefore be conceptualized as an anti-inflammatory brake on the inflammatory actions of IgG1. In certain circumstances, switching may occur quickly, leading to a response that is dominated by IgG2. This could help explain reports that IgG2 dominates the antibody

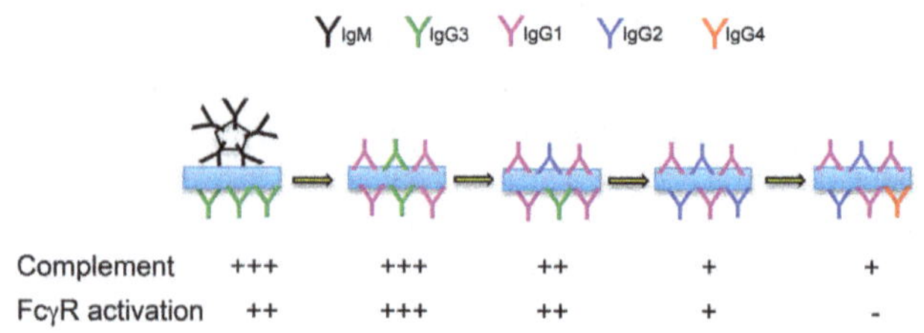

FIGURE 2 | Immune complex formation over the course of a prolonged immune response. The likely complement-fixing and FcγR-binding abilities of immune complexes formed by antibodies of mixed isotypes are indicated.

response to carbohydrates response (42). In fact similar concentrations of IgG1 and IgG2 antibodies have often been reported in response to carbohydrate antigens (43–45), and IgG2 antibodies are also a conspicuous part of the response to many protein antigens (46). It is clear that the chemistry of carbohydrate antigens cannot explain the IgG2 response.

The human IgG4 response is often described as an anti-inflammatory blocking response (47), but the apparent functions of these antibodies have been difficult to reconcile with their very low concentrations. We believe that their mode of action is revealed by the levels of mutations that are seen in IgG4-associated VDJ sequences. IgG4 is the most distal of the IgG subclass genes within the heavy chain constant region locus. In our sequence study, IgG4 antibodies carried the highest mean number of VDJ mutations of the IgG subclasses (mean: 27.1), and no unmutated IgG4-associated VDJ sequences were seen (11). This suggests to us that IgG4-committed cells are (typically) the last cell type to emerge from the germinal center reaction. They are therefore likely to be the highest affinity antibodies. This is indirectly supported by the circumstances in which IgG4 antibodies are conspicuous. Serum IgG4 concentrations are elevated in chronic helminth and other parasite infections (47). Serum IgG4 concentrations also rise during allergy desensitization therapy, after repeated exposure to low doses of allergen (47). They have also been reported in the convalescent phase of the anti-viral response (35).

IgG4 antibodies do not fix complement and bind very poorly to activating FcγR (27), but they bind to the inhibitory FcγRIIB with an affinity that is higher than that of the other three IgG isotypes (27). Critical to the blocking activity of IgG4, inhibition is only mediated via the FcγRIIB receptor when immune complexes co-engage FcγRIIB and other activating FcRs (48). Despite high concentrations of specific antibodies of other isotypes, IgG4 should therefore block FcγR-mediated processes if it is present as a modest proportion of all antibodies in an immune complex. The high affinity of IgG4 should provide it with a competitive advantage, ensuring its participation in immune complex formation, and therefore allowing it to successfully act through FcγRIIB.

The ability of IgG4 antibodies to outcompete other isotypes may also be facilitated by the phenomenon of Fab arm exchange. In reducing conditions, IgG4 antibodies have the unique ability to dissociate into monovalent heavy/light chain pairs, and to re-associate again as bivalent antibodies (49, 50). This Fab arm exchange leads frequently to the formation of bi-specific antibodies. It has been suggested that this would, in practice, lead IgG4 antibodies to be functionally monovalent, as Fab arm exchange would be unlikely between antibodies of related specificities (49). We believe an alternative explanation of the consequences of Fab arm exchange could be the formation of blocking antibodies that bind with very high avidity because of their bi-specific nature.

Bivalency gives power to the IgG molecule. It most obviously allows a single antibody molecule to aggregate two antigen molecules, but it also allows high avidity binding to suitably spaced, repeated epitopes on the surface of a complex antigen. An additional outcome of bivalency has also been identified. It was first proposed on theoretical grounds that very weak binding of one arm of a bivalent antibody molecule to a "non-target" epitope could substantially improve the avidity of binding of the antibody to its target epitope, and that the probability of such bi-specific interactions was reasonably high (51). Recently, such bi-specific heteroligation was shown to facilitate antibody binding to HIV-gp140 (52). For a number of antibodies, high affinity interactions between gp140 and one antigen-binding site were supported by low affinity binding of the second antibody arm to completely different epitopes (52).

Fab arm exchange by IgG4 antibodies could improve the likelihood of heteroligation, if exchange occurs between antibodies of related specificities. This would be likely in two situations. IgG4 antibodies are undetectable in response to many antigens, and individuals with very low serum IgG4 concentrations are likely to have a limited IgG4 repertoire. In such circumstances, Fab arm exchange between antibodies targeting associated epitopes or related antigens would be more likely. In individuals with higher IgG4 concentrations, Fab arm exchange could also take place between antibodies of related specificities through their co-localization at sites of inflammation. At such sites, appropriate redox conditions of even a transient nature could lead Fab arm exchange to "lock together" Fab arms of associated specificities. This would function to increase IgG4 binding avidity, giving bi-specific IgG4 antibodies the ability to outcompete the more inflammatory isotypes, late in a response.

In addition to its IgG1-blocking activity, it is clear that IgG4 can block IgE-mediated immune function. The IgE and IgG4 isotypes are strongly linked with one another in the literature, and in fact IgE antibodies are often said to arise by class switching of IgG4$^+$ B cells (53, 54). The mutational characteristics that we have reported clearly demonstrate that this is not always so, for both the number and patterns of mutations we have seen differ between IgE and IgG4 (11). However it is possible that IgG4 antibodies could be related to high affinity IgE, if such IgE antibodies arise late in a response. Clarification of this question, and determination of the circumstances in which such high affinity IgE might be produced by the human immune system will be necessary before late-arising IgE can be incorporated into the model.

The temporal model, as presented here, outlines sequential class switching during a first, persisting exposure to antigen. The nature of isotype expression in a recall response will clearly depend upon the tendency of class-switched cells to differentiate into memory cells during the primary response. Though IgM memory cells are now known to be an important part of the memory compartment (55, 56), there is some evidence from the early literature that IgG1 dominates the switched memory compartment. Studies of the recall response after re-challenge with keyhole limpet hemocyanin (KLH) showed little or no increase in peak concentrations of KLH-specific IgG2 and IgG3 antibodies, but a marked increase in circulating IgG1 anti-KLH antibodies (57). IgG4 antibodies were only seen upon re-challenge. The high affinity of IgG1 and its inflammatory functions make it the ideal isotype for IgG memory, and the logic of the Temporal Model suggests that memory cells of the other IgG isotypes could be either unhelpful or counterproductive.

The contributions that memory cells make to antibody isotype production in a recall response will depend upon whether memory cells re-enter germinal centers or immediately differentiate into plasmablasts and plasma cells. Studies in the mouse suggest that in a recall response, mouse IgG$^+$ memory cells (55) and IgE$^+$ memory cells (8) rapidly give rise to plasma cells, but IgM$^+$

memory cells re-enter the germinal center reaction (55). If human and mouse cells are governed by similar processes, it may therefore be that events within the human germinal center during a recall response proceed as we have outlined for earlier events. In other words, reactivated IgM memory cells within the germinal centers would give rise to new IgE-switched and IgG-switched cells through a programed process of sequential switching.

Mechanisms that could underlie the temporal emergence of different IgG subclasses from the GC reaction will need to be explored, and one possibility lies in the recently reported competitive feedback between soluble antibody from plasma cells and the GC B cells (58). Soluble antibody, produced by cells that have previously emerged and differentiated, competes with GC B cells for binding to FDC-associated antigen. This competition promotes survival of GC B cells with higher affinity than the soluble antibody, while B cells of lesser affinity die by neglect. The Temporal Model suggests that as class switching proceeds, antibodies expressing subclasses from the more distally positioned IgG genes are likely to be of higher affinity. At a particular point in the response, higher affinity antibodies that express downstream IgG genes would outcompete soluble antibody of earlier subclasses, while promoting the destruction of B cells expressing earlier subclasses that carry fewer mutations and are of lower affinity. Feedback competition may therefore promote the temporal emergence of the subclasses in their genomic order.

Many studies give credence to the Temporal Model, but certainly this is not true of all studies. Discordant observations could be the result of pathogen-directed perturbations of normal immune function, for the temporal progression of isotype switching would be as susceptible as other aspects of immune function to subversion by bacterial and viral virulence factors (59). Discordant observations are particularly seen in some early studies of antibody isotypes, but these reports might be explained by the cross-reactivity of many early "isotype-specific" reagents (60). Others might now be explained by phenomena such as Fc–Fc binding of IgG4 antibodies that were unknown until recently (50). But the resolution of the mystery of antibody function cannot come from studies of the past. It is our hope that this description of the Temporal Model will encourage the question of antibody isotype function to be revived. Having received so little attention over the last two decades, it is now time for the power of high throughput sequencing to be harnessed, to confirm the relationship between the levels of mutation and antibody isotypes in individuals of different ethnicities and states of health, and to properly address the clonal relationships between B cells producing antibodies of different isotypes. It may then be that the timing of class switching, the passage of different cell populations between anatomical compartments within the lymph node, the emergence of cells from the germinal center reaction, and the overall functions of human isotypes can finally be determined with certainty.

ACKNOWLEDGMENTS

This work was supported by a grant from the National Health and Medical Research Council.

REFERENCES

1. Ballieux RE, Bernier GM, Tominaga K, Putnam FW. Gamma globulin antigenic types defined by heavy chain determinants. *Science* (1964) **145**(3628):168–70. doi:10.1126/science.145.3628.168
2. Oxelius VA. Immunoglobulin G (IgG) subclasses and human disease. *Am J Med* (1984) **76**(3A):7–18. doi:10.1016/0002-9343(84)90314-0
3. Snapper CM, Paul WE. Interferon-gamma and B cell stimulatory factor-1 reciprocally regulate Ig isotype production. *Science* (1987) **236**(4804):944–7. doi:10.1126/science.3107127
4. Umetsu DT, Ambrosino DM, Quinti I, Siber GR, Geha RS. Recurrent sinopulmonary infection and impaired antibody response to bacterial capsular polysaccharide antigen in children with selective IgG-subclass deficiency. *N Engl J Med* (1985) **313**(20):1247–51. doi:10.1056/NEJM198511143132002
5. Erazo A, Kutchukhidze N, Leung M, Christ AP, Urban JF Jr., Curotto de Lafaille MA, et al. Unique maturation program of the IgE response in vivo. *Immunity* (2007) **26**(2):191–203. doi:10.1016/j.immuni.2006.12.006
6. Yang Z, Sullivan BM, Allen CD. Fluorescent in vivo detection reveals that IgE(+) B cells are restrained by an intrinsic cell fate predisposition. *Immunity* (2012) **36**(5):857–72. doi:10.1016/j.immuni.2012.02.009
7. Xiong H, Dolpady J, Wabl M, Curotto de Lafaille MA, Lafaille JJ. Sequential class switching is required for the generation of high affinity IgE antibodies. *J Exp Med* (2012) **209**(2):353–64. doi:10.1084/jem.20111941
8. Talay O, Yan D, Brightbill HD, Straney EE, Zhou M, Ladi E, et al. IgE(+) memory B cells and plasma cells generated through a germinal-center pathway. *Nat Immunol* (2012) **13**(4):396–404. doi:10.1038/ni.2256
9. Dahlke I, Nott DJ, Ruhno J, Sewell WA, Collins AM. Antigen selection in the IgE response of allergic and nonallergic individuals. *J Allergy Clin Immunol* (2006) **117**(6):1477–83. doi:10.1016/j.jaci.2005.12.1359
10. Kerzel S, Rogosch T, Struecker B, Maier RF, Zemlin M. IgE transcripts in the circulation of allergic children reflect a classical antigen-driven B cell response and not a superantigen-like activation. *J Immunol* (2010) **185**(4):2253–60. doi:10.4049/jimmunol.0902942
11. Wang Y, Jackson KJ, Chen Z, Gaeta BA, Siba PM, Pomat W, et al. IgE sequences in individuals living in an area of endemic parasitism show little mutational evidence of antigen selection. *Scand J Immunol* (2011) **73**(5):496–504. doi:10.1111/j.1365-3083.2011.02525.x
12. Chang B, Casali P. The CDR1 sequences of a major proportion of human germline Ig VH genes are inherently susceptible to amino acid replacement. *Immunol Today* (1994) **15**(8):367–73. doi:10.1016/0167-5699(94)90175-9
13. Snow RE, Djukanovic R, Stevenson FK. Analysis of immunoglobulin E VH transcripts in a bronchial biopsy of an asthmatic patient confirms bias towards VH5, and indicates local clonal expansion, somatic mutation and isotype switch events. *Immunology* (1999) **98**(4):646–51. doi:10.1046/j.1365-2567.1999.00910.x
14. Marshall JS. Mast-cell responses to pathogens. *Nat Rev Immunol* (2004) **4**(10):787–99. doi:10.1038/nri1460
15. Collins AM, Basil M, Nguyen K, Thelian D. Rat basophil leukaemia (RBL) cells sensitized with low affinity IgE respond to high valency antigen. *Clin Exp Allergy* (1996) **26**(8):964–70. doi:10.1046/j.1365-2222.1996.d01-387.x
16. Gieras A, Focke-Tejkl M, Ball T, Verdino P, Hartl A, Thalhamer J, et al. Molecular determinants of allergen-induced effector cell degranulation. *J Allergy Clin Immunol* (2007) **119**(2):384–90. doi:10.1016/j.jaci.2006.09.034
17. Fujieda S, Zhang K, Saxon A. IL-4 plus CD40 monoclonal antibody induces human B cells gamma subclass-specific isotype switch: switching to gamma 1, gamma 3, and gamma 4, but not gamma 2. *Mian Yi Xue Za Zhi* (1995) **155**(5):2318–28.
18. Tangye SG, Ferguson A, Avery DT, Ma CS, Hodgkin PD. Isotype switching by human B cells is division-associated and regulated by cytokines. *Mian Yi Xue Za Zhi* (2002) **169**(8):4298–306.
19. Tangye SG, Hodgkin PD. Divide and conquer: the importance of cell division in regulating B-cell responses. *Immunology* (2004) **112**(4):509–20. doi:10.1111/j.1365-2567.2004.01950.x
20. Yaish B, Mehr R. Models for the dynamics and order of immunoglobulin isotype switching. *Bull Math Biol* (2005) **67**(1):15–32. doi:10.1016/j.bulm.2004.05.007

21. Shlomchik MJ, Weisel F. Germinal center selection and the development of memory B and plasma cells. *Immunol Rev* (2012) **247**(1):52–63. doi:10.1111/j.1600-065X.2012.01124.x
22. Devey ME, Bleasdale-Barr KM, Bird P, Amlot PL. Antibodies of different human IgG subclasses show distinct patterns of affinity maturation after immunization with keyhole limpet haemocyanin. *Immunology* (1990) **70**(2):168–74. Erratum in: *Immunology* (1990) **71**(1):152.
23. Wilson KM, Di Camillo C, Doughty L, Dax EM. Humoral immune response to primary rubella virus infection. *Clin Vaccine Immunol* (2006) **13**(3):380–6. doi:10.1128/CVI.13.3.380-386.2006
24. Tobita T, Oda M, Azuma T. Segmental flexibility and avidity of IgM in the interaction of polyvalent antigens. *Mol Immunol* (2004) **40**(11):803–11. doi:10.1016/j.molimm.2003.09.011
25. Roux KH, Strelets L, Michaelsen TE. Flexibility of human IgG subclasses. *Mian Yi Xue Za Zhi* (1997) **159**(7):3372–82.
26. Schroeder HW Jr., Cavacini L. Structure and function of immunoglobulins. *J Allergy Clin Immunol* (2010) **125**(2 Suppl 2):S41–52. doi:10.1016/j.jaci.2009.09.046
27. Bruhns P. Properties of mouse and human IgG receptors and their contribution to disease models. *Blood* (2012) **119**(24):5640–9. doi:10.1182/blood-2012-01-380121
28. Morell A, Terry WD, Waldmann TA. Metabolic properties of IgG subclasses in man. *J Clin Invest* (1970) **49**(4):673–80. doi:10.1172/JCI106279
29. Barth WF, Wochner RD, Waldmann TA, Fahey JL. Metabolism of human gamma macroglobulins. *J Clin Invest* (1964) **43**:1036–48. doi:10.1172/JCI104987
30. Waldmann TA, Iio A, Ogawa M, McIntyre OR, Strober W. The metabolism of IgE. Studies in normal individuals and in a patient with IgE myeloma. *J Immunol* (1976) **117**(4):1139–44.
31. Sablitzky F, Wildner G, Rajewsky K. Somatic mutation and clonal expansion of B cells in an antigen-driven immune response. *EMBO J* (1985) **4**(2):345–50.
32. Liu YJ, Zhang J, Lane PJ, Chan EY, MacLennan IC. Sites of specific B cell activation in primary and secondary responses to T cell-dependent and T cell-independent antigens. *Eur J Immunol* (1991) **21**(12):2951–62. doi:10.1002/eji.1830211209
33. Shannon M, Mehr R. Reconciling repertoire shift with affinity maturation: the role of deleterious mutations. *J Immunol* (1999) **162**(7):3950–6.
34. Biganzoli P, Ferreyra L, Sicilia P, Carabajal C, Frattari S, Littvik A, et al. IgG subclasses and DNA detection of HHV-6 and HHV-7 in healthy individuals. *J Med Virol* (2010) **82**(10):1679–83. doi:10.1002/jmv.21880
35. Deshmukh TM, Shah RR, Gurav YK, Arankalle VA. Serum immunoglobulin G subclass responses in different phases of hepatitis E virus infection. *J Med Virol* (2013) **85**(5):828–32. doi:10.1002/jmv.23537
36. Schauer U, Stemberg F, Rieger CH, Borte M, Schubert S, Riedel F, et al. IgG subclass concentrations in certified reference material 470 and reference values for children and adults determined with the binding site reagents. *Clin Chem* (2003) **49**(11):1924–9. doi:10.1373/clinchem.2003.022350
37. Murphy SL, Li H, Mingozzi F, Sabatino DE, Hui DJ, Edmonson SA, et al. Diverse IgG subclass responses to adeno-associated virus infection and vector administration. *J Med Virol* (2009) **81**(1):65–74. doi:10.1002/jmv.21360
38. Spinsanti LI, Farias AA, Aguilar JJ, del Pilar Diaz M, Contigiani MS. Immunoglobulin G subclasses in antibody responses to St. Louis encephalitis virus infections. *Arch Virol* (2011) **156**(10):1861–4. doi:10.1007/s00705-011-1047-3
39. Pene J, Gauchat JF, Lecart S, Drouet E, Guglielmi P, Boulay V, et al. Cutting edge: IL-21 is a switch factor for the production of IgG1 and IgG3 by human B cells. *J Immunol* (2004) **172**(9):5154–7.
40. Bindon CI, Hale G, Bruggemann M, Waldmann H. Human monoclonal IgG isotypes differ in complement activating function at the level of C4 as well as C1q. *J Exp Med* (1988) **168**(1):127–42. doi:10.1084/jem.168.1.127
41. Bruggemann M, Williams GT, Bindon CI, Clark MR, Walker MR, Jefferis R, et al. Comparison of the effector functions of human immunoglobulins using a matched set of chimeric antibodies. *J Exp Med* (1987) **166**(5):1351–61. doi:10.1084/jem.166.5.1351
42. Barrett DJ, Ayoub EM. IgG2 subclass restriction of antibody to pneumococcal polysaccharides. *Clin Exp Immunol* (1986) **63**(1):127–34.
43. Hammarstrom L, Persson MA, Smith CI. Immunoglobulin subclass distribution of human anti-carbohydrate antibodies: aberrant pattern in IgA-deficient donors. *Immunology* (1985) **54**(4):821–6.
44. Morell A, Doran JE, Skvaril F. Ontogeny of the humoral response to group A streptococcal carbohydrate: class and IgG subclass composition of antibodies in children. *Eur J Immunol* (1990) **20**(7):1513–7. doi:10.1002/eji.1830200716
45. Shackelford PG, Granoff DM, Nelson SJ, Scott MG, Smith DS, Nahm MH. Subclass distribution of human antibodies to *Haemophilus influenzae* type b capsular polysaccharide. *Mian Yi Xue Za Zhi* (1987) **138**(2):587–92.
46. Xu W, Santini PA, Sullivan JS, He B, Shan M, Ball SC, et al. HIV-1 evades virus-specific IgG2 and IgA responses by targeting systemic and intestinal B cells via long-range intercellular conduits. *Nat Immunol* (2009) **10**(9):1008–17. doi:10.1038/ni.1753
47. Aalberse RC, Stapel SO, Schuurman J, Rispens T. Immunoglobulin G4: an odd antibody. *Clin Exp Allergy* (2009) **39**(4):469–77. doi:10.1111/j.1365-2222.2009.03207.x
48. Bruhns P, Fremont S, Daeron M. Regulation of allergy by Fc receptors. *Curr Opin Immunol* (2005) **17**(6):662–9. doi:10.1016/j.coi.2005.09.012
49. van der Neut Kolfschoten M, Schuurman J, Losen M, Bleeker WK, Martinez-Martinez P, Vermeulen E, et al. Anti-inflammatory activity of human IgG4 antibodies by dynamic Fab arm exchange. *Science* (2007) **317**(5844):1554–7. doi:10.1126/science.1144603
50. Rispens T, Ooijevaar-de Heer P, Bende O, Aalberse RC. Mechanism of immunoglobulin G4 Fab-arm exchange. *J Am Chem Soc* (2011) **133**(26):10302–11. doi:10.1021/ja203638y
51. Hodgkin PD. An antigen valence theory to explain the evolution and organization of the humoral immune response. *Immunol Cell Biol* (1997) **75**(6):604–18. doi:10.1038/icb.1997.95
52. Mouquet H, Scheid JF, Zoller MJ, Krogsgaard M, Ott RG, Shukair S, et al. Polyreactivity increases the apparent affinity of anti-HIV antibodies by heteroligation. *Nature* (2010) **467**(7315):591–5. doi:10.1038/nature09385
53. Jabara HH, Loh R, Ramesh N, Vercelli D, Geha RS. Sequential switching from mu to epsilon via gamma 4 in human B cells stimulated with IL-4 and hydrocortisone. *Mian Yi Xue Za Zhi* (1993) **151**(9):4528–33.
54. Aalberse RC, Platts-Mills TA. How do we avoid developing allergy: modifications of the TH2 response from a B-cell perspective. *J Allergy Clin Immunol* (2004) **113**(5):983–6. doi:10.1016/j.jaci.2004.02.046
55. Dogan I, Bertocci B, Vilmont V, Delbos F, Megret J, Storck S, et al. Multiple layers of B cell memory with different effector functions. *Nat Immunol* (2009) **10**(12):1292–9. doi:10.1038/ni.1814
56. Kurosaki T, Aiba Y, Kometani K, Moriyama S, Takahashi Y. Unique properties of memory B cells of different isotypes. *Immunol Rev* (2010) **237**(1):104–16. doi:10.1111/j.1600-065X.2010.00939.x
57. Bird P, Calvert JE, Amlot PL. Distinctive development of IgG4 subclass antibodies in the primary and secondary responses to keyhole limpet haemocyanin in man. *Immunology* (1990) **69**(3):355–60.
58. Zhang Y, Meyer-Hermann M, George LA, Figge MT, Khan M, Goodall M, et al. Germinal center B cells govern their own fate via antibody feedback. *J Exp Med* (2013) **210**(3):457–64. doi:10.1084/jem.20120150
59. Brodsky IE, Medzhitov R. Targeting of immune signalling networks by bacterial pathogens. *Nat Cell Biol* (2009) **11**(5):521–6. doi:10.1038/ncb0509-521
60. Buckley RH. Immunoglobulin G subclass deficiency: fact or fancy? *Curr Allergy Asthma Rep* (2002) **2**(5):356–60. doi:10.1007/s11882-002-0067-1

12

Secondary mechanisms of diversification in the human antibody repertoire

Bryan S. Briney[1] and James E. Crowe Jr.[1,2,3]*

[1] Department of Pathology, Microbiology and Immunology, Vanderbilt University Medical Center, Nashville, TN, USA
[2] Department of Pediatrics, Vanderbilt University Medical Center, Nashville, TN, USA
[3] The Vanderbilt Vaccine Center, Vanderbilt University Medical Center, Nashville, TN, USA

Edited by:
Harry W. Schroeder, University of Alabama at Birmingham, USA

Reviewed by:
Robert A. Eisenberg, University of Pennsylvania, USA
To-Ha Thai, Beth Deaconess Israel Medical Center, USA

***Correspondence:**
James E. Crowe Jr., Vanderbilt Vaccine Center, Vanderbilt University Medical Center, 11475 MRB IV, 2213 Garland Avenue, Nashville, TN 37232-0417, USA.
e-mail: james.crowe@vanderbilt.edu

V(D)J recombination and somatic hypermutation (SHM) are the primary mechanisms for diversification of the human antibody repertoire. These mechanisms allow for rapid humoral immune responses to a wide range of pathogenic challenges. V(D)J recombination efficiently generate a virtually limitless diversity through random recombination of variable (V), diversity (D), and joining (J) genes with diverse non-templated junctions between the selected gene segments. Following antigen stimulation, affinity maturation by SHM produces antibodies with refined specificity mediated by mutations typically focused in complementarity determining regions (CDRs), which form the bulk of the antigen recognition site. While V(D)J recombination and SHM are responsible for much of the diversity of the antibody repertoire, there are several secondary mechanisms that, while less frequent, make substantial contributions to antibody diversity including V(DD)J recombination (or D–D fusion), SHM-associated insertions and deletions, and affinity maturation and antigen contact by non-CDR regions of the antibody. In addition to enhanced diversity, these mechanisms allow the production of antibodies that are critical to response to a variety of viral and bacterial pathogens but that would be difficult to generate using only the primary mechanisms of diversification.

Keywords: VDJ rearrangement, VH replacement, B Cell Biology, human, insertion/deletion

INTRODUCTION

A diverse antibody repertoire is a principal component of humoral immunity and is critical to the development of functional adaptive immune responses. Generation of this repertoire diversity is accomplished primarily through two mechanisms: recombination and somatic hypermutation (SHM). These two mechanisms produce massive diversity within antibody complementarity determining regions (CDRs), which form the primary antigen contact site. The availability of multiple variable genes for selection at the time of recombination facilitates large combinatorial diversity, which is further expanded by a diversity of possible heavy and light chain combinations. In this review, we discuss in detail three additional mechanisms which, while less common than recombination and SHM, contribute substantially to the generation of diversity within the antibody repertoire: (1) non-standard recombinations that violate the 12/23 rule of recombination, (2) SHM-associated genetic insertions and deletions, and (3) affinity maturation and direct antigen contact by non-CDR antibody regions.

V(D)J RECOMBINATION: FOLLOWING THE 12/23 RULE

Since the discovery that recombination activating gene (RAG)-mediated recombination of variable (V), diversity (D) and joining (J) genes generates virtually unlimited sequence diversity in the antibody repertoire (Brack et al., 1978; Alt and Baltimore, 1982; Tonegawa, 1983; Schatz et al., 1989; Oettinger et al., 1990), much progress has been made in determining the genetic and mechanistic elements that participate in the antibody recombination process. It is generally understood that recombination signal sequences (RSS), which are composed of conserved AT-rich heptamer and nonamer sequences separated by spacers of either 12 or 23 nucleotides, are recognized and bound by RAG1 and RAG2 proteins at the initiation of the recombination process (Hesse et al., 1989; Alt et al., 1992). RAG binding is highly dependent on the heptamer and nonamer sequences, and alterations to either sequence results in decreased RAG binding (Cuomo et al., 1996; Difilippantonio et al., 1996; Nadel et al., 1998). The length of the spacer sequence is critical to recombination, and there is evidence of sequence conservation within the spacer region (Ramsden et al., 1994; Lee et al., 2003; Montalbano et al., 2003).

Recombination typically occurs only between RSS elements of different spacer lengths, in a model commonly referred to as the 12/23 rule of recombination (Ramsden et al., 1996; Steen et al., 1996; van Gent et al., 1996; Schatz, 2004). After binding to one 12-bp RSS and one 23-bp RSS, the RAG complex induces single-strand DNA nicks between the coding sequence and the heptamer of each RSS, resulting in hairpin formation on each of the coding ends and a blunt double-stranded break on each signal end (Roth et al., 1992; Schlissel et al., 1993; McBlane et al., 1995; Sadofsky, 2001). The hairpins are opened, nucleotides may be added to or removed from the coding ends, and the double-strand DNA breaks at the coding ends are joined into a single coding strand (Lewis, 1994; Mahajan et al., 1999; Shockett and Schatz, 1999; Walker et al., 2001; Mansilla-Soto and Cortes, 2003; Roth, 2003).

In antibody heavy chain genes, D gene segments are flanked by 12-bp RSSs on either side, while V_H and J_H gene segments are flanked by 23-bp RSSs (Early et al., 1980;

Kurosawa and Tonegawa, 1982). Recombination thus proceeds in a step-wise fashion, with D–J_H recombination preceding V_H–D recombination, resulting in a complete heavy chain variable region (Alt et al., 1987; Schatz et al., 1992). A single recombination event joins the light chain V and J gene, and pairing of recombined heavy chain and recombined light chains results in massive diversity within the unmutated antibody repertoire.

NON-12/23 RECOMBINATION: V(DD)J AND DIRECT V_H–J_H RECOMBINATION

Direct V_H–J_H joining and V(DD)J recombination (also referred to as D–D fusion) are in direct violation of the 12/23 rule, but such recombination events have been demonstrated in both *in vitro* and *in vivo* systems (Sanz, 1991; Kiyoi et al., 1992; Raaphorst et al., 1997; Koralov et al., 2005, 2006; Watson et al., 2006). Even in model systems designed to induce such recombination events, however, non-12/23 recombinations are much less efficient than recombinations that adhere to the 12/23 rule (Akira et al., 1987; Hesse et al., 1989; Akamatsu et al., 1994).

V(DD)J recombinants are the result of an aberrant recombination process by which two or more D genes are joined into a single recombinant. The joining of two D genes, which are flanked on both sides by 12-bp RSSs, can only be accomplished in clear violation of the 12/23 rule, but recombined antibody genes in this configuration have now been isolated by numerous investigators. While V(DD)J recombination typically results in an unusually long heavy chain CDR 3 (HCDR3) region, the use of two D segments is not the primary mechanism by which long HCDR3 loops are generated (Briney et al., 2012a). Long HCDR3s typically are generated by the use of longer D and J segments and long non-templated junctional regions. The precise order of events during the V(DD)J recombination process is unclear: it is not known whether V(DD)J recombinants are produced through an additional D–D recombination following the initial D–J_H recombination, or whether D–D fusion occurs before, even long before, the D–J_H recombination. V(DD)J recombinations have been estimated by some to occur in as many as 5–11% of all recombinations (Sanz, 1991; Kiyoi et al., 1992; Raaphorst et al., 1997), but the true frequency of V(DD)J recombinations is difficult to determine. Identification of V(DD)J recombinants relies on the accurate detection of two diversity genes within a single recombinant, but N-addition mimicry of diversity gene segments, which is genetically indistinguishable from true V(DD)J recombination, likely inflates many published estimates of V(DD)J recombination (Watson et al., 2006). Recent work, which leveraged high-throughput sequencing and a stringent filtering process, placed a lower bound of the frequency of V(DD)J recombinants in the human peripheral blood repertoire at approximately 1 in 800 B cells (Briney et al., 2012b).

The occurrence of direct V_H–J_H recombination, like V(DD)J recombination, requires clear violation of the 12/23 rule, since both V_H and J_H segments are flanked by 23-bp RSSs. Little is known about the frequency of direct V_H–J_H recombination in the human repertoire. Several studies of the human CDR3 repertoire that have identified D–D fusions have failed to identify V_H–J_H recombinants, indicating that if they occur, V_H–J_H recombinations are likely very rare (Sanz, 1991; Kiyoi et al., 1992; Raaphorst et al., 1997; Watson et al., 2006). This finding is somewhat surprising, since *in vitro* recombination between two 23-bp RSSs occurred much more frequently than recombination between two 12-bp RSSs (Jones and Gellert, 2002). In contrast to D–D fusions, for which there are several studies on the frequency of V(DD)J recombinants in the human peripheral blood repertoire, much of the published work describing *in vivo* V_H–J_H recombination relies on transgenic mouse models lacking D gene loci (Koralov et al., 2005, 2006). Since these model systems produce only aberrant recombinants, it is difficult to interpret the resulting data in terms of the likely occurrence and frequency of such recombinants in the naturally occurring circulating B cell repertoire. As with V(DD)J recombination, determination of the true frequency of direct V_H–J_H recombination will likely prove difficult, as extensive chewback of D genes during normal V(D)J recombination may appear genetically indistinguishable from true V_H–J_H recombination and inflate any estimates of the frequency of V_H–J_H recombination.

NON-12/23 RECOMBINATION: V_H REPLACEMENT AND RECEPTOR REVISION

V_H replacement is a process by which a secondary V_H–V(D)J recombination can occur, resulting in replacement of the variable gene while preserving the original D–J_H recombination. V_H replacement, which is though to be a form of heavy chain receptor editing, differs from light chain receptor editing, although both typically occur early in B cell development (Prak and Weigert, 1995; Nemazee and Weigert, 2000). Light chain receptor editing results in an entirely new V_L–J_L recombination through the recombination of a V_L gene segment upstream of the original recombination with a J_L gene segment downstream of the original recombination (Papavasiliou et al., 1997; Retter and Nemazee, 1998). Thus, light chain receptor editing proceeds without violating the 12/23 rule. In contrast, V_H replacement involves V_H–V(D)J recombination, which results in retention of the original D–J_H junction and replacement only of the V_H gene segment (Kleinfield and Weigert, 1989; Nemazee, 2006). V_H replacement utilizes a cryptic RSS (cRSS) found near the 3′ end of most human variable genes (Radic and Zouali, 1996), and this cRSS is used to recombine with the normal RSS at the 3′ end of the invading variable gene. The cRSS contains a heptamer sequence, but lacks an identifiable nonamer or spacer sequence, and recombination with the cRSS is inefficient, much like other forms of non-12/23 recombination (Koralov et al., 2006; Lutz et al., 2006).

V_H replacement also can be distinguished from receptor revision, which is putatively antigen-driven and has not been shown to use the conserved cRSS elements near the 3′ end of the V gene. Instead, receptor revisions are suggested to occur peripherally in mature B cells using alternate RSS-like elements that sometimes contain only the CAC motif found at the 5′ end of most RSS heptamers or the inverse GTG motif found at the 3′ end; the few examples of this phenomenon typically occurred near the middle of heavy chain framework region (FR) 3 (Itoh et al., 2000; Wilson et al., 2000; Lenze et al., 2003). Use of these alternate RSS-like elements results in formation of a hybrid V gene, retaining a substantial portion of the initially recombined V gene, as opposed to the nearly complete removal of the initially recombined V gene observed in V_H replacement. Because the observed receptor revision events occurred in stretches of sequence similarity between V genes, it has been proposed that these revisions may instead be polymerase chain reaction (PCR) artifacts caused by incomplete recombinant amplification followed by priming of a different V(D)J recombinant with the partially amplified fragment, resulting in a hybrid sequence (Darlow and Stott, 2005). In approximately half of all identified receptor revisions in these studies, the invading V gene is located downstream of the variable gene used in the initial V(D)J recombination, which would not be possible using the proposed receptor revision mechanism. Inter-chromosomal recombination has been proposed as the mechanism for these out-of-order receptor revisions (Wilson et al., 2000). More recent work has shown that receptor reversions are not observed when amplifying from single B cells (Goossens et al., 2001), providing further evidence that the previously observed receptor revisions may be an artifact of PCR amplification of multiple antibody sequences from bulk B cells.

It is thought that V_H replacement, like other forms of receptor editing, occurs primarily in the immature B cell population to rescue non-functional or autoreactive recombinants (Zhang et al., 2004; Lutz et al., 2006), but some studies suggest that V_H replacement may be possible in mature B cells (Hikida et al., 1996; Han et al., 1997; Papavasiliou et al., 1997; Hertz et al., 1998; Nussenzweig, 1998). Somewhat paradoxically, V_H replacement, which is purported to be a primary mechanism for resolving self-reactive recombinations, can itself result in antibodies with autoreactive characteristics (Klonowski and Monestier, 2000; Zhang et al., 2003). V_H replacement was observed first in transformed murine pre-B cells (Kleinfield et al., 1986; Reth et al., 1986), with subsequent studies identifying V_H replacement *in vivo* (Taki et al., 1993; Chen et al., 1995). In the most informative work done on V_H replacement in the human repertoire, a genetic fingerprint of V_H replacement was identified in the human peripheral blood repertoire (Zhang et al., 2003). Identification of V_H replacement events in the peripheral repertoire relies on detection of short pentameric sequences that are located between the cRSS and the 3′ end of V genes. These pentamers remain even after V_H replacement, providing an identifiable remnant of the replaced V gene. Short pentameric sequences are easily mimicked through random N-addition, making reliable detection of V_H replacement difficult. Therefore, estimates of V_H recombination frequency in the peripheral blood repertoire have varied widely, from 5 to 22% of the total repertoire (Zhang et al., 2003; Koralov et al., 2006; Watson et al., 2006).

SOMATIC HYPERMUTATION

In humans and in mice, diversification of the secondary antibody repertoire, which arises in response to antigenic stimulus, is accomplished primarily through SHM (Brenner and Milstein, 1966; Kelsoe, 1994). Naïve, antigen-inexperienced B cells undergo the SHM process upon recognition of an infectious agent. It is through the SHM process, which occurs primarily in secondary lymphoid tissue, that hosts mutate the variable region of their antibody genes (MacLennan et al., 1992; Li et al., 2004). Many of these mutations have no effect on antigen recognition and many have deleterious effects on either antigen recognition or proper folding of the antibody protein. Some mutations, however, produce antibodies with improved affinity for the target pathogenic epitope (Casali et al., 2006). Thus, the SHM process provides a basis for the positive selection of high-affinity antibodies that are characteristic of a mature immune response (MacLennan, 1994).

Many components of the SHM machinery are known, but the complete process and the mechanisms by which it is targeted specifically to the immunoglobulin loci are still poorly understood. SHM introduces point mutations at a frequency of approximately 10^{-3} mutations per base pair, which is about 10^6-fold higher than the rate of spontaneous mutation in other genes (Rajewsky et al., 1987). Mutations begin approximately 150-bp downstream of the transcription start site and the mutation frequency decreases exponentially with increasing distance from the transcription start site (Rada and Milstein, 2001). Activation-induced cytidine deaminase (AID) is required for SHM and initiates the SHM process by the deamination of C nucleotides (Muramatsu et al., 1999, 2000). Deamination results in a U–G mismatch, and several possible processes result in the error-prone repair of the mismatch. Although the precise mechanism(s) responsible for error-prone repair during SHM are not known, several DNA repair mechanisms have been shown to be critical to the SHM process, including base excision repair and mismatch repair (Phung et al., 1998; Rada et al., 1998; Wiesendanger et al., 2000; Di Noia and Neuberger, 2002; Zheng et al., 2005).

SOMATIC HYPERMUTATION-ASSOCIATED INSERTIONS AND DELETIONS

Although the SHM process typically results in single nucleotide substitutions, deletion of germline nucleic acids or insertion of non-germline nucleic acids does occur in association with SHM (Goossens et al., 1998; Wilson et al., 1998a; Bemark and Neuberger, 2003). These insertions and deletions (indels) are rare, with SHM-associated (SHA) indels estimated to be present in 1.3–6.5% of circulating B cells (Goossens et al., 1998; Wilson et al., 1998a; Bemark and Neuberger, 2003). Short SHA indels are much more common than long SHA indels, with most insertions and deletions being 1–2 codons in length (Goossens et al., 1998; Wilson et al., 1998a; Bemark and Neuberger, 2003). Although infrequent, SHA insertion and deletion events add substantially to the diversity of the human antibody repertoire (Wilson et al., 1998b; de Wildt et al., 1999; Reason and Zhou, 2006).

Somatic hypermutation-associated insertions and deletions also have been shown to play a critical role in the antibody response against viral and bacterial pathogens, including HIV, influenza, and *Streptococcus pneumoniae* (Zhou et al., 2004; Walker et al., 2009, 2011; Wu et al., 2010a; Krause et al., 2011; Pejchal et al., 2011). Of particular interest, structural analysis of an SHA insertion in the anti-influenza antibody 2D1 identified a substantial structural alteration induced by the insertion (Krause et al., 2011). This insertion, although located in a FRs, caused a large conformational change in a CDR and allowed antibody–antigen interactions that were sterically hindered without the insertion-induced conformational change. In addition to 2D1, the extremely broad and potently neutralizing HIV antibody VRC01 contained a six nucleotide deletion in the CDR1 of the light chain (CDR-L1; Wu et al., 2010a). This SHA deletion shortened the CDR-L1 loop, thereby removing potential clashes with loop D of the HIV envelope protein and allowing direct interaction between the HIV antigen and the CDR-L2 loop of VRC01 (Zhou et al., 2010).

ANTIBODY COMPLEMENTARITY DETERMINING REGIONS

Antibody CDRs (also referred to as hypervariable regions) are the primary region of antigen recognition, contain extensive sequence diversity even among germline genes, and are targeted preferentially for affinity maturation, making them the most variable regions of the antibody gene (Capra and Kehoe, 1975; Kabat et al., 1992). There are several structural and genetic reasons for the preferential targeting of CDRs by SHM. Genetically, SHM is known to preferentially target the WRCY hotspot motif (or its reverse complement, RGYW; Dörner et al., 1998), and the frequency of these hotspots is increased in CDRs (Wagner et al., 1995; Shapiro and Wysocki, 2002; Pham et al., 2003). Further, codon usage is biased in CDRs toward codons that are easily mutable, enhancing the likelihood that a nucleotide substitution induced by SHM results in an amino acid change (Motoyama et al., 1991; Wagner et al., 1995; Kepler, 1997). Structurally, the CDRs are largely loop-based, which make them sufficiently flexible to incorporate the substitutions and short indels introduced by SHM without compromising structural integrity. FRs, by contrast, are highly structured and less able to accommodate somatic mutations (Celada and Seiden, 1996).

AFFINITY MATURATION AND ANTIGEN CONTACT BY ANTIBODY FRAMEWORK REGIONS

While much affinity maturation is focused on the CDRs, there are other regions that are important to antigen recognition. T cell receptors (TCRs) contain a fourth hypervariable region (HV4, sometimes referred to as CDR4), which is highly variable, surface-exposed, and involved in superantigen and accessory molecule recognition (Choi et al., 1990; Garcia et al., 1996; Li et al., 1998). We have recently used high-throughput sequencing approaches to determine the sequence of thousands of antibody genes containing SHM-associated insertions and deletions (SHA indels), which revealed significant differences between the location of SHA indels and somatic mutations (Briney et al., 2012c). Further, we identified a cluster of insertions and deletions in the antibody FR3 region that corresponds to the HV4 in TCRs.

Emerging evidence suggests that an HV4-like region may exist in antibodies as well as TCRs. Recent crystallographic work on the anti-influenza antibody CR6261 has shown that the HV4-like region of FR3 was somatically mutated (Throsby et al., 2008) and directly contributed to antigen binding (Ekiert et al., 2009). The anti-influenza antibody 2D1 contains a three-codon insertion in a HV4-like region of FR3 which, while not directly involved in antigen recognition, causes a critical conformational shift in nearby CDRs that is required for antigen recognition (Krause et al., 2011). A unique example of HV4-like contribution to antigen recognition is the anti-HIV antibody 21c (Diskin et al., 2010). 21c binds to the HIV co-receptor binding pocket, which is only exposed following binding of CD4, the primary host receptor. Interestingly, while the majority of the binding surface of 21c is in contact with the HIV envelope protein, the HV4-like region of 21c binds to CD4, forming a cross-protein epitope. In addition to 21c, the broadly neutralizing anti-HIV antibody VRC03 contains a surprisingly long seven-codon insertion in the HV4-like region of FR3 (Wu et al., 2010a). Finally, the HV4-like FR3 region of antibody heavy chains of the V_H3 family has been shown to interact with Staphylococcal protein A, a known superantigen (Potter et al., 1996), mimicking the superantigen-binding activity of the HV4 region in TCRs. While the HV4-like regions that have been identified to date are not somatically mutated to the same extent as antibody CDRs, the ability of this HV4-like region to tolerate a substantial number of somatic mutations and genetic insertions suggests the existence of a somewhat flexible region that has an under-appreciated ability to accommodate affinity maturation modifications.

CONCLUSION

V(DD)J recombination, SHA indels, and antigen contact by non-CDR antibody regions, while secondary to V(D)J recombination and SHM as mechanisms of antibody diversification, contribute substantially to antibody diversity. Each of these secondary affinity maturation mechanisms allows for the generation of unique genetic or structural elements that have been shown to be important to the humoral response against a variety of viral and bacterial pathogens including HIV, influenza virus, staphylococci and pneumococci. These secondary affinity maturation events are much less common than SHM and, as a consequence, are more difficult to study effectively. The advent of next-generation sequencing technology has made it is possible to obtain thousands or millions, and soon to be billions, of antibody sequences (Boyd et al., 2009, 2010; Wu et al., 2010b; Prabakaran et al., 2011; Briney et al., 2012d). It is likely that over the coming years, this digital flood of antibody sequence data will allow a much more complete understanding of these secondary affinity maturation events. For example, current technologies for isolating antigen-specific antibodies from human blood or bone marrow cells are relatively inefficient and result in stochastic discovery of unique antibodies. High-throughput sequence analysis techniques now allow comprehensive definition of all expressed antibody sequences in samples, even to the scale of analyzing all antibody sequences in leukopacks containing most of the circulating B cells in an individual at a time point. Novel methods under current development for determining phylogenetic relationships among expressed antibody sequences may allow us to define the path of somatic mutation from unmutated ancestor sequences to the final affinity-matured antigen-specific sequence. Likely, these studies will reveal that B cell clones that develop following antigen stimulation do not follow linear paths of development, but rather diverge into complex families with multiply branched phylogenies. Such studies should greatly broaden our understanding of the molecular and genetic events occurring in the B cell repertoire following antigen stimulation.

ACKNOWLEDGMENT

This work was supported by U01 AI-078407 (NIAID, NIH), NIAID Contract HHSN272200900047C and DoD grant HDTRA1-10-1-0067.

REFERENCES

Akamatsu, Y., Tsurushita, N., Nagawa, F., Matsuoka, M., Okazaki, K., Imai, M., et al. (1994). Essential residues in V(D)J recombination signals. *J. Immunol.* 153, 4520–4529.

Akira, S., Okazaki, K., and Sakano, H. (1987). Two pairs of recombination signals are sufficient to cause immunoglobulin V-(D)-J joining. *Science* 238, 1134–1138.

Alt, F., Blackwell, T., and Yancopoulos, G. (1987). Development of the primary antibody repertoire. *Science* 238, 1079–1087.

Alt, F. W., and Baltimore, D. (1982). Joining of immunoglobulin heavy chain gene segments: implications from a chromosome with evidence of three D–J_H fusions. *Proc. Natl. Acad. Sci. U.S.A.* 79, 4118–4122.

Alt, F. W., Oltz, E. M., Young, F., Gorman, J., Taccioli, G., and Chen, J. (1992). VDJ recombination. *Immunol. Today* 13, 306–314.

Bemark, M., and Neuberger, M. S. (2003). By-products of immunoglobulin somatic hypermutation. *Genes Chromosomes Cancer* 38, 32–39.

Boyd, S. D., Gaëta, B. A., Jackson, K. J., Fire, A. Z., Marshall, E. L., Merker, J. D., et al. (2010). Individual variation in the germline Ig gene repertoire inferred from variable region gene rearrangements. *J. Immunol.* 184, 6986–6992.

Boyd, S. D., Marshall, E. L., Merker, J. D., Maniar, J. M., Zhang, L. N., Sahaf, B., et al. (2009). Measurement and clinical monitoring of human lymphocyte clonality by massively parallel VDJ pyrosequencing. *Sci. Transl. Med.* 1, 12ra23.

Brack, C., Hirama, M., Lenhard-Schuller, R., and Tonegawa, S. (1978). A complete immunoglobulin gene is created by somatic recombination. *Cell* 15, 1–14.

Brenner, S., and Milstein, C. (1966). Origin of antibody variation. *Nature* 211, 242–243.

Briney, B. S., Willis, J. R., and Crowe, J. E. (2012a). Human peripheral blood antibodies with long HCDR3s are established primarily at original recombination using a limited subset of germline genes. *PLoS ONE* 7:e36750. doi: 10.1371/journal.pone.0036750

Briney, B. S., Willis, J. R., Hicar, M. D., Thomas, J. W., and Crowe, J. E. (2012b). Frequency and genetic characterization of V(DD)J recombinants in the human peripheral blood antibody repertoire. *Immunology* 137, 56–64.

Briney, B. S., Willis, J. R., and Crowe, J. E. Jr. (2012c). Location and length distribution of somatic hypermutation-associated DNA insertions and deletions reveals regions of antibody structural plasticity. *Genes Immun.* 13, 523–529.

Briney, B. S., Willis, J. R., McKinney, B. A., and Crowe, J. E. Jr. (2012d). High-throughput antibody sequencing reveals genetic evidence of global regulation of the naïve and memory repertoires that extends across individuals. *Genes Immun.* 13, 469–473.

Capra, J. D., and Kehoe, J. M. (1975). Hypervariable regions, idiotypy, and the antibody-combining site. *Adv. Immunol.* 20, 1–40.

Casali, P., Pal, Z., Xu, Z., and Zan, H. (2006). DNA repair in antibody somatic hypermutation. *Trends Immunol.* 27, 313–321.

Celada, F., and Seiden, P. E. (1996). Affinity maturation and hypermutation in a simulation of the humoral immune response. *Eur. J. Immunol.* 26, 1350–1358.

Chen, C., Nagy, Z., Prak, E., and Weigert, M. (1995). Immunoglobulin heavy chain gene replacement: a mechanism of receptor editing. *Immunity* 3, 747–755.

Choi, Y. W., Herman, A., Digiusto, D., Wade, T., Marrack, P., and Kappler, J. (1990). Residues of the variable region of the T-cell-receptor beta-chain that interact with *S. aureus* toxin superantigens. *Nature* 346, 471–473.

Cuomo, C. A., Mundy, C. L., and Oettinger, M. A. (1996). DNA sequence and structure requirements for cleavage of V(D)J recombination signal sequences. *Mol. Cell. Biol.* 16, 5683–5690.

Darlow, J. M., and Stott, D. I. (2005). V(H) replacement in rearranged immunoglobulin genes. *Immunology* 114, 155–165.

de Wildt, R. M., van Venrooij, W. J., Winter, G., Hoet, R. M., and Tomlinson, I. M. (1999). Somatic insertions and deletions shape the human antibody repertoire. *J. Mol. Biol.* 294, 701–710.

Difilippantonio, M. J., McMahan, C. J., Eastman, Q. M., Spanopoulou, E., and Schatz, D. G. (1996). RAG1 mediates signal sequence recognition and recruitment of RAG2 in V(D)J recombination. *Cell* 87, 253–262.

Di Noia, J., and Neuberger, M. S. (2002). Altering the pathway of immunoglobulin hypermutation by inhibiting uracil-DNA glycosylase. *Nature* 419, 43–48.

Diskin, R., Marcovecchio, P. M., and Bjorkman, P. J. (2010). Structure of a clade C HIV-1 gp120 bound to CD4 and CD4-induced antibody reveals anti-CD4 polyreactivity. *Nat. Struct. Mol. Biol.* 17, 608–613.

Dörner, T., Foster, S., Farner, N., and Lipsky, P. (1998). Somatic hypermutation of human immunoglobulin heavy chain genes: targeting of RGYW motifs on both DNA strands. *Eur. J. Immunol.* 28, 3384–3396.

Early, P., Huang, H., Davis, M., Calame, K., and Hood, L. (1980). An immunoglobulin heavy chain variable region gene is generated from three segments of DNA: VH, D and JH. *Cell* 19, 981–992.

Ekiert, D. C., Bhabha, G., Elsliger, M.-A., Friesen, R. H. E., Jongeneelen, M., Throsby, M., et al. (2009). Antibody recognition of a highly conserved influenza virus epitope. *Science* 324, 246–251.

Garcia, K., Degano, M., Stanfield, R., Brunmark, A., Jackson, M., Peterson, P., et al. (1996). An alpha beta T cell receptor structure at 2.5 angstrom and its orientation in the TCR-MHC complex. *Science* 274, 209–219.

Goossens, T., Bräuninger, A., Klein, U., Küppers, R., and Rajewsky, K. (2001). Receptor revision plays no major role in shaping the receptor repertoire of human memory B cells after the onset of somatic hypermutation. *Eur. J. Immunol.* 31, 3638–3648.

Goossens, T., Klein, U., and Küppers, R. (1998). Frequent occurrence of deletions and duplications during somatic hypermutation: implications for oncogene translocations and heavy chain disease. *Proc. Natl. Acad. Sci. U.S.A.* 95, 2463–2468.

Han, S., Dillon, S. R., Zheng, B., Shimoda, M., Schlissel, M. S., and Kelsoe, G. (1997). V(D)J recombinase activity in a subset of germinal center B lymphocytes. *Science* 278, 301–305.

Hertz, M., Kouskoff, V., Nakamura, T., and Nemazee, D. (1998). V(D)J recombinase induction in splenic B lymphocytes is inhibited by antigen-receptor signalling. *Nature* 394, 292–295.

Hesse, J., Lieber, M., Mizuuchi, K., and Gellert, M. (1989). V(D)J recombination – a functional definition of the joining signals. *Genes Dev.* 3, 1053–1061.

Hikida, M., Mori, M., Takai, T., Tomochika, K., Hamatani, K., and Ohmori, H. (1996). Reexpression of RAG-1 and RAG-2 genes in activated mature mouse B cells. *Science* 274, 2092–2094.

Itoh, K., Meffre, E., Albesiano, E., Farber, A., Dines, D., Stein, P., et al. (2000). Immunoglobulin heavy chain variable region gene replacement As a mechanism for receptor revision in rheumatoid arthritis synovial tissue B lymphocytes. *J. Exp. Med.* 192, 1151–1164.

Jones, J. M., and Gellert, M. (2002). Ordered assembly of the V(D)J synaptic complex ensures accurate recombination. *EMBO J.* 21, 4162–4171.

Kabat, E. A., Wu, T. T., Gottesman, K. S., and Foeller, C. (1992). *Sequences of Proteins of Immunological Interest.* Darby: Diane Books Publishing Company.

Kelsoe, G. (1994). B cell diversification and differentiation in the periphery. *J. Exp. Med.* 180, 5–6.

Kepler, T. B. (1997). Codon bias and plasticity in immunoglobulins. *Mol. Biol. Evol.* 14, 637–643.

Kiyoi, H., Naoe, T., Horibe, K., and Ohno, R. (1992). Characterization of the immunoglobulin heavy chain complementarity determining region (CDR)-III sequences from human B cell precursor acute lymphoblastic leukemia cells. *J. Clin. Invest.* 89, 739–746.

Kleinfield, R., Hardy, R. R., Tarlinton, D., Dangl, J., Herzenberg, L. A., and Weigert, M. (1986). Recombination between an expressed immunoglobulin heavy-chain gene and a germline variable gene segment in a Ly 1+ B-cell lymphoma. *Nature* 322, 843–846.

Kleinfield, R. W., and Weigert, M. G. (1989). Analysis of VH gene replacement events in a B cell lymphoma. *J. Immunol.* 142, 4475–4482.

Klonowski, K. D., and Monestier, M. (2000). Heavy chain revision in MRL mice: a potential mechanism for the development of autoreactive B cell precursors. *J. Immunol.* 165, 4487–4493.

Koralov, S. B., Novobrantseva, T. I., Hochedlinger, K., Jaenisch, R., and Rajewsky, K. (2005). Direct *in vivo* VH to JH rearrangement violating the 12/23 rule. *J. Exp. Med.* 201, 341–348.

Koralov, S. B., Novobrantseva, T. I., Königsmann, J., Ehlich, A., and Rajewsky, K. (2006). Antibody repertoires generated by VH replacement and direct VH to JH joining. *Immunity* 25, 43–53.

Krause, J. C., Ekiert, D. C., Tumpey, T. M., Smith, P. B., Wilson, I. A., and Crowe, J. E. (2011). An insertion mutation that distorts antibody binding site architecture enhances function of a human antibody. *MBio* 2, e00345-10.

Kurosawa, Y., and Tonegawa, S. (1982). Organization, structure, and assembly of immunoglobulin heavy chain diversity DNA segments. *J. Exp. Med.* 155, 201–218.

Lee, A. I., Fugmann, S. D., Cowell, L. G., Ptaszek, L. M., Kelsoe, G., and Schatz, D. G. (2003). A functional analysis of the spacer of V(D)J recombination signal sequences. *PLoS Biol.* 1:e1. doi: 10.1371/journal.pbio.0000001

Lenze, D., Greiner, A., Knörr, C., Anagnostopoulos, I., Stein, H., and Hummel, M. (2003). Receptor revision of immunoglobulin heavy chain genes in human MALT lymphomas. *Mol. Pathol.* 56, 249–255.

Lewis, S. M. (1994). The mechanism of V(D)J joining: lessons from molecular, immunological, and comparative analyses. *Adv. Immunol.* 56, 27–150.

Li, H., Llera, A., and Mariuzza, R. (1998). Structure-function studies of T-cell receptor superantigen interactions. *Immunol. Rev.* 163, 177–186.

Li, Z., Woo, C. J., Iglesias-Ussel, M. D., Ronai, D., and Scharff, M. D. (2004). The generation of antibody diversity through somatic hypermutation and class switch recombination. *Genes Dev.* 18, 1–11.

Lutz, J., Müller, W., and Jäck, H.-M. (2006). VH replacement rescues progenitor B cells with two nonproductive VDJ alleles. *J. Immunol.* 177, 7007–7014.

MacLennan, I. C. (1994). Germinal centers. *Annu. Rev. Immunol.* 12, 117–139.

MacLennan, I. C., Liu, Y. J., and Johnson, G. D. (1992). Maturation and dispersal of B-cell clones during T cell-dependent antibody responses. *Immunol. Rev.* 126, 143–161.

Mahajan, K. N., Gangi-Peterson, L., Sorscher, D. H., Wang, J., Gathy, K. N., Mahajan, N. P., et al. (1999). Association of terminal deoxynucleotidyl transferase with Ku. *Proc. Natl. Acad. Sci. U.S.A.* 96, 13926–13931.

Mansilla-Soto, J., and Cortes, P. (2003). VDJ Recombination: Artemis and its in vivo role in hairpin opening. *J. Exp. Med.* 197, 543–547.

McBlane, J. F., van Gent, D. C., Ramsden, D. A., Romeo, C., Cuomo, C. A., Gellert, M., et al. (1995). Cleavage at a V(D)J recombination signal requires only RAG1 and RAG2 proteins and occurs in two steps. *Cell* 83, 387–395.

Montalbano, A., Ogwaro, K. M., Tang, A., Matthews, A. G. W., Larijani, M., Oettinger, M. A., et al. (2003). V(D)J recombination frequencies can be profoundly affected by changes in the spacer sequence. *J. Immunol.* 171, 5296–5304.

Motoyama, N., Okada, H., and Azuma, T. (1991). Somatic mutation in constant regions of mouse lambda 1 light chains. *Proc. Natl. Acad. Sci. U.S.A.* 88, 7933–7937.

Muramatsu, M., Kinoshita, K., Fagarasan, S., Yamada, S., Shinkai, Y., and Honjo, T. (2000). Class switch recombination and hypermutation require activation-induced cytidine deaminase (AID), a potential RNA editing enzyme. *Cell* 102, 553–563.

Muramatsu, M., Sankaranand, V. S., Anant, S., Sugai, M., Kinoshita, K., Davidson, N. O., et al. (1999). Specific expression of activation-induced cytidine deaminase (AID), a novel member of the RNA-editing deaminase family in germinal center B cells. *J. Biol. Chem.* 274, 18470–18476.

Nadel, B., Tang, A., Lugo, G., Love, V., Escuro, G., and Feeney, A. J. (1998). Decreased frequency of rearrangement due to the synergistic effect of nucleotide changes in the heptamer and nonamer of the recombination signal sequence of the V kappa gene A2b, which is associated with increased susceptibility of Navajos to Haemophilus influenzae type b disease. *J. Immunol.* 161, 6068–6073.

Nemazee, D. (2006). Receptor editing in lymphocyte development and central tolerance. *Nat. Rev. Immunol.* 6, 728–740.

Nemazee, D., and Weigert, M. (2000). Revising B cell receptors. *J. Exp. Med.* 191, 1813–1817.

Nussenzweig, M. C. (1998). Immune receptor editing: revise and select. *Cell* 95, 875–878.

Oettinger, M., Schatz, D., Gorka, C., and Baltimore, D. (1990). RAG-1 and RAG-2, adjacent genes that synergistically activate V(D)J recombination. *Science* 248, 1517–1523.

Papavasiliou, F., Casellas, R., Suh, H., Qin, X. F., Besmer, E., Pelanda, R., et al. (1997). V(D)J recombination in mature B cells: a mechanism for altering antibody responses. *Science* 278, 298–301.

Pejchal, R., Doores, K. J., Walker, L. M., Khayat, R., Huang, P.-S., Wang, S.-K., et al. (2011). A potent and broad neutralizing antibody recognizes and penetrates the HIV glycan shield. *Science* 334, 1097–1103.

Pham, P., Bransteitter, R., Petruska, J., and Goodman, M. F. (2003). Processive AID-catalysed cytosine deamination on single-stranded DNA simulates somatic hypermutation. *Nature* 424, 103–107.

Phung, Q. H., Winter, D. B., Cranston, A., Tarone, R. E., Bohr, V. A., Fishel, R., et al. (1998). Increased hypermutation at G and C nucleotides in immunoglobulin variable genes from mice deficient in the MSH2 mismatch repair protein. *J. Exp. Med.* 187, 1745–1751.

Potter, K. N., Li, Y., and Capra, J. D. (1996). Staphylococcal protein A simultaneously interacts with framework region 1, complementarity-determining region 2, and framework region 3 on human VH3-encoded Igs. *J. Immunol.* 157, 2982–2988.

Prabakaran, P., Chen, W., Singarayan, M. G., Stewart, C. C., Streaker, E., Feng, Y., et al. (2011). Expressed antibody repertoires in human cord blood cells: 454 sequencing and IMGT/HighV-QUEST analysis of germline gene usage, junctional diversity, and somatic mutations. *Immunogenetics* 64, 337–350.

Prak, E. L., and Weigert, M. (1995). Light chain replacement: a new model for antibody gene rearrangement. *J. Exp. Med.* 182, 541–548.

Raaphorst, F. M., Raman, C. S., Tami, J., Fischbach, M., and Sanz, I. (1997). Human Ig heavy chain CDR3 regions in adult bone marrow pre-B cells display an adult phenotype of diversity: evidence for structural selection of DH amino acid sequences. *Int. Immunol.* 9, 1503–1515.

Rada, C., Ehrenstein, M. R., Neuberger, M. S., and Milstein, C. (1998). Hot spot focusing of somatic hypermutation in MSH2-deficient mice suggests two stages of mutational targeting. *Immunity* 9, 135–141.

Rada, C., and Milstein, C. (2001). The intrinsic hypermutability of antibody heavy and light chain genes decays exponentially. *EMBO J.* 20, 4570–4576.

Radic, M., and Zouali, M. (1996). Receptor editing, immune diversification, and self-tolerance. *Immunity* 5, 505–511.

Rajewsky, K., Förster, I., and Cumano, A. (1987). Evolutionary and somatic selection of the antibody repertoire in the mouse. *Science* 238, 1088–1094.

Ramsden, D. A., Baetz, K., and Wu, G. E. (1994). Conservation of sequence in recombination signal sequence spacers. *Nucleic Acids Res.* 22, 1785–1796.

Ramsden, D. A., McBlane, J. F., van Gent, D. C., and Gellert, M. (1996). Distinct DNA sequence and structure requirements for the two steps of V(D)J recombination signal cleavage. *EMBO J.* 15, 3197–3206.

Reason, D. C., and Zhou, J. (2006). Codon insertion and deletion functions as a somatic diversification mechanism in human antibody repertoires. *Biol. Direct* 1, 24.

Reth, M., Gehrmann, P., Petrac, E., and Wiese, P. (1986). A novel VH to VHDJH joining mechanism in heavy-chain-negative (null) pre-B cells results in heavy-chain production. *Nature* 322, 840–842.

Retter, M. W., and Nemazee, D. (1998). Receptor editing occurs frequently during normal B cell development. *J. Exp. Med.* 188, 1231–1238.

Roth, D. B. (2003). Restraining the V(D)J recombinase. *Nat. Rev. Immunol.* 3, 656–666.

Roth, D. B., Menetski, J. P., Nakajima, P. B., Bosma, M. J., and Gellert, M. (1992). V(D)J recombination: broken DNA molecules with covalently sealed (hairpin) coding ends in scid mouse thymocytes. *Cell* 70, 983–991.

Sadofsky, M. J. (2001). The RAG proteins in V(D)J recombination: more than just a nuclease. *Nucleic Acids Res.* 29, 1399–1409.

Sanz, I. (1991). Multiple mechanisms participate in the generation of diversity of human H chain CDR3 regions. *J. Immunol.* 147, 1720–1729.

Schatz, D. G. (2004). V(D)J recombination. *Immunol. Rev.* 200, 5–11.

Schatz, D. G., Oettinger, M. A., and Baltimore, D. (1989). The V(D)J recombination activating gene, RAG-1. *Cell* 59, 1035–1048.

Schatz, D. G., Oettinger, M. A., and Schlissel, M. S. (1992). V(D)J recombination: molecular biology and regulation. *Annu. Rev. Immunol.* 10, 359–383.

Schlissel, M., Constantinescu, A., Morrow, T., Baxter, M., and Peng, A. (1993). Double-strand signal sequence breaks in V(D)J recombination are blunt, 5′-phosphorylated, RAG-dependent, and cell cycle regulated. *Genes Dev.* 7, 2520–2532.

Shapiro, G., and Wysocki, L. (2002). DNA target motifs of somatic mutagenesis in antibody genes. *Crit. Rev. Immunol.* 22, 183–200.

Shockett, P. E., and Schatz, D. G. (1999). DNA hairpin opening mediated by the RAG1 and RAG2 proteins. *Mol. Cell. Biol.* 19, 4159–4166.

Steen, S., Gomelsky, L., and Roth, D. (1996). The 12/23 rule is enforced at the cleavage step of V(D)J recombination *in vivo*. *Genes Cells* 1, 543–553.

Taki, S., Meiering, M., and Rajewsky, K. (1993). Targeted insertion of a variable region gene into the immunoglobulin heavy chain locus. *Science* 262, 1268–1271.

Throsby, M., van den Brink, E., Jongeneelen, M., Poon, L. L. M., Alard, P., Cornelissen, L., et al. (2008). Heterosubtypic neutralizing monoclonal antibodies cross-protective against H5N1 and H1N1 recovered from human IgM+ memory B cells. *PLoS ONE* 3:e3942. doi: 10.1371/journal.pone.0003942

Tonegawa, S. (1983). Somatic generation of antibody diversity. *Nature* 302, 575–581.

van Gent, D. C., Ramsden, D. A., and Gellert, M. (1996). The RAG1 and RAG2 proteins establish the 12/23 rule in V(D)J recombination. *Cell* 85, 107–113.

Wagner, S. D., Milstein, C., and Neuberger, M. S. (1995). Codon bias targets mutation. *Nature* 376, 732.

Walker, J. R., Corpina, R. A., and Goldberg, J. (2001). Structure of the Ku heterodimer bound to DNA and its implications for double-strand break repair. *Nature* 412, 607–614.

Walker, L. M., Huber, M., Doores, K. J., Falkowska, E., Pejchal, R., Julien, J.-P., et al. (2011). Broad neutralization coverage of HIV by multiple highly potent antibodies. *Nature* 477, 466–470.

Walker, L. M., Phogat, S. K., Chan-Hui, P.-Y., Wagner, D., Phung, P., Goss, J. L., et al. (2009). Broad and potent neutralizing antibodies from an African donor reveal a new HIV-1 vaccine target. *Science* 326, 285–289.

Watson, L. C., Moffatt-Blue, C. S., McDonald, R. Z., Kompfner, E., Ait-Azzouzene, D., Nemazee, D., et al. (2006). Paucity of V-D-D-J rearrangements and VH replacement events in lupus prone and nonautoimmune TdT−/− and TdT+/+ mice. *J. Immunol.* 177, 1120–1128.

Wiesendanger, M., Kneitz, B., Edelmann, W., and Scharff, M. D. (2000). Somatic hypermutation in MutS homologue (MSH)3-, MSH6-, and MSH3/MSH6-deficient mice reveals a role for the MSH2–MSH6 heterodimer in modulating the base substitution pattern. *J. Exp. Med.* 191, 579–584.

Wilson, P. C., de Bouteiller, O., Liu, Y., Potter, K., Banchereau, J., Capra, J. D., et al. (1998a). Somatic hypermutation introduces insertions and deletions into immunoglobulin genes. *J. Exp. Med.* 187, 59–70.

Wilson, P. C., Liu, Y. J., Banchereau, J., Capra, J. D., and Pascual, V. (1998b). Amino acid insertions and deletions contribute to diversify the human Ig repertoire. *Immunol. Rev.* 162, 143–151.

Wilson, P. C., Wilson, K., Liu, Y. J., Banchereau, J., Pascual, V., and Capra, J. D. (2000). Receptor revision of immunoglobulin heavy chain variable region genes in normal human B lymphocytes. *J. Exp. Med.* 191, 1881–1894.

Wu, X., Yang, Z.-Y., Li, Y., Hogerkorp, C.-M., Schief, W. R., Seaman, M. S., et al. (2010a). Rational design of envelope identifies broadly neutralizing human monoclonal antibodies to HIV-1. *Science* 329, 856–861.

Wu, Y.-C., Kipling, D., Leong, H. S., Martin, V., Ademokun, A. A., and Dunn-Walters, D. K. (2010b). High-throughput immunoglobulin repertoire analysis distinguishes between human IgM memory and switched memory B-cell populations. *Blood* 116, 1070–1078.

Zhang, Z., Burrows, P. D., and Cooper, M. D. (2004). The molecular basis and biological significance of VH replacement. *Immunol. Rev.* 197, 231–242.

Zhang, Z., Zemlin, M., Wang, Y.-H., Munfus, D., Huye, L. E., Findley, H. W., et al. (2003). Contribution of Vh gene replacement to the primary B cell repertoire. *Immunity* 19, 21–31.

Zheng, N.-Y., Wilson, K., Jared, M., and Wilson, P. C. (2005). Intricate targeting of immunoglobulin somatic hypermutation maximizes the efficiency of affinity maturation. *J. Exp. Med.* 201, 1467–1478.

Zhou, J., Lottenbach, K. R., Barenkamp, S. J., and Reason, D. C. (2004). Somatic hypermutation and diverse immunoglobulin gene usage in the human antibody response to the capsular polysaccharide of *Streptococcus pneumoniae* Type 6B. *Infect. Immun.* 72, 3505–3514.

Zhou, T., Georgiev, I., Wu, X., Yang, Z.-Y., Dai, K., Finzi, A., et al. (2010). Structural basis for broad and potent neutralization of HIV-1 by antibody VRC01. *Science* 329, 811–817.

13

HSP60: issues and insights on its therapeutic use as an immunoregulatory agent

Verônica Coelho[1,2] and Ana M. C. Faria[2,3]*

[1] Laboratório de Imunologia, Instituto do Coração, Universidade de São Paulo, São Paulo, Brazil
[2] Instituto de Investigação em Imunologia, Instituto Nacional de Ciência e Tecnologia, São Paulo, Brazil
[3] Departamento de Bioquímica e Imunologia, Instituto de Ciências Biológicas, Universidade Federal de Minas Gerais, Belo Horizonte, Brasil

Edited by:
Cristina Bonorino, Pontificia Universidade Catolica do Rio Grande do Sul, Brazil

Reviewed by:
Irun R. Cohen, The Weizmann Institute of Science, Israel
Thiago J. Borges, Pontifícia Universidade Católica do Rio Grande do Sul, Brazil

***Correspondence:**
Ana M. C. Faria, Departamento de Bioquímica e Imunologia, Instituto de Ciências Biológicas, Universidade Federal de Minas Gerais, Av. Antonio Carlos, 6627, Belo Horizonte, Brazil.
e-mail: afaria@icb.ufmg.br

Heat shock proteins 60 (HSP60) is one of the most well studied member of the HSP family. Although found to be a target self antigen in pathological autoimmunity and HSP60-reactive T and B cells are part of immune responses in several infectious diseases, there is consistent experimental evidence that HSP60 displays dominant immunoregulatory properties. There are a series of reports on animal models showing that the administration of HSP60 can modulate inflammatory diseases. However, HSP60 has both immune-regulatory and inflammatory properties placing it as an essentially homeostatic antigen, but with potentially harmful effects as well. There have been a series of reports on the successful use of HSP60 and its peptides as immune-modulatory agent for several models of autoimmune diseases and in some clinical trials as well. We believe that the potential risks of HSP60 as a therapeutic agent can be controlled by addressing important factors determining its effects. These factors would be route of administration, appropriate peptides, time point of administration in the course of the disease, and possible association with other modulatory agents.

Keywords: heat shock proteins, HSP60, homeostasis, inflammation, immunoregulation

HSP60 AS AN IMMUNODOMINANT HOMEOSTATIC ANTIGEN

Heat shock proteins (HSP) are highly conserved proteins during evolution. Besides being upregulated in stress conditions, they are constitutively and abundantly present in all living beings and are profoundly involved in various intracellular and systemic homeostatic functions in different species (Hemmingsen et al., 1988; Karlin and Brocchieri, 2000). This feature can be illustrated by their capacity to prevent protein degradation in salamanders or in tropical trees that live exposed to very high temperatures (Kusukawa and Yura, 1988), or by their capacity to interact with the immune system in mammalians, contributing to the fine tuning of inflammation (Pockley et al., 2009), and participating in cell survival signaling pathways (Chun et al., 2010). These robust homeostatic properties and their marked evolutionary conservation lead us to think that HSP can be considered as dominant homeostatic molecules in evolution. Taken the diversity of HSP families (classified according to their molecular weight), it is possible that different HSP families play differential roles in the complex integrated homeostatic network.

Heat shock proteins 60 is one of the most well studied HSP, especially in the interaction with the immune system. It was first described as intracellular chaperone, assisting the folding of polypeptides into proteins and the transporting of proteins (Bukau et al., 2006), but later it was found to be a dominant antigen recognized during infections, together with HSP70 (Kaufmann, 1990; Zügel and Kaufmann, 1999). These properties place these two proteins in a special category as antigens. Indeed, HSP60 has been intensely studied in various immunologic contexts such as in autoimmune diseases (Danielle et al., 1992; Tanaka et al., 1999; Dieude et al., 2004; Quintana et al., 2004, 2008; Van Eden et al., 2005) – often considered as an important target molecule in the pathogenesis – in tumors (Michaluart et al., 2008; Victora et al., 2009) and in transplantation (Qian et al., 1995; Birk et al., 1999; Granja et al., 2004). But, HSP60 does not seem to be a relevant antigen only in pathological conditions. Autoreactivity to HSP60 is also found in health and a high frequency of B and T cell clones reactive to self HSP60 is found in physiological conditions in mammalians (Munk et al., 1989; Fischer et al., 1992; Abulafia-Lapid et al., 1999; Pockley et al., 1999).

Heat shock proteins have been considered by Irun Cohen (Cohen and Young, 1991) as immunodominant antigens for self immune responses and as key players in physiological autoimmunity, likely to be involved in homeostasis (Cohen and Lohse, 1991; Cohen, 1992). In line with this idea, self-HSP-reactive T and B cell clones can be seen as an important part of a network of regulatory cells and molecules in the immune system engaged in homeostatic activities (Cohen, 2007). These activities would include tissue maintenance and repair, but also limiting clonal expansion and controlling inflammation.

Since the discovery of AIRE and its role in the expression of various tissue specific antigens by thymic medullary epithelial cells (MEC; Anderson et al., 2002), it became clear that the different levels of expression of these antigens placed them at a hierarchical order of relevance for central tolerance (Kyewski and Klein, 2006). All highly expressed antigens would compose a particular set of "dominant" antigens relevant for the immune homeostasis (Coutinho and Haas, 2001). In this sense, HSPs can be considered as strong candidates to be part of this immunodominant homeostatic self. They are ubiquitous antigens expressed both in housekeeping as well as in stressed circumstances, and they are highly expressed in the thymus (Mamalaki et al., 1996). Taken that transgenic expression of HSP60 in the thymus does not lead to the deletion of HSP60 specific T cell clones (Minter and Osborne, 2003), it is possible that central tolerance to HSPs relies on the generation of natural regulatory T cells (nTregs) akin to the way tolerance is imposed to many other self antigens (Coutinho et al., 2005; Aschenbrenner et al., 2007). Indeed, nTregs do recognize self antigens and HSPs, including HSP60, are likely to be among these self antigens. In addition, HSP60 has a strong effect in the survival and function of CD4+CD25+Foxp3+ regulatory T cells (Zanin-Zhorov et al., 2006) and they were shown to efficiently drive the differentiation of CD4+CD25− T cell clones derived from Juvenile idiopathic arthritis (JIA) patients into CD4+CD25^{high} regulatory T cells expressing GITR, CTLA-4, and Foxp3 (de Kleer et al., 2004).

In addition to the reported immunomodulatory effect of HSP60, it is clear that this molecule also displays inflammatory actions. HSP60 activates both innate and adaptive arms of the immune response being considered as a danger signal that amplifies inflammation and influence a wide range of immune reactions (Chen et al., 1999; Wallin et al., 2002; Habich and Burkat, 2007). Anti-HSP antibodies and HSP60-reactive T cells are part of immune responses in several infectious diseases (Kaufmann, 1990). Approximately 10–20% of the specific T cells in mice immunized with *Mycobacterium tuberculosis* are against the bacterial HSP65 (Kaufmann et al., 1987). Antibodies to HSP60 of *Chlamydia trachomatis* have been detected at high levels in the sera of infected patients (Sanchez-Campillo et al., 1999), and immunodominant responses to HSP60 are present in other fungal infections (Matthews et al., 1998). This strong immune response directed to HSP60 during infection can be explained by its critical role in cellular homeostasis and by its upregulation in host tissues as a result of stress during infection. In addition, antibodies as well as effector pathological T cells reactive to self HSP60 were found in different autoimmune and inflammatory diseases including type 1 diabetes (Elias et al., 1991; Birk et al., 1996; Abulafia-Lapid et al., 1999) rheumatoid arthritis (RA), multiple sclerosis (Quintana et al., 2008), lupus erythematosus (Dieude et al., 2004), atherosclerosis (Xu et al., 1993), Behcet's disease (Tanaka et al., 1999), inflammatory bowel disease (Stevens et al., 1992), and inflammatory skin disorders (Bayramgurler et al., 2004).

Although HSP60 was first found to be a mitochondrial protein (McMullin and Hallberg, 1988), it is now known that, in eukaryotes, it can also locate in the cytosol (Chandra et al., 2007), at the cell surface (Wand-Wurttenberger et al., 1991; Soltys and Gupta, 1997), in the extracellular space (Davies et al., 2006), and soluble in the peripheral blood (Cappello et al., 2008). In addition, HSP60 peptides can be also be presented in MHC class I and class II molecules (Koga et al., 1989; Anderton et al., 1995), activating specific CD8+ and CD4+ T cells (Van Eden et al., 2005). Thus, we believe that many of its immunologic functions may be triggered/modulated by soluble HSP60 and its peptides present in the microenvironment. In this respect, several synthetic HSP60 peptides have been shown to be immunologically active *in vitro* (Paul et al., 2000; Caldas et al., 2004; Van Eden et al., 2005) and *in vivo* (Elias and Cohen, 1995; Huurman et al., 2007), but the repertoire of HSP60 peptides actually generated *in vivo* in different physio and pathological contexts is still unknown.

Immunologic activation induced by any type of stimulus triggers a variety of both inflammatory and anti-inflammatory mechanisms, and the capacity to both induce and control inflammation is critical to homeostasis. HSP60 has both properties placing it as an essentially homeostatic antigen, but with potentially harmful effects as well. Thus, we think it is crucial to always look at both functional sides of the immune response in any given immunologic context. We have proposed the term REG/INFLAMMA to denote functional activities predominantly immunoregulatory or proinflammatory of any given immune molecule. In our descriptive model, a REG/INFLAMMA molecular panel of immunologically relevant transcription factors (such as GATA-3, RORγt, T-bet, Foxp3) and cytokines (such as IL-6, TGF-β, IL-10, IFN-γ, TNF-α) is used as a way to evaluate the overall immunologic activity of a given molecule or of a particular pathological context (Moraes-Vieira et al., 2012). We believe this may be a useful strategy to evaluate the functional activities of HSP60 peptides, for selecting adequate candidates for clinical application. As a matter of fact, for the specific selection of HSP60 peptides, the REG/INFLAMMA panel could be expanded to also include relevant innate molecules, since HSP60 and its derived peptides also interact with a variety of these molecules.

Some of the HSP60-autoreactive T cell clones have been already isolated from mice (Birk et al., 1996), rats (Feige and Cohen, 1991), and humans (Caldas et al., 2006), under a variety of inflammatory conditions, showed REG and INFLAMMA properties *in vitro* and *in vivo*. This dual immunologic activity places Hsp60 and its derived peptides in a privileged position as potential therapeutic immunomodulators, to either amplify or control inflammation. On the other hand, the same duality also poses a concern for clinical application because it is still unclear what determines a predominant REG or INFLAMMA outcome induced by HSP60 and derived peptides, as previously discussed (Coelho et al., 2008).

HSP60 REGULATORY ACTIVITY IN INFLAMMATORY DISEASES

Although found to be a target self antigen in pathological autoimmunity, there is consistent experimental evidence that HSP60 displays dominant immunoregulatory properties. There are a series of reports on animal models showing that the administration of HSP60 can generate T cell responses that modulate inflammatory diseases (arthritis, type 1 diabetes, atherosclerosis, EAE, asthma, lupus, dermatomyositis; Quintana and Cohen, 2011).

Administration of HSP60 and its peptides by oral, nasal, intraperitoneal, and subcutaneous routes has been extensively studied in experimental models of arthritis in rats (Van Eden et al., 2005). The protective effects of these protocols lead some groups to explore the reactivity of T cells of patients with JIA and RA to HSP60. Interestingly, HSP60-reactive T cells isolated from JIA, but not from AR, patients display a regulatory phenotype and secrete predominantly cytokines such as IL-10 e TGF-beta (de Kleer et al., 2004).

Intranasal and oral administration of HSP65 from *Mycobacterium tuberculosis* has been also tested with success in the

Ldlr−/− mice which develop atherosclerosis upon feeding a hypercholesterolemic diet (Harats et al., 2002; Maron et al., 2002). HSP65-treated mice showed a co-relation between plaque reduction and IL-10 expression at the aortic arch (Maron et al., 2002).

In the NOD mice, a type 1 diabetes model, systemic treatment with HSP65 from Mycobacteria as well as with HSP60 p277 peptide trigger immunoregulatory pathways that result in suppression of disease (Elias et al., 1991; Elias and Cohen, 1995; Birk et al., 1996). Phases II and III clinical trials using HSP60 p277 in patients with type 1 diabetes have been successful in the preservation of islet beta-cell function (Raz et al., 2001, 2007) and, more recently, also in a randomized phase III trial with over 400 newly diagnosed type 1 diabetes patients. Other clinical trials employing HSP60 peptides arrested the autoimmune destruction in patients with RA (van Roon et al., 1997; de Kleer et al., 2004), and autoimmune uveitis (Stanford et al., 2004).

The capacity of HSP60 to control inflammation in the context of transplantation seems to be a harder task. May be this is related to the more robust inflammatory response, simultaneously triggered by multiple alloantigens, in an already highly inflammatory milieu induced by surgery, in contrast to the more insidious development of inflammation in autoimmune diseases, together with the insidious occurrence of epitope spreading to newly exposed self antigens. Nonetheless, our group has been investing on the identification of potent HSP60 immunoregulatory peptides for use in allotransplantation. We have been able to prolong allograft survival across both minor (Luna et al., 2007) and major (unpublished data from V. Coelho laboratory) alloantigen disparities but so far, we have been unsuccessful in inducing transplantation tolerance. Nevertheless, other investigators have been able to induce transplantation tolerance in a mouse model of skin allograft (Birk et al., 1999), but publications in this field are scarcer. Despite the difficulties, we believe it is worth investing on the use of HSP60 peptides as immunomodulators in allotransplantation; may be not alone, but in combination with other drugs and immunoregulatory molecules. If HSP60 and its peptides are, indeed, endogenous immunoregulators, we should find ways to enhance/activate endogenous immunoregulatory networks, in a synergic manner with other therapies. This strategy seems particularly relevant to transplantation, due to the multicity of antigens involved in triggering inflammation; each pair of donor/recipient comprise a different set of alloantigens inducing aggression against the graft. If we are able to identify combinations of conserved dominantly immunoregulator HSP60 peptides, they could be used in allotransplantation, alone or in combination with other immunoregulatory therapies, irrespective of specific alloantigen disparities. A broad immunoregulatory effect is likely to occur once human HSP60 DNA vaccination has been able to control disease in NOD diabetes, inducing a Th2-like immune response not only to HSP60 but also to other relevant target self antigens, such as GAD (glutamic acid decarboxylase) and insulin (Quintana et al., 2002).

IMMUNOREGULATORY MECHANISMS INDUCED BY HSP60

Heat shock proteins 60 and derived peptides are able to exert an important role in the fine balance between promoting and controlling inflammation through a variety of mechanisms. It is very likely even that HSP60's REG and INFLAMMA functional activities occur simultaneously within an inflammatory microenvironment, probably also mediated by its different peptides, affecting different cell types, and mobilizing different molecular pathways. However, it is not known whether specific molecular signals, either immune cell or tissue-derived, influence HSP60's functional activity in the course of inflammation. Maybe there is also a time course difference – a proinflammatory predominance at the initial phase of inflammation and a regulatory one at a later time point – as we previously suggested in the context of human renal transplantation (Granja et al., 2004).

Heat shock proteins 60 can be viewed as a protein antigen that will be processed and presented to T cells inducing a typical lymphocyte reaction. However, HSP60 and its various peptides have the capacity to interact with a variety of immune molecules, intracellularly (Cappello et al., 2008; Chun et al., 2010) and at the cell surface such as with TLR2, TLR4 (Vabulas et al., 2001), and MHC molecules (Newcomb and Cresswell, 1993), bridging innate and adaptive immune responses. Therefore, plasticity and multiple connectivity are also striking immunologic properties of HSP60.

An important issue that may be raised regarding this plasticity is the relationship between the dual role (regulatory and inflammatory) of HSP60 with its binding molecules. The signaling of an endogenous protein expressed in low amounts chronically may lead to distinct patterns of activation of TRL-expressing cells such as dendritic cells, macrophages, and T cells. In this respect, we would like to highlight the complex diversity of effects triggered by different molecules through the same receptor on different cell types. For instance, it has been shown that both HSP60 and HSP70 signaling, through TLR2 and NF-κB activation, on murine cardiomyocytes induce, *in vitro*, contractile dysfunction and cell death (Mathur et al., 2011). The treatment of human CD4+CD25+ Tregs with human HSP60 or its p277 peptide before anti-CD3 activation also enhanced their ability to downregulate proliferation and production of IFN-γ and TNF-α by CD4+CD25− or CD8+ target T cells. In addition, the enhancing effects of HSP60 costimulation on Tregs involved innate signaling via TLR2, led to activation of PKC, PI3K, and p38, and were further enhanced by the inhibition of ERK. HSP60-treated Tregs suppressed target T cells both by cell-to-cell contact and by secretion of TGF-β and IL-10 (Zanin-Zhorov et al., 2006). HSP60 is also a ligand that activates B cells via TLR4. Simultaneous ligation of TLR4 and BCR in HSP60 specific B cells induces antibody secretion (Cohen-Sfady et al., 2005; Herlands et al., 2008) and this may be an important way to induce the anti-HSP60 IgM autoantibodies that are prevalent in physiologic conditions (Merbl et al., 2007). TLR4 ligation in epithelial cells are also known to play a protective role in the intestinal mucosa. On the other hand, high concentrations of HSP60 usually trigger TLR4 signaling and inflammatory activation of monocytes (Pockley et al., 2009).

Adding more complexity to the plethoric immunobiology of HSP60, it was recently reported that HSP60 interacts with beta-catenin, increasing its transcriptional activity and protein expression, and favoring metastasis (Tsai et al., 2009). Taken that beta-catenin also enhances cell survival of several cell types including Tregs (Ding et al., 2008), it is plausible that this may represent an additional pathway by which HSP60 and derived peptides promote immunoregulatory activity.

THERAPEUTIC USE OF HSP60 FOR INFLAMMATORY DISEASES: ADVANTAGES AND RISKS

Since administration of Hsp60 has a well documented regulatory effect in inflammatory disease models, it has been proposed by several groups that this antigen may be used as a therapeutic tool in diseases where inflammation is undesirable such as autoimmune and allergic diseases and transplantation.

Despite the concerns about the potential risks of inducing inflammatory undesirable effects, different formulations of HSP60 and derived peptides have been used for immunoregulation in a variety of animal models, and no evidence of pathological autoimmunity was detected. Accordingly, we have not found histopathological signs of inflammation in over 10 tissues following the use of the HSP65-DNA vaccine, in mice (Lima et al., 2009). Nevertheless, we believe that the use of HSP60 peptides displaying a predominant immunoregulatory function, instead of the whole molecule, may reduce potentially harmful effects. In addition, this strategy may provide an opportunity to combine different peptides which trigger distinct immunoregulatory mechanisms. Nonetheless, depending on the route of administration, the quantity of peptides required may be a limiting issue for clinical application.

Another risk that can be foreseen for the use of HSP60 is a possibility of immunosuppression to protective responses against infection. Experiments carried out by our group have shown that mice treated with HSP65 by the oral route for 4 days have decrease immune responses to HSP65 but show a normal response to *Salmonella* infection (Rezende et al., unpublished results). The course of infection was not altered by the treatment suggesting that protective responses to infectious agents may rely on other potent pathogen-associated antigens.

On the contrary, in infectious contexts, immune response to bacterial antigens might benefit from the fact that there is a high frequency of self-HSP-reactive T and B cell clones in a normal repertoire. These HSP-reactive lymphocytes would be recruited and take part in the ongoing immune response, exerting mainly a regulatory role and contribute to reestablishing homeostasis (Cohen and Young, 1991). Indeed, immunomodulation of inflammatory responses during infection is critical for the outcome of the infectious disease. There are several examples of infectious diseases in which severity of disease is mostly related to a high prevalence of proinflammatory cytokines (especially TNF-α) and poor immune-regulatory components (such as IL-10 or Tregs). This is true for Chagas disease (Vitelli-Avelar et al., 2008), Schistosomiasis (Wamachi et al., 2004), and Leishmaniasis (Oliveira et al., 2011).

It has been shown that effector CD4+ T cells that secrete large amounts of IL-2 are able to efficiently recruit CD4+CD25+Foxp3+ regulatory T cells (Curotto de Lafaille et al., 2004; Almeida et al., 2006). IL-2 is a critical cytokine for Treg function and this is one of the mechanisms triggered during inflammatory events capable of modulating the degree of tissue damage without compromising needed inflammatory responses. Therefore, the REG/INFLAMMA balance is an essential part of all inflammatory responses. HSPs fit very well to this picture since they are self proteins ubiquitously expressed and also they are upregulated in stress conditions.

The fact that HSP60 is an ubiquitous molecule, on the other hand, may represent another benefit. Its use would circumvent the need for the identification of the target antigens involved in the induction of each inflammatory disease. In this regard, it has been demonstrated that tolerance induced to an antigen can recruit regulatory T cells and molecules that would spread their effect in a bystander fashion (Miller et al., 1991). This bystander effect depends on the antigen presenting cells that induce the regulatory T cells and it recruits for the modulatory immune network most the antigens presented in the same context.

In view of these potential risks and benefits, we believe that some issues have to be addressed on the therapeutic use of HSP60 as an immunoregulatory agent: route of administration, form of the protein (whole molecule, peptides), time point in the course of the disease, possible association with other modulatory agents.

ROUTE OF ADMINISTRATION

The majority of studies on the use of HSPs and HSP60 as modulatory agents in several models of inflammatory diseases have used the parenteral (subcutaneous, intraperitoneal, intravenous, and intramuscular) route of administration (Van Eden et al., 2005), probably because of its easy translation into a later clinical setting. However, we believe it is time to reexamine the pros and contras of the routes in the light of new knowledge on HSP60 immunobiology.

It has been extensively described that the oral route is a very efficient way to induce peripheral tolerance in animal models (Faria and Weiner, 2006) and also in humans (Mestecky et al., 1996). Oral tolerance is a well known phenomenon that probably accounts for the robust balance that keeps the homeostasis of the gut mucosa to the daily challenge of microbiota and dietary antigens (Faria and Weiner, 2005). Indeed, we are all tolerant to the food proteins we ingest and also to our microbiota and this has been documented in mice and humans (Andrade et al., 2006; Round et al., 2010). This is especially interesting regarding HSP because bacterial components of our microbiota do express HSPs and they are likely to be involved in immunoregulatory networks in the gut. Although many of these proteins are intracellular, we now know that HSP60 can also be expressed at the cell surface and in the extra cellular space, therefore providing a variety of molecular forms and pathways by which HSP60 could affect the immunologic milieu in the gut. In addition, it is plausible that some of the luminal contents (including dead bacteria) in contact with the abundant lymphoid tissue of the gut mucosa would induce regulatory T cells and oral tolerance. Therefore, oral tolerance to our microbiota can be envisaged as a peripheral form of homeostasis reinforcement of tolerance involving HSPs.

Of all the feeding regimens already tested for oral tolerance, continuous feeding has been shown to be the most efficient way to induce tolerance. Continuous feeding of antigen, but not gavage, can render otherwise refractory animals, such as aged mice, tolerant. Moreover, oral tolerance induced by continuous feeding of antigen lasts longer and, in mice, do not require any type of reinforcement during their lifetime (Faria et al., 1998, 2003).

Since continuous feeding protocols are very cumbersome for human studies, the use of a probiotic vehicle has been designed to continuously deliver *Mycobacterium leprae* HSP65 in the gut mucosa upon a single administration daily. This strategy associates the immunomodulatory and tolerogenic potential of HSP65 and of the gut mucosa. We observed that oral administration of Hsp65-producing *Lactococcus lactis* prevented EAE in mice (Rezende et al., unpublished results). Histological analysis showed no inflammatory cell infiltrate and no tissue destruction in the spinal cord of HSP65-treated mice. Moreover, increased frequency of regulatory T cells correlated with the treatment. Thus, this strategy may constitute a promising alternative therapy for the treatment of autoimmune and inflammatory diseases.

Nasal administration of antigens is also an effective form of inducing long living tolerance (Mestecky et al., 1996; Faria and Weiner, 2006). Regulatory elements triggered by nasal versus oral administration of antigen may be distinct but both routes have been described as efficient ways to modulate inflammatory diseases by HSP60, including reducing atherosclerotic plaque formation in the Ldlr−/− mice (Maron et al., 2002) and prolonging allograft survival in mice (Luna et al., 2007). We would like to point that other forms of continuous delivery of HSP60 have been explored with success. Accordingly, intranasal administration of HSP60 peptide p277 encapsulated into polylactide-co-glycolide acid microspheres resulted in increased skin graft survival in two combinations of murine strains with minor H-2 disparities (Luna et al., 2007).

We believe that the use of strategies such as continuous delivery of antigen by mucosal routes is an appropriate way to favor anti-inflammatory activities of HSPs by mimicking natural routes of tolerance induction and should be further explored.

WHOLE PROTEIN OR PEPTIDES?

An important caveat regarding the *in vitro* functional studies using recombinant HSP60 is endotoxin contamination which, even at very low concentrations, may still influence cytokine production and immune cell functional activity. This seems particularly important because HSP60 and its derived peptides bind to TLRs, including TLR4 which is also a ligand to endotoxin, raising controversies regarding HSP60 specific immunologic effects. This issue has been extensively discussed in the literature and several investigators claim that there is sufficient evidence to support HSP60 specific signaling actions (Henderson et al., 2010). Indeed, working with low-endotoxin HSP60 recombinant preparations has minimized the effect of bacterial contaminants. However, we believe this issue will only be clearly solved when HSP60 produced in endotoxin-free systems is used for functional assays. Taking this into consideration, as well as HSP60 REG/INFLAMMA properties, several groups and ours have been exploring the immunologic functions of HSP60 synthetic peptides in a variety of pathological and physiological (Prakken et al., 1997; Luna et al., 2007) contexts, and have identified immunologically active peptides, effective in, at least partially, downregulating inflammation in animal models (Elias et al., 1991; Thompson et al., 1998; Luna et al., 2007) and in humans in the context of diabetes (Raz et al., 2001, 2007).

Using a panel of HSP60 synthetic peptides and a gene panel of predominantly REG/INFLAMMA molecules, we have found several peptides displaying the capacity to simultaneously modify the gene expression of a variety of immune molecules, *in vitro*, and have identified some predominantly REG and others INFLAMMA, using both mouse splenocytes and human peripheral blood mononuclear cells (PBMC; unpublished data from V. Coelho's laboratory). Interestingly, some predominantly regulatory HSP60 peptides were shared by the two species, suggesting evolutionary functional conservation.

TIME POINT OF THE DISEASE

For oral administration protocols, it is well established that the regulatory mechanisms of oral tolerance is very efficiently triggered before inflammation onset and their efficiency declines progressively after sensitization. Therefore, for oral administration of hsp65, early diagnosis and treatment would be the ideal protocol. This will be critical for HSP60 administration considering the dual functional properties of the antigen (REG–INFLAMMA). Another way to circumvent this caveat of oral treatment with HSP60 might be the association with a delivery system that could act as a modulatory adjuvant boosting the tolerogenic effect of HSP60.

As mentioned before, it is not known whether specific molecular signals from the tissues influence HSP60's functional activity in the course of inflammation. It is possible that a time course difference exists as we have observed in patients who had renal transplants (Granja et al., 2004). Autoreactivity to HSP60 displayed a proinflammatory effect at the initial phase of transplantation and a regulatory one at a later time point.

ASSOCIATION WITH OTHER MODULATORY AGENTS

Since immune tolerance mediated by HSP60 could be more difficult to induce in sensitized diseased individuals, the use of modulatory adjuvants might be helpful. If the oral route is chosen, probiotic bacteria would be excellent candidates since they are well known as agents with immunomodulatory properties. Several probiotic bacteria are already in use for this purpose (*Lactobacillus, Bifidobacteria, Lactococcus*) and the ones that were genetically engineered to express immune-relevant proteins are specially interesting (Pontes et al., 2011). A trial on IL-10-producing *L. lactis* is currently been carried out after promising results in animals models of inflammatory bowel disease (Braat et al., 2006). Hsp65-producing *L. lactis* would also fulfill these requirements since the bacteria *L. lactis* has modulatory properties on its own (unpublished data) besides their effect as delivery agent.

Another interesting strategy recently reported is the use of a pathologically relevant antigen along with HSP60 to induce immunomodulation. Nemirovsky and coworkers used amyloid beta peptide Aβ1–15 conjugated with HSP60 peptide p458 in a subcutaneous vaccination protocol for a murine experimental model of Alzheimer disease. The combined peptide vaccine resulted in a significant decrease in cerebral amyloid burden and inflammation in the brain (Nemirovsky et al., 2011). A similar approach could be designed for autoimmune diseases such as type 1 diabetes, arthritis, myasthenia gravis, and others for which a target self molecule has already been identified.

CONCLUDING REMARKS

The dual immunologic role of HSP60 and derived peptides – inflammatory and regulatory – can be viewed as an advantage for multiple clinical applications, either boosting effector responses or controlling inflammation. On the other hand, it also raises concerns, since it is still unclear what determines HSP60's immune-regulatory or inflammatory activities. We believe that critical factors such as route of administration, time course of the disease in which it will be used, dosage, HSP60 peptides chosen, and the combination with other modulatory molecules may circumvent the putative risks posed by its inflammatory potential.

REFERENCES

Abulafia-Lapid, R., Elias, D., Raz, I., Keren-Zur, Y., Atlan, H., and Cohen, I. R. (1999). T cell proliferative responses of type 1 diabetes patients and healthy individuals to human hsp60 and its peptides. *J. Autoimmun.* 12, 121–129.

Almeida, A. R., Zaragoza, B., and Freitas, A. A. (2006). Indexation as a novel mechanism of lymphocyte homeostasis: the number of CD4+CD25+ regulatory T cells is indexed to the number of IL-2-producing cells. *J. Immunol.* 177, 192–200.

Anderson, M. S., Venanzi, E. S., Klein, L., Chen, Z., Berzins, S. P., Turley, S. J., von Boehmer, H., Bronson, R., Dierich, A., Benoist, C., and Mathis, D. (2002). Projection of an immunological self shadow within the thymus by the Aire protein. *Science* 298, 1395–1401.

Anderton, S. M., Van der Zee, R., Prakken, B., Noordzij, A., van Eden, W. (1995). Activation of T cells recognizing self 60-kD heat shock protein can protect against experimental arthritis. *J. Exp. Med.* 181, 943–952.

Andrade, M. C., Menezes, J. S., Cassali, G. D., Martins-Filho, O. A., Cara, D. C., and Faria, A. M. (2006). Alcohol-induced gastritis prevents oral tolerance induction in mice. *Clin. Exp. Immunol.* 146, 312–322.

Aschenbrenner, K., D'Cruz, L. M., Vollmann, E. H., Hinterberger, M., Emmerich, J., Swee, L. K., Rolink, A., and Klein, L. (2007). Selection of Foxp3+ regulatory T cells specific for self antigen expressed and presented by Aire+ medullary thymic epithelial cells. *Nat. Immunol.* 8, 351–358.

Bayramgurler, D., Ozkara, S. K., Apaydin, R., Ercin, C., and Bilen, N. (2004). Heat shock proteins 60 and 70 expression of cutaneous lichen planus: comparison with normal skin and psoriasis vulgaris. *J. Cutan. Pathol.* 31, 586–594.

Birk, O. S., Elias, D., Weiss, A. S., Rosen, A., van-der Zee, R., Walker, M. D., and Cohen, I. R. (1996). NOD mouse diabetes: the ubiquitous mouse hsp60 is a beta-cell target antigen of autoimmune T cells. *J. Autoimmun.* 9, 159–166.

Birk, O. S., Gur, S. L., Elias, D., Margalit, R., Mor, F., Carmi, P., Bockova, J., Altmann, D. M., and Cohen, I. R. (1999). The 60-kDa heat shock protein modulates allograft rejection. *Proc. Natl. Acad. Sci. U.S.A.* 96, 5159–5163.

Braat, H., Rottiers, P., Hommes, D. W., Huyghebaert, N., Remaut, E., Remon, J. P., van Deventer, S. J., Neirynck, S., Peppelenbosch, M. P., and Steidler, L. (2006). A phase I trial with transgenic bacteria expressing interleukin-10 in Crohn's disease. *Clin. Gastroenterol. Hepatol.* 4, 754–759.

Bukau, B. J., and Weissman, J., and Horwich, A. (2006). Molecular chaperones and protein quality control. *Cell* 125, 443–451.

Caldas, C., Luna, E., Spadafora-Ferreira, M., Porto, G., Iwai, L. K., Oshiro, S. E., Monteiro, S. M., Fonseca, J. A., Lemos, F., Hammer, J., Ho, P. L., Kalil, J., and Coelho, V. (2006). Cellular autoreactivity against heat shock protein 60 in renal transplant patients: peripheral and graft-infiltrating responses. *Clin. Exp. Immunol.* 146, 66–75.

Caldas, C., Spadafora-Ferreira, M., Fonseca, J. A., Luna, E., Iwai, L. K., Kalil, J., and Coelho, V. (2004). T-cell response to self HSP60 peptides in renal transplant recipients: a regulatory role? *Transplant Proc.* 36, 833–835.

Cappello, F., Conway de Macario, E., Marasà, L., Zummo, G., and Macario, A. J. (2008). Hsp60 expression, new locations, functions and perspectives for cancer diagnosis and therapy. *Cancer Biol. Ther.* 7, 801–809.

Chandra, D., Choy, G., and Tang, D. G. (2007). Cytosolic accumulation of HSP60 during apoptosis with or without apparent mitochondrial release: evidence that its pro-apoptotic or pro-survival functions involve differential interactions with caspase-3. *J. Biol. Chem.* 282, 31289–31301.

Chen, W., Syldath, U., Bellmann, K., Burkart, V., and Kolb, H. (1999). Human 60-kDa heat-shock protein: a danger signal to the innate immune system. *J. Immunol.* 162, 3212–3219.

Chun, J. N., Choi, B., Lee, K. W., Lee, D. J., Kang, D. H., Lee, J. Y., Song, I. S., Kim, H. I., Lee, S. H., Kim, H. S., Lee, N. K., Lee, S. Y., Lee, K. J., Kim, J., and Kang, S. W. (2010). Cytosolic Hsp60 is involved in the NF-kappaB-dependent survival of cancer cells via IKK regulation. *PLoS ONE* 5, e9422. doi:10.1371/journal.pone.0009422

Coelho, V., Broere, F., Binder, R. J., Shoenfeld, Y., and Moudgil, K. D. (2008). Heat-shock proteins: inflammatory versus regulatory attributes. *Cell Stress Chaperones* 13, 119–125.

Cohen, I. R. (1992). Autoimmunity to hsp65 and the immunologic paradigm. *Adv. Intern. Med.* 37, 295–311.

Cohen, I. R. (2007). Real and artificial immune systems: computing the state of the body. *Nat. Rev. Immunol.* 7, 569–574.

Cohen, I. R., and Lohse, A. W. (1991). Physiology and pathophysiology of autoimmunity. *Semin. Liver Dis.* 11, 183–186.

Cohen, I. R., and Young, D. B. (1991). Autoimmunity, microbial immunity and the immunological homunculus. *Immunol. Today* 12, 105–110.

Cohen-Sfady, M., Nussbaum, G., Pevsner-Fischer, M., Mor, F., Carmi, P., Zanin-Zhorov, A., Lider, O., and Cohen, I. R. (2005). Heat shock protein 60 activates B cells via the TLR4-MyD88 pathway. *J. Immunol.* 175, 3594–3602.

Coutinho, A., Caramalho, I., Seixas, E., and Demengeot, J. (2005). Thymic commitment of regulatory T cells is a pathway of TCR-dependent selection that isolates repertoires undergoing positive or negative selection. *Curr. Top. Microbiol. Immunol.* 293, 43–71.

Coutinho, A., and Haas, W. (2001). In vivo models of dominant T-cell tolerance: where do we stand today? *Trends Immunol.* 22, 350–351.

Curotto de Lafaille, M. A., Lino, A. C., Kutchukhidze, N., and Lafaille, J. J. (2004). CD25- T cells generate CD25+Foxp3+ regulatory T cells by peripheral expansion. *J. Immunol.* 173, 7259–7268.

Danieli, M. G., Markovits, D., Gabrielli, A., Corvetta, A., Giorgi, P. L., van der Zee, R., van Embden, J. D., Danieli, G., and Cohen, I. R. (1992). Juvenile rheumatoid arthritis patients manifest immune reactivity to the mycobacterial 65-kDa heat shock protein, to its 180-188 peptide, and to a partially homologous peptide of the proteoglycan link protein. *Clin. Immunol. Immunopathol.* 64, 121–128.

Davies, E. L., Bacelar, M. M., Marshall, M. J., Johnson, E., Wardle, T. D., Andrew, S. M., and Williams, J. H. (2006). Heat shock proteins form part of a danger signal cascade in response to lipopolysaccharide and GroEL. *Clin. Exp. Immunol.* 145, 183–189.

de Kleer, I. M., Wedderburn, L. R., Taams, L. S., Patel, A., Varsani, H., Klein, M., de Jager, W., Pugayung, G., Giannoni, F., Rijkers, G., Albani, S., Kuis, W., and Prakken, B. (2004). CD4+CD25bright regulatory T cells actively regulate inflammation in the joints of patients with the remitting form of juvenile idiopathic arthritis. *J. Immunol.* 172, 6435–6443.

Dieude, M., Senécal, J. L., and Raymond, Y. (2004). Induction of endothelial cell apoptosis by heatshock protein 60-reactive antibodies from anti-endothelial cell autoantibody-positive systemic lupus erythematosus patients. *Arthritis Rheum.* 50, 3221–3231.

Ding, Y., Shen, S., Lino, A. C., Curotto de Lafaille, M. A., and Lafaille, J. J. (2008). Beta-catenin stabilization extends regulatory T cell survival and induces anergy in nonregulatory T cells. *Nat. Med.* 14, 162–169.

Elias, D., and Cohen, I. R. (1995). Treatment of autoimmune diabetes and insulitis in NOD mice with heat shock protein 60 peptide p277. *Diabetes* 44, 1132–1138.

Elias, D., Reshef, T., Birk, O. S., Van der Zee, R., Walker, M. D., and Cohen, I. R. (1991). Vaccination against autoimmune mouse diabetes with a T-cell epitope of the human 65-kDa heat shock protein. *Proc. Natl. Acad. Sci. U.S.A.* 88, 3088–3091.

Faria, A. M., Maron, R., Ficker, S. M., Slavin, A. J., Spahn, T., and Weiner, H. L. (2003). Oral tolerance induced by continuous feeding: enhanced up-regulation of transforming growth factor-beta/interleukin-10 and suppression of experimental autoimmune encephalomyelitis. *J. Autoimmun.* 20, 135–145.

Faria, A. M., and Weiner, H. L. (2005). Oral tolerance. *Immunol. Rev.* 206, 232–259.

Faria, A. M., and Weiner, H. L. (2006). Oral tolerance: therapeutic implications for autoimmune diseases. *Clin. Dev. Immunol.* 13, 143–145.

Faria, A. M. C., Ficker, S. M., Speziali, E., Menezes, J. S., Stransky, B., Silva Rodrigues, V., and Vaz, N. M. (1998). Aging affects oral tolerance induction but not its maintenance in mice. *Mech. Ageing Dev.* 102, 67–80.

Feige, U., and Cohen, I. R. (1991). The 65-kDa heat-shock protein in the pathogenesis, prevention and therapy of autoimmune arthritis and diabetes-mellitus in rats and mice. *Springer Semin. Immunopathol.* 13, 99–113.

Fischer, H. P., Sharrock, C. E., and Panayi, G. S. (1992). High frequency of cord blood lymphocytes against mycobacterial 65-kDa heat-shock protein. *Eur. J. Immunol.* 22, 1667–1669.

Granja, C., Moliterno, R. A., Ferreira, M. S., Fonseca, J. A., Kalil, J., and Coelho, V. (2004). T-cell autoreactivity to Hsp in human transplantation may involve both proinflammatory and regulatory functions. *Hum. Immunol.* 65, 124–134.

Habich, C., and Burkat, V. (2007). Heat shock protein 60: regulatory role on innate immune cells. *Cell. Mol. Life Sci.* 64, 742–751.

Harats, D., Yacov, N., Gilburd, B., Shoenfeld, Y., and George, J. (2002). Oral tolerance with heat shock protein 65 attenuates *Mycobacterium tuberculosis*-induced and highfat-diet-driven atherosclerotic lesions. *J. Am. Coll. Cardiol.* 40, 1333–1338.

Hemmingsen, S. M., Woolford, C., Van der Vies, S. M., Tilly, K., Dennis, D. T., Georgopoulos, C. P., Hendrix, R. W., and Ellis, R. J. (1988). Homologous plant and bacterial proteins chaperone oligomeric protein assembly. *Nature* 333, 330–334.

Henderson, B., Calderwood, S. K., Coates, A. R., Cohen, I., van Eden, W., Lehner, T., and Pockley, A. G. (2010). Caught with their PAMPs down? The extracellular signalling actions of molecular chaperones are not due to microbial contaminants. *Cell Stress Chaperones* 15, 123–141.

Herlands, R. A., Christensen, S. R., Sweet, R. A., Hershberg, U., and Shlomchik, M. J. (2008). T cell-independent and toll-like receptor dependent antigen-driven activation of autoreactive B cells. *Immunity* 29, 249–260.

Huurman, V. A., Decochez, K., Mathieu, C., Cohen, I. R., and Roep, B. O. (2007). Therapy with the hsp60 peptide DiaPep277(trade mark) in C-peptide positive type 1 diabetes patients. *Diabetes Metab. Res. Rev.* 23, 269–275.

Karlin, S., and Brocchieri, L. (2000). Heat shock protein 60 sequence comparisons: duplications, lateral transfer, and mitochondrial evolution. *Proc. Natl Acad. Sci. USA* 97, 11348–11353.

Kaufmann, S. H. (1990). Heat shock proteins and the immune response. *Immunol. Today* 11, 129–136.

Kaufmann, S. H., Vath, U., Thole, J. E., Van Embden, J. D., and Emmrich, F. (1987). Enumeration of T cells reactive with *Mycobacterium tuberculosis* organisms and specific for the recombinant mycobacterial 64-kDa protein. *Eur. J. Immunol.* 17, 351–357.

Koga, T., Wand-Württenberger, A., DeBruyn, J., Munk, M. E., Schoel, B., and Kaufmann, S. H. (1989). T cells against a bacterial heat shock protein recognize stressed macrophages. *Science* 245, 1112–1115.

Kusukawa, N., and Yura, T. (1988). Heat shock protein GroE of *Escherichia coli*: key protective roles against thermal stress. *Genes Dev.* 2, 874–882.

Kyewski, B., and Klein, L. (2006). A central role for central tolerance. *Annu. Rev. Immunol.* 2006;24, 571–606.

Lima, D. S., Zárate-Blades, C. R., Souza, P. R. M., Trombonr, A. P., Santos-Junior, R. R., Brandao, I. T., Masson, A. P., Bonato, V. L. D., Sartori, A., Vendramini, M., Soares, E. G., Soares, E. G., Benvenutti, L. A., Silva, C. L., and Coelho, V. (2009). No evidence of pathological autoimmunity following *Mycobacterium leprae* heat-shock protein 56-DNA vaccination in mice. *Eur. J. Inflam.* 7, 75–78.

Luna, E., Postol, E., Caldas, C., Benvenuti, L. A., Rodrigues, J. M. Jr., Lima, K., Kalil, J., and Coelho, V. (2007). Treatment with encapsulated Hsp60 peptide (p277) prolongs skin graft survival in a murine model of minor antigen disparity. *Scand. J. Immunol.* 66, 62–70.

Mamalaki, C., Murdjeva, M., Tolaini, M., Norton, T., Chandler, P., Townsend, A., Simpson, E., and Kioussis, D. (1996). Tolerance in TCR/cognate antigen double-transgenic mice mediated by incomplete thymic deletion and peripheral receptor downregulation. *Dev. Immunol.* 4, 299–315.

Maron, R., Sukhova, G., Faria, A. M., Hoffmann, E., Mach, F., Libby, P., and Weiner, H. L. (2002). Mucosal administration of heat shock protein-65 decreases atherosclerosis and inflammation in aortic arch of low-density lipoprotein receptor-deficient mice. *Circulation* 106, 1708–1715.

Mathur, S., Walley, K. R., Wang, Y., Indrambarya, T., and Boyd, J. H. (2011). Extracellular heat shock protein 70 induces cardiomyocyte inflammation and contractile dysfunction via TLR2. *Circ. J.* 75, 2445–2452.

Matthews, R. C., Maresca, B., Burnie, J. P., Cardona, A., Carrutu, L., Conti, S., Deepe, G. S., Florez, A. M., Franceschelli, S., Garcia, E., Gargano, L. S., Kobayashi, G. S., McEwen, J. G., Ortiz, B. L., Oviedo, A. M., Polonelli, L., Ponton, J., and Restrepo, A. (1998). Stress proteins in fungal diseases. *Med. Mycol.* 36(Suppl. 1), 45–51.

McMullin, T. W., and Hallberg, R. L. (1988). A highly evolutionarily conserved mitochondrial protein is structurally related to the protein encoded by the *Escherichia coli* groEL gene. *Mol. Cell. Biol.* 8, 371–380.

Merbl, Y., Zucker-Toledano, M., Quintana, F. J., and Cohen, I. R. (2007). Newborn humans manifest autoantibodies to defined self molecules detected by antigen microarray informatics. *J. Clin. Invest.* 117, 712–718.

Mestecky, J., Husby, S., Moldoveanu, Z., Waldo, F. B., van den Wall Bake, A. W., and Elson, C. O. (1996). Induction of tolerance in humans: effectiveness of oral and nasal immunization routes. *Ann. N. Y. Acad. Sci.* 778, 194–201.

Michaluart, P., Abdallah, K. A., Lima, F. D., Smith, R., Moysés, R. A., Coelho, V., Victora, G. D., Socorro-Silva, A., Volsi, E. C., Zárate-Bladés, C. R., Ferraz, A. R., Barreto, A. K., Chammas, M. C., Gomes, R., Gebrim, E., Arakawa-Sugueno, L., Fernandes, K. P., Lotufo, P. A., Cardoso, M. R., Kalil, J., and Silva, C. L. (2008). Phase I trial of DNA-hsp65 immunotherapy for advanced squamous cell carcinoma of the head and neck. *Cancer Gene Ther.* 15, 676–684.

Miller, A., Lider, O., and Weiner, H. L. (1991). Antigen-driven bystander suppression after oral administration of antigens. *J. Exp. Med.* 174, 791–798.

Minter, L. M., and Osborne, B. A. (2003). Cell death in the thymus – it's all a matter of contacts. *Semin. Immunol.* 15, 135–144.

Moraes-Vieira, P. M., Takenaka, M. C., Silva, H. M., Monteiro, S. M., Agena, F., Lemos, F., Saitovitch, D., Kalil, J., and Coelho, V. (2012). GATA3 and a dominant regulatory gene expression profile discriminate operational tolerance in human transplantation. *Clin. Immunol.* [Ahead of print].

Munk, M. E., Schoel, B., Modrow, S., Karr, R. W., Young, R. A., and Kaufmann, S. H. (1989). T lymphocytes from healthy individuals with specificity to self-epitopes shared by the mycobacterial and human 65-kilodalton heat shock protein. *J. Immunol.* 143, 2844–2849.

Nemirovsky, A., Fisher, Y., Baron, R., Cohen, I. R., and Monsonego, A. (2011). Amyloid beta-HSP60 peptide conjugate vaccine treats a mouse model of Alzheimer's disease. *Vaccine* 29, 4043–4050.

Newcomb, J. R., and Cresswell, P. (1993). Characterization of endogenous peptides bound to purified HLA-DR molecules and their absence from invariant chain-associated αβ dimers. *J. Immunol.* 150, 499–507.

Oliveira, F., Bafica, A., Rosato, A. B., Favali, C. B., Costa, J. M., Cafe, V., Barral-Netto, M., and Barral, A. (2011). Lesion size correlates with Leishmania antigen-stimulated TNF-levels in human cutaneous leishmaniasis. *Am. J. Trop. Med. Hyg.* 85, 70–73.

Paul, A. G., Van der Zee, R., Taams, L. S., and van Eden, W. (2000). A self-hsp60 peptide acts as a partial agonist inducing expression of B7-2 on mycobacterial hsp60-specific T cells: a possible mechanism for inhibitory T cell regulation of adjuvant arthritis? *Int. Immunol.* 12, 1041–1050.

Pockley, A. G., Bulmer, J., Hanks, B. M., and Wright, B. H. (1999). Identification of human heat shock protein 60 (Hsp60) and anti-Hsp60 antibodies in the peripheral circulation of normal individuals. *Cell Stress Chaperones* 4, 29–35.

Pockley, A. G., Muthana, M., and Calderwood, S. K. (2009). The dual immunoregulatory roles of stress proteins. *Trends Biochem. Sci.* 33, 71–79.

Pontes, D. S., de Azevedo, M. S., Chatel, J. M., Langella, P., Azevedo, V., and Miyoshi, A. (2011). *Lactococcus lactis* as a live vector: heterologous protein production and DNA delivery systems. *Protein Expr. Purif.* 79, 165–175.

Prakken, B. J., Van der Zee, R., Anderton, S. M., van Kooten, P. J., Kuis, W., and van Eden, W. (1997). Peptide-induced nasal tolerance for a mycobacterial heat shock protein 60 T cell epitope in rats suppresses both adjuvant arthritis and nonmicrobially induced experimental arthritis. *Proc. Natl. Acad. Sci. U.S.A.* 94, 3284–3289.

Qian, J., Moliterno, R., Donovan-Peluso, M. A., Liu, K., Suzow, J., Valdivia, L., Pan, F., and Duquesnoy, R. J. (1995). Expression of stress proteins and lymphocyte reactivity in heterotopic cardiac allografts undergoing cellular rejection. *Transpl. Immunol.* 3, 114–123.

Quintana, F. J., Carmi, P., and Cohen, I. R. (2002). DNA vaccination with heat shock protein 60 inhibits cyclophosphamide-accelerated diabetes. *J. Immunol.* 169, 6030–6035.

Quintana, F. J., Farez, M. F., Viglietta, V., Iglesias, A. H., Merbl, Y., Izquierdo, G., Lucas, M., Basso, A. S., Khoury, S. J., Lucchinetti, C. F., Cohen, I. R., and Weiner, H. L. (2008). Antigen microarrays identify unique serum autoantibody signatures in clinical and pathologic subtypes of multiple sclerosis. *Proc. Natl. Acad. Sci. U.S.A.* 105, 18889–18894.

Quintana, F. J., Hagedorn, P. H., Elizur, G., Merbl, Y., Domany, E., and Cohen, I. R. (2004). Functional immunomics: microarray analysis of IgG autoantibody repertoires predicts the future response of mice to induced diabetes. *Proc. Natl. Acad. Sci. U.S.A.* 101(Suppl. 2), 14615–14621.

Quintana, F. J., and Cohen, I. (2011). HSP60 immune system network. *Trends Immunol.* 32, 89–95.

Raz, I., Avron, A., Tamir, M., Metzger, M., Symer, L., Eldor, R., Cohen, I. R., and Elias, D. (2007). Treatment of new-onset type 1 diabetes with peptide DiaPep277 is safe and associated with preserved beta-cell function: extension of a randomized, double-blind, phase II trial. *Diabetes Metab. Res. Rev.* 23, 292–298.

Raz, I., Elias, D., Avron, A., Tamir, M., Metzger, M., and Cohen, I. R. (2001). Beta-cell function in new-onset type 1 diabetes and immunomodulation with a heat-shock protein peptide (DiaPep277): a randomised, double-blind, phase II trial. *Lancet* 358, 1749–1753.

Round, J. L., O'Connell, R. M., and Mazmanian, S. K. (2010). Coordination of tolerogenic immune responses by the commensal microbiota. *J. Autoimmun.* 34, J220–J225.

Sanchez-Campillo, M., Bini, L., Comanducci, M., Raggiaschi, R., Marzocchi, B., Pallini, V., and Ratti, G. (1999). Identification of immunoreactive proteins of *Chlamydia trachomatis* by Western blot analysis of a two-dimensional electrophoresis map with patient sera. *Electrophoresis* 20, 2269–2279.

Soltys, B. J., and Gupta, R. S. (1997). Cell surface localization of the 60 kDa heat shock chaperonin protein (hsp60) in mammalian cells. *Cell Biol. Int.* 21, 315–320.

Stanford, M., Whittall, T., Bergmeier, L. A., Lindblad, M., Lundin, S., Shinnick, T., Mizushima, Y., Holmgren, J., and Lehner, T. (2004). Oral tolerization with peptide 336–351 linked to cholera toxin B subunit in preventing relapses of uveitis in Behcet's disease. *Clin. Exp. Immunol.* 137, 201–208.

Stevens, T. R., Winrow, V. R., Blake, D. R., and Rampton, D. S. (1992). Circulating antibodies to heat-shock protein 60 in Crohn's disease and ulcerative colitis. *Clin. Exp. Immunol.* 90, 271–274.

Tanaka, T., Yamakawa, N., Koike, N., Suzuki, J., Mizuno, F., and Usui, M. (1999). Behcet's disease and antibody titers to various heat-shock protein 60 s. *Ocul. Immunol. Inflamm.* 7, 69–74.

Thompson, S. J., Francis, J. N., Siew, L. K., Webb, G. R., Jenner, P. J., Colston, M. J., and Elson, C. J. (1998). An immunodominant epitope from mycobacterial 65-kDa heat shock protein protects against pristane-induced arthritis. *J. Immunol.* 160, 4628–4634.

Tsai, Y. P., Yang, M. H., Huang, C. H., Chang, S. Y., Chen, P. M., Liu, C. J., Teng, S. C., and Wu, K. J. (2009). Interaction between HSP60 and beta-catenin promotes metastasis. *Carcinogenesis* 30, 1049–1057.

Vabulas, R. M., Ahmad-Nejad, P., da Costa, C., Miethke, T., Kirschning, C. J., Häcker, H., and Wagner, H. (2001). Endocytosed HSP60s use toll-like receptor 2 (TLR2) and TLR4 to activate the toll/interleukin-1 receptor signaling pathway in innate immune cells. *J. Biol. Chem.* 276, 31332–31339.

Van Eden, W., Van der Zee, R., and Prakken, B. (2005). Heat-shock proteins induce T-cell regulation of chronic inflammation. *Nat. Rev.* 5, 318–330.

van Roon, J. A., van Eden, W., van Roy, J. L., Lafeber, F. J., and Bijlsma, J. W. (1997). Stimulation of suppressive T cell responses by human but not bacterial 60-kD heat-shock protein in synovial fluid of patients with rheumatoid arthritis. *J. Clin. Invest.* 100, 459–463.

Victora, G. D., Socorro-Silva, A., Volsi, E. C., Abdallah, K., Lima, F. D., Smith, R. B., Moyses, R. A., Zárate-Bladés, C. R., Michaluart, P., Silva, C. L., Kalil, J., and Coelho, V. (2009). Immune response to vaccination with DNA-Hsp65 in a phase I clinical trial with head and neck cancer patients. *Cancer Gene Ther.* 16, 598–608.

Vitelli-Avelar, D. M., Sathler-Avelar, R., Teixeira-Carvalho, A., Pinto Dias, J. C., Gontijo, E. D., Faria, A. M., Elói-Santos, S. M., and Martins-Filho, O. A. (2008). Strategy to assess the overall cytokine profile of circulating leukocytes and its association with distinct clinical forms of human Chagas disease. *Scand. J. Immunol.* 68, 516–525.

Wallin, R. P. A., Lundqvist, A., Mor, S. H., von Bonin, A., Kiessling, R., and Ljunggren, H. G. (2002). Heat-shock proteins as activators of the innate immune system. *Trends Immunol.* 23, 130–135.

Wamachi, A. N., Mayadev, J. S., Mungai, P. L., Magak, P. L., Ouma, J. H., Magambo, J. K., Muchiri, E. M., Koech, D. K., King, C. H., and King, C. L. (2004). Increased ratio of tumor necrosis factor-alpha to interleukin-10 production is associated with Schistosoma haematobium-induced urinary-tract morbidity. *J. Infect. Dis.* 190, 2020–2030.

Wand-Wurttenberger, A., Schoel, B., Ivanyi, J., and Kaufmann, S. H. E. (1991). Surface expression by mononuclear phagocytes of an epitope shared with mycobacterial heat-shock protein-60. *Eur. J. Immunol.* 21, 1089–1092.

Xu, Q., Willeit, J., Marosi, M., Kleindienst, R., Oberhollenzer, F., Kiechl, S., Stulnig, T., Luef, G., and Wick, G. (1993). Association of serum antibodies to heat-shock protein 65 with carotid atherosclerosis. *Lancet* 341, 255–259.

Zanin-Zhorov, A., Cahalon, L., Tal, G., Margalit, R., Lider, O., and Cohen, I. R. (2006). Heat shock protein 60 enhances CD4+ CD25+ regulatory T cell function via innate TLR2 signaling. *J. Clin. Invest.* 116, 2022–2032.

Zügel, U., and Kaufmann, S. H. (1999). Role of heat shock proteins in protection from and pathogenesis of infectious diseases. *Clin. Microbiol. Rev.* 12, 19–39.

14

Age-related changes in human peripheral blood *IGH* repertoire following vaccination

Yu-Chang Bryan Wu[1], David Kipling[2] and Deborah K. Dunn-Walters[1]*

[1] Department of Immunobiology, King's College London School of Medicine, London, UK
[2] Institute of Cancer and Genetics, School of Medicine, Cardiff University, Cardiff, UK

Edited by:
Harry W. Schroeder, University of Alabama, USA

Reviewed by:
Kishore Alugupalli, Thomas Jefferson University, USA
Harry W. Schroeder, University of Alabama, USA
Kay L. Medina, Mayo Clinic, USA

***Correspondence:**
Deborah K. Dunn-Walters, Reader in Immunology, Department of Immunobiology, King's College London School of Medicine, Guy's Campus, London SE1 9RT, UK.
e-mail: deborah.dunn-walters@kcl.ac.uk

Immune protection against pulmonary infections, such as seasonal flu and invasive pneumonia, is severely attenuated with age, and vaccination regimes for the elderly people often fail to elicit effective immune response. We have previously shown that influenza and pneumococcal vaccine responses in the older population are significantly impaired in terms of serum antibody production, and have shown repertoire differences by CDR-H3 spectratype analysis. Here we report a detailed analysis of the B cell repertoire in response to vaccine, including a breakdown of sequences by class and subclass. Clustering analysis of high-throughput sequencing data enables us to visualize the response in terms of expansions of clonotypes, changes in CDR-H3 characteristics, and somatic hypermutation as well as identifying the commonly used *IGH* genes. We have highlighted a number of significant age-related changes in the B cell repertoire. Interestingly, in light of the fact that IgG is the most prevalent serum antibody and the most widely used as a correlate of protection, the most striking age-related differences are in the IgA response, with defects also seen in the IgM repertoire. In addition there is a skewing toward IgG2 in the IgG sequences of the older samples at all time points. This analysis illustrates the importance of antibody classes other than IgG and has highlighted a number of areas for future consideration in vaccine studies of the elderly.

Keywords: B cell repertoire, aging, vaccine, immunoglobulin, IgA

INTRODUCTION

Until recently the methods available to study B cell repertoire were limited by the fact that the diversity of the repertoire was far greater than the number of sequences that could feasibly be studied. A random sampling of cells responding to vaccine would pick up the most prevalent Ig genes but would not give any indication of the diversity of cells responding to challenge. In mice the T-dependent NP response is a widely used and versatile tool for the study of immune responses, it tends to be restricted to use of the V186.2 heavy chain. In humans the isolation of rearranged Ig genes with more than one type of *IGHV* gene has indicated that there might be diversity in the response, but the numbers of sequences studied in these experiments have been low. One of the best examples of repertoire analysis was by Kolibab et al. (2005a) who looked at approximately 1300 sequences from 40 different donors after immunization by the pneumococcal vaccine and identified the major *IGHV* genes in use. With the advent of high-throughput sequencing methods we can now study the human immune response in much more detail.

A perennial problem in vaccination is that of vaccine inefficiency in older people. Vaccine-specific antibodies in older people are quantitatively and qualitatively impaired. For example, anti-pneumococcal polysaccharide (PPS) antibodies have lower opsonophagocytic index and affinity in the elderly than in healthy young adults (Kolibab et al., 2005b; Park and Nahm, 2011). *Streptococcus pneumoniae* infection is a serious complication secondary to influenza, and together these two diseases comprise a substantial infectious burden for children aged under two, the elderly and immunocompromised individuals (McCullers, 2006). In the UK and many other countries, co-administration of trivalent-influenza and pneumococcal vaccines has been recommended as the routine immunization schedule to protect these at-risk groups. Although influenza vaccines appear effective in most groups with nearly 70% vaccine efficacy (Osterholm et al., 2012), less than half of the older adults are protected by influenza vaccines (Nichol et al., 2007). While the immunogenicity of PPS vaccines in the protein-conjugated form (PCV) is much improved for young children, neither PCV nor 23-valent PPS vaccine (PPV-23) is able to confer an effective protection in the older population (Baxendale et al., 2010).

We have previously seen that there may be changes in the selection process during affinity maturation of B cells (Banerjee et al., 2002), and also that the B cell repertoire is often less diverse in old age with evidence of non-pathogenic clonal expansions (Gibson et al., 2009). This loss of diversity correlated with the health of the individual. Further investigation as to whether loss of diversity in the B cell repertoire correlated with poor vaccine responses against influenza and pneumonia indicated that it may be a contributory factor, but that other factors were likely also involved (Ademokun et al., 2011). These two vaccines generate different responses; influenza is believed to mainly induce IgG1/IgG3/IgA1 T-dependent responses (Brown et al., 1985; Hocart et al., 1990;

Powers, 1994), while pneumococcal responses are thought to be T-independent and can lead to significant elevation of IgA2/IgG2 antibodies in the serum and mucosa (Lue et al., 1988; Carson et al., 1995; Sanal et al., 1999; Simell et al., 2006; Benckert et al., 2011).

To investigate the diversity of the response to these vaccines in more detail we have analyzed high-throughput sequencing data in order to characterize the response with respect to Ig gene usage and hypermutation whilst paying particular attention to the subclasses of antibodies involved. There are significant differences in the older vaccine response with respect to class and subclass of antibody, extent and timing of clonal expansions and focusing of the repertoire toward Ig sequences with higher mutation and shorter CDR-H3 regions.

MATERIALS AND METHODS

VOLUNTEERS AND SAMPLE COLLECTION

Six young (aged 19–45) and six older (aged 70–89) healthy volunteers were recruited as a part of the 2009/10 influenza vaccination program in Lambeth Walk GP Practice. Blood and serum samples were collected after obtaining written consent as approved by the Guy's Hospital Research ethics committee, prior to vaccination at day 0 (D0) with the influenza (Influvac; Solvay, Southampton, UK), and 23-valent pneumococcal (Pneumovax II; Sanofi Pasteur MSD, Maidenhead, UK) vaccines and post vaccination at day 7 (D7) and day 28 (D28). PBMCs were isolated using Ficoll-Paque Plus (GE Healthcare, Buckinghamshire, UK) in conjunction with Leucosep tubes (Greiner Bio-One Ltd., Gloucestershire, UK), according to manufacturer's instructions.

TOTAL RNA EXTRACTION AND cDNA CONVERSION

Total RNA was extracted from 2×10^7 PBMCs per donor per time point using the RNeasy Mini Kit (Qiagen, UK). The SuperScript III First-Strand cDNA Synthesis System (Invitrogen, UK) was then used to convert RNA into cDNA according to the manufacturer's protocol. In brief, a 200-μL cDNA reaction mix contained extracted total RNA, 500 ng Oligo(dT)$_{20}$, 500 μM dNTPs, 400 U RNaseOut, 10 mM DTT, and 2000 U SuperScript III RT in 1× First-Stand RT buffer. The cDNA reaction was carried out as follows: 65°C for (5 min), 4°C (60 s); 50°C (1 h); 70°C (15 min).

HIGH-THROUGHPUT SEQUENCING OF *IgH* GENES

Ig genes were isolated by semi-nested, isotype-specific PCR reactions, as previously reported (Wu et al., 2010). Briefly, a 25-μL PCR1 reaction mix contained 6.25 μL of cDNA, 0.625 U Phusion DNA polymerase (NEB, UK), 200 μM each dNTP, 41.75 nM each of 6 *IGHV* gene family primers in conjunction with 250 nM of either IgM, pan-IgA, or pan-IgG constant region primers. Two microliters of PCR1 products were subsequently re-amplified using multiplex identifier (MID)-containing primers in a semi-nested reaction consisting of 0.5 U Phusion DNA polymerase, 200 μM each dNTPs, 41.75 nM each of the *IGHV* gene family/MID primers, and 250 nM of the nested constant region/MID primers in a 20-μL reaction volume. PCR conditions are as follows: 98°C for (30 s), 15 (PCR1), or 20 (PCR2) cycles of 98°C (10 s); 58°C (15 s); 72°C (45 s), and 1 cycle of 72°C (10 min). In order to produce sufficient quantity for high-throughput sequencing on the GS FLX System (Roche, Germany), eight different PCR1 for each sample, followed by 16 PCR2 (two per initial PCR1 round) reactions were performed for each isotype. This total sampling of cDNA was approximately equivalent to that from 2×10^5 B cells. The downstream preparation of PCR products and data processing are as previously published (Wu et al., 2010).

DETECTION OF ANTI-PPS IgA ANTIBODIES

Serum anti-PPS IgA antibodies from immunized young (age 18–49, $n = 39$) and older (age 65–89, $n = 27$) healthy volunteers were measured by ELISA, as previous reported (Ademokun et al., 2011). In brief, the 89-SF standard (Bethesda, MD, USA) or serum samples were pre-absorbed with 10 μg/mL cell wall polysaccharide (CPS; Statens Serum Institute, Copenhagen, Denmark) or 10 μg/mL CPS in conjunction with 10 μg/mL 22F polysaccharide, respectively, before being serial diluted and incubated with microtiter plates coated with 100 μL per well of a combination of seven polysaccharide serotypes (4, 6B, 9, 14, 18C, 19F, and 23F, 1 μg/mL each; ATCC, Rockville, MD, USA) overnight at 4°C. After washing with TBS containing 0.1% Brij 35 (Sigma-Aldrich, St. Louis, MO, USA), HRP-conjugated goat anti-human IgA (Invitrogen) diluted at 1/4000 in PBS with 0.05% Tween-20 was added to the plates and incubated for 2 h, followed by another 2 h of incubation with TMB chromogen substrate (Invitrogen) in diethanolamine buffer, before terminating the reaction with 3 M NaOH. Serum anti-PPS IgA levels were read at OD 450 nM on an ELISA microplate reader and then compared with the 89-SF standard.

SEQUENCE ANALYSIS

Ig gene usage and CDR-H3 junction regions between the conserved first (cysteine) and last amino acid (tryptophan) were determined using IMGT V-QUEST (Wilkins et al., 1999). Internal isotype motifs in the constant regions of each sequence further identified subclasses of sequences. ProtParam was used to determine the physicochemical properties of the CDR-H3 peptide (Brochet et al., 2008). The grand average of hydropathicity (GRAVY) and aliphatic indices are positive indicators for peptide hydrophobicity and structural thermostability respectively (Ikai, 1980; Wilkins et al., 1999). The percentage match of each IGHV sequence to germline gene was returned by IMGT V-QUEST, and the level of hypermutation was calculated to be the percentage difference from the corresponding germline gene.

The DNA sequences of the CDR-H3 were used for clonotype clustering by a distance-matrix between all pairwise comparisons, as previously reported (Ademokun et al., 2011). When necessary, clonally related IGH sequences were aligned with putative germline genes and edited to remove homopolymer tract errors using DNAstar software (Laser Gene). Mutational phylogenetic trees of the edited IGH sequences were constructed by the multiple sequence alignment modes (MUSCLE 3.7) using the Phylogeny Analysis program (Dereeper et al., 2010).

STATISTICS

Statistics were performed with GraphPad Prism 5.0. Most statistical analyses were one-way or repeated measures ANOVA (with Bonferroni post-test) and Kruskal–Wallis comparisons (with Dunn's post-test). Wherever necessary, Chi-squared test (with

Bonferroni post-test), paired t-test, and Mann–Whitney U-test was performed. To test association between different metrics, Pearson correlation analysis in conjunction with linear regression was performed.

RESULTS

IGH REPERTOIRE CHANGES IN RESPONSE TO VACCINATION

High-throughput sequencing of samples from peripheral blood B cells in six young and six old donors in the course of vaccination produced 45,784 *IGH* sequences, which were grouped into 17,962 different clonotypes (i.e., a representative clone for that particular Ig gene rearrangement, **Table 1**). In order to investigate the effect of vaccination on the underlying repertoire without the influence of *in vivo* and *in vitro* clonal expansion, only clonotypes were included for this analysis. In general, the repertoire displayed resilience in that at D28 post vaccination it showed similar characteristics to D0 (before vaccination) despite significant changes at day 7 post vaccination. These changes at D7 included a change in expression of some *IGHV* and *IGHJ* genes such that significant differences were seen in IGH gene family usage (**Figure 1A**). Most notably, at D7 after vaccination there is a significant increase in the proportion of clonotypes that use *IGHV6-1*, *IGHV1-46*, and several *IGHV3* genes with a decrease in those using *IGHV2*, *IGHV4* gene families, and *IGHV3-21* (**Figure 1B**). An increased usage of the shorter *IGHJ4* genes by 4.5% with a concomitant decrease in use of the longer *IGHJ6* gene (**Figure 1C**; $p < 0.05$) at D7 may explain the overall reduction in the CDR-H3 size by 2 nt (**Figure 1D**; $p < 0.0005$, Kruskal–Wallis test). The D7 population also has a more hydrophilic CDR-H3, as shown by a more negative GRAVY index (**Figure 1E**; $p < 0.0005$), and is also less aliphatic (**Figure 1F**; $p < 0.0005$).

AGE-RELATED DIFFERENCES IN VACCINE-INDUCED CLONAL EXPANSION

It has been shown that clonal expansion after challenge is delayed and persists longer in old mice (Szabo et al., 2004). More recently, Lindner et al. (2012) reported that the intestinal IgA repertoire has fewer large, expanded, clones in old mice. In humans, we have previously shown vaccine-induced changes in CDR-H3 size and hydrophobicity in expanded clones of young people, but the changes are less obvious in the older group (Ademokun et al., 2011). Here we aim to investigate age and challenge-related changes in *IGH* gene usage. To ensure that our comparative analyses of clonal expansion reflect the effects of *in vivo* clonal expansion, rather than *in vitro* amplification from PCR, the *IGH* sequences were produced using the same number of cells in each sample. In the overall repertoire, large clones containing up to 687 member sequences appear at D7 and are seen less frequently at D28 in the young group, whereas in the older group the largest clone that appears at D7 has only 242 sequence members and some large clones are also observed at D28 (**Figure 2A**). Intraclonal variations in *IGHV* sequences indicate that these large clones likely represent *in vivo* expansion (**Figure 6**). To understand how clonal expansion occurs in different classes of B cells, *IGH* sequences were grouped by isotype for further analyses of clone size (**Figures 2B–D**). Significant increases in the average clone size at D7, as result of increased proportion of large clones, are seen in all isotypes in both age groups, although the increase in IgM clones is not as great as that seen in IgA and IgG clones. The pattern of vaccine responses in IgG and IgM clones, as indicated by changes in the average clone size, is similar between the two age groups (**Figure 2B**). The increase in average clone size was usually related to the accumulation of greater numbers of larger clone sizes, except in the case of IgA, where the young and old samples had comparable numbers of clones larger than 3, but the average clone size in young IgA clones at D7 is twice that of the old clones at D7 (**Figure 2B**; $p < 0.005$) This implies that the IgA clones in the young are larger than in the old. Consistent with this, the largest clones at D7 in the young in **Figure 2A** were IgA. Interestingly, the clone size is 2.5-fold larger in old IgA clones at D28 as compared with the young (**Figure 2B**; $p < 0.005$), and is larger than it was in the old at D7. So there may be a more delayed clonal expansion in IgA cells with age; while the young showed expansion at D7 and contraction back to D0 levels at D28, the level of expansion in the old may not yet have reached a peak by D28.

The vaccine response at D7 is very diverse at all ages in that changes in the average clone size are not restricted to particular *IGHV* family *IGHJ* gene combinations (**Figure 2C**). We calculated the fold difference in clone size between D7/D0 and D28/D7 for individual *IGHV* genes. At D7 there were 24 different *IGHV* genes of the IgA isotype and 16 different *IGHV* genes of the IgG isotype that had more than twofold increases in their average clone size

Table 1 | Numbers of *IGH* sequence and clonotypes produced by high-throughput sequencing.

Ages	Days	IgA	IgG	IgM	Unknown[3]	Total
Young (6 donors)	D0	886[1]/1424[2]	1035/1651	847/1208	413/737	3181/5020
	D7	976/5922	717/2707	641/1214	4912750	2825/12593
	D28	1070/1777	1298/2085	1036/1280	626/1059	4030/6201
Old (6 donors)	D0	928/1747	675/1528	809/1109	474/1175	2886/5559
	D7	644/1994	988/3801	579/998	418/1825	2629/8618
	D28	1223/5099	475/901	322/400	391/1393	2411/7793

[1]*The numbers of clonotypes refer to unique sequences, where only one example of a clonal expansion is counted after CDR-H3 clonotype clustering.*

[2]*The numbers of IGH sequences, generated from approximately 2 × 10^5 B cells per sample, represent those that passed quality control with full immunoglobulin VDJ gene rearrangement.*

[3]*Unknown isotype refers to sequences that do not extend far enough to the constant region for isotype identification.*

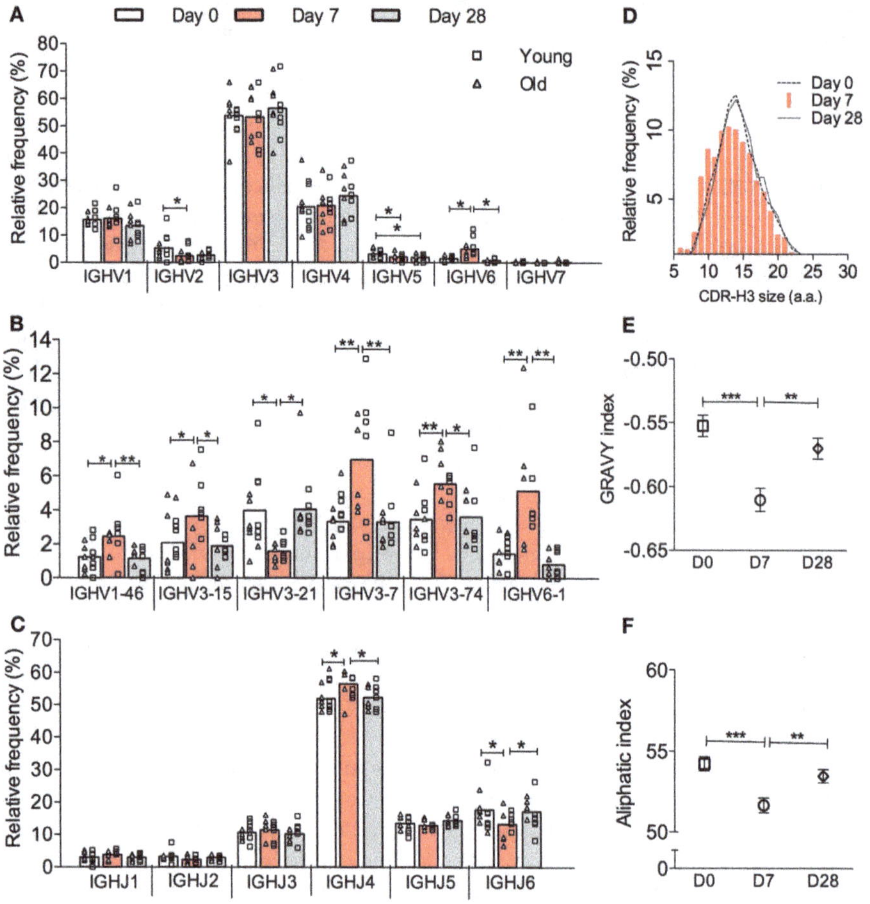

FIGURE 1 | Vaccine-induced changes in the overall *IGH* clonotype repertoire. *IGH* genes in each sequence were analyzed by IMGT V-QUEST and then clustered into clones by CDR-H3 DNA sequence similarity. Only one sequence example per clone was chosen to represent its clonotype. The relative frequency (*y*-axis) of all clonotypes (IgA, IgG, and IgM combined) by **(A)** *IGHV* gene family, **(B)** individual *IGHV* gene, and **(C)** *IGHJ* gene usage (*x*-axis) was calculated for six young (squares) and six old (triangles) donors individually before being grouped as a whole cohort of 12 donors for repeated measures ANOVA comparison between D0 (open bars), D7 (red bars) and D28 (grey bars). Bars indicate MEAN. **(D)** CDR-H3 virtual spectratypes, showing the relative frequency (*y*-axis) of a particular CDR-H3 size (*x*-axis in amino acid numbers) within the whole CDR-H3 repertoire, was calculated using all clonotypes from 12 donors at D0 (dotted line), D7 (red bars), and D28 (solid line). The GRAVY and aliphatic indices for each CDR-H3 peptide was determined by ProtParam. The overall GRAVY **(E)** and aliphatic **(F)** indices all clonotypes from 12 donors were compared by Kruskal–Wallis comparisons with Dunn's post-test between D0 (squares), D7 (circles), and D28 (diamonds). Error bars indicate ±SEM. $^{*}p < 0.05$, $^{**}p < 0.005$, and $^{***}p < 0.0005$.

(**Figure 2D**). The above age-related differences in the average clone size for IgA clones at D7 and D28 (**Figure 2B**) are a reflection of a diverse response, involving many different *IGHV* family *IGHJ* combinations and individual *IGHV* genes rather than any particular *IGH* genes (**Figures 2C,D**). The changes in the average clone size and serum anti-PPS IgA antibodies at D7 from D0 were also negatively correlated with age (**Figures 2E,F**).

AGE-RELATED DIFFERENCES IN CDR-H3 CHARACTERISTICS OF EXPANDED CLONES

CDR-H3 regions have been regarded as indispensible Ig structures for antigen recognition, therefore alterations in the physiochemical properties of CDR-H3 peptides could potentially affect BCR binding ability and selection and expansion of antigen specific cells within a population may be detectable by changes in the CDR-H3 characteristics (Romero-Steiner et al., 1999; Kolibab et al., 2005b; Park and Nahm, 2011). We therefore compared CDR-H3 characteristics in *IGH* sequences from clones of different sizes at D7 after challenge. The clonotypes were divided into those seen four or less times in the sample (small clones) and those seen five or more times (large clones). The overall hydrophobicity and aliphatic index of CDR-H3 regions from large clones does not significantly differ between ages when all isotypes are considered together (data not shown). However, there are significant age-related changes in CDR-H3 size in IgA and IgM clonotypes from large clones (**Figure 3A**) that was not seen in IgG clonotypes (data not shown). IgM clonotypes show significantly larger CDR-H3 sizes in all clones regardless of clone size in the old samples than in the young at both D0 and D7 (**Figure 3A**). The differences in the CDR-H3 size are mainly due to an increase in the total length of *IGHD* genes (**Figure 3B**), not *IGHJ* (data not shown), and an increase in the numbers of N-nucleotides that reaches significance

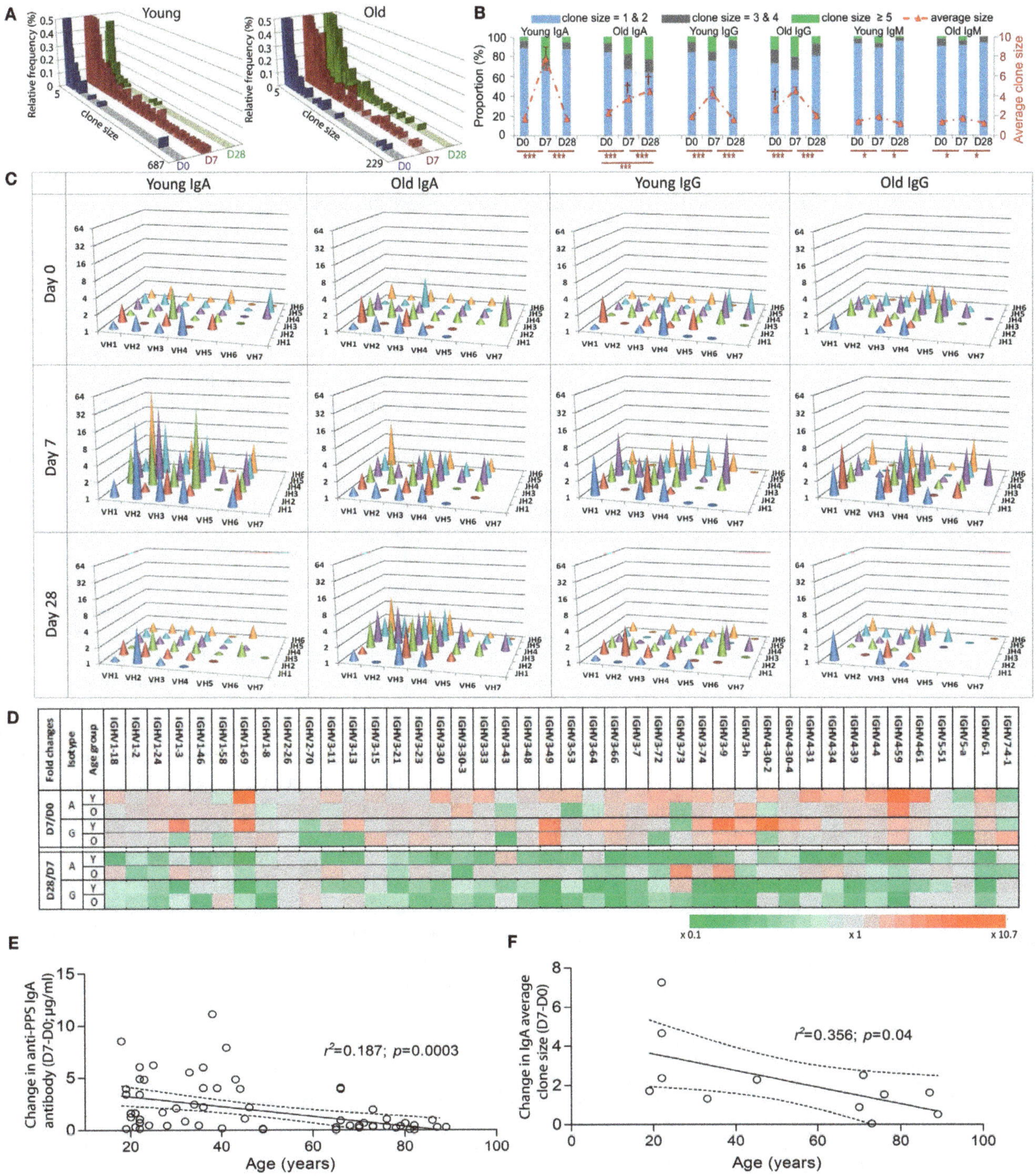

FIGURE 2 | Age-related differences in clonal expansion and serum anti-PPS IgA antibodies after vaccination. The size of each clone was determined. **(A)** The relative proportion (*y*-axis; %) of clones of different sizes (*x*-axis) was calculated using a collection of total clonotypes (IgA + IgG + IgM) from six young and six old donors at D0 (blue bars), D7 (red bars), and D28 (green bars). **(B)** Clonotypes were grouped by isotype and size (clone size = 1 and 2 in blue bars, 3 and 4 in grey bars; 5 and above in green bars; Left *y*-axis in %), and the proportion of each group was calculated for six young and six old donors at D0, D7, and D28. The average clone size (red line; Right *y*-axis) was calculated for each donor individually to be the ratio of total sequence numbers to total clonotype numbers, before being compared between different days ($*p < 0.05$ and $***p < 0.0005$; repeated measures ANOVA comparison) or between ages ($^{\dagger}\mathbf{p} < 0.005$; one-way ANOVA comparisons). Bars indicate ±SEM. **(C)** IgA and IgG clonotypes from six young and six old donors at different days were grouped by *IGHV* family (*x*-axis) and *IGHJ* (*z*-axis) gene usage, and the average clone size (*y*-axis) for each group was calculated. **(D)** IgA and IgG clonotypes from six young (Y) and

(Continued)

FIGURE 2 | Continued
six old (O) donors at different days were grouped by individual *IGHV* gene usage, and the average clone size for each group was calculated. The fold change of the average clone size at D0 from D7 (D7/D0) and at D28 from D7 (D28/D7) was calculated and is shown by different colors (grey as unchanged, green as fold decrease and red as fold increase). Serum levels of IgA antibodies specific for seven serotypes combined were determined using ELISA. Pearson correlation analysis was used to test the correlative relationship of age (*x*-axis in years) with changes in **(E)** serum anti-PPS IgA antibodies ($n = 66$) and **(F)** the average clone size (D7-D0, $n = 12$), r^2 and p values indicated. The Goodness-of-Fit (solid lines) was analyzed by linear regression with 95% CI indicated (dashed lines).

in expanded large clones (**Figure 3C**). There is also a significant age-related increase in the CDR-H3 size and CDR-H3 components in IgA clonotypes, although this is restricted to D7 and D28 post-challenge and is mainly in the larger clones (**Figures 3A–C**).

AGE- AND CHALLENGE-RELATED CHANGES IN HYPERMUTATION

Since the level of hypermutation accumulated in the Ig variable region often reflects the history of affinity maturation in B cell clones specific for a particular type of antigen, we compared *IGHV* mutation levels over the course of vaccination and in different age groups. The average mutation frequency is significantly increased in IgM clonotypes from both age groups at D7 after vaccination (**Figure 4A**), although the change at D7 from D0 in old IgM clones was threefold smaller than that in the young. Changes in overall *IGHV* mutation levels in IgM clones in response to vaccines and with age can also be demonstrated by the proportional alteration between unmutated versus heavily mutated IgM clones (**Figures 4B,C**).

A higher mutational frequency is observed with age in IgG clonotypes at all time points ($p = 0.0003$, Mann–Whitney *U*-test; data not shown). We did not see an increase in the overall mutation levels in IgA clonotypes after challenge in either age group (data not shown). Since IgA populations are reflective of prior challenge and hypermutation this perhaps would not be expected. However, looking solely at the large clones (five sequences or more per clone), presumably enriched for the ones responding to vaccination as opposed to those that were historically mutated, we saw that IgA clonotypes from old donors had a lower average frequency of mutation than the young ($p = 0.0025$, Mann–Whitney *U*-test). This may be due to the reduction in the proportion of heavily mutated, large IgA clonotypes with age (**Figures 4D,E**). A similar trend is also observed in IgM clonotypes (**Figure 4F**).

AGE AND CHALLENGE-RELATED CHANGES IN CLONOTYPES AND CLONAL EXPANSION BY *IGH* SUBCLASS

We previously reported that isotype-switched and innate-like IgM+ memory cells have distinct *IGHV* repertoires, and later that there are some similarities between the innate-like IgM+ memory cell repertoire and that of IgG2 and (to a lesser extent) IgA2 memory cells. Therefore we proposed that a large proportion of IgG2 and IgM (and possibly IgA2) memory cells may be subject to a different selection process from that imposed on other classes and subclasses of memory cells (Wu et al., 2010, 2011). In order to compare the vaccine response in B cells of different subclasses we stratified the overall clonotype repertoire by subclass. This was done by searching for subclass-specific motifs upstream of the pan-IgA or pan-IgG primer sequences, so that any difference in subclass within a particular class is not due to a difference in primer binding efficiency. In line with previous reports (Wu et al., 2010, 2011), over-representation of *IGHV3* and under-representation of *IGHV1* genes are seen in IgM, IgG2, and IgA2 clonotypes in both age groups at all time points analyzed when compared to IgG1, IgG3, and IgA1 clonotypes (data not shown). Within the IgA and IgG compartments the proportions of the subclasses vary with challenge, with a significant increase in the proportion of IgA2 and IgG2 clonotypes being seen in both age groups at D7 compared to D0 (**Figure 5A**; $p < 0.005$, repeated measures ANOVA). Although we failed to detect any age-related differences in Ig gene usage in IgA and IgG subclasses (data not shown), there is a significant difference in IgG subclass distribution with age at both D0 and D7, with the older group having an increased proportion of IgG2 compared with the young (**Figure 5A**; $p < 0.0005$, Mann–Whitney *U*-test). The increased proportion of IgA2 and IgG2 subclasses after vaccination are also observed when clone relatives (i.e., all sequences not just clonotypes) are included for analysis (**Figure 5B**).

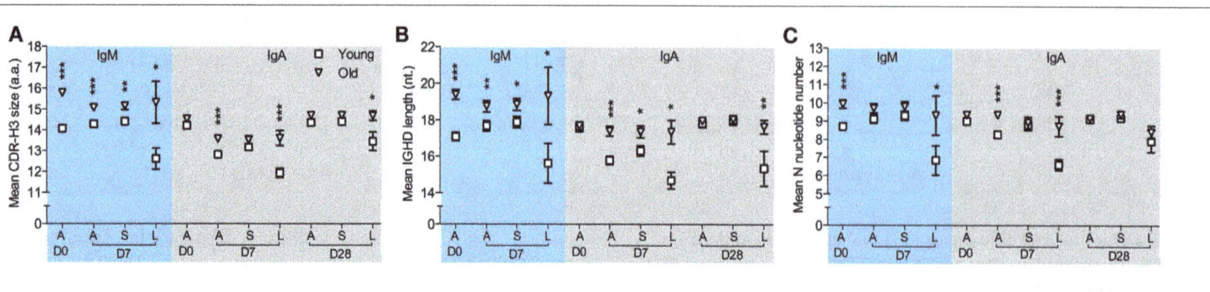

FIGURE 3 | Age-related changes in CDR-H3 characteristics from clonotypes in different sizes. IMGT V-QUEST was used to determine the size of the CDR-H3 region and its components, i.e., N-nucleotide numbers and *IGHD* genes, in each *IGH* sequence. After clustered by CDR-H3 sequence motifs, IgM, and IgA clonotypes were sorted by clone sizes. **(A)** The mean size of CDR-H3 regions (in amino acids), **(B)** the mean length of overall *IGHD* genes (in nucleotides), and **(C)** the mean number of N-nucleotides from all clonotypes **(A)**, clonotypes ≤4 (S) and clonotypes ≥5 in size (L) were compared between six young (square) and six old (triangle) donors at D0, D7, and D28, using Mann-Whitney *U*-tests (*$p < 0.05$, **$p < 0.005$, and ***$p < 0.0005$). Error bars indicate ±SEM.

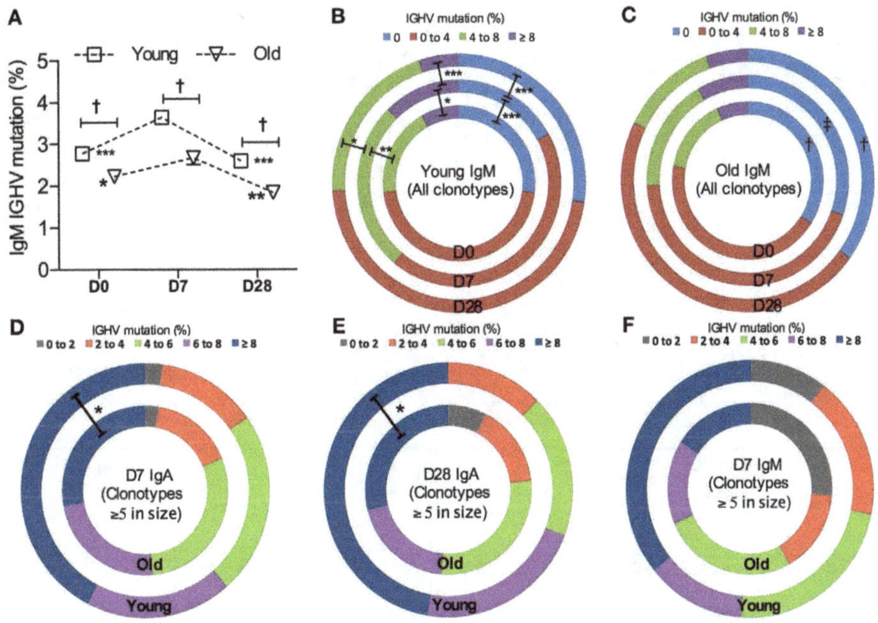

FIGURE 4 | Vaccine-induced changes in *IGHV* mutations. (A) The frequency of *IGHV* mutations in each sequence was calculated to be the percentage difference from germline identity, determined by IMGT V-QUEST. Kruskal–Wallis comparisons were used to compare the mean *IGHV* mutation between IgM clonotypes from six young (squares) and six old (triangle) donors (age-related differences: $^{‡}<0.0005$) and between D0, D7, and D28 (temporal differences: $^{*}p<0.05$, $^{**}p<0.005$, and $^{***}p<0.0005$, as compared with D7). Error bars indicate ±SEM. All IgM clonotypes were grouped by the level of *IGHV* mutation and the proportion of each group was compared using Chi-squared tests between days (D0: inner circles, D7: middle circles, and D28: outer circles; $^{*}p<0.05$, $^{**}p<0.005$, and $^{***}p<0.0005$) and between six young **(B)** and six old **(C)** donors [$^{†}p<0.05$ and $^{‡}p<0.005$, as indicated in **(C)**]. For clones ≥5 in size, IgM clonotypes at D7 **(D)**, IgA clonotypes at D7 **(E)**, and IgA clonotypes at D28 **(F)** were grouped by the level of *IGHV* mutations and the proportion of each group was compared between six young (outer circles) and six old (inner circles) donors, using Chi-squared tests ($^{*}p<0.05$).

Generally the differences in clonotype subclass distribution (**Figure 5A**) are mirrored in sequence subclass distribution (**Figure 5B**). However, in IgG there appears to be a greater bias toward IgG2 in sequences compared to clonotypes, indicating that in the young the IgG2 clonotypes belong to larger clones. Differences in IgA and IgG average clone size at the different time points are shown in **Figures 5C,E** respectively, with details of the distribution of clones in the different subclasses in **Figures 5D,F**. Significant age-related differences in the average IgA clone size (**Figure 2B**) are seen at D7 and D28, and appear to be mainly due to the IgA1 subclass having a smaller clone size at D7 but bigger at D28 in the old as compared with the young (**Figure 5C**). Although the average clone size in IgA2 does not seem to change with age, more detailed analysis of IgA2 clone size distribution shows that the frequency of large clones, containing over 20 sequence members, is lower at D7 ($p=0.002$; Chi-squared test) but higher at D28 in old repertoires, as compared with the young (**Figure 5E**). In both age groups the average clone size of IgG2 is significantly bigger than IgG1 at D7 ($p=0.0008$, paired t-test; **Figure 5D**). Thus, in addition to there being an increase in the number of different IgG2 clonotypes in the sampled repertoire at D7, the individual IgG2 clonotypes are expanded more than IgG1 clonotypes. The age-related increase in the proportion of IgG2 clonotypes at D7 and D28 (**Figure 5A**) is not accompanied by any significant difference in the clone size (**Figure 5D**). So although the older repertoire has a greater representation of IgG2 sequences these are not expanded any more than in the younger group. The IgG1 and IgG2 clone distribution is illustrated in more detail in **Figure 5F**.

CLONAL EXPANSION AS A RESULT OF RECALL IMMUNE RESPONSES

Previous studies show that influenza-specific cells (Wrammert et al., 2008) and anti-PPS plasma cells (Baxendale et al., 2010) can be detected in the serum prior to vaccination and their frequencies are increased at D7 following vaccination. Although our sequences were produced using unsorted PBMCs, large sequence numbers allowed us to track responding clones sampled at D7 back to their clone relatives sampled at D0 prior to vaccination, using mutational phylogeny analysis (Dereeper et al., 2010). We find a total of 648 different clonotypes (3.6% of all clonotypes) containing clonally related *IGH* sequences that represent cells sampled at different days (**Table 2**). 71% of these clones are of a single isotype, being significantly more frequent than those having *IGHM* sequences related to *IGHG* and *IGHA* sequences (12.8%; Chi-squared test, $p<0.0001$). As expected, the proportion of clonotypes that share sequences across different time points increases to 20%, when only large clones are considered (**Table 2**). Out of these larger clones, 57 clonotypes (4.6%) contain *IGH* sequences that have already switched to IgA and IgG isotypes at D0 prior to vaccination (**Figure 6A**), suggesting a recall immune response by pre-existing memory B cells. Similarly, there are also clones that contain mutated IgM+ sequences at D0 (**Figure 6B**). Mutational phylogenetic trees show great diversification within

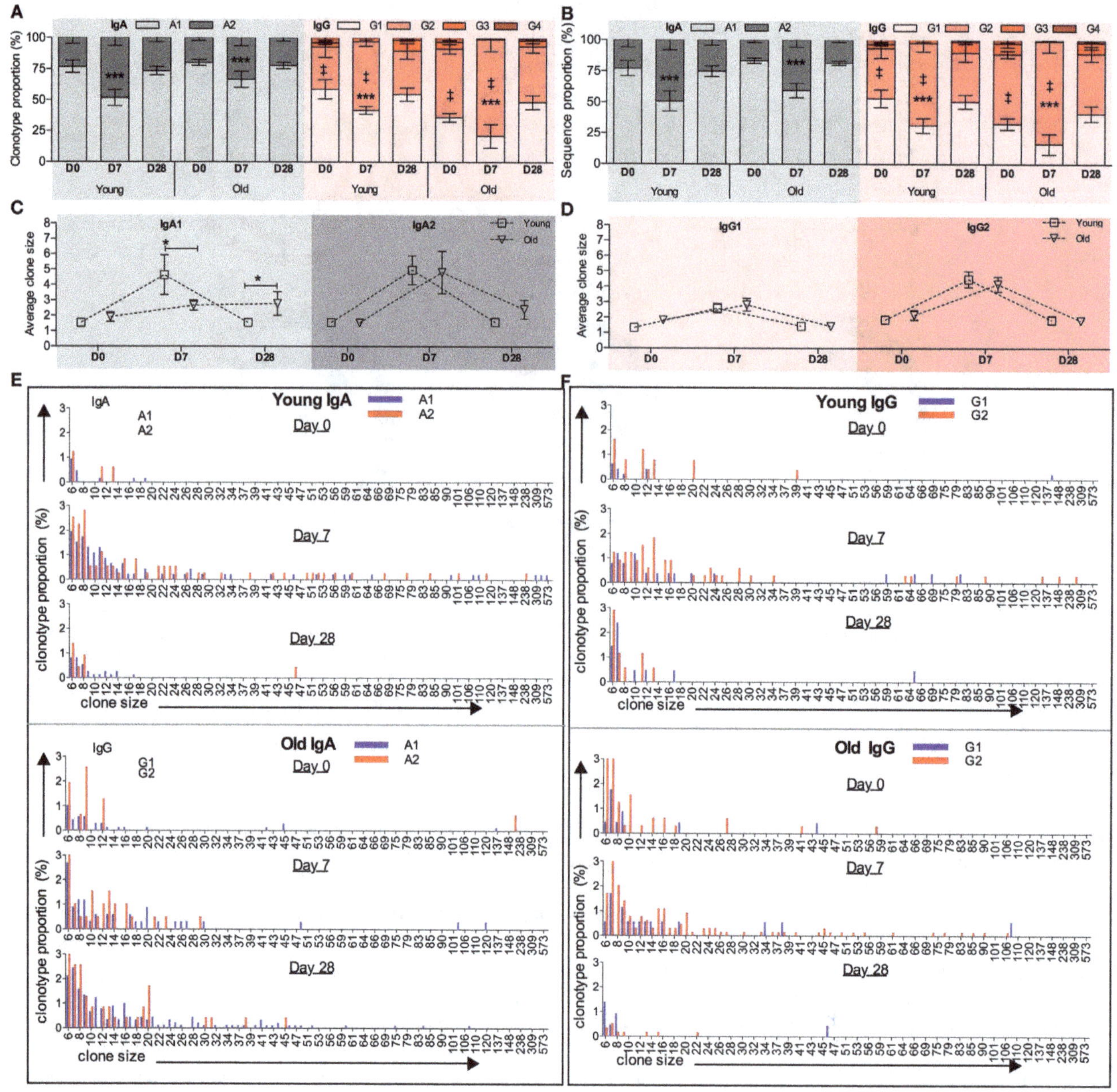

FIGURE 5 | Age and challenge-related changes in *IGH* subclass. Internal motifs in the constant region were used to identify subclasses (IgA1, IgA2, IgG1, IgG2, IgG3, and IgG4) in each *IGH* sequence. The proportion (*y*-axis) of clonotypes clustered by CDR-H3 **(A)** and total sequences **(B)** of different IgA or IgG subclasses at D0, D7, and D28 was calculated for each donor individually before being collectively analyzed (temporal differences: $^{***}p < 0.0005$ using repeated measures ANOVA when compared with D7; age-related differences: $^{‡}p < 0.005$ using Mann–Whitney *U*-tests). Error bars indicate ±SEM. The average clone size (*y*-axis) of IgA1 and IgA2 clonotypes **(C)** and IgG1 and IgG2 clonotypes **(D)** was calculated to be the ratio of total sequences over total clonotypes for each donor individually, before being compared between young versus old ages ($^{*}p < 0.05$; one-way ANOVA comparison). Bars indicate ±SEM. Clonotypes of **(E)** IgA subclasses (IgA1: blue bars and IgA2: red bars) and **(F)** IgG subclasses (IgG1: blue bars and IgG2: red bars) were grouped by their clone sizes (*x*-axis), and the proportion of each groups (*y*-axis) was calculated at D0, D7, and D28. Clones containing fewer than five sequences are not shown.

expanded clones. Interestingly we also observe that sequences sampled at D0 do not always appear less mutated than those at D7 and D28. Similarly, *IGHM* sequences do not always appear before *IGHA*/*IGHG* sequences in the lineage tree. These observations have important consequences for future interpretation of data based on analysis of phylogenetic trees.

DISCUSSION

Improving the immunogenicity of vaccines against *S. pneumoniae* and influenza in the older person is a challenge (Artz et al., 2003; Hannoun et al., 2004). Effective antibody production is impaired in older people but the exact causes of this impairment have not been fully elucidated. An earlier study showed that affinity

Table 2 | Numbers of clones with clonality between *IGH* sequences sampled at different days[1].

					All clonotypes[2]					
Day[1]	**Old ($n = 7926$[3]; 6 donors)**					**Young ($n = 9774$[3]; 6 donors)**				
ISO[5]	**AG**	**AGM**	**AM**	**GM**	**Single[6]**	**AG**	**AGM**	**AM**	**GM**	**Single**
0 and 28	3	1	1	1	94	17	0	3	7	94
0 and 7	4	3	7	4	47	8	3	20	1	38
0 and 7 and 28	4	1	2	0	16	5	3	2	0	4
7 and 28	23	4	3	3	93	38	6	8	0	77
					Clonotypes ≥5 in size					
Day	**Old ($n = 671$[4]; 6 donors)**					**Young ($n = 572$[4]; 6 donors)**				
ISO	**AG**	**AGM**	**AM**	**GM**	**Single**	**AG**	**AGM**	**AM**	**GM**	**Single**
0 and 28			1	1	25	11	0	0	1	22
0 and 7	3	3	1	1	19	5	2	13	1	9
0 and 7 and 28	4	1	1	0	12	4	3	1	0	2
7 and 28	20	4	2	0	36	32	6	3	0	24

[1] *CDR-H3 sequence motifs are used to identify clones containing IGH sequences that that have the same VDJ rearrangement but are sampled at Day 0, 7, and 28.*

[2] *All clonotype refers to all clones in various sizes.*

[3] *Numbers refers to all clonotypes produced by high-throughput sequencing.*

[4] *Numbers refer to clonotypes ≥5 in size produced by high-throughput sequencing.*

[5] *Iso refers to clones containing IGH sequences sharing the same CDR-H3 region but are of different isotypes (A for IgA, G for IgG, and M for IgM).*

[6] *Single refer to clones containing IGH sequences of only one isotype.*

selection in the germinal center may be altered with age, this may be partly due to lack of appropriate help, for example from T cells, as well as intrinsic differences in the B cell affecting its ability to express AID (Banerjee et al., 2002; Frasca et al., 2008). We later showed that B cell diversity decreases with age and is associated with poor health (Gibson et al., 2009). Kolibab et al. (2005a) also suggest that changes in Ig gene usage may account for the different affinity of vaccine-specific antibodies between young and older populations. Thus there may be a causal relationship between the distortion of B cell repertoires and vaccine hypo-responsiveness with age. However, previous repertoire analyses to investigate similar subjects are restricted to certain genes and isotypes due to the small numbers of sequences available (Kolibab et al., 2005a; Smithson et al., 2005).

We have performed high-throughput sequence analysis of *IGH* repertoires in human peripheral blood in order to investigate B cell responses following vaccination with the pneumococcal and influenza vaccines. In contrast to the oligoclonal response previously reported in response to the pneumococcal vaccine (Zhou et al., 2004; Kolibab et al., 2005a), here we report a very diverse and resilient vaccine response, with increased clone sizes at D7 and normal repertoire resumed at D28 (**Figures 2** and **5**). The discrepancy in diversity with previous reports may reflect the number of sequences analyzed and/or the fact that the influenza vaccine was included in this study in addition to the pneumococcal vaccine. Since the peak of the plasmablast response is generally between days 6 and 8 (Cox et al., 1994; Wrammert et al., 2008), and plasma cells and plasmablasts have many more copies of immunoglobulin RNA per cell than B cells (Kuo et al., 2007), it is reasonable to assume that the clonal expansions seen at D7 represent the cells that are responding to vaccine. We can also see vaccine-induced changes in the CDR-H3 repertoire despite the fact that there are a large number of different antigens in this challenge. We previously showed that memory B cells in general have shorter CDR-H3 regions that are more hydrophilic (Wu et al., 2010), implying that Ig genes with these characteristics are preferentially selected in many different responses. These changes are also seen at D7 here (**Figures 1E,F**) and these data together strongly imply that the antibody immune response to challenge is skewed toward antibodies with certain characteristics of the antigen binding region even though the antigens themselves can be quite variable.

Many studies use specific serum IgG levels as a correlate of vaccine protection, although this metric is not always the best indicator. There are no age-related differences in anti-PPS IgG serology, but there is a significant age-related decrease in serum antibody function as determined by the opsonophagocytic assay (Anttila et al., 1999). Recent evidence suggests that this is due to a decrease in IgM antibody, since depletion of IgM from serum results in decreased opsonophagocytic activity (Park and Nahm, 2011; Sasaki et al., 2011). Our repertoire analysis does not show any age-related changes in IgG, except for a higher mutational frequency in the older group that is likely due to longer prior exposures to challenge with age. Nor do we see any significant age-related differences in the level of clonal expansion of IgM sequences. We do, however, see significant age-related differences

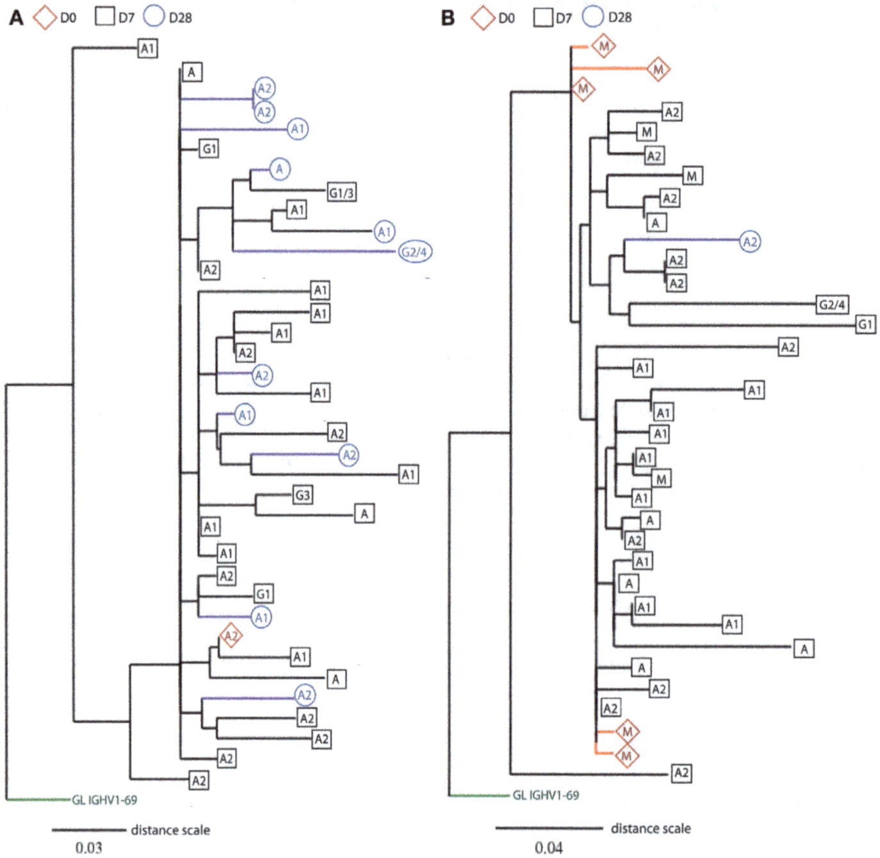

FIGURE 6 | Rooted phylograms show clonally related *IGH* sequences sampled at different days. CDR-H3 sequence motifs were used to identify clone relatives of *IGH* sequences found across D0, D7, and D28. After editing and aligning *IGH* sequences with germline gene using DNAstar software, mutational phylogenetic trees were generated using the online Phylogeny Analysis program (Dereeper et al., 2010). Leaves represent *IGH* sequences sampled at different days (D0: red diamonds, D7: black squares, and D28: blue circles), and the putative germline (GL) genes are indicated at the base of trees in green. The class (IgG, IgA, and IgM) or subclass (indicated by numbers) of *IGH* genes is indicated in the shapes. Internal nodes represent hypothetical intermediates of *IGH* sequences, and the branch lengths indicate percentage mutation differences between *IGH* sequences in proportion to the distance scale. Only two illustrations of phylogenetic trees are shown **(A)** from an old donor aged 71 years and **(B)** from a young donor aged 22 years. For space consideration, sequences in the two clones are randomly chosen for illustration.

in the CDR-H3 characteristics (**Figure 4**) and levels of mutation in the IgM repertoire (**Figure 3**), with generally less mutation and longer CDR-H3 in the old (both these factors being more characteristic of naïve B cell repertoires rather than memory B cell repertoires). The differences were significant at all time points so may not necessarily be confined to a change in the response. The IgM repertoire includes the naïve B cell population as well as IgM memory cells, so a change in the proportions of these two populations would also have an effect on our repertoire observations; thus, a decrease in IgM memory cells such as has been previously suggested may account for some difference (Shi et al., 2005). However, both age groups did show an increased level of mutation at D7 and a decrease at D28, although to a lesser extent in the old group. In order to look at the differences between age groups in the response without the background of naïve cells we split the data to look at sequences that were part of large clones in isolation, on the assumption that if a clone has expanded it is part of the IgM memory response rather than the naïve B cells in the background. The older IgM response repertoire had longer CDR-H3 and less mutation (**Figures 3** and **4**), which would strongly suggest that there is an age-related defect in the normal mechanisms of selection and hypermutation in IgM memory. We do not know what the specificity of these expanded IgM clones is, although based on previous literature we would hypothesize that they are T-independent responders to the polysaccharide antigen (Lortan et al., 1992). IgG2 antibodies are also thought to respond to T-independent polysaccharide antigens (Lortan et al., 1992) so it is interesting that alongside the defect in IgM memory repertoire there is a skewing in favor of IgG2 use in the IgG repertoire of older people.

A role for IgA in the protective vaccine response against influenza and pneumonia has not previously been highlighted, and the removal of IgA from serum was not shown to have any effect on the opsonophagocytic capability of post-vaccine serum. Since these respiratory diseases originate at mucosal surfaces it would seem plausible that IgA has some vital function, even if not in the circulation. It is clear from our data that there are significant differences in the IgA response in older people. In a similar manner to the IgM memory cells there is less hypermutation in the expanded clones and they have larger CDR-H3 regions. The degree of clonal expansion is less overall and takes much longer, to the extent that is still appears to be occurring at D28 after the younger group has contracted the response. The IgA serum antibody response is short lived. In contrast to IgG and IgM antibodies, which increase in serum with maximum values at D28, the maximal serum level of IgA is at D7 in the normal young population and it decreases by D28 (Ademokun et al., 2011). The clonal expansions of all three isotypes peaks at D7 and contracts at D28 in the blood (**Figure 2B**). Thus for IgG and IgM one can envisage a scenario where cells have left the blood to reside in a niche where they continue to secrete antibody into the circulation. However the serum IgA antibody concentration seems to mirror the clonal expansion data, which may indicate that the cells are short lived and do not go on to secrete antibody in survival niches, or perhaps they do survive but secrete IgA antibody at mucosal surfaces rather than into the circulation.

Since the most striking age-related difference in these data was in the IgA response we split the data into IgA1 and IgA2 sequences. IgA1 has previously been associated with serum responses and IgA2 with mucosal responses (Russell et al., 1992). It is clear from our lineage tree analysis that IgA1 and IgA2 can be quite closely related, since we find many clones containing both subclasses (**Figure 6**). However in **Figure 5C** we see that the main age-related difference in clonal expansions that we saw at D7 and D28 is mainly due to IgA1 rather than IgA2, and we also find clones which do not mix the subclasses, so it is possible that certain types of antigens/responses may elicit one subclass only.

The existence of many clones with relatives in both pre- and post-vaccination samples (**Table 2**) indicates that some of these clones may be very large even before vaccination. The chances of finding a particular clonotype in a sample are dependent on the number of cells sampled, the total number of cells in the blood, and the total number of clone members in the blood. We would not expect to find a particular clonotype more than once if it were not part of an expanded clone. In the simplest terms, if we assume that there are 10^8 B cells in the blood, and we have found two related sequences in a sample of 5000, then there could be approximately $(10^8/5000)^2$, or 40,000, related sequences in that one clone in the blood altogether. Also, if we assume that an expansion at D7 originated from a single unique precursor in the blood at D0, the chances of sampling and sequencing that precursor would be 1 in 10^8. Since we see nearly 400 examples of clones where there are related sequences at D0 then we can provisionally conclude that many expanded precursors of cells with specificity for these vaccines are already present in the blood pre-challenge. Whether these pre-existing specificities are mono-specific for the antigens in the vaccine or are cross-reactive from a prior, related, challenge cannot be determined since it was impossible to determine the prior extent of exposure to influenza or *S. pneumoniae* in the participants. These high-throughput data have also shown that we need to be careful about interpretation of lineage trees with respect to inference of chronological ordering since the trees can be quite complex (**Figure 6**). If there has been extensive prior expansion of cells in the blood it cannot be assumed that all clones in the expansion will have mutated at the same rate or in the same reaction. Hence a random sampling will not always result in the samples from the earlier time points appearing at the top of the lineage trees (i.e., with less mutations from germline). Similarly, extensive expansion followed by random switching and sampling may result in a seemingly impossible succession of switching events, such as *IGHM* sequences appearing downstream of *IGHA* sequences. However this could simply mean that a cell has expanded without mutation, 50% of them have switched and the sampling has picked up one of the switched parents together with offspring of one of the unswitched parents.

In conclusion, our high-throughput *IGH* repertoire analyses have demonstrated that we can visualize an immune response to vaccine by the expansion of clonotypes expressing particular Ig genes, and with particular CDR-H3 characteristics. The large clonal expansions indicate a complex recall response. There are significant age-related differences in the response with respect to subclass distribution, particularly in the extent and timing of IgA clonal expansion and skewing toward greater use of IgG2. Older responding IgM and IgA clonotypes are also less mutated and use a longer CDR-H3, which might affect antigen recognition. Although much more now needs to be done to explore the significance of the age-related changes in IgA responses described here, our work does highlight the critical need to consider different classes and subclasses of antibody in vaccine studies in general.

AUTHOR CONTRIBUTION

Yu-Chang Bryan Wu designed and carried out experiments, analyzed data and wrote the manuscript; David Kipling designed and ran the data handling and analysis scripts, analyzed data, and wrote the manuscript; Deborah K. Dunn-Walters, oversaw the project, designed experiments and analytical tools, carried out data analysis and wrote the manuscript.

ACKNOWLEDGMENTS

This work was funded by the Human Frontiers Science program and Research into Aging, Age UK. The authors would like to thank all our volunteers for their blood donation.

REFERENCES

Ademokun, A., Wu, Y. C., Martin, V., Mitra, R., Sack, U., Baxendale, H., Kipling, D., and Dunn-Walters, D. K. (2011). Vaccination-induced changes in human B-cell repertoire and pneumococcal IgM and IgA antibody at different ages. *Aging Cell* 10, 922–930.

Anttila, M., Voutilainen, M., Jantti, V., Eskola, J., and Kayhty, H. (1999). Contribution of serotype-specific IgG concentration, IgG subclasses and relative antibody avidity to opsonophagocytic activity against *Streptococcus pneumoniae. Clin. Exp. Immunol.* 118, 402–407.

Artz, A. S., Ershler, W. B., and Longo, D. L. (2003). Pneumococcal vaccination and revaccination of older adults. *Clin. Microbiol. Rev.* 16, 308–318.

Banerjee, M., Mehr, R., Belelovsky, A., Spencer, J., and Dunn-Walters, D. K. (2002). Age- and tissue-specific differences in human germinal center B cell selection revealed by analysis of IgVH gene hypermutation and lineage trees. *Eur. J. Immunol.* 32, 1947–1957.

Baxendale, H. E., Keating, S. M., Johnson, M., Southern, J., Miller, E., and Goldblatt, D. (2010). The early kinetics of circulating pneumococcal-specific memory B cells following pneumococcal conjugate and plain polysaccharide vaccines in the elderly. *Vaccine* 28, 4763–4770.

Benckert, J., Schmolka, N., Kreschel, C., Zoller, M. J., Sturm, A., Wiedenmann, B., and Wardemann, H. (2011). The majority of intestinal IgA+ and IgG+ plasmablasts in the human gut are antigen-specific. *J. Clin. Invest.* 121, 1946–1955.

Brochet, X., Lefranc, M. P., and Giudicelli, V. (2008). IMGT/V-QUEST: the highly customized and integrated system for IG and TR standardized V-J and V-D-J sequence analysis. *Nucleic Acids Res.* 36, W503–W508.

Brown, T. A., Murphy, B. R., Radl, J., Haaijman, J. J., and Mestecky, J. (1985). Subclass distribution and molecular form of immunoglobulin A hemagglutinin antibodies in sera and nasal secretions after experimental secondary infection with influenza A virus in humans. *J. Clin. Microbiol.* 22, 259–264.

Carson, P. J., Schut, R. L., Simpson, M. L., O'Brien, J., and Janoff, E. N. (1995). Antibody class and subclass responses to pneumococcal polysaccharides following immunization of human immunodeficiency virus-infected patients. *J. Infect. Dis.* 172, 340–345.

Cox, R. J., Brokstad, K. A., Zuckerman, M. A., Wood, J. M., Haaheim, L. R., and Oxford, J. S. (1994). An early humoral immune response in peripheral blood following parenteral inactivated influenza vaccination. *Vaccine* 12, 993–999.

Dereeper, A., Audic, S., Claverie, J. M., and Blanc, G. (2010). BLAST-EXPLORER helps you building datasets for phylogenetic analysis. *BMC Evol. Biol.* 10, 8. doi:10.1186/1471-2148-10-8

Frasca, D., Landin, A. M., Lechner, S. C., Ryan, J. G., Schwartz, R., Riley, R. L., and Blomberg, B. B. (2008). Aging down-regulates the transcription factor E2A, activation-induced cytidine deaminase, and Ig class switch in human B cells. *J. Immunol.* 180, 5283–5290.

Gibson, K. L., Wu, Y. C., Barnett, Y., Duggan, O., Vaughan, R., Kondeatis, E., Nilsson, B. O., Wikby, A., Kipling, D., and Dunn-Walters, D. K. (2009). B-cell diversity decreases in old age and is correlated with poor health status. *Aging Cell* 8, 18–25.

Hannoun, C., Megas, F., and Piercy, J. (2004). Immunogenicity and protective efficacy of influenza vaccination. *Virus Res.* 103, 133–138.

Hocart, M. J., Mackenzie, J. S., and Stewart, G. A. (1990). Serum IgG subclass responses of humans to inactivated and live influenza A vaccines compared to natural infections with influenza A. *J. Med. Virol.* 30, 92–96.

Ikai, A. (1980). Thermostability and aliphatic index of globular proteins. *J. Biochem.* 88, 1895–1898.

Kolibab, K., Smithson, S. L., Rabquer, B., Khuder, S., and Westerink, M. A. (2005a). Immune response to pneumococcal polysaccharides 4 and 14 in elderly and young adults: analysis of the variable heavy chain repertoire. *Infect. Immun.* 73, 7465–7476.

Kolibab, K., Smithson, S. L., Shriner, A. K., Khuder, S., Romero-Steiner, S., Carlone, G. M., and Westerink, M. A. (2005b). Immune response to pneumococcal polysaccharides 4 and 14 in elderly and young adults. I. Antibody concentrations, avidity and functional activity. *Immun. Ageing* 2, 10.

Kuo, T. C., Shaffer, A. L., Haddad, J. Jr., Choi, Y. S., Staudt, L. M., and Calame, K. (2007). Repression of BCL-6 is required for the formation of human memory B cells in vitro. *J. Exp. Med.* 204, 819–830.

Lindner, C., Wahl, B., Fohse, L., Suerbaum, S., Macpherson, A. J., Prinz, I., and Pabst, O. (2012). Age, microbiota, and T cells shape diverse individual IgA repertoires in the intestine. *J. Exp. Med.* 209, 365–377.

Lortan, J. E., Vellodi, A., Jurges, E. S., and Hugh-Jones, K. (1992). Class- and subclass-specific pneumococcal antibody levels and response to immunization after bone marrow transplantation. *Clin. Exp. Immunol.* 88, 512–519.

Lue, C., Tarkowski, A., and Mestecky, J. (1988). Systemic immunization with pneumococcal polysaccharide vaccine induces a predominant IgA2 response of peripheral blood lymphocytes and increases of both serum and secretory anti-pneumococcal antibodies. *J. Immunol.* 140, 3793–3800.

McCullers, J. A. (2006). Insights into the interaction between influenza virus and pneumococcus. *Clin. Microbiol. Rev.* 19, 571–582.

Nichol, K. L., Nordin, J. D., Nelson, D. B., Mullooly, J. P., and Hak, E. (2007). Effectiveness of influenza vaccine in the community-dwelling elderly. *N. Engl. J. Med.* 357, 1373–1381.

Osterholm, M. T., Kelley, N. S., Sommer, A., and Belongia, E. A. (2012). Efficacy and effectiveness of influenza vaccines: a systematic review and meta-analysis. *Lancet Infect. Dis.* 12, 36–44.

Park, S., and Nahm, M. H. (2011). Older adults have a low capacity to opsonize pneumococci due to low IgM antibody response to pneumococcal vaccinations. *Infect. Immun.* 79, 314–320.

Powers, D. C. (1994). Effect of age on serum immunoglobulin G subclass antibody responses to inactivated influenza virus vaccine. *J. Med. Virol.* 43, 57–61.

Romero-Steiner, S., Musher, D. M., Cetron, M. S., Pais, L. B., Groover, J. E., Fiore, A. E., Plikaytis, B. D., and Carlone, G. M. (1999). Reduction in functional antibody activity against *Streptococcus pneumoniae* in vaccinated elderly individuals highly correlates with decreased IgG antibody avidity. *Clin. Infect. Dis.* 29, 281–288.

Russell, M. W., Lue, C., Van Den Wall Bake, A. W., Moldoveanu, Z., and Mestecky, J. (1992). Molecular heterogeneity of human IgA antibodies during an immune response. *Clin. Exp. Immunol.* 87, 1–6.

Sanal, O., Ersoy, F., Yel, L., Tezcan, I., Metin, A., Ozyurek, H., Gariboglu, S., Fikrig, S., Berkel, A. I., Rijkers, G. T., and Zegers, B. J. (1999). Impaired IgG antibody production to pneumococcal polysaccharides in patients with ataxia-telangiectasia. *J. Clin. Immunol.* 19, 326–334.

Sasaki, S., Sullivan, M., Narvaez, C. F., Holmes, T. H., Furman, D., Zheng, N. Y., Nishtala, M., Wrammert, J., Smith, K., James, J. A., Dekker, C. L., Davis, M. M., Wilson, P. C., Greenberg, H. B., and He, X. S. (2011). Limited efficacy of inactivated influenza vaccine in elderly individuals is associated with decreased production of vaccine-specific antibodies. *J. Clin. Invest.* 121, 3109–3119.

Shi, Y., Yamazaki, T., Okubo, Y., Uehara, Y., Sugane, K., and Agematsu, K. (2005). Regulation of aged humoral immune defense against pneumococcal bacteria by IgM memory B cell. *J. Immunol.* 175, 3262–3267.

Simell, B., Kilpi, T., and Kayhty, H. (2006). Subclass distribution of natural salivary IgA antibodies against pneumococcal capsular polysaccharide of type 14 and pneumococcal surface adhesin A (PsaA) in children. *Clin. Exp. Immunol.* 143, 543–549.

Smithson, S. L., Kolibab, K., Shriner, A. K., Srivastava, N., Khuder, S., and Westerink, M. A. (2005). Immune response to pneumococcal polysaccharides 4 and 14 in elderly and young adults: analysis of the variable light chain repertoire. *Infect. Immun.* 73, 7477–7484.

Szabo, P., Li, F., Mathew, J., Lillvis, J., and Weksler, M. E. (2004). Evolution of B-cell clonal expansions with age. *Cell. Immunol.* 231, 158–167.

Wilkins, M. R., Gasteiger, E., Bairoch, A., Sanchez, J. C., Williams, K. L., Appel, R. D., and Hochstrasser, D. F. (1999). Protein identification and analysis tools in the ExPASy server. *Methods Mol. Biol.* 112, 531–552.

Wrammert, J., Smith, K., Miller, J., Langley, W. A., Kokko, K., Larsen, C., Zheng, N. Y., Mays, I., Garman, L., Helms, C., James, J., Air, G. M., Capra, J. D., Ahmed, R., and Wilson, P. C. (2008). Rapid cloning of high-affinity human monoclonal antibodies against influenza virus. *Nature* 453, 667–671.

Wu, Y. C., Kipling, D., Leong, H. S., Martin, V., Ademokun, A. A., and Dunn-Walters, D. K. (2010). High-throughput immunoglobulin repertoire analysis distinguishes between human IgM memory and switched memory B-cell populations. *Blood* 116, 1070–1078.

Wu, Y.-C. B., Kipling, D., and Dunn-Walters, D. K. (2011). The relationship between CD27 negative and positive B cell populations in human peripheral blood. *Front. Immunol.* 2:81. doi:10.3389/fimmu.2011.00081

Zhou, J., Lottenbach, K. R., Barenkamp, S. J., and Reason, D. C. (2004). Somatic hypermutation and diverse immunoglobulin gene usage in the human antibody response to the capsular polysaccharide of *Streptococcus pneumoniae* type 6B. *Infect. Immun.* 72, 3505–3514.

15

ER stress proteins in autoimmune and inflammatory diseases

Daisuke Morito and Kazuhiro Nagata*

Faculty of Life Sciences, Kyoto Sangyo University, Kyoto, Japan

Edited by:
Willem Van Eden, Utrecht University, Netherlands

Reviewed by:
Rik Lories, Katholieke Universiteit Leuven, Belgium
Cristina Bonorino, Pontificia Universidade Catolica do Rio Grande do Sul, Brazil
Ruurd Van Der Zee, Universiteit Utrecht, Netherlands

***Correspondence:**
Kazuhiro Nagata, Laboratory of Molecular and Cellular Biology, Faculty of Life Sciences, Kyoto Sangyo University, Kamigamo Motoyama, Kyoto, Kyoto 603-8555, Japan.
e-mail: nagata@cc.kyoto-su.ac.jp

Over the past two decades, heat shock proteins (HSPs) have been implicated in inflammatory responses and autoimmunity. HSPs were originally believed to maintain protein quality control in the cytosol. However, they also exist extracellularly and appear to act as inflammatory factors. Recently, a growing body of evidence suggested that the other class of stress proteins such as, endoplasmic reticulum (ER) stress proteins, which originally act as protein quality control factors in the secretory pathway and are induced by ER stress in inflammatory lesions, also participate in inflammation and autoimmunity. The immunoglobulin heavy-chain binding protein (Bip)/glucose-regulated protein 78 (GRP78), calnexin, calreticulin, glucose-regulated protein 94 (GRP94)/gp96, oxygen regulated protein 150 (ORP150)/glucose-regulated protein 170 (GRP170), homocysteine-induced ER protein (Herp) and heat shock protein 47 (hsp47)/Serpin H1, which are expressed not only in the ER but also occasionally at the cell surface play pathophysiological roles in autoimmune and inflammatory diseases as pro- or anti-inflammatory factors. Here we describe the accumulating evidence of the participation of ER stress proteins in autoimmunity and inflammation and discuss the critical differences between the two classes of stress proteins.

Keywords: autoimmunity, inflammation, ER stress, ERAD, molecular chaperone

INTRODUCTION

Inflammation is a typical sign of autoimmune diseases. Misdirected immune responses target self-antigens and induce severe inflammatory responses, which sometimes cause death. In addition to numerous components in autoimmune responses, heat shock proteins (HSPs) have been implicated in autoimmune and inflammatory diseases over the past two decades (Hauet-Broere et al., 2006; Van Eden et al., 2007). Many HSPs are so-called molecular chaperones and folding enzymes, which maintain protein folding in a cell (Bukau et al., 2006; Hartl, 2011). Because protein folding is easily impaired by various cytotoxic stresses, such as heat shock, cytotoxic chemicals, hypoxia, and inflammation, prokaryotic to higher eukaryotic organisms have evolved stress responses and HSPs. The transcription of HSPs and their subsequent protein expression are stimulated by cytotoxic stresses, and they immediately restore protein folding and cellular homeostasis to counter toxic stresses (Morimoto, 1998). Thus, HSPs could be postulated to act as intracellular protein homeostasis maintenance factors. However, HSPs have also been reported to be observed in the extracellular fluid (Njemini et al., 2011), and act as pro- and anti-inflammatory factors especially in autoimmune and inflammatory diseases in diverse manners. In inflammatory lesions, HSPs are upregulated by inflammatory stress and are released into the extracellular fluid. Then, the extracellular HSPs specifically induce proinflammatory cytokines and enhance the antigenicity of autoantigens through modulations of antigen presentation (Multhoff, 2006; Yokota and Fujii, 2010). However, the extracellular HSPs can also stimulate anti-inflammatory regulatory T cell responses, thereby inducing the negative feedback control of inflammation (Hauet-Broere et al., 2006; Van Eden et al., 2007). Indeed, immunization with HSP peptides prevents disease development in autoimmune model animals, such as adjuvant arthritis and collagen-induced arthritis (CIA; van Eden et al., 1988; Jorgensen et al., 1998; Wendling et al., 2000). Presently, besides HSPs, another class of stress proteins is also known to exist in eukaryotic cells. Endoplasmic reticulum (ER) stress proteins, the specialized factors involved in protein quality control in the secretory pathway (Hoseki et al., 2010; Araki and Nagata, 2011; Smith et al., 2011), are induced by ER stress, which is very different from cytosolic stress (Mori, 2000; Walter and Ron, 2011). However, similar to HSPs, ER stress proteins are also induced by inflammatory stress (Yoshida, 2007), suggesting that ER stress proteins might also participate in autoimmune and inflammatory responses. Here, we discuss the accumulating evidence that ER stress proteins and their autoantibodies play roles in autoimmune and inflammatory diseases.

REGULAR FUNCTIONS OF ER STRESS PROTEINS

Before discussing the relevance of ER stress proteins in autoimmune diseases, we have briefly sketched the regular functions of ER stress proteins in a cell. Although the boundary between the two is ambiguous, ER stress proteins can be classified into two groups. The first group consists of molecular chaperones and folding enzymes, which assist the folding and assembly of newly synthesized proteins and prevent misfolding and aggregation of preexisting proteins. The other group consists of protein degradation factors, which mediate the clearance of proteins that should be degraded, such as misfolded proteins. The latter protein clearance pathway is called the ER-associated degradation (ERAD) pathway (McCracken and Brodsky, 1996; Brodsky and McCracken, 1997).

The ER is located at the starting point of the protein secretory pathway. Secretory or membrane proteins are first cotranslationally transported into the ER from cytosolic ribosomes, modified and properly folded, and then translocated to the next step of the secretory pathway (**Figures 1A,B**; Ni and Lee, 2007; Araki and Nagata, 2011). After the ER, proteins pass through the Golgi apparatus and are finally secreted to the cell surface through a secretory vesicle. In the ER, most proteins are glycosylated and covalently crosslinked with disulfide bonds. Such protein modifications are believed necessary for the structural stabilization of the proteins destined to be secreted into the extracellular environment (Ni and Lee, 2007; Araki and Nagata, 2011). Calnexin and calreticulin are lectin-like chaperones that specifically maintain the folding of glycosylated proteins (Williams, 2006). Protein disulfide isomerase (PDI) is an oxidoreductase that mediates protein disulfide bond formation and isomerization (Tu and Weissman, 2004; Ellgaard and Ruddock, 2005). The immunoglobulin heavy-chain binding protein (Bip)/glucose-regulated protein 78 (GRP78) is a hsp70-type molecular chaperone that maintains protein folding (Ni and Lee, 2007; Araki and Nagata, 2011). Glucose-regulated protein 94 (GRP94)/gp96 and oxygen regulated protein 150 (ORP150) are hsp90 and hsp70 family molecular chaperones, respectively; their functions remain unclear (Ni and Lee, 2007; Araki and Nagata, 2011). Another characteristic stress protein in the ER is heat shock protein 47 (hsp47)/Serpin H1, the only heat shock regulated protein in the ER, is the collagen-specific molecular chaperone (Nagata, 2003; Ishida and Nagata, 2011). Using these molecular chaperones and folding enzymes, secretory and membrane proteins are properly folded in the ER and then transported to the Golgi apparatus. Other chaperones and enzymes were precisely described in a recent article (Araki and Nagata, 2011).

Improperly folded proteins are strictly retained in the ER via anchoring by ER chaperones and enter the ERAD pathway (Araki and Nagata, 2011; Smith et al., 2011). ERAD is a multi-step mechanism, which can be divided into the following three steps: (1) the substrate is recognized and isolated, (2) the substrate is dislocated from the ER into the cytosol, and (3) the substrate is then degraded by the ubiquitin proteasome system in the cytosol (**Figures 1C–E**; Hershko and Ciechanover, 1998). Thereby, the clearance of the proteins from the ER is completed. Among these steps, the first step is mediated by ERAD-enhancing mannosidase-like protein 1 (EDEM-1), ERdj5, Bip, Osteosarcoma 9 (OS9), XTP3 transactivating gene B (XTP3B), and SEL1L (Hosokawa et al., 2001; Ushioda et al., 2008; Hagiwara et al., 2011; Ushioda and Nagata, 2011). The substrate is directly transferred from the calnexin/calreticulin-mediated folding cycle to the EDEM-1-containing degradation recognition complex (Molinari et al., 2003; Oda et al., 2003). The substrate is then transferred from EDEM-1 and SEL1L to the so-called ERAD complex, postulated to form a protein dislocation channel (Mueller et al., 2006, 2008; Christianson et al.,

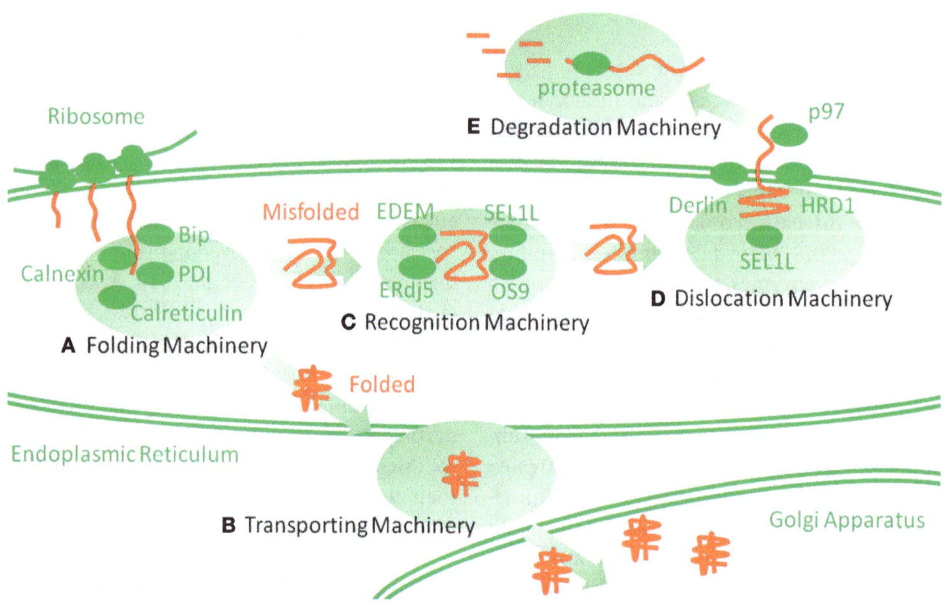

FIGURE 1 | Schematic representation of endoplasmic reticulum (ER) protein folding and ER-associated degradation (ERAD). Secretory and membrane proteins are cotranslationally transported into the ER by cytosolic ribosomes. Newly synthesized unfolded polypeptide are then captured by molecular chaperones and protein folding enzymes **(A)**, which involve immunoglobulin heavy-chain binding protein (Bip), calnexin, calreticulin, protein disulfide isomerase (PDI) and heat shock protein 47 (hsp47), and are properly folded. The folded polypeptides are transported into the Golgi apparatus through transporting machinery **(B)**. However, the proteins that are improperly folded are specifically recognized and isolated by ERAD recognition machinery **(C)**, which involves ERAD-enhancing mannosidase-like protein (EDEM), ERdj5, Bip, SEL1L, osteosarcoma 9 (OS9), and XBP1. The misfolded proteins are then transferred to the dislocation machinery **(D)**, which involves HRD1, Derlin, Herp, and p97. Then, the proteins are dislocated into the cytosol through a putative narrow pore. The dislocated proteins are ubiquitinated by ERAD ubiquitin ligases, such as HRD1, and are finally degraded by huge cytosolic protease complexes, the proteasome **(E)**, into peptides.

2008). ER stress proteins, such as HRD1/synoviolin, Derlin, and homocysteine-induced ER protein (Herp), are involved in this supramolecular complex (Lilley and Ploegh, 2004, 2005; Oda et al., 2006). The substrate is then dislocated into the cytosol from the ER. During dislocation, the substrate is ubiquitinated by the ER ubiquitin ligase and pulled by p97/VCP from the cytosolic side (Ye et al., 2001, 2003; Tsai et al., 2002). Finally, in the third step, the ubiquitinated substrate is degraded by the cytosolic complex protease, the proteasome. Detailed comprehensive descriptions of the ERAD pathways can be found elsewhere (Araki and Nagata, 2011; Smith et al., 2011).

ER STRESS

The stress response for HSPs, called heat shock response, is mediated by transcription factors called heat shock factors (HSFs; Morimoto, 1998). Similarly, the stress response for ER stress proteins, called the unfolded protein response (UPR), is mediated by the unconventional transcription factors, ATF6 and XBP1, and a translation and apoptosis regulating factor, PERK (**Figure 2**; Mori, 2000; Walter and Ron, 2011). The UPR can be experimentally stimulated by chemical compounds that specifically interfere with protein glycosylation and disulfide bond formation because these protein modifications are necessary for the structural stability of secretory and membrane proteins. In addition, perturbation of calcium storage in the ER causes impairments in the quality of ER proteins because the ER has a high calcium concentration, and many of the ER proteins need calcium ions. Alternatively, the UPR is physiologically activated during plasma cell differentiation in order to expand the protein folding capacity for massive production of immunoglobulins. The activation of the UPR has been observed in various neurodegenerative diseases, inflammatory diseases, and viral infections (Yoshida, 2007). Thus, the UPR can be postulated as a completely independent pathway from cytosolic stresses. Both cytosolic and ER stresses are commonly stimulated by inflammation. Although several studies suggest that ER stress protein levels correlate with inflammatory pathogenesis, the roles of ER stress and ER stress proteins in autoimmune and inflammatory diseases remain unclear. Thus, in addition to the heat shock response, the other axis of the cellular stress response might provide new insights into disease mechanisms and clinical treatments.

BIP/GRP78

The 68-kDa glycoprotein was identified through exploration of autoantigens that predominantly immunoreact with sera from rheumatoid arthritis (RA) patients and thus expected to be associated with RA pathogenesis (Blass et al., 1995, 1997, 1998). Subsequently, the 68-kDa antigen was demonstrated to be identical to the ER resident hsp70 family chaperone Bip (Blass et al., 2001; Corrigall et al., 2001). This crucial ER resident stress protein appears to be expressed at the cell surface and acts as an autoantigen in RA. Indeed, 30–75% of RA patients exhibit Bip overexpression in synovial fluid or autoantibodies to Bip in serum (Blass et al., 2001; Corrigall et al., 2001; Shoda et al., 2011). Although the exact roles of extracellular Bip and anti-Bip autoantibodies in RA pathogenesis remain debatable, three possible functions can be considered. First, extracellular Bip and its antibody may result

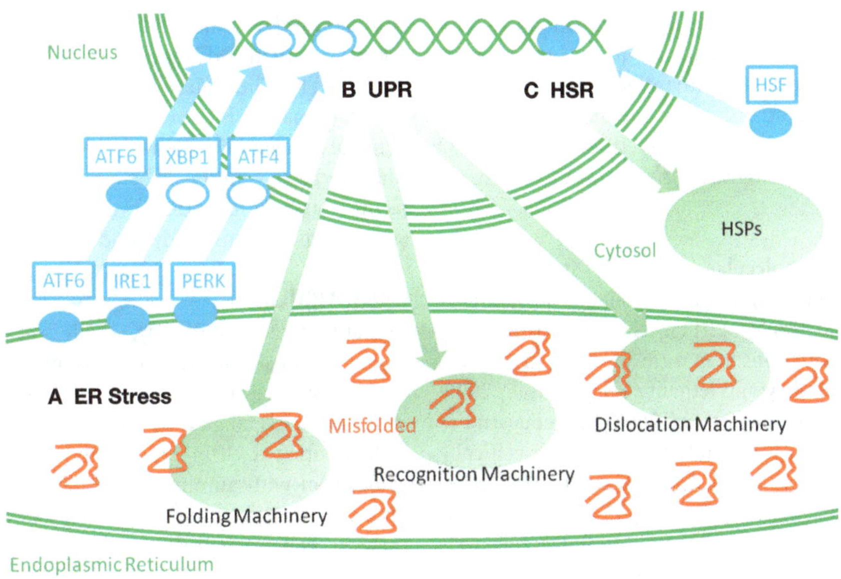

FIGURE 2 | Schematic representation of two distinct stress responses. When misfolded proteins accumulate in the ER, they perturb ER protein homeostasis and organelle functions. Such perturbations are called ER stressors **(A)**. ER stress leads to the activation of membrane spanning stress sensors. ATF6 is a membrane spanning transcription factor that is processed and released from the ER membrane under ER stress, and the stress signal is then transmitted to the nucleus. IRE1 and PERK activate the transcription factors, XBP1 and ATF4, and stimulate a stress response. Such stress responses are called an unfolded protein response (UPR) **(B)**. UPR leads to an upregulation of ER stress proteins, which consist of molecular chaperones and folding enzymes, and ERAD recognition and dislocation factors. Such cross-membrane signal transduction is very different from the heat shock response (HSR) **(C)**. When the cytosolic stresses perturb the cytosolic protein homeostasis, heat shock factor (HSF) is activated and transmits the signal into the nucleus. Then, an upregulation of HSPs is induced. It is a challenge to recover cytosolic protein homeostasis.

from inflammatory stress during RA progression, and they might have no pathophysiological roles. Because the UPR is stimulated through inflammation and ER stress proteins, including Bip, are subsequently induced (Yoshida, 2007), Bip could be simply a specific and abundant autoantigen in the inflammatory lesion that is unrelated to RA pathogenesis. Second, the autoantigen might act as an anti-inflammatory factor, similar to HSPs. Several studies suggested that extracellular Bip stimulates the production of the anti-inflammatory cytokines, IL-4 and IL-10, through specific T lymphocytes (Blass et al., 2001; Corrigall et al., 2001, 2004; Bodman-Smith et al., 2003; Brownlie et al., 2006; Panayi and Corrigall, 2006). Furthermore, the pre-administration of Bip protein to mice prevents the *in vivo* induction of adjuvant arthritis or CIA, both of which are well-known artificial models of autoimmune diseases (Corrigall et al., 2001; Brownlie et al., 2006). Third, the Bip antigen could act as a proinflammatory factor. Bip positively causes immunological responses and inflammation. Recently, Shoda et al. (2011) reported that in addition to the intact Bip antibody, anti-citrullinated Bip (ctBip) antibody is frequently detected in RA patients. The ctBip protein, but not intact Bip, enhances anti-citrullin antibodies and worsens arthritis symptoms in a mouse model of adjuvant arthritis. Citrullination is protein modification in which an arginine residue is converted into a citrulline residue by a specific intracellular enzyme, peptidylarginine deiminase (PAD; Vossenaar et al., 2003). The anti-citrullinated peptide/protein antibody (ACPA) is frequently detected in RA patients (Vincent et al., 2005; Suzuki et al., 2007; van Venrooij et al., 2011). Although the reasons why citrullination is frequently observed and how it participates in RA pathogenesis remains unclear, the relationship between stress proteins and this specific protein modification suggests an undescribed crosstalk between inflammatory stress and disease-specific protein modifications in RA pathogenesis. In addition to RA, the anti-Bip autoantibody is also detected in another autoimmune and inflammatory disease, systemic lupus erythematosus (SLE; Casciola-Rosen et al., 1994; Weber et al., 2010), in which its pathophysiological role remains unknown.

HSP47

Hsp47 is an ER resident molecular chaperone; it is the only HSP in the ER. Hsp47 specifically maintains collagen biosynthesis (Nagata, 2003; Ishida and Nagata, 2011). Its gene disruption in mice causes significant reductions in mature collagens in connective tissues, resulting in embryonic lethality (Nagai et al., 2000; Marutani et al., 2004; Matsuoka et al., 2004). Several studies showed that the levels of anti-hsp47 autoantibody are specifically increased in RA patients (Hattori et al., 1998, 2000, 2001, 2003, 2005). However, little is known about how hsp47 and its autoantibody correlate with RA pathogenesis. In addition to RA, the levels of the autoantibody to hsp47 are also increased in other autoimmune diseases, such as SLE, Sjögren's syndrome (SjS), mixed connective tissue disease (MCTD), systemic sclerosis (SSc), and non-specific idiopathic pneumonia (Yokota et al., 2003; Fujimoto et al., 2004; Kakugawa et al., 2008). Most of these diseases can be considered connective tissue diseases in which an upregulation of various types of collagen is observed. The expression profiles of collagens and hsp47 are fully consistent in both healthy (Masuda et al., 1998; Yamamura et al., 1998; Hirata et al., 1999; Yasuda et al., 2002) and diseased conditions (Masuda et al., 1994; Naitoh et al., 2001; Sato et al., 2008). Hsp47 might be the protein that stands at the junction of stress, the extracellular matrix (ECM) biogenesis, and autoimmune/connective tissue diseases.

HERP

Lupus nephritis, which is a kidney inflammatory disorder, is one of the manifestations of SLE, a complex autoimmune disease. Among the variety of autoantibodies that are detected in SLE patients, the anti-double-stranded DNA (dsDNA) antibody, which is a type of anti-nuclear antibody (ANA), is most characteristic of SLE and appears to significantly contribute to the pathogenesis of lupus nephritis (Isenberg et al., 2007). Although administration of dsDNA failed to initiate antibody production (Madaio et al., 1984), nucleosome-forming dsDNA elicited the anti-dsDNA antibody production (Rumore and Steinman, 1990; Casciola-Rosen et al., 1994; Voynova et al., 2005), suggesting that proteins like histone can work as an adjuvant for enhancing the antigenicity of dsDNA. Another possibility for anti-dsDNA antibody production is elicitation by cross-reactive protein antigens. Several proteins have been reported to cross-react with the anti-dsDNA antibody (Isenberg et al., 2007). Among them, α-actinin, which is an actin-associated protein, might be a potent candidate for the original antigen, which evokes anti-dsDNA antibody production (Mostoslavsky et al., 2001; Deocharan et al., 2002). However, a dysregulation of the negative selection of B-cell clones, which produce autoantibodies, occurs in these diseases.

Recently, Herp was suggested as a possible cross-reactive antigen of the anti-dsDNA antibody (Hirabayashi et al., 2010). Herp is an ER resident membrane protein that is involved in the ERAD complex and is induced by UPR (Kokame et al., 2000, 2001; Okuda-Shimizu and Hendershot, 2007; Kny et al., 2011; Marutani et al., 2011). Thus, Herp is an ER stress protein, can be induced by inflammatory ER stress. Among the known candidates for the original antigen of the anti-dsDNA antibody including α-actinin, only Herp can be induced by inflammatory stress. Thus, Herp can be the key component that connects inflammatory stress responses and anti-dsDNA antibody production in SLE.

CALRETICULIN

The anti-Ro/SS-A antibody, which is also considered an ANA, is one of the most studied and crucial markers in many autoimmune diseases, such as SLE, Sjs, SSc, and RA (Anderson et al., 1962; Clark et al., 1969; Alspaugh and Tan, 1975; Schulte-Pelkum et al., 2009; Defendenti et al., 2011). Although it has a strong, well-established association with autoimmune diseases, especially with neonatal lupus, it is unclear how it participates in autoimmune diseases (Schulte-Pelkum et al., 2009; Defendenti et al., 2011). Recently, it was shown that the anti-Ro/SS-A antibody can be categorized into two types, each of which specifically recognizes the 52-kDa (Ro52) and 60-kDa (Ro60) antigens. Ro52 and Ro60 form a Ro ribonucleoprotein (RNP) complex with a couple of other proteins, while the intracellular functions and pathogenic relevancies of those antigens remain unclear (Schulte-Pelkum et al., 2009; Defendenti et al., 2011).

Calreticulin is an essential ER resident lectin-like chaperone, which is induced by ER stress (Yoshida et al., 1998; Mesaeli et al.,

1999; Williams, 2006). Calreticulin was first postulated as the Ro/SS-A autoantigen (Collins et al., 1989; McCauliffe et al., 1990). However, it was later demonstrated that calreticulin itself was not an antigen (Lu et al., 1993; Boehm et al., 1994), but it maintained Ro RNP complex formation through its chaperone activity and modulated the antigenicity of the complex (Cheng et al., 1996; Staikou et al., 2003). Although it was shown that calreticulin was not the autoantigen for the Ro/SS-A autoantibody, the anti-calreticulin autoantibody has been independently observed in SLE patients (Boehm et al., 1994), complete congenital heart block (CCHB; Orth et al., 1996), which is one of the manifestations of SLE, and inflammatory bowel disease (Watanabe et al., 2006).

CALNEXIN, GRP94, AND ORP150

Calnexin is an ER resident lectin-like chaperone (Wada et al., 1991, 1997; Hebert et al., 1995; Deprez et al., 2005), which is not induced or is only mildly induced by ER stress (Kamauchi et al., 2005). An autoantibody to calnexin is observed in SLE patients, while its biological relevance remains unknown (Weber et al., 2010).

GRP94 is an essential ER resident hsp90 family chaperone, which is induced by cytosolic and ER stress (Wanderling et al., 2007; Eletto et al., 2010). Anti-GRP94 autoantibodies have been observed in SLE patients (Boehm et al., 1994), RA (Weber et al., 2010), and myasthenia gravis (MG; Suzuki et al., 2011). In addition, cell surface expression of GRP94 itself is detected in patients with type I diabetes (Pagetta et al., 2003) and in GRP94 transgenic mice (Liu et al., 2003). In GRP94 transgenic mice, lupus-like autoimmune disorder and systemic inflammation are induced, suggesting that extracellular GRP94 and its autoantibody have proinflammatory effects in autoimmune diseases.

ORP150 is an essential ER resident hsp70 chaperone that is induced by ER stress and hypoxia (Kitao et al., 2001; Ni and Lee, 2007). An autoantibody to ORP150 is detected in patients with atherosclerosis and type I diabetes (Tsukamoto et al., 1996; Nakatani et al., 2006), but it remains unclear if they have a pathophysiological role in autoimmune responses.

REGULATION OF ER STRESS PROTEIN DISTRIBUTION

As discussed above, the critical difference between HSPs and ER stress proteins is based on the stress pathway they are induced through. One is through a heat shock response, and the other is through the UPR. However, another striking difference exists, i.e., HSPs are originally distributed in the cytosol. In patients with inflammatory diseases, HSPs are observed in extracellular fluid; this could be due to the destruction of the plasma membrane that accompanies stress-induced apoptosis, necrosis, and phagocytosis or alternative active secretion through exosomes. On the other hand, ER stress proteins are originally located in the secretory pathway. Thus, ER stress proteins can potentially be secreted into the cell surface, after which they escape from the ER retention mechanism. Indeed, some ER stress proteins are expressed on the cell surface without any cell destruction, e.g., calnexin (Okazaki et al., 2000), calreticulin (Jeffery et al., 2011), Bip (Delpino and Castelli, 2002), GRP94 (Altmeyer et al., 1996), and hsp47 (Hebert et al., 1999). How they escape, how they are retained, and whether this leaky expression correlates with autoimmune pathogenesis remains unknown. However, this apparent difference between the two types of stress proteins might cause physiological differences, therefore, this should be examined in autoimmune and inflammatory diseases.

CONCLUSION

Several studies suggested that ER stress proteins are potent immunomodulating components in autoimmune and inflammatory diseases. Although their pathogenic relevancies remain unclear, some of them appear to participate in disease progression. Their inducibility by inflammatory stress and their original distribution in the secretory pathway could be advantageous for participation in autoimmune and inflammatory responses. Until now, the major evidence of the involvement of ER stress proteins in autoimmune diseases appears to be autoantigens. This situation can be compared to that of HSPs two decades ago. Since then, much has been revealed about the functions of HSPs in addition to being autoantigens. Because HSPs and ER stress proteins share several properties as molecular chaperones, we may be able to expect unidentified and important roles of ER stress proteins in autoimmune response as well as HSPs. Indeed, another issue of the stress proteins in autoimmune responses is their potential immunomodulating abilities. Because chaperones can broadly associate with other proteins, including autoantigens and recruit antigen presentation pathway, they can work as endogenous adjuvants in immune responses. In this review, we focused on the roles of ER stress proteins as autoantigens. However, several other issues that are related to ER stress are also important, e.g., HLA-B27 misfolding in ankylosing spondylitis and anti-apoptotic function of HRD1/synoviolin in synovial cells in RA (Yoshida, 2007; Todd et al., 2008; Yagishita et al., 2008; Colbert et al., 2010). At the moment, the features of ER stress proteins in autoimmunity remain largely unclear. The potential relevance of ER stress proteins in many autoimmune and inflammatory diseases makes them potential clinical targets.

ACKNOWLEDGMENTS

We thank Dr. Shinichi Yokota (Sapporo Medical University) for critical reading of the manuscript. This work was supported by Grant-in-Aid for Creative Scientific Research (19G50314; to Kazuhiro Nagata), Grant-in-Aid for Young Scientists (B) (22710193), and Grant-in-Aid for Scientific Research on Innovative Areas (23122520; to Daisuke Morito).

REFERENCES

Alspaugh, M. A., and Tan, E. M. (1975). Antibodies to cellular antigens in Sjogren's syndrome. *J. Clin. Invest.* 55, 1067–1073.

Altmeyer, A., Maki, R. G., Feldweg, A. M., Heike, M., Protopopov, V. P., Masur, S. K., and Srivastava, P. K. (1996). Tumor-specific cell surface expression of the-KDEL containing, endoplasmic reticular heat shock protein gp96. *Int. J. Cancer* 69, 340–349.

Anderson, J. R., Gray, K. G., Beck, J. S., Buchanan, W. W., and Mc, E. A. (1962). Precipitating auto-antibodies in the connective tissue diseases. *Ann. Rheum. Dis.* 21, 360–369.

Araki, K., and Nagata, K. (2011). Protein folding and quality control in the ER. *Cold Spring Harb. Perspect. Biol.* 3.

Blass, S., Haferkamp, C., Specker, C., Schwochau, M., Schneider, M., and Schneider, E. M. (1997). Rheumatoid arthritis: autoreactive T cells recognising a novel 68k autoantigen. *Ann. Rheum. Dis.* 56, 317–322.

Blass, S., Meier, C., Vohr, H. W., Schwochau, M., Specker, C., and Burmester, G. R. (1998). The p68 autoantigen characteristic of rheumatoid arthritis is reactive with carbohydrate epitope specific autoantibodies. *Ann. Rheum. Dis.* 57, 220–225.

Blass, S., Specker, C., Lakomek, H. J., Schneider, E. M., and Schwochau, M. (1995). Novel 68 kDa autoantigen detected by rheumatoid arthritis specific antibodies. *Ann. Rheum. Dis.* 54, 355–360.

Blass, S., Union, A., Raymackers, J., Schumann, F., Ungethum, U., Muller-Steinbach, S., De Keyser, F., Engel, J. M., and Burmester, G. R. (2001). The stress protein BiP is overexpressed and is a major B and T cell target in rheumatoid arthritis. *Arthritis Rheum.* 44, 761–771.

Bodman-Smith, M. D., Corrigall, V. M., Kemeny, D. M., and Panayi, G. S. (2003). BiP, a putative autoantigen in rheumatoid arthritis, stimulates IL-10-producing CD8-positive T cells from normal individuals. *Rheumatology (Oxford)* 42, 637–644.

Boehm, J., Orth, T., Van Nguyen, P., and Soling, H. D. (1994). Systemic lupus erythematosus is associated with increased auto-antibody titers against calreticulin and grp94, but calreticulin is not the Ro/SS-A antigen. *Eur. J. Clin. Invest.* 24, 248–257.

Brodsky, J. L., and McCracken, A. A. (1997). ER-associated and proteasomemediated protein degradation: how two topologically restricted events came together. *Trends Cell Biol.* 7, 151–156.

Brownlie, R. J., Myers, L. K., Wooley, P. H., Corrigall, V. M., Bodman-Smith, M. D., Panayi, G. S., and Thompson, S. J. (2006). Treatment of murine collagen-induced arthritis by the stress protein BiP via interleukin-4-producing regulatory T cells: a novel function for an ancient protein. *Arthritis Rheum.* 54, 854–863.

Bukau, B., Weissman, J., and Horwich, A. (2006). Molecular chaperones and protein quality control. *Cell* 125, 443–451.

Casciola-Rosen, L. A., Anhalt, G., and Rosen, A. (1994). Autoantigens targeted in systemic lupus erythematosus are clustered in two populations of surface structures on apoptotic keratinocytes. *J. Exp. Med.* 179, 1317–1330.

Cheng, S. T., Nguyen, T. Q., Yang, Y. S., Capra, J. D., and Sontheimer, R. D. (1996). Calreticulin binds hYRNA and the 52-kDa polypeptide component of the Ro/SS-A ribonucleoprotein autoantigen. *J. Immunol.* 156, 4484–4491.

Christianson, J. C., Shaler, T. A., Tyler, R. E., and Kopito, R. R. (2008). OS-9 and GRP94 deliver mutant alpha1-antitrypsin to the Hrd1-SEL1L ubiquitin ligase complex for ERAD. *Nat. Cell Biol.* 10, 272–282.

Clark, G., Reichlin, M., and Tomasi, T. B. Jr. (1969). Characterization of a soluble cytoplasmic antigen reactive with sera from patients with systemic lupus erythmatosus. *J. Immunol.* 102, 117–122.

Colbert, R. A., Delay, M. L., Klenk, E. I., and Layh-Schmitt, G. (2010). From HLA-B27 to spondyloarthritis: a journey through the ER. *Immunol. Rev.* 233, 181–202.

Collins, J. H., Xi, Z. J., Alderson-Lang, B. H., Treves, S., and Volpe, P. (1989). Sequence homology of a canine brain calcium-binding protein with calregulin and the human Ro/SS-A antigen. *Biochem. Biophys. Res. Commun.* 164, 575–579.

Corrigall, V. M., Bodman-Smith, M. D., Brunst, M., Cornell, H., and Panayi, G. S. (2004). Inhibition of antigen-presenting cell function and stimulation of human peripheral blood mononuclear cells to express an anti-inflammatory cytokine profile by the stress protein BiP: relevance to the treatment of inflammatory arthritis. *Arthritis Rheum.* 50, 1164–1171.

Corrigall, V. M., Bodman-Smith, M. D., Fife, M. S., Canas, B., Myers, L. K., Wooley, P., Soh, C., Staines, N. A., Pappin, D. J., Berlo, S. E., Van Eden, W., Van Der Zee, R., Lanchbury, J. S., and Panayi, G. S. (2001). The human endoplasmic reticulum molecular chaperone BiP is an autoantigen for rheumatoid arthritis and prevents the induction of experimental arthritis. *J. Immunol.* 166, 1492–1498.

Defendenti, C., Atzeni, F., Spina, M. F., Grosso, S., Cereda, A., Guercilena, G., Bollani, S., Saibeni, S., and Puttini, P. S. (2011). Clinical and laboratory aspects of Ro/SSA-52 autoantibodies. *Autoimmun. Rev.* 10, 150–154.

Delpino, A., and Castelli, M. (2002). The 78 kDa glucose-regulated protein (GRP78/BIP) is expressed on the cell membrane, is released into cell culture medium and is also present in human peripheral circulation. *Biosci. Rep.* 22, 407–420.

Deocharan, B., Qing, X., Lichauco, J., and Putterman, C. (2002). Alpha-actinin is a cross-reactive renal target for pathogenic anti-DNA antibodies. *J. Immunol.* 168, 3072–3078.

Deprez, P., Gautschi, M., and Helenius, A. (2005). More than one glycan is needed for ER glucosidase II to allow entry of glycoproteins into the calnexin/calreticulin cycle. *Mol. Cell* 19, 183–195.

Eletto, D., Dersh, D., and Argon, Y. (2010). GRP94 in ER quality control and stress responses. *Semin. Cell Dev. Biol.* 21, 479–485.

Ellgaard, L., and Ruddock, L. W. (2005). The human protein disulphide isomerase family: substrate interactions and functional properties. *EMBO Rep.* 6, 28–32.

Fujimoto, M., Hamaguchi, Y., Yazawa, N., Komura, K., Takehara, K., and Sato, S. (2004). Autoantibodies to a collagen-specific molecular chaperone, heat-shock protein 47, in systemic sclerosis. *Clin. Exp. Immunol.* 138, 534–539.

Hagiwara, M., Maegawa, K., Suzuki, M., Ushioda, R., Araki, K., Matsumoto, Y., Hoseki, J., Nagata, K., and Inaba, K. (2011). Structural basis of an ERAD pathway mediated by the ER-resident protein disulfide reductase ERdj5. *Mol. Cell* 41, 432–444.

Hartl, F. U. (2011). Chaperone-assisted protein folding: the path to discovery from a personal perspective. *Nat. Med.* 17, 1206–1210.

Hattori, T., Fujisawa, T., Sasaki, K., Yutani, Y., Nakanishi, T., Takahashi, K., and Takigawa, M. (1998). Isolation and characterization of a rheumatoid arthritis-specific antigen (RA-A47) from a human chondrocytic cell line (HCS-2/8). *Biochem. Biophys. Res. Commun.* 245, 679–683.

Hattori, T., Kawaki, H., Kubota, S., Yutani, Y., De Crombrugghe, B., Von Der Mark, K., and Takigawa, M. (2003). Downregulation of a rheumatoid arthritis-related antigen (RA-A47) by ra-a47 antisense oligonucleotides induces inflammatory factors in chondrocytes. *J. Cell. Physiol.* 197, 94–102.

Hattori, T., Kubota, S., Yutani, Y., Fujisawa, T., Nakanishi, T., Takahashi, K., and Takigawa, M. (2001). Change in cellular localization of a rheumatoid arthritis-related antigen (RA-A47) with downregulation upon stimulation by inflammatory cytokines in chondrocytes. *J. Cell. Physiol.* 186, 268–281.

Hattori, T., Takahash, K., Yutani, Y., Fujisawa, T., Nakanishi, T., and Takigawa, M. (2000). Rheumatoid arthritis-related antigen 47kDa (RA-A47) is a product of colligin-2 and acts as a human HSP47. *J. Bone Miner. Metab.* 18, 328–334.

Hattori, T., Von Der Mark, K., Kawaki, H., Yutani, Y., Kubota, S., Nakanishi, T., Eberspaecher, H., De Crombrugghe, B., and Takigawa, M. (2005). Downregulation of rheumatoid arthritis-related antigen RA-A47 (HSP47/colligin-2) in chondrocytic cell lines induces apoptosis and cell-surface expression of RA-A47 in association with CD9. *J. Cell. Physiol.* 202, 191–204.

Hauet-Broere, F., Wieten, L., Guichelaar, T., Berlo, S., Van Der Zee, R., and Van Eden, W. (2006). Heat shock proteins induce T cell regulation of chronic inflammation. *Ann. Rheum. Dis.* 65(Suppl. 3), iii65–iii68.

Hebert, C., Norris, K., Della Coletta, R., Reynolds, M., Ordonez, J., and Sauk, J. J. (1999). Cell surface colligin/Hsp47 associates with tetraspanin protein CD9 in epidermoid carcinoma cell lines. *J. Cell. Biochem.* 73, 248–258.

Hebert, D. N., Foellmer, B., and Helenius, A. (1995). Glucose trimming and reglucosylation determine glycoprotein association with calnexin in the endoplasmic reticulum. *Cell* 81, 425–433.

Hershko, A., and Ciechanover, A. (1998). The ubiquitin system. *Annu. Rev. Biochem.* 67, 425–479.

Hirabayashi, Y., Oka, Y., Ikeda, T., Fujii, H., Ishii, T., Sasaki, T., and Harigae, H. (2010). The endoplasmic reticulum stress-inducible protein, Herp, is a potential triggering antigen for anti-DNA response. *J. Immunol.* 184, 3276–3283.

Hirata, H., Yamamura, I., Yasuda, K., Kobayashi, A., Tada, N., Suzuki, M., Hirayoshi, K., Hosokawa, N., and Nagata, K. (1999). Separate cis-acting DNA elements control cell type- and tissue-specific expression of collagen binding molecular chaperone HSP47. *J. Biol. Chem.* 274, 35703–35710.

Hoseki, J., Ushioda, R., and Nagata, K. (2010). Mechanism and components of endoplasmic reticulum-associated degradation. *J. Biochem.* 147, 19–25.

Hosokawa, N., Wada, I., Hasegawa, K., Yorihuzi, T., Tremblay, L. O., Herscovics, A., and Nagata, K. (2001). A novel ER alpha-mannosidase-like protein accelerates ER-associated degradation. *EMBO Rep.* 2, 415–422.

Isenberg, D. A., Manson, J. J., Ehrenstein, M. R., and Rahman, A. (2007). Fifty years of anti-ds DNA antibodies: are we approaching journey's end? *Rheumatology (Oxford)* 46, 1052–1056.

Ishida, Y., and Nagata, K. (2011). Hsp47 as a collagen-specific molecular chaperone. *Meth. Enzymol.* 499, 167–182.

Jeffery, E., Peters, L. R., and Raghavan, M. (2011). The polypeptide binding conformation of calreticulin facilitates its cell-surface expression under conditions of endoplasmic reticulum stress. *J. Biol. Chem.* 286, 2402–2415.

Jorgensen, C., Gedon, E., Jaquet, C., and Sany, J. (1998). Gastric administration of recombinant 65 kDa heat shock protein delays the severity of type II collagen induced arthritis in mice. *J. Rheumatol.* 25, 763–767.

Kakugawa, T., Yokota, S., Mukae, H., Kubota, H., Sakamoto, N., Mizunoe, S., Matsuoka, Y., Kadota, J., Fujii, N., Nagata, K., and Kohno, S. (2008). High serum concentrations of autoantibodies to HSP47 in nonspecific interstitial pneumonia compared with idiopathic pulmonary fibrosis. *BMC Pulm. Med.* 8, 23. doi:10.1186/1471-2466-8-23

Kamauchi, S., Nakatani, H., Nakano, C., and Urade, R. (2005). Gene expression in response to endoplasmic reticulum stress in *Arabidopsis thaliana*. *FEBS J.* 272, 3461–3476.

Kitao, Y., Ozawa, K., Miyazaki, M., Tamatani, M., Kobayashi, T., Yanagi, H., Okabe, M., Ikawa, M., Yamashima, T., Stern, D. M., Hori, O., and Ogawa, S. (2001). Expression of the endoplasmic reticulum molecular chaperone (ORP150) rescues hippocampal neurons from glutamate toxicity. *J. Clin. Invest.* 108, 1439–1450.

Kny, M., Standera, S., Hartmann-Petersen, R., Kloetzel, P. M., and Seeger, M. (2011). Herp regulates Hrd1-mediated ubiquitylation in a ubiquitin-like domain-dependent manner. *J. Biol. Chem.* 286, 5151–5156.

Kokame, K., Agarwala, K. L., Kato, H., and Miyata, T. (2000). Herp, a new ubiquitin-like membrane protein induced by endoplasmic reticulum stress. *J. Biol. Chem.* 275, 32846–32853.

Kokame, K., Kato, H., and Miyata, T. (2001). Identification of ERSE-II, a new cis-acting element responsible for the ATF6-dependent mammalian unfolded protein response. *J. Biol. Chem.* 276, 9199–9205.

Lilley, B. N., and Ploegh, H. L. (2004). A membrane protein required for dislocation of misfolded proteins from the ER. *Nature* 429, 834–840.

Lilley, B. N., and Ploegh, H. L. (2005). Multiprotein complexes that link dislocation, ubiquitination, and extraction of misfolded proteins from the endoplasmic reticulum membrane. *Proc. Natl. Acad. Sci. U.S.A.* 102, 14296–14301.

Liu, B., Dai, J., Zheng, H., Stoilova, D., Sun, S., and Li, Z. (2003). Cell surface expression of an endoplasmic reticulum resident heat shock protein gp96 triggers MyD88-dependent systemic autoimmune diseases. *Proc. Natl. Acad. Sci. U.S.A.* 100, 15824–15829.

Lu, J., Willis, A. C., and Sim, R. B. (1993). A calreticulin-like protein co-purifies with a "60 kD" component of Ro/SSA, but is not recognized by antibodies in Sjogren's syndrome sera. *Clin. Exp. Immunol.* 94, 429–434.

Madaio, M. P., Hodder, S., Schwartz, R. S., and Stollar, B. D. (1984). Responsiveness of autoimmune and normal mice to nucleic acid antigens. *J. Immunol.* 132, 872–876.

Marutani, T., Maeda, T., Tanabe, C., Zou, K., Araki, W., Kokame, K., Michikawa, M., and Komano, H. (2011). ER-stress-inducible Herp, facilitates the degradation of immature nicastrin. *Biochim. Biophys. Acta* 1810, 790–798.

Marutani, T., Yamamoto, A., Nagai, N., Kubota, H., and Nagata, K. (2004). Accumulation of type IV collagen in dilated ER leads to apoptosis in Hsp47-knockout mouse embryos via induction of CHOP. *J. Cell. Sci.* 117, 5913–5922.

Masuda, H., Fukumoto, M., Hirayoshi, K., and Nagata, K. (1994). Coexpression of the collagen-binding stress protein HSP47 gene and the alpha 1(I) and alpha 1(III) collagen genes in carbon tetrachloride-induced rat liver fibrosis. *J. Clin. Invest.* 94, 2481–2488.

Masuda, H., Hosokawa, N., and Nagata, K. (1998). Expression and localization of collagen-binding stress protein Hsp47 in mouse embryo development: comparison with types I and II collagen. *Cell Stress Chaperones* 3, 256–264.

Matsuoka, Y., Kubota, H., Adachi, E., Nagai, N., Marutani, T., Hosokawa, N., and Nagata, K. (2004). Insufficient folding of type IV collagen and formation of abnormal basement membrane-like structure in embryoid bodies derived from Hsp47-null embryonic stem cells. *Mol. Biol. Cell* 15, 4467–4475.

McCauliffe, D. P., Zappi, E., Lieu, T. S., Michalak, M., Sontheimer, R. D., and Capra, J. D. (1990). A human Ro/SS-A autoantigen is the homologue of calreticulin and is highly homologous with onchocercal RAL-1 antigen and an aplysia "memory molecule." *J. Clin. Invest.* 86, 332–335.

McCracken, A. A., and Brodsky, J. L. (1996). Assembly of ER-associated protein degradation in vitro: dependence on cytosol, calnexin, and ATP. *J. Cell Biol.* 132, 291–298.

Mesaeli, N., Nakamura, K., Zvaritch, E., Dickie, P., Dziak, E., Krause, K. H., Opas, M., Maclennan, D. H., and Michalak, M. (1999). Calreticulin is essential for cardiac development. *J. Cell Biol.* 144, 857–868.

Molinari, M., Calanca, V., Galli, C., Lucca, P., and Paganetti, P. (2003). Role of EDEM in the release of misfolded glycoproteins from the calnexin cycle. *Science* 299, 1397–1400.

Mori, K. (2000). Tripartite management of unfolded proteins in the endoplasmic reticulum. *Cell* 101, 451–454.

Morimoto, R. I. (1998). Regulation of the heat shock transcriptional response: cross talk between a family of heat shock factors, molecular chaperones, and negative regulators. *Genes Dev.* 12, 3788–3796.

Mostoslavsky, G., Fischel, R., Yachimovich, N., Yarkoni, Y., Rosenmann, E., Monestier, M., Baniyash, M., and Eilat, D. (2001). Lupus anti-DNA autoantibodies cross-react with a glomerular structural protein: a case for tissue injury by molecular mimicry. *Eur. J. Immunol.* 31, 1221–1227.

Mueller, B., Klemm, E. J., Spooner, E., Claessen, J. H., and Ploegh, H. L. (2008). SEL1L nucleates a protein complex required for dislocation of misfolded glycoproteins. *Proc. Natl. Acad. Sci. U.S.A.* 105, 12325–12330.

Mueller, B., Lilley, B. N., and Ploegh, H. L. (2006). SEL1L, the homologue of yeast Hrd3p, is involved in protein dislocation from the mammalian ER. *J. Cell Biol.* 175, 261–270.

Multhoff, G. (2006). Heat shock proteins in immunity. *Handb. Exp. Pharmacol.* 172, 279–304.

Nagai, N., Hosokawa, M., Itohara, S., Adachi, E., Matsushita, T., Hosokawa, N., and Nagata, K. (2000). Embryonic lethality of molecular chaperone hsp47 knockout mice is associated with defects in collagen biosynthesis. *J. Cell Biol.* 150, 1499–1506.

Nagata, K. (2003). HSP47 as a collagen-specific molecular chaperone: function and expression in normal mouse development. *Semin. Cell Dev. Biol.* 14, 275–282.

Naitoh, M., Hosokawa, N., Kubota, H., Tanaka, T., Shirane, H., Sawada, M., Nishimura, Y., and Nagata, K. (2001). Upregulation of HSP47 and collagen type III in the dermal fibrotic disease, keloid. *Biochem. Biophys. Res. Commun.* 280, 1316–1322.

Nakatani, Y., Kaneto, H., Hatazaki, M., Yoshiuchi, K., Kawamori, D., Sakamoto, K., Matsuoka, T., Ogawa, S., Yamasaki, Y., and Matsuhisa, M. (2006). Increased stress protein ORP150 autoantibody production in Type 1 diabetic patients. *Diabet. Med.* 23, 216–219.

Ni, M., and Lee, A. S. (2007). ER chaperones in mammalian development and human diseases. *FEBS Lett.* 581, 3641–3651.

Njemini, R., Bautmans, I., Onyema, O. O., Van Puyvelde, K., Demanet, C., and Mets, T. (2011). Circulating heat shock protein 70 in health, aging and disease. *BMC Immunol.* 12, 24. doi:10.1186/1471-2172-12-24

Oda, Y., Hosokawa, N., Wada, I., and Nagata, K. (2003). EDEM as an acceptor of terminally misfolded glycoproteins released from calnexin. *Science* 299, 1394–1397.

Oda, Y., Okada, T., Yoshida, H., Kaufman, R. J., Nagata, K., and Mori, K. (2006). Derlin-2 and Derlin-3 are regulated by the mammalian unfolded protein response and are required for ER-associated degradation. *J. Cell Biol.* 172, 383–393.

Okazaki, Y., Ohno, H., Takase, K., Ochiai, T., and Saito, T. (2000). Cell surface expression of calnexin, a molecular chaperone in the endoplasmic reticulum. *J. Biol. Chem.* 275, 35751–35758.

Okuda-Shimizu, Y., and Hendershot, L. M. (2007). Characterization of an ERAD pathway for nonglycosylated BiP substrates, which require Herp. *Mol. Cell* 28, 544–554.

Orth, T., Dorner, T., Meyer Zum Buschenfelde, K. H., and Mayet, W. J. (1996). Complete congenital heart block is associated with increased autoantibody titers against calreticulin. *Eur. J. Clin. Invest.* 26, 205–215.

Pagetta, A., Folda, A., Brunati, A. M., and Finotti, P. (2003). Identification and purification from the plasma of Type 1 diabetic subjects of a proteolytically active Grp94Evidence that Grp94 is entirely responsible for plasma proteolytic activity. *Diabetologia* 46, 996–1006.

Panayi, G. S., and Corrigall, V. M. (2006). BiP regulates autoimmune inflammation and tissue damage. *Autoimmun. Rev.* 5, 140–142.

Rumore, P. M., and Steinman, C. R. (1990). Endogenous circulating DNA in systemic lupus erythematosus. Occurrence as multimeric complexes bound to histone. *J. Clin. Invest.* 86, 69–74.

Sato, Y., Murase, K., Kato, J., Kobune, M., Sato, T., Kawano, Y., Takimoto, R., Takada, K., Miyanishi, K., Matsunaga, T., Takayama, T., and Niitsu, Y. (2008). Resolution of liver cirrhosis using vitamin A-coupled liposomes to deliver siRNA against a collagen-specific chaperone. *Nat. Biotechnol.* 26, 431–442.

Schulte-Pelkum, J., Fritzler, M., and Mahler, M. (2009). Latest update on the Ro/SS-A autoantibody system. *Autoimmun. Rev.* 8, 632–637.

Shoda, H., Fujio, K., Shibuya, M., Okamura, T., Sumitomo, S., Okamoto, A., Sawada, T., and Yamamoto, K. (2011). Detection of autoantibody to citrullinated BiP in rheumatoid arthritis patients and pro-inflammatory roles of citrullinated BiP in collagen-induced arthritis. *Arthritis Res. Ther.* 13, R191.

Smith, M. H., Ploegh, H. L., and Weissman, J. S. (2011). Road to ruin: targeting proteins for degradation in the endoplasmic reticulum. *Science* 334, 1086–1090.

Staikou, E. V., Routsias, J. G., Makri, A. A., Terzoglou, A., Sakarellos-Daitsiotis, M., Sakarellos, C., Panayotou, G., Moutsopoulos, H. M., and Tzioufas, A. G. (2003). Calreticulin binds preferentially with B cell linear epitopes of Ro60 kD autoantigen, enhancing recognition by anti-Ro60 kD autoantibodies. *Clin. Exp. Immunol.* 134, 143–150.

Suzuki, A., Yamada, R., and Yamamoto, K. (2007). Citrullination by peptidylarginine deiminase in rheumatoid arthritis. *Ann. N. Y. Acad. Sci.* 1108, 323–339.

Suzuki, S., Utsugisawa, K., Iwasa, K., Satoh, T., Nagane, Y., Yoshikawa, H., Kuwana, M., and Suzuki, N. (2011). Autoimmunity to endoplasmic reticulum chaperone GRP94 in myasthenia gravis. *J. Neuroimmunol.* 237, 87–92.

Todd, D. J., Lee, A. H., and Glimcher, L. H. (2008). The endoplasmic reticulum stress response in immunity and autoimmunity. *Nat. Rev. Immunol.* 8, 663–674.

Tsai, B., Ye, Y., and Rapoport, T. A. (2002). Retro-translocation of proteins from the endoplasmic reticulum into the cytosol. *Nat. Rev. Mol. Cell Biol.* 3, 246–255.

Tsukamoto, Y., Kuwabara, K., Hirota, S., Ikeda, J., Stern, D., Yanagi, H., Matsumoto, M., Ogawa, S., and Kitamura, Y. (1996). 150-kD oxygen-regulated protein is expressed in human atherosclerotic plaques and allows mononuclear phagocytes to withstand cellular stress on exposure to hypoxia and modified low density lipoprotein. *J. Clin. Invest.* 98, 1930–1941.

Tu, B. P., and Weissman, J. S. (2004). Oxidative protein folding in eukaryotes: mechanisms and consequences. *J. Cell Biol.* 164, 341–346.

Ushioda, R., Hoseki, J., Araki, K., Jansen, G., Thomas, D. Y., and Nagata, K. (2008). ERdj5 is required as a disulfide reductase for degradation of misfolded proteins in the ER. *Science* 321, 569–572.

Ushioda, R., and Nagata, K. (2011). The endoplasmic reticulum-associated degradation and disulfide reductase ERdj5. *Meth. Enzymol.* 490, 235–258.

van Eden, W., Thole, J. E., Van Der Zee, R., Noordzij, A., Van Embden, J. D., Hensen, E. J., and Cohen, I. R. (1988). Cloning of the mycobacterial epitope recognized by T lymphocytes in adjuvant arthritis. *Nature* 331, 171–173.

Van Eden, W., Wick, G., Albani, S., and Cohen, I. (2007). Stress, heat shock proteins, and autoimmunity: how immune responses to heat shock proteins are to be used for the control of chronic inflammatory diseases. *Ann. N. Y. Acad. Sci.* 1113, 217–237.

van Venrooij, W. J., Van Beers, J. J., and Pruijn, G. J. (2011). Anti-CCP antibodies: the past, the present and the future. *Nat. Rev. Rheumatol.* 7, 391–398.

Vincent, C., Nogueira, L., Clavel, C., Sebbag, M., and Serre, G. (2005). Autoantibodies to citrullinated proteins: ACPA. *Autoimmunity* 38, 17–24.

Vossenaar, E. R., Zendman, A. J., Van Venrooij, W. J., and Pruijn, G. J. (2003). PAD, a growing family of citrullinating enzymes: genes, features and involvement in disease. *Bioessays* 25, 1106–1118.

Voynova, E. N., Tchorbanov, A. I., Todorov, T. A., and Vassilev, T. L. (2005). Breaking of tolerance to native DNA in nonautoimmune mice by immunization with natural protein/DNA complexes. *Lupus* 14, 543–550.

Wada, I., Kai, M., Imai, S., Sakane, F., and Kanoh, H. (1997). Promotion of transferrin folding by cyclic interactions with calnexin and calreticulin. *EMBO J.* 16, 5420–5432.

Wada, I., Rindress, D., Cameron, P. H., Ou, W. J., Doherty, J. J. II, Louvard, D., Bell, A. W., Dignard, D., Thomas, D. Y., and Bergeron, J. J. (1991). SSR alpha and associated calnexin are major calcium binding proteins of the endoplasmic reticulum membrane. *J. Biol. Chem.* 266, 19599–19610.

Walter, P., and Ron, D. (2011). The unfolded protein response: from stress pathway to homeostatic regulation. *Science* 334, 1081–1086.

Wanderling, S., Simen, B. B., Ostrovsky, O., Ahmed, N. T., Vogen, S. M., Gidalevitz, T., and Argon, Y. (2007). GRP94 is essential for mesoderm induction and muscle development because it regulates insulin-like growth factor secretion. *Mol. Biol. Cell* 18, 3764–3775.

Watanabe, K., Ohira, H., Orikasa, H., Saito, K., Kanno, K., Shioya, Y., Obara, K., and Sato, Y. (2006). Anti-calreticulin antibodies in patients with inflammatory bowel disease. *Fukushima J. Med. Sci.* 52, 1–11.

Weber, C. K., Haslbeck, M., Englbrecht, M., Sehnert, B., Mielenz, D., Graef, D., Distler, J. H., Mueller, R. B., Burkhardt, H., Schett, G., Voll, R. E., and Furnrohr, B. G. (2010). Antibodies to the endoplasmic reticulum-resident chaperones calnexin, BiP and Grp94 in patients with rheumatoid arthritis and systemic lupus erythematosus. *Rheumatology (Oxford)* 49, 2255–2263.

Wendling, U., Paul, L., Van Der Zee, R., Prakken, B., Singh, M., and Van Eden, W. (2000). A conserved mycobacterial heat shock protein (hsp) 70 sequence prevents adjuvant arthritis upon nasal administration and induces IL-10-producing T cells that cross-react with the mammalian self-hsp70 homologue. *J. Immunol.* 164, 2711–2717.

Williams, D. B. (2006). Beyond lectins: the calnexin/calreticulin chaperone system of the endoplasmic reticulum. *J. Cell. Sci.* 119, 615–623.

Yagishita, N., Yamasaki, S., Nishioka, K., and Nakajima, T. (2008). Synoviolin, protein folding and the maintenance of joint homeostasis. *Nat. Clin. Pract. Rheumatol.* 4, 91–97.

Yamamura, I., Hirata, H., Hosokawa, N., and Nagata, K. (1998). Transcriptional activation of the mouse HSP47 gene in mouse osteoblast MC3T3-E1 cells by TGF-beta 1. *Biochem. Biophys. Res. Commun.* 244, 68–74.

Yasuda, K., Hirayoshi, K., Hirata, H., Kubota, H., Hosokawa, N., and Nagata, K. (2002). The Kruppel-like factor Zf9 and proteins in the Sp1 family regulate the expression of HSP47, a collagen-specific molecular chaperone. *J. Biol. Chem.* 277, 44613–44622.

Ye, Y., Meyer, H. H., and Rapoport, T. A. (2001). The AAA ATPase Cdc48/p97 and its partners transport proteins from the ER into the cytosol. *Nature* 414, 652–656.

Ye, Y., Meyer, H. H., and Rapoport, T. A. (2003). Function of the p97-Ufd1-Npl4 complex in retrotranslocation from the ER to the cytosol: dual recognition of nonubiquitinated polypeptide segments and polyubiquitin chains. *J. Cell Biol.* 162, 71–84.

Yokota, S., and Fujii, N. (2010). Immunomodulatory activity of extracellular heat shock proteins and their autoantibodies. *Microbiol. Immunol.* 54, 299–307.

Yokota, S., Kubota, H., Matsuoka, Y., Naitoh, M., Hirata, D., Minota, S., Takahashi, H., Fujii, N., and Nagata, K. (2003). Prevalence of HSP47 antigen and autoantibodies to HSP47 in the sera of patients with mixed connective tissue disease. *Biochem. Biophys. Res. Commun.* 303, 413–418.

Yoshida, H. (2007). ER stress and diseases. *FEBS J.* 274, 630–658.

Yoshida, H., Haze, K., Yanagi, H., Yura, T., and Mori, K. (1998). Identification of the cis-acting endoplasmic reticulum stress response element responsible for transcriptional induction of mammalian glucose-regulated proteins. Involvement of basic leucine zipper transcription factors. *J. Biol. Chem.* 273, 33741–33749.

16

Natural and man-made V-gene repertoires for antibody discovery

William J. J. Finlay[1] and Juan C. Almagro[2]*

[1] Global Biotherapeutics Technologies, Pfizer, Dublin, Ireland
[2] Centers for Therapeutic Innovation, Pfizer, Boston, MA, USA

Edited by:
Harry W. Schroeder, University of Alabama at Birmingham, USA

Reviewed by:
Laurence Morel, University of Florida, USA
Wenxia Song, University of Maryland, USA

***Correspondence:**
Juan C. Almagro, CTI-Boston, Pfizer, 3 Blackfan Circle - 18th Floor, Boston, MA 02115, USA.
e-mail: juan.c.almagro@pfizer.com

Antibodies are the fastest-growing segment of the biologics market. The success of antibody-based drugs resides in their exquisite specificity, high potency, stability, solubility, safety, and relatively inexpensive manufacturing process in comparison with other biologics. We outline here the structural studies and fundamental principles that define how antibodies interact with diverse targets. We also describe the antibody repertoires and affinity maturation mechanisms of humans, mice, and chickens, plus the use of novel single-domain antibodies in camelids and sharks. These species all utilize diverse evolutionary solutions to generate specific and high affinity antibodies and illustrate the plasticity of natural antibody repertoires. In addition, we discuss the multiple variations of man-made antibody repertoires designed and validated in the last two decades, which have served as tools to explore how the size, diversity, and composition of a repertoire impact the antibody discovery process.

Keywords: therapeutic antibodies, antigen-binding site, antibody structure, structure-function relationship

INTRODUCTION

In recent decades, rodent monoclonal antibodies obtained by hybridoma technology and engineered by molecular biology techniques, or human antibodies obtained by display technologies or B-cell cloning, have become the treatment of choice in diverse diseases such as multiple sclerosis, rheumatoid arthritis, and several types of cancers, making a significant component of the pharmaceuticals market (Nelson et al., 2010). The success of therapeutic antibodies, with as many as 28 antibodies and antibody fragments marketed in The United States or The European Union (Reichert, 2012), resides in their exquisite specificity, high potency, stability, solubility, clinical tolerability, and relatively inexpensive manufacturing process in comparison with other biologics.

The factors contributing to the specificity and potency of antibodies have intrigued scientists since their discovery in the late 1800s and only in the last three decades has a clear picture of how antibodies work emerged. The current knowledge base has been assembled by combining insights from multiple disciplines such as: structural biology—studying hundreds of x-ray crystallography antibody structures from different species (Davies and Metzger, 1983; Chothia and Lesk, 1987; Wilson and Stanfield, 1994; Stanfield and Wilson, 2010) free and in complex with a wide variety of ligands (MacCallum et al., 1996; Ragunathan et al., 2012); immunogenetics—by fully characterizing the germline gene antibody repertoire of humans and other species (Lefranc et al., 2005) and by deciphering the molecular mechanisms used to generate functional antibody molecules starting from diverse gene families (Tonegawa, 1983); and cellular immunology—dissecting the process by which *in vivo* selection of specific antibodies occurs during an immune response and understanding the mechanisms that allow the affinity and specificity of the selected antibodies to mature as the immune response progresses (Noia and Neuberger, 2007).

The accumulation of this knowledge has potentiated several technological advances in the antibody engineering field, such as humanization of non-human antibodies to increase their human content and to enhance their manufacturability profile (Gilliland et al., 2012), the development of display technologies to select specific human antibodies *in vitro* (Hoogenboom, 2005), and the engineering of antibody characteristics such as affinity, cross-reactivity with target orthologs, stability, and solubility. Each of these great leaps forward have relied directly on a core of fundamental immunological knowledge and made it possible to create close to 30 antibody-based drugs, at the time of writing.

Here, we first provide an overview of the antibody structure and outline the fundamental principles that define how antibodies interact with diverse ligands. In the second section, we review the current knowledge of the antibody repertoire of humans and experimental species commonly used to generate monoclonal antibodies such as mice, chickens, and camelids. Each of these species possess distinct germline gene repertoires, have differing mechanisms of generating and affinity maturing their antibody molecules and, therefore, offer alternative sources of specific variable regions for therapeutic antibody development. In the third section, multiple variations of man-made antibody repertoires are described, from their inception to the current state of the art. These designer repertoires have applied the compound knowledge derived from both structural and repertoire studies, serving as tools to test hypotheses on how the size of a repertoire, its diversity and composition impact the selection of more specific and higher affinity antibodies. These repertoires have also been used extensively by academic laboratories and biotech companies to discover and optimize human antibodies *in vitro*. At the end of the article, a section with conclusions and future directions is included.

THE ANTIBODY MOLECULE

The IgG isotype is the most abundant form of circulating antibody and the molecular format of choice for most marketed therapeutic antibodies (Reichert, 2012), as it is stable, soluble, readily expressed in heterologous systems such as Chinese hamster ovary (CHO) cells and can potentially engage effector functions such as antibody-dependent cell-mediated cytotoxicity (ADCC) and complement-dependent cytotoxicity (CDC). IgGs are Y-shaped glycoproteins of approximately 150 kDa composed of two identical polypeptide heavy (H) chains and two identical light (L) chains. The most abundant classes of L chains are κ and λ, which are functionally indistinguishable, but structurally different and vary in proportion in different species. For instance, the human repertoire is approximately 40:60 λ:κ, whereas, the mouse repertoire is ~95% κ-type. The H chain divides Igs into five classes, IgG, IgD, IgE, IgA, and IgM, each with a unique role in the adaptive immune system.

By digesting IgGs with papain, two fractions can be obtained, one containing the so-called crystallizable fragment (Fc) and the other containing two identical antigen-binding fragments or Fabs (**Figure 1**). In the Fc resides the effector functions, whereas, the Fab, as its name indicates, binds the antigen and thus defines the specificity of antibodies. Each Fab has two variable domains, one from the H chain (V_H) and another from the L chain (V_L), in addition to two C domains: C_H1 and C_L. The Fc is a dimer made of four C domains, two C_H2 and two C_H3 domains.

The first antibody structures, solved in the 1970s [for early reviews see (Padlan, 1977; Amzel and Poljak, 1979; Davies and Metzger, 1983) and for more current reviews see (Wilson and Stanfield, 1994; Stanfield and Wilson, 2010)], revealed that V- and C-domains have a conserved and similar structure, termed "immunoglobulin (Ig) fold." The Ig fold is also the building block of a large number of other proteins with diverse functions, which are collectively called the Ig superfamily (Williams and Barclay, 1988). The Ig fold consists of two anti-parallel β-sheets that are tightly packed together. In the C domain, one of the β-sheets is formed by four β-strands A to D, whereas, the other β-sheet is formed by three β-strands C to G (**Figure 2**). A conserved intra-domain disulfide bridge, formed between cysteine residues in the B and F β-strands, stabilizes the C domain. The V-domain have an insertion with respect to the C domain of two extra β-strands, identified as C' and C'', present between β-strands C and D (**Figure 2**). As in the C domain, an intra-domain disulfide bridge is formed between cysteine residues in β-strands B and F. The V-domains are in general less compact than the C domains with some longer loops connecting the β-strands. This flexibility and the longer loops contribute to the mechanism of antigen binding, thus defining the capability of antibodies to recognize diverse antigens.

THE ANTIGEN-BINDING SITE

The antigen binding site is principally defined by the Complementarity-Determining Regions (CDRs). These regions were originally identified by amino acid sequence variability analysis (Wu and Kabat, 1970; Kabat and Wu, 1971) as highly variable regions within the V-domains. The CDRs were defined prior to our knowledge of the mechanisms by which antibodies are generated and predated the three-dimensional structure solution of antibodies. Once the first Fab structures were solved, it was realized that the CDRs approximately correspond to loops that vary in structure, called hypervariable loops (HVLs). Each V-domain contributes three CDRs to the antigen-binding site: CDR-L1, CDR-L2, and CDR-L3 from the V_L and CDR-H1,

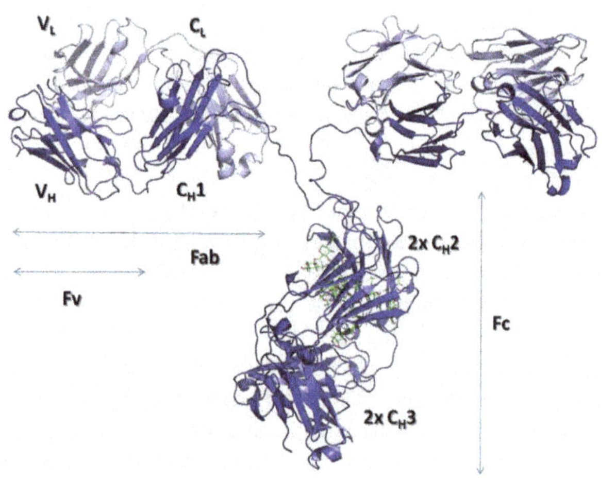

FIGURE 1 | Ribbon representation of an intact IgG molecule (PDBID: 1IGT). The heavy chains are shown in dark blue, while the Light chains are colored in light blue. The carbohydrate moieties attached to the C_H2 domains are represented with sticks. The figure was produced using PyMol (DeLano, 2002. *The PyMOL molecular graphics system.* Delano Scientific, San Carlos, CA).

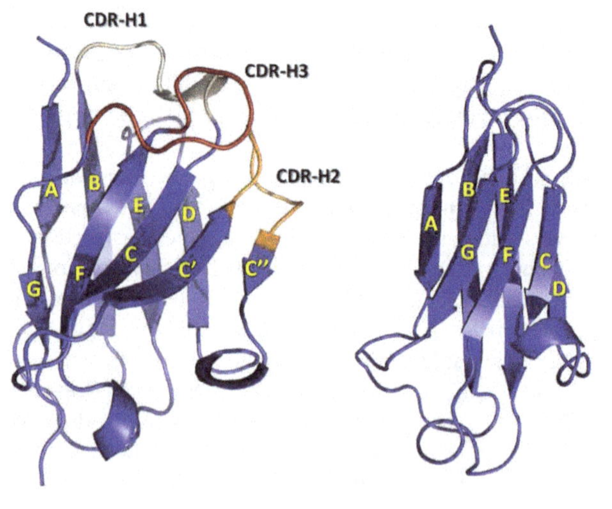

FIGURE 2 | Ribbon representation of a V_H (left) domain and a C_H1 (right) domain. CDRs are colored in yellow (CDR-1), orange (CDR-2), and red (CDR-3). Note the insertion in the V_H domain with respect to the C_H1 domain of two β-strands, C' and C'', and the loop linking them, which contains the CDR-H2. The coordinates used to produce the Figure were the same as in **Figure 1**. The figure was generated with PyMol.

CDR-H2, and CDR-H3 from the V_H. The three CDRs from V_H and the three from V_L are brought together by non-covalent association of the V-domains at the N-terminal region of the Fv (**Figure 3**). The remaining portion of the V-domain, i.e., the two β-sheets and non-HVLs, generally provide structural support to the antigen-binding site, rather than making contact with antigen and are thus referred to as framework regions (FRs). However, the sequence variability observed in the FRs is not irrelevant to functional binding diversity, as it can directly affect CDR loop conformation and the orientation of V_H–V_L pairing (Foote and Winter, 1992; Abhinandan and Martin, 2010).

Given the essential variability of the antigen-binding site, which must be capable of recognizing a large array of diverse antigens to fulfill its remit, it was initially thought that each antibody possesses a unique conformation at the antigen-binding site. Nevertheless, analysis (Chothia and Lesk, 1987; Chothia et al., 1989) in the late 1980s of a small set of structures of immunoglobulin fragments available at the time revealed that, although the HVLs vary in sequence, five out of the six HVLs (CDR-L1, CDR-L2, CDR-L3, CDR-H1, and CDR-H2) had a limited set of main-chain conformations or "canonical structures." The canonical structure model implied a paradigm shift in the field, replacing the notion that each antibody has unique HVL conformations and thus overall unique antigen-binding site structure. The limited set of canonical structures helped to develop 3D modeling structure strategies (Martin and Thornton, 1996) and suggested that structural constraints are at work in antigen recognition.

A canonical structure is defined by the HVL length and conserved residues located in the HVL and FR (Chothia and Lesk, 1987). Overall, the structural repertoire generated by λ-type chains is broader than that of κ-type chains (Chailyan et al., 2011). In the latter, all the canonical structures at CDR-L1 follow a similar pattern, which consists of an extended conformation between residues 26 and 29 [Chothia's numbering; (Al-Lazikani et al., 1997)], and hairpin loops of different lengths encompassing residues 30–32, with up to seven insertions in this segment of the loop. The CDR-L2 adopts a single conformation. Most (~70%) of the CDR-L3 loops have a single canonical structure. In contrast, the CDR-L1 of λ-type chains adopts a helical structure with up to eight conformations and an average root mean square deviation (RMSD) between loops of 2.3 Å (Chailyan et al., 2011). The λ-type CDR-L2 usually adopts a similar hairpin loop conformation to that of κ-type, but can in some instances have an insertion of four residues, which leads to another canonical structure. The CDR-L3 in λ-type antibodies has a broader variety of lengths and conformations than κ-type antibodies, with only a small fraction of the loops following a defined canonical structure (Chailyan et al., 2011).

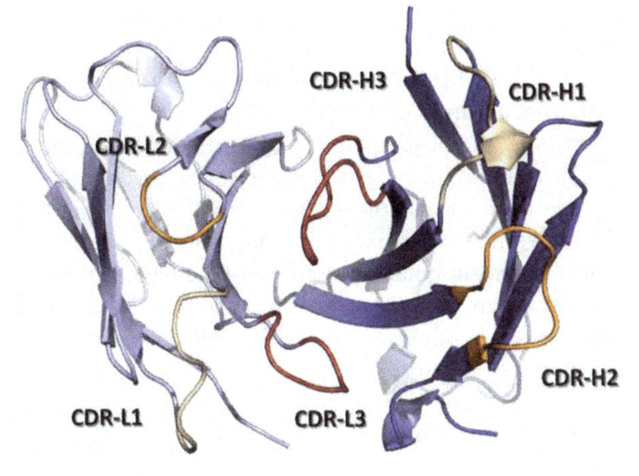

FIGURE 3 | Ribbon representation of a Fv fragment seen from the antigen perspective. V_H is colored in dark blue, while V_L is colored in light blue. CDRs are colored in yellow (CDR-1), orange (CDR-2), and red (CDR-3). The coordinates used to produce the Figure are the same as in **Figure 1**. The Figure was generated with PyMol.

The CDR-H1, similar to the CDR-L1, has an extended conformation linking β-strands from the two β-sheets that form the Ig fold. However, it is less diverse than its counterpart in V_L, with three canonical structures and a strong bias (~85%) (Ragunathan et al., 2012) toward the shortest loop (seven residues). The repertoire of canonical structures of CDR-H2 is less skewed than that for CDR-L3 and CDR-H1, with six canonical structures. Still, 59–70% of the antibodies (Ragunathan et al., 2012) have a six-residue canonical structure.

Recently, the application of clustering algorithms (North et al., 2011) on 300 non-redundant antibody structures has further stratified the canonical structure combinations by identifying 28 HVL combinations of lengths for the loops with canonical structures, whereas, previous analysis (Al-Lazikani et al., 1997) covered only 20. Only four of these clusters had more than one conformation, of which two could be distinguished by gene source (mouse/human; κ/λ) and one could be distinguished solely by the presence and position of Proresidues in the CDR-L3. Of the 28 CDR-lengths, 15 have multiple conformational clusters, including 10 for which previous analysis had only one canonical structure combination.

The CDR-H3, localized at the center of the antigen-binding site, is by far the most variable loop in length and sequence of the CDRs (Chothia and Lesk, 1987; Wu et al., 1993; Zemlin et al., 2003). The diversity of the CDR-H3 comes from the recombination of three germline genes: IGHV, IGHD, and IGHJ (Tonegawa, 1983), imprecise recombination of these genes, i.e., junctional diversity (Alt and Baltimore, 1982), the possibility of using three reading frames for translation of the IGHD gene (Sanz, 1991), and further diversification during somatic hypermutation process (see below).

Human CDR-H3 loops have an average length of 15.2 (±4.1) residues (IMGT CDR definition) (Zemlin et al., 2003), with a range of lengths between 1–35 residues, and a length distribution resembling a Gaussian process. While extensive analysis of antibody structures has identified sequence patterns to predict the conformation of the residues at the base of the CDR-H3 (Shirai et al., 1996; Morea et al., 1998), the enormous variability in amino acid sequence and length of this loop, as well as its flexibility, has precluded delineation of rules for predicting its overall conformation. Thus, structural modeling of CDR-H3 is still challenging (Almagro et al., 2011), using either comparative methods that rely on templates chosen based on sequence homology, or knowledge-based methods such as the canonical structure model.

STRUCTURE-FUNCTION RELATIONSHIPS AT THE ANTIGEN-BINDING SITE

Since antibodies have a small subset of canonical structures in five of the six loops that define the antigen-binding site, it is reasonable to hypothesize that only a limited subset of antigen-binding site geometries exists, and the arising questions are whether the general architecture of the antigen-binding site can be predicted and whether it correlates with antigen recognition (Vargas-Madrazo et al., 1995). Finding structure-function correlations at the antigen-biding site holds the promise of providing insights into the mechanism of the molecular recognition process used by antibodies to bind diverse antigens and thereby to assist the rational design of antibodies of desired specificity.

Initial work (Vargas-Madrazo et al., 1995) showed that from a total of 300 possible canonical structure combinations described at that time, only 10 exist in 90% of the sequences analyzed. The existing canonical structure combinations were classified in two sets: one with preference for some specific types of antigens like proteins, peptides or haptens, and other with multi-specific binding capabilities. In the specific classes, the length of CDR-H2 and CDR-L1 was found to correlate with the type of antigen, whereas, in the multi-specific classes, such a correlation could not be established. A recent study (Ragunathan et al., 2012) of 140 unique antigen-antibody complexes has corroborated that most of the anti-protein antibodies have canonical structures determined by short CDR-L1 loops (6–8 residues). This is in contrast to anti-peptide and anti-hapten antibodies, which predominantly have canonical structures made of long CDR-L1 loops (11–13 residues). The remaining loops show little difference in the canonical structure distribution across anti-protein, anti-peptide, and anti-hapten antibodies.

Figure 4 overlays 99 unique mid to high resolution (≤3.0 Å) antibody structures, including 30 in complex with proteins, 34 with peptides, and 35 with haptens. As can be seen, the topography of the antigen-binding site tends to determine the size of the antigen with which the antibody interacts. Anti-protein antibodies tend to have flatter binding sites than anti-peptide antibodies. The antigen-binding of anti-peptide antibodies is grooved, mainly determined by the long CDR-L1, which accommodates the peptides at the center of the antigen-binding site. Anti-hapten antibodies have a smaller antigen-biding site with contacts with haptens being buried deeper in the V_H:V_L interface where proteins and peptides cannot reach.

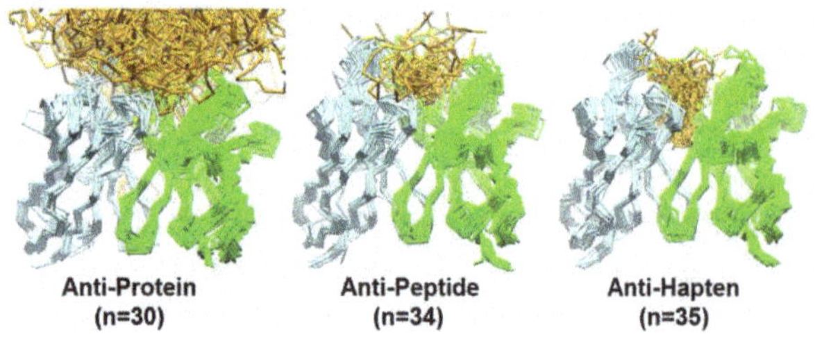

FIGURE 4 | Trace representation of 99 unique mid to high resolution (= 3.0 Å) Fv structures, including 30 in complex with proteins, 34 with peptides, and 35 with haptens. V_H colored in dark blue. V_L colored in light blue. Ligands are colored in orange. The coordinates used to generate the Figure are listed in Ragunathan et al. (2012). The structures were superposed in Discovery Studio using the FR Cα atoms.

In non-specific classes, the CDR-H3 plays a predominant role in defining the topography of the binding site (Vargas-Madrazo et al., 1995). Short CDR-H3 loops can create a cavity in the antigen-binding site to accommodate peptides. Long CDR-H3 loops are found in antibodies associated with chronic viral infections, in contrast to antibodies from acute viral infections, which have relatively short CDR-H3 loops (Breden et al., 2011). Long and extended CDR-H3 loops can generate a definite type of structure, called finger-like topography (Saphire et al., 2001), which differ from the typical flat anti-protein binding-site. This finger-like topography allows antibodies to access recessed epitopes in the viral proteins.

The number of residues in contact with antigens also differs in antibodies recognizing proteins, peptides and haptens (MacCallum et al., 1996; Almagro, 2004; Ragunathan et al., 2012). The average number of contact residues in V_L for the anti-protein, anti-peptide, and anti-hapten antibodies is 9, 9, and 7, respectively (Ragunathan et al., 2012). The corresponding values for V_H are 14, 12, and 10. A more detailed analysis of the solvent accessible surface (SAS) that is buried upon antigen binding and the location and frequency of contacts (called specificity-determining residues usage, SDRUs) of antibodies in complex with proteins, peptides or haptens also show distinctive patterns (Almagro, 2004). Anti-protein antibodies have an average (±SD) SAS value of 737 (±272) $Å^2$ with hotspots of SDRUs located at the edge of the antigen-binding site (Ragunathan et al., 2012). Anti-hapten antibodies have a roughly 2-fold smaller SAS value of 374 (±117) $Å^2$ with hotspots of SDRUs placed in the interior of the antigen-binding site or even buried in the V_L:V_H interface. Anti-peptide antibodies have a SAS value of 544 (±158) $Å^2$, which is in between anti-protein and anti-hapten antibodies. The SDRU hotspots of anti-peptide antibodies are located in the interior of the antigen-binding site but not buried in the V_L:V_H interface as with anti-hapten antibodies.

Combining the SDRU patterns with the distinctive shape of the antigen-binding site of antibodies recognizing different types of antigens lead to the conclusion that anti-protein antibodies tend to have flatter and larger binding sites than anti-peptide and anti-hapten antibodies. The antigen-binding of anti-peptides is grooved, whereas, anti-hapten antibodies have a smaller and deeper antigen-biding site, with SDRU hotspots buried in the V_H:V_L interface (**Figure 5**).

Since SDRUs are a measure of the likelihood of establishing contacts with the antigen, they can provide a definition of the antigen-binding site in absence of the antigen-antibody complex structure. A definition of the antigen-binding site based on SDRUs could thus guide the selection of residues to transfer the specificity from a given antibody into a different scaffold, either to produce a molecule with enhanced biophysical profile such as increased stability (Ewert et al.,

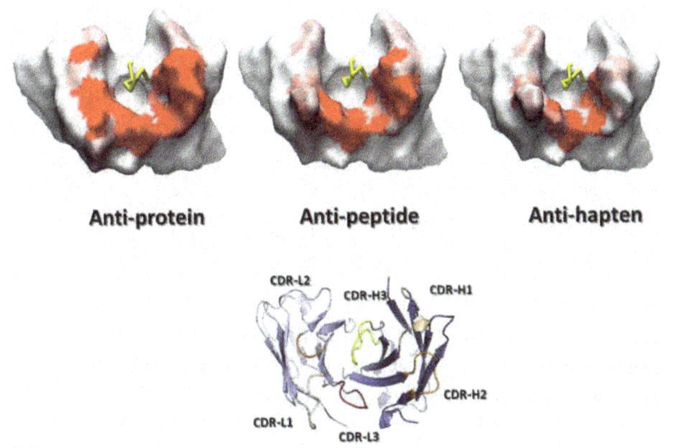

FIGURE 5 | Connolly (1983) surfaces of representative anti-protein, anti-peptide and anti-hapten Fvs, shown from the antigen perspective. A gradient from red (contact) to white (no contact) represents the SDRUs of antibodies recognizing generic ligands. The surfaces were generated by running a 7.0-Å radius probe over the Fv after removing the CDR-H3 loop (yellow ribbon) to better represent the surface common to all antibodies. Note the variation in size of the surface from anti-protein, a large surface, to anti-hapten antibodies, a small one. On the bottom, a ribbon representation of a Fv in the same orientation as the Fvs displaying the Connolly surface to indicate the position of the CDRs. Also note the protruding CDR-L1 in the anti-peptide and anti-hapten Fvs, which modulates the topography of the antigen-binding site. The ribbon figure was generated with PyMol, while the Connolly surface figures were produced using Discovery Studio.

2004) and/or to humanize a nonhuman antibody (Almagro and Fransson, 2008). Importantly, protocols using SDRUs can tailor humanization of antibodies recognizing different types of ligands, thereby minimizing the region of the non-human antibody grafted into the human context and hence potential immunogenicity.

Not all amino acids are equally used to contact antigens and the types of antibody residues involved in contacts with proteins, peptides, and haptens also differ. Tyrosine (Y), arginine (R), asparagine (N), aspartic acid (D), histidine (H), serine (S), and threonine (T) make more contacts than other amino acids in all the three antigen types. Of particular interest is Y, which has been found in a high proportion in the antigen-binding site of antibodies. For instance, Lo Conte et al. (1999) observed that Y contributed to 16.6% of all amino acids in contact in the 19 antigen-antibody complexes available at that time. Similarly, an earlier report by Mian et al. (1991) based on the analysis of only six antibody–antigen complexes reported the overuse of Y to contact antigens. Cysteine (C), proline (P), glutamine (Q), glutamic acid (E) and hydrophobic amino acids such as alanine (A), valine (V), isoleucine (I), leucine (L), methionine (M) and phenylalanine (F) make significantly fewer contacts. Thus, hydrophilic amino acids predominate over hydrophobic ones. In the CDR-L1, N, and D are the most frequent residues in contacts. R is rare and tryptophan (W) does not occur. CDR-L2 has less diversity than CDR-L1 and CDR-L3, and in the latter, most contacts involve amino acids S, T, W, and Y, whereas, R, N, G, and H make fewer contacts.

A detailed analysis of the contribution of each amino acid called Specificity-Determining Residues Matrix (SDRM) to each SDRU depending upon the type of antigen the antibody interacts with have been described by Ragunathan et al. (2012). Briefly, there are more D and T contacts in anti-protein antibodies in CDR-L1 than anti-peptide and anti-hapten antibodies. In CDR-L3, anti-protein antibodies have more R and W contacts, whereas, anti-hapten antibodies have more Q, G, and H contacts. Similar to V_L, S, T, and Y dominate the contacts for V_H. Likewise, C, P, Q, D and hydrophobic amino acids are significantly underrepresented at contact residues. Interestingly, V_H has more contacts involving negatively charged amino acids and fewer K residues in comparison to V_L. In CDR-H1, N, G, S, T, and Y predominant in contact sites for all antibodies. In addition, D occurs frequently in anti-protein and anti-peptide antibodies. The detailed picture of the contribution of each amino acid (SDRM) to each SDRU depending upon the type of antigen the antibody interacts with has practical applications to design antibody repertoires.

THE ANTIBODY REPERTOIRE IN HUMANS AND IMMUNIZATION OF HOST SPECIES

In addition to the structural studies outlined above, antibody repertoire analyses and comparative immunogenetics have been highly informative approaches to understanding how antibodies evolved to recognize diverse antigen structures. Indeed, the lessons learned from such studies have been critical factors in the progress of antibody engineering. For example, a profound understanding of the biases inherent in the functional repertoire of human antibodies, in comparison to those of other species (Schroeder et al., 1995; Zemlin et al., 2003; Schroeder, 2006) inspired experimental work to define the critical biochemical characteristics required to form a functional synthetic antibody repertoire (Fellouse et al., 2006; Birtalan et al., 2008, 2010). To further illustrate the important influence these studies, below we outline what has been learned about the human antibody repertoire and several other species of interest in antibody discovery and highlight how this knowledge is impacting the antibody engineering field.

THE HUMAN ANTIBODY REPERTOIRE

The primary repertoire of antibodies is produced via the combinatorial rearrangement of IG (H, K, or L)V with IGHD (only in V_H) and IG (H, K, or L)J germline genes, followed by pairing of V_H and V_L domains (Tonegawa, 1983). This repertoire should be diverse and versatile enough to recognize any antigen with a low or medium affinity during the primary immune response (Neuberger and Milstein, 1995). The physical maps of the human IGH and IGL gene loci were elucidated in the 1990s (Tomlinson et al., 1992; Schäble et al., 1994; Matsuda et al., 1998) and the information has been compiled and annotated at The ImmunoGenetics Database (IMGT; http://www.imgt.org/). This information has provided the foundations to understand the mechanisms of generation of diversity in human antibodies and has shed light on the evolution of the antibody repertoire.

Overall, the human IGK locus contains approximately 30 functional IGKV genes distributed in six families, and five IGKJ segments which recombine to form the primary Vκ repertoire. There are 30–36 functional IGLV genes arranged in three distinct clusters containing 11 IGLV gene families and four functional Cλ domains, each with its own IGLJ gene. The IGH locus contains approximately 39 functional IGHV genes distributed in seven IGHV gene families, approximately 30 IGHD segments classified also in seven families and six IGHJ genes. As more human germline genes from diverse individuals have been sequenced and studied, an increasing number of alleles have been compiled at IMGT (Lefranc et al., 2005).

Analysis of the antibody genes amplified from diverse sources (Cox et al., 1994; Huang et al., 1996; Ignatovich et al., 1997; Brezinschek et al., 1998; de Wildt et al., 1999; Farner et al., 1999; Glanville et al., 2009) indicates a strong bias in gene usage. For instance, only five IGHV genes (5–51, 1–69, 1–2, 4–59/61, and 3–30/33) make 50% of the rearranged antibodies and only 24 out of 39 functional genes (~60%) are expressed with a frequency above 1% (Glanville et al., 2009). For IGVK the bias is more dramatic. Only three IGVK genes (3–20, 1–39, and 3–15) make 50% of the rearranged antibody repertoire and only 16 out of 30 genes are expressed with a frequency of more than 1%. Pairing of heavy and light chains in B cells (de Wildt et al., 1999) and in recombinant libraries (Glanville et al., 2009) appears to be a random process, reflecting the relative abundance of the IGHV and IGLV gene family members. The bias in the gene usage is due to a number of factors including position in the locus, ontogenetic regulation of the immune response, gene copy and binding properties of the antibodies encoded by certain genes (Dal-Bo et al., 2011; Lerner, 2011; Zhu et al., 2011).

After antibody exposure to antigen, an affinity maturation process generates diversity from which antibodies with higher affinity are selected, as the antigen concentration decreases during the secondary immune response. Affinity maturation mechanisms include somatic hypermutation (in most mammalian systems) and gene conversion (in certain species, see below). The somatic hypermutation process takes place in the germinal centers with the help of T-cells. The V-genes in activated B cells undergo activation-induced (cytidine) deaminase (AID)-catalyzed somatic hypermutation at a rate of up to 10^{-3} changes per base pair per cell cycle (Rajewsky et al., 1987). Two separate mechanisms are involved in the mutation process (Maizels, 2005); one targets mutation hotspots with the RGYW (R = purine, Y = pyrimidine, W = A or T) motif (Dörner et al., 1998) which includes the reverse complement of the preferential substrate site for AID, while the second incorporates an error-prone DNA synthesis that can lead to a nucleotide mismatch between the original template and the mutated DNA strand (Rada et al., 1998). The overall process favors single-base transitions over transversions at a 3:1 ratio (Betz et al., 1993).

The frequency of mutations in V_H and V_L are qualitatively similar, following an exponential distribution with as much as 15–20% of the V-regions showing no mutations at the amino acid level (Tomlinson et al., 1996; Ramirez-Benitez and Almagro, 2001). The average number of mutations per V-region has been estimated for humans and mice to be around 8 and 5 mutations for V_H and V_L, respectively (Tomlinson et al., 1996; Ramirez-Benitez and Almagro, 2001; Clark et al., 2006). Although the mutations are spread throughout the V-domains, they occur at a proportion of 3:2:1 mutations at the antigen-binding site, surface of the V-domains and V_L:V_H interface, and core of the V-domain, respectively (Clark et al., 2006). The relatively high proportion of mutations in the CDRs with respect to FRs is explained in part by a higher concentration of mutation hotspots in the former. It also reflects the selection for affinity improvement, although it has been found that somatic mutations in residues in direct contact with antigen are less frequent than in residues adjacent to the residues in contact (Ramirez-Benitez and Almagro, 2001), suggesting that the residues selected during the primary immune response do not change during the affinity maturation. Insertions and deletions also occur but at a lower rate (Wilson et al., 1998; Zhao and Lu, 2010), implying that the overall geometry of the antigen-binding site as defined by the canonical structures does not change significantly during the affinity maturation process either.

The amino acid content and length distribution of the CDR-H3 region is of critical importance to antibody repertoire function and the diversity encoded in this loop in humans has been extensively characterized to aid synthetic mimicry of human diversity (Schroeder et al., 1987; Zemlin et al., 2003; Schroeder, 2006; Glanville et al., 2009). These studies have shown very clearly that the human CDR-H3 repertoire is distinctly different from that of the mouse, particularly in length distribution. The human loops tend to be significantly longer, at 15.2 (±4.1) residues, while mice average at only 11.5 (±2.7) (Zemlin et al., 2003). Both species exhibit common conserved motifs at the stem of the loop, but the biases in amino acids used overall and, indeed, in a positional sense, show distinct differences. While humans and mice both show a strong preference for the use of Y, S, and G residues, this phenomenon is much more pronounced in mice (26% Y), than humans (14% Y) and in both species this trend toward high Y use increases proportionally with loop length. In humans in particular, longer CDR-H3 loops are associated with increased use of the IGHJ-6 segment, which encodes a series of contiguous Y residues, increasing the frequency of Y content overall (Prassler et al., 2011; Zhai et al., 2011). In addition, humans use more P and do not exhibit the clear hallmarks of hydrogen bond ladder formation in the loop as often as mice, suggesting more complex overall loop topology in humans. This phenomenon may be directly correlated with increased length in human CDR-H3, with an associated higher use of cysteine via germline-encoded "D2" DH sequences. These long D-segments encode for cysteine residues spaced four amino acids apart, allowing disulphide loop formation that can be critical to CDR secondary structure and rigidity (Almagro et al., 2012). While these disulphide-stabilized loops are relatively rare in humans (C = 1.21% of all amino acid use in human CDR-H3), (Zemlin et al., 2003) they are a commonly used motif in the antibodies of both chickens and camelids, as outlined later.

HARNESSING NON-HUMAN ANTIBODY V-GENE REPERTOIRES

Species such as mouse, chicken and camelids (such as llama) are all used as immune sources of antibodies with therapeutic potential. While antibodies from human libraries theoretically contain "fully human" amino acid sequence in their FRs, antibodies from immune animal repertoires do not. Nonhuman-derived antibodies may initially have their immunogenicity reduced by cloning the V-genes onto a set of human C regions, to form a "chimeric" antibody (Morrison et al., 1984). Even the small amount of "foreign" amino acid content with respect to humans in the V-domain FRs of a chimeric IgG may be enough to provoke an anti-idiotypic antibody response, however, especially patients that receive repeated doses of antibody as therapy (Stephens et al., 1995). As a result, before clinical use, antibodies derived from animals usually undergo a process of "humanization," whereby recombinant DNA technology is used to "graft" the CDRs of the clone of interest onto human V-gene framework scaffolds (Jones et al., 1986). It is typically necessary to carry out subsequent V-gene engineering, e.g., via "back mutations" in the FRs, to return the target binding affinity of the parental clone (Almagro and Fransson, 2008). For this humanization process to be efficient, it is helpful not only to be able to predict which human FRs might be optimal to accept the grafted CDRs from a lead clone, but also to understand the nuances of the structural characteristics of the repertoire from which the clone was derived. Armed with sufficient prior knowledge of each species' repertoires, we can confidently predict the likely engineering path that will be required to derive a fully active, but maximally humanized product.

THE MOUSE ANTIBODY REPERTOIRE

The mouse (*Mus muscullus*) is the most widely used model organism in immunology and perhaps in biology and medicine. For the study of antibodies, the development of hybridoma technology, first described by Köhler and Milstein (1975) and awarded the Nobel Prize in 1984, was the key advancement that ultimately led to development of antibody-based drugs. Hybridoma technology involves the immunization of rodents with an antigen of interest and once a satisfactory immune response against the antigen has been obtained, the antibody-producing B cells are harvested and fused to a murine myeloma cell line. The resulting hybrid cells can be sub-cloned to generate clonal cell lines in which every cell secretes antibodies with a single specificity. Thus, hybridoma technology became an efficient means to produce unlimited amounts of single-specificity antibodies which enabled the biochemical and structural characterization of antibodies and the production of sufficient quantities of high quality protein for therapeutic settings.

The physical maps of the mouse IGH and IGL gene loci were elucidated in the second half of the 1990s (Tomlinson et al., 1992; Schäble et al., 1994, 1999; Matsuda et al., 1998; Thiebe et al., 1999) and, as for humans, the information is compiled and annotated at IMGT (http://www.imgt.org/). The total number of mouse (*M. musculus)* IGK genes per haploid genome is 164 (174 if the orphons are included), of which 99 are functional, belonging to 18 subgroups (Martinez-Jean et al., 2001). Eighty-one are in opposite orientation of transcription, 59 of them are functional and must rearrange by a mechanism of inversion. These genes are recombined with five IGKJ genes. The IGL locus contains only three IGLV genes each with one associated IGLJ gene. The reduced contribution of the IGL locus to the mouse germline repertoire is consistent with the approximately 8-fold reduction in the prevalence of lambda-bearing IgG in the serum of mice compared to humans.

The IGH locus is both larger and more diverse than that of the humans (Schroeder, 2006). IMGT reported as of August 2012 two tables for the mouse IGVH germline gene repertoire. One with IGHV genes compiled from diverse sources, which represent genes characterized in several strains and thus some genes may be alleles. The other table compiles data from the C57BL/6 Mouse Genome Sequencing and is provisional since not all the genes have been mapped and confirmed. It lists 170 IGVH germline genes distributed in 15 IGHV gene families. One hundred one out of the one hundred seventy known genes (~60%) are functional genes. These IGHV genes recombine with 21 functional IGDH genes assorted in four families and four IGHJ functional genes.

Interestingly enough, comparisons of the canonical structure repertoire encoded in mouse and humans IGHV genes (Almagro et al., 1997; Bono et al., 2004) indicate that the human structural repertoire has two additional classes (1–1 and 1–3). Thus, the human repertoire is more diverse in structural terms than that of mouse. In addition, the canonical structure class 1–2 is more prevalent in mouse (~60%), while in humans the dominant class is 1–3 (~40%) (Almagro et al., 1997). This divergence, together with phylogenetic analysis of the human and mouse IGHV genes (Bono et al., 2004), indicates that most of the sequences in the human and mouse IGHV loci have arisen subsequent to the divergence of the two organisms from their common ancestor. Identifying these differences between human and mouse genes, which are perhaps a reflection of functional and/or structural constraints at work to balance the free diversification of the antibody repertoire in humans and mice (Almagro et al., 1997), could be useful to select the most human-like genes for humanization of mouse antibodies.

THE CHICKEN REPERTOIRE

Gallus gallus, the domestic chicken, is a classic model for immunological study. Indeed, "B-cell" derives from the term "Bursal cell," as B-cells were first recognized as products of the Bursa of Fabricius, a cloaca-associated organ that is critical to immune development in birds (Ratcliffe, 2006). The antibody repertoire of chickens has also been extensively characterized in functional isotype content and at the genomic level (Reynaud et al., 1985, 1989; Ratcliffe, 2006). Their immunoglobulin system is distinct from that of humans and mice as they have structural equivalents of mammalian IgM, IgA, and IgG, but not IgE or IgD. IgM is the major isotype expressed on the surface of their B-cells (Ratcliffe, 2006). Additionally, all chicken antibodies use λ isotype light chains, exclusively (Reynaud et al., 1987). Chicken IgG has 4 Cγ domains, however, and is thought to be a structural relative of both mammalian IgG and IgE subclasses (Parvari et al., 1988). Chicken IgG is also found in a "short" form, lacking the CH3 and CH4 regions. Avian IgG is often described as "IgY" as it can be found at high concentration in egg yolk, but it has been proposed that the full-length form should be called IgG and the short form IgY, to aid their differentiation (Ratcliffe, 2006).

The avian V-gene germline repertoire is extremely simple, with single functional V-genes in both the light and heavy chains, that contain unique V_L-J_L and V_H-D-J_H segments (Reynaud et al., 1989, 1991; Parvari et al., 1990). The chicken V_L and V_H germline domains are highly homologous to stable and soluble human V_λ and V_H3 families (Ewert et al., 2002, 2003), respectively, and this is maintained across the fully mature repertoire (Wu et al., 2011). The uniformity of chicken V-gene FW sequences renders them highly predictable in humanization (Tsurushita et al., 2004; Nishibori et al., 2006). Despite this simple V-gene system (Reynaud et al., 1983; Parvari et al., 1987a,b, 1988; Ratcliffe, 2006), chickens have a broadly adaptable repertoire that generates high affinity antibodies to protein, peptide and hapten antigens (Yamanaka et al., 1996; Finlay et al., 2005, 2006; Nishibori et al., 2006).

The chicken V-gene system is in stark contrast to that found in humans, mice and primates, which all utilize a large set of V-gene sequences that are highly diverse in both sequence and structure (Schroeder et al., 1990; Schroeder, 2006). In chickens, as in rabbits (Weill and Reynaud, 1992), a distinctly different set of diversification mechanisms are used, including gene conversion (Reynaud et al., 1987, 1989). Gene conversion relies on a single template V-gene being diversified via the incorporation of segments from upstream pseudogenes that lack recombination signal sequences. This process is used to diversify both the heavy and light chains, with mutations being introduced into both CDRs and FRs. For the process to be efficient, it relies on high sequence homology between the pseudogene and the germline gene which acts as the acceptor (Ratcliffe, 2006). A recent chicken V_H repertoire analysis suggests the requirement for sequence homology between germline and pseudogene leads to a low level of mutagenesis in the FWs, but hypervariability in the CDRs (Wu et al., 2011). Interestingly, this was coupled with strong maintenance of common CDR structural residues that have also been observed in mammals (Rader et al., 2000; Zemlin et al., 2003; Lee et al., 2004), but modulation of residues that affect V_H–V_L interaction (Padlan, 1994) and CDR structure (Foote and Winter, 1992). The chicken V_H repertoire therefore adds significant variability at select FW positions to increase structural diversity, e.g., by changing the angle of interaction between the V_H and V_L domains (Abhinandan and Martin, 2010).

The CDR-H3 repertoire of chickens differs distinctly from that of humans and mice, in both length distribution and amino acid content. Surprisingly, chickens have only 15 functional D-segments, all of which are highly homologous and some (e.g., D9/12/13, plus D4/8/11) are even identical in amino acid sequence (Reynaud et al., 1991). Additionally, reading frame 1 predominates in chickens (Raaphorst et al., 1997), as reading frames 2 and 3 create sequences containing stretches of hydrophobic residues and stop codons, respectively (Reynaud et al., 1991; Weill and Reynaud, 1992). This form of reading frame control appears to be universal and has also been observed (albeit in different reading frames) for; rabbits, sharks, mice, primates, and humans (Raaphorst et al., 1997; Schroeder et al., 1998; Schroeder, 2006). In reading frame 1, chicken D-segments are biased toward the use of G, S, and Y, as observed in all other vertebrate species studied to date (Zemlin et al., 2003; Schroeder, 2006). In contrast to humans and mice however, chicken D-segments obligately contain C, with the consensus sequence G-S- (A/G)-Y-C- (G/C)- (S/W)-X-A- (Y/E) (X = non-conserved) (Reynaud et al., 1991). This limited initial V_H CDR3 repertoire is hyper-diversified both by somatic mutation and the insertion of new sequences via gene conversion. These D-like sequences are donated by pseudogenes and may replace the entire D-segment or only a small section, leading to the creation of "mosaic CDRs" (Reynaud et al., 1989, 1991).

Analyses of CDR-H3 amino acid content in the chicken shows very different paratope chemical composition in comparison to humans and mice (Wu et al., 2011). There is a distinct bias toward small amino acids G/S/A/C/T (but not P), while large aromatic and hydrophobic residues are strongly disfavored, including an unusually low representation of Y, the dominant residue in the repertoires of mice and humans (Zemlin et al., 2003). This observation may be important, as synthetic antibody repertoire studies have suggested that Y is a critical amino acid for target binding (Fellouse et al., 2004, 2005, 2006, 2007). Additionally, the chicken CDR3 repertoire has low representation of positively charged residues (K/R). This may be of practical importance, as excess positive charge in the V_H CDR3 is associated with polyreactivity (Li et al., 2001) and poor pK profile *in vivo* (Boswell et al., 2010).

The use of C in the CDR-H3 of >50% of all B-cell clones in the chicken repertoire is suggestive that it plays an important functional role. While humans and rhesus make functional CDR-H3 sequences containing a pair of cysteines (Zemlin et al., 2003; Schroeder, 2006), these are found at low frequency in mature human B-cells, and they are very rare in mice (Raaphorst et al., 1997; Zemlin et al., 2003). The high incorporation rate of C in the chicken CDR-H3 is rendered functional by two mechanisms: (1) frequent use of D-D junctions (Reynaud et al., 1991) to create CDR3s with intra-CDR disulphide bridges and (2) insertion of single C residues in the V_H CDRs 1 and 2 for inter-CDR disulphide bonding. These covalent bonds between CDRs are structurally analogous to those observed at high frequency in the immunoglobulins of other species such as camelids (Harmsen et al., 2000), sharks (Dooley et al., 2003; Stanfield et al., 2004), cows (Aitken et al., 1997; Sinclair et al., 1997; O'Brien et al., 1999), pigs (Li and Aitken, 2004), and even the duckbilled platypus (Johansson et al., 2002). It seems likely that the increased use of disulphide binding in long CDRs, by several species, may be highly beneficial to stabilize longer loops that have greater sequence diversity, but could suffer from a lack of structural rigidity that leads to an entropic penalty during binding interactions (Wong et al., 2011; Hackel et al., 2010). Mutagenesis studies have shown that these disulphides, in either IgG or single-domain antibodies, are essential for both V-domain stability and binding function (Lee et al., 2006; Fennell et al., 2010; Govaert et al., 2012).

BEYOND STANDARD IGG STRUCTURES—NATURAL 'DOMAIN ANTIBODIES'

Despite being the main format for many successful therapeutics, IgG molecules have some practical limitations as they are large (~150 kDa), covalently-linked tetrameric structures that classically contain two antigen-binding sites. The necessity for two V-regions to combine and stabilize each other makes it technically challenging to reduce antibodies to anything smaller than the dual-domain single chain Fv (scFv) antibody fragment (~30 kDa). The desire for smaller, more stable and monomeric binding modalities in appropriate indications has led to the investigation of a logical alternative; modular therapeutics built from naturally-occurring binding proteins that can be used as a source of "domain antibodies." As outlined below, comparative immunogenetics led to the discovery of non-classical immune proteins such as the camelid VHH and the shark V_{NAR} (variable domain of the IgNAR), which can both be isolated as soluble, stable, monomeric V-domains (**Figure 6**) (Flajnik and Dooley, 2009; Wesolowski et al., 2009; Flajnik et al., 2011). These single domain proteins are only ~12–15 kDa in size and have been the subject of significant academic and industrial research to characterize their origins and utilities (Muyldermans et al., 2009; Flajnik et al., 2011). Humanization of VHH antibodies is facile, as the isolated antibodies are typically close to a human VH germline sequence. Together with high stability and low aggregation, this gives the humanized VHH antibody theoretically low immunogenicity risk. To date, the less heavily investigated IgNAR has not been extensively characterized in humanization studies and may represent a different challenge from VHH. The VNAR domain is actually more structurally related to a T-cell receptor α-domain and has much lower a.a. identity to human homologous domains. As a result, in this section we concentrate on the more experimentally advanced VHH.

Domain antibodies, lacking an Fc region, suffer from fast renal clearance and without protein engineering they have short *in vivo* half-lives. Luckily, the stable, soluble nature of isolated domain antibodies renders then relatively simple to engineer in a modular fashion. Modifications at the N- or C-terminus are typically possible without loss of function, allowing fusion to common half-life extension molecules such as serum albumin or immunoglobulin Fc and covalent conjugation to natural or non-natural polymers that expand the hydrodynamic radius of the proteins, greatly reducing renal clearance. Domain antibodies have also been extensively exploited as modular units to create bispecific molecules for targeting multiple disease mediators with a single polypeptide (Gill and Damle, 2006; Harmsen and De Haard, 2007). A final exciting avenue open to domain antibodies is the possibility of oral administration, e.g., via strains of *Lactobacillus* expressing a TNF-specific VHH antibody, which was efficacious in a murine gut inflammation model (Vandenbroucke et al., 2010). In the following sections we outline the current state of knowledge surrounding these molecules and the influence that combined repertoire and structural analyses have had on their understanding and application.

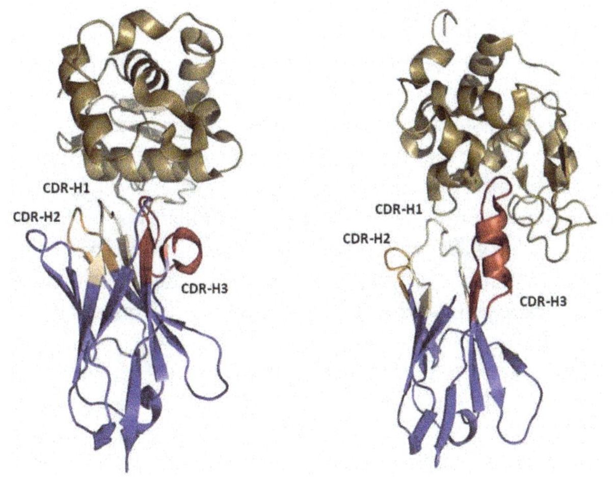

FIGURE 6 | Ribbon representation of Llama VHH (left) and Shark IgNAR (right) in complex with Hen Egg White Lysozyme (HEL). PDBID 1OP6 was used to represent the VHH:HEL complex. PDBID 2I26 was used to represent the IgNAR:HEL complex. Note the protruding IgNAR CDR-H3 blocking the active site of HEL, which contrasts with the bended VHH CDR-H3 that recognizes a flat epitope. The Figure was generated using PyMOL.

THE CAMEL ANTIBODY REPERTOIRE AND VHH

In 1993, the Hamers' group identified a previously unknown immunoglobulin form observed in camel serum (Hamers-Casterman et al., 1993). This new immunoglobulin was found not only to lack a light chain, but to have also deleted the CH1 domain in the heavy chain, following the loss of the splice consensus site (Nguyen et al., 1999). These unique, "heavy chain antibodies" were shown to have a VHH-Hinge-CH2-CH3 structure and performed their antigen binding function exclusively via a stable and soluble VH domain, subsequently dubbed "VHH." VHH antibodies were found to be fully functional constituents of the immune repertoire of camels, representing >50% of the total Ig population in serum samples (Muyldermans and Lauwereys, 1999; Nguyen et al., 2001). Later studies have shown that other camelids such as llama and alpaca also share these unusual immunoglobulins (Harmsen et al., 2000). The VHH and IgG camel antibodies can be separated by isotype, with IgG1 using architecture of conventional antibodies, whereas the IgG2 and IgG3 isotypes are associated with VHH antibodies (Flajnik et al., 2011).

While they are simple in structure, immunogenetics studies have shown that rather than being a rudimentary evolutionary form of immunoglobulin, the VHH antibody in camelids was actually derived from the genes of a conventional IgH locus by a relatively recent adaptation (Nguyen et al., 2002). Multiple contributory selection pressures have been postulated that might have driven this evolutionary event including; amyloidosis associated with a key light-chain sequence, a virus that targeted a light-chain as a co-receptor, or a simple biophysical pressure to develop high frequency antibodies with a "protruding" CDR structure that is highly appropriate for probing cryptic epitopes (Flajnik et al., 2011). Indeed, multiple co-crystal structures of both VHH (De Genst et al., 2006) and IgNAR (Stanfield et al., 2004, 2007) in complex with enzymes have shown the CDRs to protrude into the active site cleft of the enzyme, neutralizing its function.

Despite relying on a single variable domain for antigen recognition, it has been shown that the VHH repertoire is as complex in sequence diversity as its VH counterpart in camelid IgG1 (De Genst et al., 2006). Indeed, although camelid VHH and VH domains are encoded by distinct sets of V-gene segments, both forms of antibody share some D segments and an identical JH region (Nguyen et al., 2001). Similar to chickens, sequence analysis of camelid VHH domains has shown very close homology to the human V_H3 family, which is also associated with relatively high stability and solubility (Ewert et al., 2002, 2003). Comparative analyses of VHH and VH germline and repertoire sequences have shown clearly important differences in their respective structures (Riechmann and Muyldermans, 1999; Harmsen et al., 2000), with VHH exhibiting higher frequency of hypermutation hotspots, leading to greater diversity in CDR-H1 and CDR-H2 sequences and length, plus the frequent observation of clones with long CDRs 1 and 3. In another convergence with chickens, VHH antibodies frequently use non-canonical C residues in their CDRs (Govaert et al., 2012). While the disulphide bonding patterns seen in camelids are not as varied as those observed for chickens (Wu et al., 2011), they do lead to disulphide bonding within the CDR-H3, between CDR-H3 and CDR-H1, or between CDR-H3 and FR-2, with the cysteine groups outside the CDR3 typically being placed in very similar positions to those observed in chickens (IMGT positions 38, 55) (Harmsen et al., 2000).

Most critical of all known VHH characteristics, are the hydrophobic to hydrophilic substitutions of four critical residues in the FR-2, known as the "VHH tetrad." These residues in the FW2 are in critical positions where the V_H of a conventional IgG would pack against the V_L (Abhinandan and Martin, 2010), providing hydrophobic binding affinity between the two domains. The classic substitutions V37F/Y, G44E, L45R, and W47G lead to a major increase in hydrophilicity of the VHH, allowing it to fold and function independently, without the need for a stabilizing V_L partner (Harmsen and De Haard, 2007). This adaptation is essential for biotechnological use, as it allows expression of VHH antibodies at high concentration. While some conventional V_H domains can be expressed, they will typically become insoluble at concentrations above 1 mg/ml (Davies and Riechmann, 1994).

Importantly, while long CDR-H3 loops may be common for some VHH sub-types (particularly in camels) and can contribute to solubility by folding over the FR-2, in llama VHH the average CDR-H3 length has been shown to not exceed that observed for humans (Harmsen et al., 2000). Indeed, experimental analyses of independent V_H domains derived from chicken IgGs, which do use long CDRs (Wu et al., 2011) but do not contain the FR-2 "tetrad" substitutions, have shown that these domains do not exhibit high solubility and do lose binding affinity when separated from a light chain partner (Finlay et al., unpublished observations). Long CDR-H3 sequences are therefore not a guarantee of FR-2 coverage or solubility in VHH and the FR-2 tetrad appears to be an essential factor in achieving solubility. Studies on the "camelization" of VH domains isolated from monoclonal IgG antibodies have corroborated this, by showing that the addition of the FR-2 tetrad mutations can significantly improve the solubility of those domains (Davies and Riechmann, 1994; Riechmann and Muyldermans, 1999). Nonetheless, camelized and/or CDR-solubilized human antibody domains struggle to replicate the qualities of natural VHH, (Barthelemy et al., 2008) suggesting that combined FR and CDR repertoire content may also play a major role. At the time of writing, no major repertoire analyses have been performed for VHH in the way they have for humans, mice and chickens (Zemlin et al., 2003; Wu et al., 2011).

MAN-MADE ANTIBODY REPERTOIRES

Phage display technology was developed by George Smith in 1985 (Smith, 1985) to display peptides on the surface of the filamentous bacteriophage M13. In an effort to isolate "fully human" antibodies and thus bypass humanization, phage display was adapted at the beginning of 1990s (McCafferty et al., 1990) to display antibody V-domain repertoires and to isolate antibodies of interest *in vitro*. During the 1990s and the last decade, several academic laboratories and biotechnology companies have designed and implemented human antibody phage-displayed libraries for antibody discovery (Hoogenboom, 2005; Bradbury, 2010). Such libraries have enabled the isolation of high affinity and specific antibodies against a wide range of molecules and the antibody library design and implementation process continues to evolve.

Since phage display bypasses immunization, it is especially useful for obtaining antibodies against targets that are highly conserved across species and those that may be toxic, where *in vivo* methods are ineffective and/or impractical. In addition, since phage display technology allows access to the repertoire of genes intended for expression and display on the phage surface, the number of genes and variants can be designed or chosen to bias the repertoire toward genes with predefined characteristics, opening up the possibility of testing hypotheses on how the size of a repertoire, its diversity and composition impact the selection of specific, stable, soluble, and high affinity antibodies. Overviews of different man-made repertoires and how their performance has enhanced our knowledge of the evolution of the antibody repertoire are provided below.

NATURAL (NAÏVE) REPERTOIRES

Originally, human antibody phage-displayed libraries for *in vitro* discovery were implemented either by cloning the natural repertoire of rearranged antibody genes (Marks et al., 1991) or by rearranging human antibody germ-line genes *in vitro* (Griffiths et al., 1994). This first generation of natural or naïve repertoires contained the diversity harvested from the total B-cell repertoire by RT-PCR and thus suffered from a lack of control over FR usage and mutation rate (Sidhu and Fellouse, 2006). This can be a significant issue in antibody therapeutic development, as not all human FRs are used at high frequency in the B-cell repertoire (see above) and, importantly, not all will express well in heterologous systems or be stable in delivery formulations (Ewert et al., 2003). Additionally, antibodies from naïve libraries may contain somatic mutations leading to FR or CDR based T-cell epitopes and/or aggregation-prone sequences that could potentially lead to immunogenicity (Harding et al., 2010). As a result, several research groups have developed fully synthetic antibody repertoires in which a few well-expressed and well-behaved scaffolds are used for the repertoire synthesis and diversity is restricted to the CDRs (Pini et al., 1998; Sidhu et al., 2004).

SYNTHETIC REPERTOIRES

The earliest experimental synthetic antibody repertoire was based on single V_H and V_L scaffolds, introduced limited diversity into the CDR-H3 alone and was used to generate moderate affinity hits against haptens (Barbas et al., 1992, 1993). This library exploited basic knowledge of antibody structure and diversity by placing random amino acid diversity into the exposed regions of the CDR-H3. Amino acid randomization was made possible by the use of PCR and oligonucleotides containing degenerate DNA sequence in the appropriate CDR-encoding codons. The simplest forms of degenerate codons used are based on random incorporation in the first two bases, followed by restricted incorporation in the third position to either G/T ("NNK" codon) or G/C ("NNS" codon). Both of these schemes predominantly incorporate functional diversity, as they encode for 32 codons total, including only one of the three stop codons (amber) and encoding all 20 amino acids, although not at equal ratio. These codons therefore incorporate a reasonable number of translatable polypeptide sequences, so long as the number of contiguous codons used is not so many that one stop codon would be expected per clone. One complicating factor is the obligate encoding of cysteine by each of these codons, leading to a significant number of clones in which thiol groups are presented unpaired, leading to loop malfunction and reducing the overall functional content of the library.

This very simple method of diversification of key CDR loops was exploited by a series of teams (Griffiths et al., 1993, 1994; Viti et al., 2000; Silacci et al., 2005), who used similar methods to diversify both the CDRs H3 and L3 in a variety of FRs, while maintaining key loop stem residues in the CDR-H3 such as Kabat 93, 94, 101, and 102. Despite the simple nature of these repertoires, they have been highly successful at generating antibodies to proteins, peptides, and haptens. The isolated antibodies have proven utility as immunochemical reagents (Neri et al., 1998) and some have even been applied successfully in therapeutic settings (Neri et al., 1995; Carnemolla et al., 1996; Borsi et al., 1998; Brack et al., 2006; Silacci et al., 2006). This antibody construction style was then progressed by examining the additional benefit of adding synthetic diversity in the CDRs 1 and 2 of V_H and exploiting the use of a variety of tailored (A.K.A. "parsimonious") degenerate codons that encoded a smaller number of amino acids at key positions. This improved the quality of the resulting libraries, so they encoded a larger proportion of functionally folded clones and the avoidance of stop codons allowed the incorporation of greater length diversity in the CDR-H3 (Lee et al., 2004; Sidhu et al., 2004).

Further examination of the amino acid content of the mature human, primate and rodent V-gene repertoires, coupled with expanded structural understanding of antibody-antigen interactions, as outlined above, subsequently created highly defined knowledge of positional amino acid usage in CDRs. These studies strongly suggested that the key amino acids used in making functional contacts with protein antigens were highly biased and the adoption of TRInucleotide, or "TRIM" technology (Virnekas et al., 1994) allowed the first opportunities for this knowledge to be fully exploited. TRIM technology is a method based on classical oligonucleotide synthesis chemistry, but at positions of randomization, mixes of trinucleotide phosphoramidites (A.K.A. trimers) are added instead of a series of single base mixes. Each trimer is a fully synthetic codon and the use of precise combinations of these trimers therefore allows the incorporation of positional bias in amino acid mutagenesis libraries (Virnekas et al., 1994).

The earliest use of TRIM technology in antibody repertoire construction did not exploit its full capability, only introducing fully random amino acid diversity into the CDR-H3 of a single framework pair and selecting the library successfully against a series of haptens (Braunagel and Little, 1997). Subsequent landmark studies, however, took the use of trinucleotides to its logical conclusion and attempted to closely mimic the natural human immune repertoire in synthetic form (Knappik et al., 2000; Rothe et al., 2008; Prassler et al., 2011). Knappik et al. (2000) generated the first iteration of the HuCal© libraries, in which they first recognized that 95% of all human antibody diversity is represented in only seven V_H and seven V_L germline gene families. This observation inspired them to create a library of V-genes built on consensus FRs derived via alignment of each of these families. Into these FRs they placed double-stranded CDR diversity "cassettes" that had been built using trinucleotides to represent each of the amino acids naturally found at all positions in CDRs H3 and L3. They also included length diversity in the CDR3s and canonical structural determinants for the L3, approximately mimicking the natural biases observed in the human repertoire. In the CDR-H3, the natural dominance of G and Y in the human repertoire was closely reflected, with those two residues making up approximately 15% each, of the encoded residues between Kabat 95 and 100s. All other residues were included at ~4% other than cysteine, which was allowed at only ~1% to allow potential generation of the disulphide-constrained loops that are occasionally observed in the human repertoire. Stem loop biases in both the CDRs H3 and L3 were also closely maintained and limited diversity was introduced at several key positions in the structurally conserved Vκ and Vλ L3 loops. This repertoire design was highly effective in generating nM-affinity clones with specificity for a selection of proteins and peptides (Knappik et al., 2000; Marget et al., 2000).

The methods used by Knappik et al. (2000) have since been elaborated upon in a number of reports. Rothe et al. (2008), reported the construction of the next-generation library HuCal Gold™ in which the design strategy was refined to change the CDR design complexity, the structural format of the library (to Fab fragment) and also to move to "CysDisplay" in which the expressed antibody is tethered to the phage via a disulphide bond with a mutant p3 protein. In this library, the CDR diversity was extended to the CDRs 1 and 2 of both V-domains, in addition to the CDR3s. The CDR cassettes were again based on trinucleotide technology and were built to accurately reflect the canonical structures and diversity found in the families upon which each of the consensus frameworks were built, consciously including structures known to be preferred in the recognition of peptides. The finalized library was found to be of very high practical utility, routinely generating antibody specificities and affinities in the single digit nM range that were useful for both therapeutic and reagent purposes (Jarutat et al., 2006, 2007; Ohara et al., 2006; Prassler et al., 2009). This library design had, however, made a critical concession to optimize its function in *E. coli* expression and phage display technology: the FRs were codon optimized specifically to maximize for *E. coli* periplasmic expression rate. In addition, this function had been aggressively selected for by pre-screening all antibody sequences for periplasmic transport as β–lactamase fusions before inclusion in the final library. This resulted in a high frequency of antibodies being selected that performed very well in prokaryotic expression, but poorly in mammalian cell lines used for industrial production of IgGs. As a result, a third iteration "HuCal Platinum™" has since been made which further updated the design and performance of these synthetic libraries, by optimizing codon use to suit both prokaryotic and eukaryotic expression systems (Prassler et al., 2011). This library also further refined the FR use and CDR content to minimize T-cell epitope content and maximize similarity to the human repertoire, by adding length-dependent positional amino acid bias in the CDR-H3 and by switching some V_H gene families to fully germline (e.g., VH3-23). These changes made the library higher performing than the HuCal Gold™library in diversity of hits generated, average affinity and expression rate in mammalian cells. Similar libraries that have recently been generated by separate groups have also strongly supported the broad utility and quality of libraries that naturally mimic the human immune system and that these libraries are flexible in display format as they can be selected by alternative phage display systems such as pIX display (Shi et al., 2010).

The overall HuCal™ story is therefore a clear paradigm and example of the intrinsic attraction of synthetic antibody libraries: they can be designed to add positive attributes and to minimize negatives. While fully human natural cDNA-derived libraries are simple to construct and highly functional, negative attributes such as unwanted FR use, somatic hypermutation in frameworks and potential liability sequences such as aggregation motifs, deamidation sites, N-linked glycosylation motifs, oxidation sensitivities and non-canonical disulphide content cannot be avoided as a rule. The very latest libraries make use of a novel DNA synthesis technology known as Slonomics, which has been shown to be an excellent method for the synthesis of molecular diversity, as it allows the production of precise amino acid/codon biases and low dysfunctional sequence content at any given position (Zhai et al., 2011). Analysis of the first large library generated using this technology strongly supports another benefit of carefully designed synthetic antibody libraries: the removal of segmental linkage within the CDR-H3 that limits paratope structural diversity. While natural CDR-H3 sequences have the benefit of being selected for function in the B-cell, synthetic versions are not generated by IGV-D-IGJ recombination mechanisms and therefore, escape potential limitations on self-reactivity that may be imposed by natural tolerance mechanisms (Zhai et al., 2011). Such synthetic antibody libraries are clearly a mature technology and have become an important section of the armamentarium currently in use for therapeutic human antibody discovery.

MINIMALIST REPERTOIRES

A series of illuminating studies set out to examine the validity of the suggestion that only certain amino acids, with particular emphasis on Y (see above), are essential in the formation of a functional antibody repertoire (Fellouse et al., 2004, 2005, 2006, 2007; Birtalan et al., 2008, 2010; Fisher et al., 2010). It was postulated that antibody critical contacts were predominantly mediated by Y and that small amino acids played a critical support role in creating conformational flexibility and diversity, especially in the CDR-H3 (Koide and Sidhu, 2009). To examine this hypothesis, large phage libraries of human Fabs on a single FR combination were synthesized containing only four amino acids; Y, A, D, and S in solvent-exposed CDR positions, including CDR-H3 (Fellouse et al., 2004). These libraries were capable of generating high affinity and specific antibodies, including antibodies of 2 nM affinities for VEGF. Remarkably, when the four amino acid code was reduced to only Y and S, highly functional repertoires could still be generated, (Fellouse et al., 2005, 2007) with structural studies subsequently showing that Y was indeed the key residue for making critical contacts with antigen, while serine predominantly provided structural flexibility and "space" to accommodate the bulky Y side-chains (Fellouse et al., 2006).

Importantly, Birtalan et al. (2010) have since progressed these studies and demonstrated that W is the only natural amino acid that can be used as a functional alternative to Y in experimental synthetic antibody libraries based on binary diversity (Birtalan et al., 2010). Indeed, co-crystal structure analysis of an antibody from a W/S-containing repertoire with its target HER2 showed clearly that W is a key determinant of the binding specificity (Fisher et al., 2010). Additionally, these investigators have shown that excess content of highly charged residues such as R is a significant risk factor for the high frequency generation of polyreactive clones (Birtalan et al., 2008, 2010). A subsequent study performed using a set of libraries of synthetic single-domain binding proteins has provided supporting evidence for the idea that minimal diversity can be genuinely functional, but that increased amino acid diversity overall is still the best for high function (Hackel and Wittrup, 2010). Synthetic antibody libraries have, therefore, not only allowed the interrogation of fundamental antibody structure/function relationships, but have illustrated what library design elements are critical to maximal function. Future studies will most likely continue to advance this field to make synthetic diversity as reliable as possible.

RATIONAL REPERTOIRES

Finally, based on the finding that the anatomy of the antigen-binding site determines the propensity to recognize a defined type of generic antigen such as a peptide or a hapten, it has been hypothesized that by biasing an antibody repertoire toward the recognition of predefined antigens the probability of obtaining more specific and higher affinity antibodies may increase. This can be rationalized in terms that, when general purpose repertoires, such as naïve or synthetic repertoires, are used to obtain antibodies to a given target, a vast region of the shape space has to be explored to produce specific antibodies. Provided that only an infinitesimally small fraction of all possible functional antigen-binding sites can be explored by using enrichment technologies, such an exploration should be sparse. Consequently, the probability of selecting specific antibodies of higher affinity should increase in repertoires that have been designed to be focused on predefined regions of the shape space.

Rational repertoires of antibodies are built by selecting genes encoding combinations of canonical structures that resemble the structural features of antibodies that bind the desired type of ligands. Sequence diversity is then introduced at residues typically involved in recognition of those types of targets. For instance, two antibody repertoires have been designed and tested for peptide recognition (Cobaugh et al., 2008). First, a human anti-peptide repertoire was constructed by pairing the human IGVH germ line gene 3–23 with a variant of the IGVK germline gene 3–20. The CDR-L1 of the gene 3–20 was modified to encode a long loop, typical of anti-peptide antibodies (**Figure 7**) and diversity was engineered in V_H SDRUs of anti-protein and anti-peptide antibodies (see above). Another repertoire was generated using the V-regions of the murine antibody 26–10, which was originally isolated, based on its affinity to the hapten digoxin, but also binds peptides and exhibits a canonical structure pattern typical of anti-peptide antibodies. As in the first repertoire, diversity was introduced in V_H only, using the profile of amino acid found at positions that frequently contact peptide antigens. Both repertoires yielded binders to two model peptides, angiotensin and neuropeptide Y, following screening by solution phage panning. The repertoire built onto the 26–10 scaffold yielded antibodies with affinities below 20 nM to both targets.

Another example of a rational repertoire (Persson et al., 2006) was designed using as scaffold the antibody FITC8, which has a cavity in the antigen-binding site, common to anti-hapten antibodies. In five CDRs, diversity was designed on the basis of a 3D model structure of FITC8 and anti-hapten SDRUs. In addition, length variation was introduced into the CDR-H2, as longer versions of this loop have been shown to correlate with increased hapten binding. The repertoire was cloned, phage-displayed and screened against a panel of five haptens, yielding diverse and highly specific binders to four of the selectors. Parallel selections were performed with a repertoire having diversity in more peripherally located residues, which are more often found in contact with protein than haptens. The binders selected from the control (anti-protein) repertoire were not able to bind to the soluble hapten in the absence of the carrier protein, in contrast to the clones selected from the anti-hapten repertoire. Thus, although more validation is needed in order to conclude that rational repertoires increase the probability of obtaining more specific and higher affinity antibodies, these two examples have shown the feasibility and potential advantages of designing repertoires to recognize predefined generic ligands.

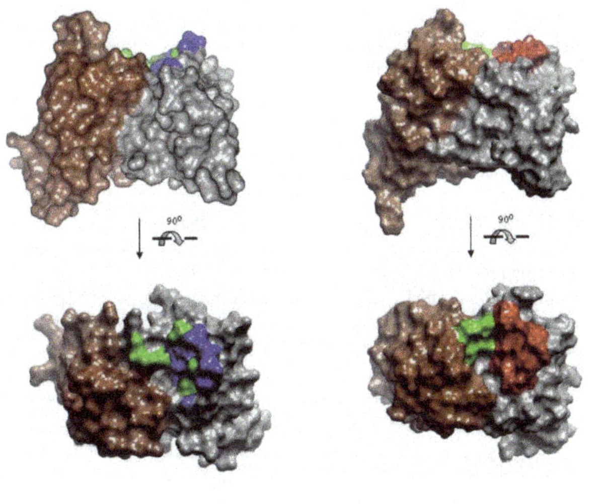

FIGURE 7 | Model of the human anti-peptide (left) and mouse anti-peptide (right) repertoires. On the **top**, side view of the Connolly surface of the models. **Bottom**, models seen from the antigen perspective. Invariant V_Ls are colored in brown. V_Hs are colored in gray. Within the antigen-binding site, green represents fully randomized positions, i.e., 20 amino acids; blue positions diversified to Tyr, Asp, Ala, and Ser; red positions diversified to incorporate the most common anti-peptide SDRs. PDBID: 1MCP and 2IGF were used as template for modeling human V_L and V_H, respectively. Coordinates of the antibody 26-10 (PDBID 1IGI) were used for modeling the mouse anti-peptide repertoire. The models and Figures were created in Discovery Studio.

CONCLUSIONS AND FUTURE DIRECTIONS

In this review, we have outlined the importance of the continuum of knowledge that runs through antibody structural studies, species repertoire analyses and experimental exploitation of this information to design antibody repertoires and advance antibody-based drug discovery. Study of hundreds of x-ray crystallography antibody structures free and bound to wide variety of ligands have provided a detailed picture of how antibodies recognize diverse types of ligands with exquisite specificity and high affinity. It has also shown that, although the antigen-binding site is very diverse in sequence and structure, it has predictable geometrical features that determine the types of generic ligands with which the antibody interacts. This knowledge has been critical to understand the mechanisms of the immune response mediated by antibodies and the evolution of the antibody repertoire. Its application has led to the development of engineering methods such as humanization, antigen-affinity optimization and effector function enhancement, which have made possible the approval of more than 30 antibody-based medicines in the last two decades.

The knowledge gained on the antibody structure has been complemented with the study of the antibody repertoire of several species. In addition to humans, we described in previous sections the repertoires and the affinity maturation mechanisms of mice and chickens, plus the use of novel single-domain antibodies in camelids and sharks. These species all utilize diverse evolutionary solutions to generate specific and high affinity antibodies and illustrate the plasticity of natural antibody repertoires. Their comparative study has raised fundamental questions about the evolutionary factors shaping the antibody repertoire such as: has the evolution of the antibody repertoire been a stochastic process or has it been shaped by functional and/or structural constraints? What is the optimal size and diversity of a repertoire that can be generated *in vitro* in order to generate specific and high affinity antibodies to a wide variety of antigen types?

Multiple variations of man-made antibody repertoires have been designed and validated in the last two decades, which have served as tools to explore the above conundrums on how the evolution, size, diversity, and composition of a repertoire impact the selection of more specific and higher affinity antibodies to any given target. A first generation of man-made antibodies included all the antibody genes encoding the repertoire of circulating antibodies, but a relatively limited subset of the genes predominated the panning of the repertoires, showing that many genes are dispensable. A second generation of synthetic repertoires followed. Learning the lesson from the study of natural and man-made naïve repertoires, the new generation of synthetic human antibody repertoires was built on single or a few well-behaved scaffolds. The diversity in these libraries was designed to mimic that of the natural antibodies. These repertoires produced antibodies to a vast array of the diverse antigens. In a further round of design and testing, minimalist repertoires have been designed and validated. These repertoires have been designed to display antigen-binding sites made of very few amino acids or even only binary Y/S and W/S mixes, again yielding antibodies specific against diverse antigens. Finally, rational repertoires encoding genes with predefined recognition features have been tested, which hold the promise of increasing the probability of obtaining more specific and higher affinity antibodies.

Looking forward into the future, new technologies such as next generation sequencing (NGS) are providing the means to study whole natural (Weinstein et al., 2009; Jiang et al., 2011) and man-made repertoires (Glanville et al., 2009) in expedited ways and at relatively low costs (Fischer, 2011; Benichou et al., 2012). Having access to the complete information encoded in repertoires before and after selection under diverse selection pressures, combined with faster and more accurate 3D modeling methods (Almagro et al., 2011; Kuroda et al., 2012) and indeed new conceptual tools and algorithms such as network analysis, may reveal new features of antibody repertoires. These findings will hopefully further impact the theories addressing the origin and evolution of antibody binding specificity. It will also inform the design and optimization of man-made repertoires to isolate more potent, stable, safe and efficacious antibody-based therapeutics, at a lower cost.

REFERENCES

Abhinandan, K. R., and Martin, A. C. (2010). Analysis and prediction of VH/VL packing in antibodies. *Protein Eng. Des. Sel.* 23, 689–697.

Aitken, R., Gilchrist, J., and Sinclair, M. C. (1997). A single diversified VH gene family dominates the bovine immunoglobulin repertoire. *Biochem. Soc. Trans.* 25, 326S.

Al-Lazikani, B., Lesk, A. M., and Chothia, C. (1997). Standard conformations for the canonical structures of immunoglobulins. *J. Mol. Biol.* 273, 927–948.

Almagro, J. C. (2004). Identification of differences in the specificity-determining residues of antibodies that recognize antigens of different size: implications for the rational design of antibody repertoires. *J. Mol. Recognit.* 17, 132–143.

Almagro, J. C., Beavers, M., Hernandez-Guzman, F., Maier, J., Shaulsky, J., Butenhof, K., et al. (2011). Antibody modeling assessment. *Proteins* 79, 3050–3066.

Almagro, J. C., and Fransson, J. (2008). Humanization of antibodies. *Front. Biosci.* 13, 1619–1633.

Almagro, J. C., Hernandez I., del Carmen Ramirez, M., and Vargas-Madrazo, E. (1997). The differences between the structural repertoires of IGHV germ-line gene segments of mice and humans: implication for the molecular mechanism of the immune response. *Mol. Immunol.* 34, 1199–1214.

Almagro, J. C., Raghunathan, G., Beil, E., Janecki, D. J., Chen, Q., Dinh, T., et al. (2012). Characterization of a high-affinity human antibody with a disulfide bridge in the third complementarity-determining region of the heavy chain. *J. Mol. Recognit.* 25, 125–135.

Alt, F., and Baltimore, D. (1982). Joining of immunoglobulin heavy chain gene segments: implications from a chromosome with evidence of three D-JH fusions. *Proc. Natl. Acad. Sci. U.S.A.* 79, 4118–4122.

Amzel, L. M., and Poljak, R. J. (1979). Three-dimensional structure of immunoglobulins. *Annu. Rev. Biochem.* 48, 961–997.

Barbas, C. F. 3rd., Amberg, W., Simoncsits, A., Jones, T. M., and Lerner, R. A. (1993). Selection of human anti-hapten antibodies from semisynthetic libraries. *Gene* 137, 57–62.

Barbas, C. F. 3rd., Bain, J. D., Hoekstra, D. M., and Lerner, R. A. (1992). Semisynthetic combinatorial antibody libraries: a chemical solution to the diversity problem. *Proc. Natl. Acad. Sci. U.S.A.* 89, 4457–4461.

Barthelemy, P. A., Raab, H., Appleton, B. A., Bond, C. J., Wu, P., Wiesmann, C., et al. (2008). Comprehensive analysis of the factors contributing to the stability and solubility of autonomous human VH domains. *J. Biol. Chem.* 283, 3639–3654.

Benichou, J., Ben-Hamo, R., Louzoun, Y., and Efroni, S. (2012). Rep-Seq: uncovering the immunological repertoire through next-generation sequencing. *Immunology* 135, 183–191.

Betz, A. G., Rada, C., Pannell, R., Milstein, C., and Neuberger, M. S. (1993). Passenger transgenes reveal intrinsic specificity of the antibody hypermutation mechanism: clustering, polarity, and specific hot spots. *Proc. Natl. Acad. Sci. U.S.A.* 90, 2385–2388.

Birtalan, S., Fisher, R. D., and Sidhu, S. S. (2010). The functional capacity of the natural amino acids for molecular recognition. *Mol. Biosyst.* 6, 1186–1194.

Birtalan, S., Zhang, Y., Fellouse, F. A., Shao, L., Schaefer, G., and Sidhu, S. S. (2008). The intrinsic contributions of tyrosine, serine, glycine and arginine to the affinity and specificity of antibodies. *J. Mol. Biol.* 377, 1518–1528.

Bono, B. D., Madera, M., and Chothia, C. (2004). VH gene segments in the mouse and human genomes. *J. Mol. Biol.* 342, 131–143.

Borsi, L., Castellani, P., Allemanni, G., Neri, D., and Zardi, L. (1998). Preparation of phage antibodies to the ED-A domain of human fibronectin. *Exp. Cell Res.* 240, 244–251.

Boswell, C. A., Tesar, D. B., Mukhyala, K., Theil, F. P., Fielder, P. J., and Khawli, L. A. (2010). Effects of charge on antibody tissue distribution and pharmacokinetics. *Bioconjug. Chem.* 21, 2153–2163.

Brack, S. S., Silacci, M., Birchler, M., and Neri, D. (2006). Tumor-targeting properties of novel antibodies specific to the large isoform of tenascin-C. *Clin. Cancer Res.* 12, 3200–3208.

Bradbury, A. R. (2010). The use of phage display in neurobiology. *Curr. Protoc. Neurosci.* Chapter 5, Unit 5. 12.

Braunagel, M., and Little, M. (1997). Construction of a semisynthetic antibody library using trinucleotide oligos. *Nucleic Acids Res.* 25, 4690–4691.

Breden, F., Lepik, C., Longo, N., Montero, M., Lipsky, P., and Scott, J. (2011). Comparison of antibody repertoires produced by HIV-1 infection, other chronic and acute infections, and systemic autoimmune disease. *PLoS ONE* 6:e16857. doi: 10.1371/journal.pone.0016857

Brezinschek, H. P., Foster, S. J., Dorner, T., Brezinschek, R. I., and Lipsky, P. E. (1998). Pairing of variable heavy and variable kappa chains in individual naive and memory B cells. *J. Immunol.* 160, 4762–4767.

Carnemolla, B., Neri, D., Castellani, P., Leprini, A., Neri, G., Pini, A., et al. (1996). Phage antibodies with pan-species recognition of the oncofoetal angiogenesis marker fibronectin ED-B domain. *Int. J. Cancer* 68, 397–405.

Chailyan, A., Marcatili, P., Cirillo, D., and Tramontano, A. (2011). Structural repertoire of immunoglobulin λ light chains. *Proteins* 79, 1513–1524.

Chothia, C., and Lesk, A. M. (1987). Canonical structures for the hypervariable regions of immunoglobulins. *J. Mol. Biol.* 196, 901–917.

Chothia, C., Lesk, A. M., Gherardi, E., Tomlinson, I. M., Walter, G., Marks, J. D., et al. (1992). Structural repertoire of the human VH segments. *J. Mol. Biol.* 227, 799–817.

Chothia, C., Lesk, A. M., Tramontano, A., Levitt, M., Smith-Gill, S. J., Air, G., et al. (1989). Conformations of immunoglobulin hypervariable regions. *Nature* 342, 877–883.

Clark, L. A., Ganesan, S., Papp, S., and Vlijmen, H. W. V. (2006). Trends in antibody sequence changes during the somatic hypermutation process. *J. Immunol.* 177, 333–340.

Cobaugh, C., Almagro, J., Pogson, M., Iverson, B., and Georgiou, G. (2008). Synthetic antibody libraries focused towards peptide ligands. *J. Mol. Biol.* 378, 622–633.

Connolly, M. L. (1983). Solvent-accessible surfaces of proteins and nucleic acids. *Science* 221, 709–713.

Cox, J. P., Tomlinson, I. M., and Winter, G. (1994). A directory of human germ-line V kappa segments reveals a strong bias in their usage. *Eur. J. Immunol.* 24, 827–836.

Dal-Bo, M., Giudice, I. D., Bomben, R., Capello, D., Bertoni, F., Forconi, F., et al. (2011). B-cell receptor, clinical course and prognosis in chronic lymphocytic leukaemia: the growing saga of the IGHV3 subgroup gene usage. *Br. J. Haematol.* 153, 3–14.

Davies, D. R., and Metzger, H. (1983). Structural basis of antibody function. *Annu. Rev. Immunol.* 1, 87–117.

Davies, J., and Riechmann, L. (1994). 'Camelising' human antibody fragments: NMR studies on VH domains. *FEBS Lett.* 339, 285–290.

De Genst, E., Saerens, D., Muyldermans, S., and Conrath, K. (2006). Antibody repertoire development in camelids. *Dev. Comp. Immunol.* 30, 187–198.

De Genst, E., Silence, K., Decanniere, K., Conrath, K., Loris, R., Kinne, J., et al. (2006). Molecular basis for the preferential cleft recognition by dromedary heavy-chain antibodies. *Proc. Natl. Acad. Sci. U.S.A.* 103, 4586–4591.

de Wildt, R. M., Hoet, R. M., van Venrooij, W. J., Tomlinson, I. M., and Winter, G. (1999). Analysis of heavy and light chain pairings indicates that receptor editing shapes the human antibody repertoire. *J. Mol. Biol.* 285, 895–901.

Dooley, H., Flajnik, M. F., and Porter, A. J. (2003). Selection and characterization of naturally occurring single-domain (IgNAR) antibody fragments from immunized sharks by phage display. *Mol. Immunol.* 40, 25–33.

Dörner, T., Foster, S. J., Farner, N. L., and Lipsky, P. E. (1998). Somatic hypermutation of human immunoglobulin heavy chain genes: targeting of RGYW motifs on both DNA strands. *Eur. J. Immunol.* 28, 3384–3396.

Ewert, S., Cambillau, C., Conrath, K., and Pluckthun, A. (2002). Biophysical properties of camelid V (HH) domains compared to those of human V (H)3 domains. *Biochemistry* 41, 3628–3636.

Ewert, S., Honegger, A., and Pluckthun, A. (2004). Stability improvement of antibodies for extracellular and intracellular applications: CDR grafting to stable frameworks and structure-based framework engineering. *Methods* 34, 184–199.

Ewert, S., Huber, T., Honegger, A., and Pluckthun, A. (2003). Biophysical properties of human antibody variable domains. *J. Mol. Biol.* 325, 531–553.

Farner, N. L., Dorner, T., and Lipsky, P. E. (1999). Molecular mechanisms and selection influence the generation of the human V lambda J lambda repertoire. *J. Immunol.* 162, 2137–2145.

Fellouse, F. A., Barthelemy, P. A., Kelley, R. F., and Sidhu, S. S. (2006). Tyrosine plays a dominant functional role in the paratope of a synthetic antibody derived from a four amino acid code. *J. Mol. Biol.* 357, 100–114.

Fellouse, F. A., Esaki, K., Birtalan, S., Raptis, D., Cancasci, V. J., Koide, A., et al. (2007). High-throughput generation of synthetic antibodies from highly functional minimalist phage-displayed libraries. *J. Mol. Biol.* 373, 924–940.

Fellouse, F. A., Li, B., Compaan, D. M., Peden, A. A., Hymowitz, S. G., and Sidhu, S. S. (2005). Molecular recognition by a binary code. *J. Mol. Biol.* 348, 1153–1162.

Fellouse, F. A., Wiesmann, C., and Sidhu, S. S. (2004). Synthetic antibodies from a four-amino-acid code: a dominant role for tyrosine in antigen recognition. *Proc. Natl. Acad. Sci. U.S.A.* 101, 12467–12472.

Fennell, B. J., Darmanin-Sheehan, A., Hufton, S. E., Calabro, V., Wu, L., Muller, M. R., et al. (2010). Dissection of the IgNAR V domain: molecular scanning and orthologue database mining define novel IgNAR hallmarks and affinity maturation mechanisms. *J. Mol. Biol.* 400, 155–170.

Finlay, W. J., deVore, N. C., Dobrovolskaia, E. N., Gam, A., Goodyear, C. S., and Slater, J. E. (2005). Exploiting the avian immunoglobulin system to simplify the generation of recombinant antibodies to allergenic proteins. *Clin. Exp. Allergy* 35, 1040–1048.

Finlay, W. J., Shaw, I., Reilly, J. P., and Kane, M. (2006). Generation of high-affinity chicken single-chain Fv antibody fragments for measurement of the Pseudonitzschia pungens toxin domoic acid. *Appl. Environ. Microbiol.* 72, 3343–3349.

Fischer, N. (2011). Sequencing antibody repertoires: the next generation. *MAbs* 3, 17–20.

Fisher, R. D., Ultsch, M., Lingel, A., Schaefer, G., Shao, L., Birtalan, S., et al. (2010). Structure of the complex between HER2 and an antibody paratope formed by side chains from tryptophan and serine. *J. Mol. Biol.* 402, 217–229.

Flajnik, M. F., Deschacht, N., and Muyldermans, S. (2011). A case of convergence: why did a simple alternative to canonical antibodies arise in sharks and camels? *PLoS Biol.* 9:e1001120. doi: 10.1371/journal.pbio.1001120

Flajnik, M. F., and Dooley, H. (2009). The generation and selection of single-domain, v region libraries from nurse sharks. *Methods Mol. Biol.* 562, 71–82.

Foote, J., and Winter, G. (1992). Antibody framework residues affecting the conformation of the hypervariable loops. *J. Mol. Biol.* 224, 487–499.

Gill, D. S., and Damle, N. K. (2006). Biopharmaceutical drug discovery using novel protein scaffolds. *Curr. Opin. Biotechnol.* 17, 653–658.

Gilliland, G., Luo, J., Vafa, O., and Almagro, J. (2012). Leveraging SBDD in protein therapeutic development: antibody engineering. *Methods Mol. Biol.* 841, 321–349.

Glanville, J., Zhai, W., Berka, J., Telman, D., Huerta, G., Mehta, G. R., et al. (2009). Precise determination of the diversity of a combinatorial antibody library gives insight into the human immunoglobulin repertoire. *Proc. Natl. Acad. Sci. U.S.A.* 106, 20216–20221.

Govaert, J., Pellis, M., Deschacht, N., Vincke, C., Conrath, K., Muyldermans, S., et al. (2012). Dual beneficial effect of interloop disulfide bond for single domain antibody fragments. *J. Biol. Chem.* 287, 1970–1979.

Griffiths, A. D., Malmqvist, M., Marks, J. D., Bye, J. M., Embleton, M. J., McCafferty, J., et al. (1993). Human anti-self antibodies with high specificity from phage display libraries. *EMBO J.* 12, 725–734.

Griffiths, A. D., Williams, S. C., Hartley, O., Tomlinson, I. M., Waterhouse, P., Crosby, W. L., et al. (1994). Isolation of high affinity human antibodies directly from large synthetic repertoires. *EMBO J.* 13, 3245–3260.

Hackel, B. J., Ackerman, M. E., Howland, S. W., and Wittrup, K. D. (2010). Stability and CDR composition biases enrich binder functionality landscapes. *J. Mol. Biol.* 401, 84–96.

Hackel, B. J., and Wittrup, K. D. (2010). The full amino acid repertoire is superior to serine/tyrosine for selection of high affinity immunoglobulin G binders from the fibronectin scaffold. *Protein Eng. Des. Sel.* 23, 211–219.

Hamers-Casterman, C., Atarhouch, T., Muyldermans, S., Robinson, G., Hamers, C., Songa, E. B., et al. (1993). Naturally occurring antibodies devoid of light chains. *Nature* 363, 446–448.

Harding, F. A., Stickler, M. M., Razo, J., and Dubridge, R. B. (2010). The immunogenicity of humanized and fully human antibodies: residual immunogenicity resides in the CDR regions. *MAbs* 2, 256–265.

Harmsen, M. M., and De Haard, H. J. (2007). Properties, production, and applications of camelid single-domain antibody fragments. *Appl. Microbiol. Biotechnol.* 77, 13–22.

Harmsen, M. M., Ruuls, R. C., Nijman, I. J., Niewold, T. A., Frenken, L. G., and de Geus, B. (2000). Llama heavy-chain V regions consist of at least four distinct subfamilies revealing novel sequence features. *Mol. Immunol.* 37, 579–590.

Hoogenboom, H. R. (2005). Selecting and screening recombinant antibody libraries. *Nat. Biotechnol.* 23, 1105–1116.

Huang, S. C., Jiang, R., Glas, A. M., and Milner, E. C. (1996). Non-stochastic utilization of Ig V region genes in unselected human peripheral B cells. *Mol. Immunol.* 33, 553–560.

Ignatovich, O., Tomlinson, I. M., Jones, P. T., and Winter, G. (1997). The creation of diversity in the human immunoglobulin V (lambda) repertoire. *J. Mol. Biol.* 268, 69–77.

Jarutat, T., Frisch, C., Nickels, C., Merz, H., and Knappik, A. (2006). Isolation and comparative characterization of Ki-67 equivalent antibodies from the HuCAL phage display library. *Biol. Chem.* 387, 995–1003.

Jarutat, T., Nickels, C., Frisch, C., Stellmacher, F., Hofig, K. P., Knappik, A., et al. (2007). Selection of vimentin-specific antibodies from the HuCAL phage display library by subtractive panning on formalin-fixed, paraffin-embedded tissue. *Biol. Chem.* 388, 651–658.

Jiang, N., Weinstein, J., Penland, L., White, R. R., Fisher, D., and Quake, S. R. (2011). Determinism and stochasticity during maturation of the zebrafish antibody repertoire. *Proc. Natl. Acad. Sci. U.S.A.* 108, 5348–5353.

Johansson, J., Aveskogh, M., Munday, B., and Hellman, L. (2002). Heavy chain V region diversity in the duck-billed platypus (*Ornithorhynchus anatinus*): long and highly variable complementarity-determining region 3 compensates for limited germline diversity. *J. Immunol.* 168, 5155–5162.

Jones, P. T., Dear, P. H., Foote, J., Neuberger, M. S., and Winter, G. (1986). Replacing the complementarity-determining regions in a human antibody with those from a mouse. *Nature* 321, 522–525.

Kabat, E. A., and Wu, T. T. (1971). Attempts to locate complementarity-determining residues in the variable positions of light and heavy chains. *Ann. N.Y. Acad. Sci.* 190, 382–393.

Knappik, A., Ge, L., Honegger, A., Pack, P., Fischer, M., Wellnhofer, G., et al. (2000). Fully synthetic human combinatorial antibody libraries (HuCAL) based on modular consensus frameworks and CDRs randomized with trinucleotides. *J. Mol. Biol.* 296, 57–86.

Köhler, G., and Milstein, C. (1975). Continuous cultures of fused cells secreting antibody of predefined specificity. *Nature* 256, 495–497.

Koide, S., and Sidhu, S. S. (2009). The importance of being tyrosine: lessons in molecular recognition from minimalist synthetic binding proteins. *ACS Chem. Biol.* 4, 325–334.

Kuroda, D., Shirai, H., Jacobson, M., and Nakamura, H. (2012). Computer-aided antibody design. *Protein Eng. Des. Sel.* 25, 507–522.

Lee, C. V., Hymowitz, S. G., Wallweber, H. J., Gordon, N. C., Billeci, K. L., Tsai, S. P., et al. (2006). Synthetic anti-BR3 antibodies that mimic BAFF binding and target both human and murine B cells. *Blood* 108, 3103–3111.

Lee, C. V., Liang, W. C., Dennis, M. S., Eigenbrot, C., Sidhu, S. S., and Fuh, G. (2004). High-affinity human antibodies from phage-displayed synthetic Fab libraries with a single framework scaffold. *J. Mol. Biol.* 340, 1073–1093.

Lefranc, M. P., Giudicelli, V., Kaas, Q., Duprat, E., Jabado-Michaloud, J., Scaviner, D., et al. (2005). IMGT, the international ImMunoGeneTics information system. *Nucleic Acids Res.* 33, D593–D597.

Lerner, R. (2011). Rare antibodies from combinatorial libraries suggests an S.O.S. component of the human immunological repertoire. *Mol. Biosyst.* 7, 1004–1012.

Li, F., and Aitken, R. (2004). Cloning of porcine scFv antibodies by phage display and expression in *Escherichia coli*. *Vet. Immunol. Immunopathol.* 97, 39–51.

Li, H., Jiang, Y., Prak, E. L., Radic, M., and Weigert, M. (2001). Editors and editing of anti-DNA receptors. *Immunity* 15, 947–957.

Lo Conte, L. L., Chothia, C., and Janin, J. (1999). The atomic structure of protein-protein recognition sites. *J. Mol. Biol.* 285, 2177–2198.

MacCallum, R., Martin, A., and Thornton, J. (1996). Antibody-antigen interactions: contact analysis and binding site topography. *J. Mol. Biol.* 262, 732–745.

Maizels, N. (2005). Immunoglobulin gene diversification. *Annu. Rev. Genet.* 39, 23–46.

Marget, M., Sharma, B. B., Tesar, M., Kretzschmar, T., Jenisch, S., Westphal, E., et al. (2000). Bypassing hybridoma technology: HLA-C reactive human single-chain antibody fragments (scFv) derived from a synthetic phage display library (HuCAL) and their potential to discriminate HLA class I specificities. *Tissue Antigens* 56, 1–9.

Marks, J., Hoogenboom, H., Bonnert, T., McCafferty, J., Griffiths, A., and Winter, G. (1991). By-passing immunization. Human antibodies from V-gene libraries displayed on phage. *J. Mol. Biol.* 222, 581–597.

Martin, A. C., and Thornton, J. M. (1996). Structural families in loops of homologous proteins: automatic classification, modelling and application to antibodies. *J. Mol. Biol.* 263, 800–815.

Martinez-Jean, C., Folch, G., and Lefranc, M. (2001). Nomenclature and overview of the mouse (Mus musculus and Mus sp.) immunoglobulin kappa (IGK) genes. *Exp. Clin. Immunogenet.* 18, 255–279.

Matsuda, F., Ishii, K., Bourvagnet, P., Kuma, K., Hayashida, H., Miyata, T., and Honjo, T. (1998). The complete nucleotide sequence of the human immunoglobulin heavy chain variable region locus. *J. Exp. Med.* 188, 2151–2162.

McCafferty, J., Griffiths, A. D., Winter, G., and Chiswell, D. J. (1990). Phage antibodies: filamentous phage displaying antibody variable domains. *Nature* 348, 552–554.

Mian, I., Bradwell, A., and Olson, A. (1991). Structure, function and properties of antibody binding sites. *J. Mol. Biol.* 217, 133–151.

Morea, V., Tramontano, A., Rustici, M., Chothia, C., and Lesk, A. M. (1998). Conformations of the third hypervariable region in the VH domain of immunoglobulins. *J. Mol. Biol.* 275, 269–294.

Morrison, S. L., Johnson, M. J., Herzenberg, L. A., and Oi, V. T. (1984). Chimeric human antibody molecules: mouse antigen-binding domains with human constant region domains. *Proc. Natl. Acad. Sci. U.S.A.* 81, 6851–6855.

Muyldermans, S., Baral, T. N., Retamozzo, V. C., De Baetselier, P., De Genst, E., Kinne, J., et al. (2009). Camelid immunoglobulins and nanobody technology. *Vet. Immunol. Immunopathol.* 128, 178–183.

Muyldermans, S., and Lauwereys, M. (1999). Unique single-domain antigen binding fragments derived from naturally occurring camel heavy-chain antibodies. *J. Mol. Recognit.* 12, 131–140.

Nelson, A., Dhimolea, E., and Reichert, J. (2010). Development trends for human monoclonal antibody therapeutics. *Nat. Rev. Drug Discov.* 9, 767–774.

Neri, D., Petrul, H., and Roncucci, G. (1995). Engineering recombinant antibodies for immunotherapy. *Cell Biophys.* 27, 47–61.

Neri, D., Pini, A., and Nissim, A. (1998). Antibodies from phage display libraries as immunochemical reagents. *Methods Mol. Biol.* 80, 475–500.

Neuberger, M. S., and Milstein, C. (1995). Somatic hypermutation. *Curr. Opin. Immunol.* 7, 248–254.

Nguyen, V. K., Desmyter, A., and Muyldermans, S. (2001). Functional heavy-chain antibodies in Camelidae. *Adv. Immunol.* 79, 261–296.

Nguyen, V. K., Hamers, R., Wyns, L., and Muyldermans, S. (1999). Loss of splice consensus signal is responsible for the removal of the entire C (H)1 domain of the functional camel IGG2A heavy-chain antibodies. *Mol. Immunol.* 36, 515–524.

Nguyen, V. K., Su, C., Muyldermans, S., and van der Loo, W. (2002). Heavy-chain antibodies in Camelidae; a case of evolutionary innovation. *Immunogenetics* 54, 39–47.

Nishibori, N., Horiuchi, H., Furusawa, S., and Matsuda, H. (2006). Humanization of chicken monoclonal antibody using phage-display system. *Mol. Immunol.* 43, 634–642.

Noia, J. D., and Neuberger, M. (2007). Molecular mechanisms of antibody somatic hypermutation. *Annu. Rev. Biochem.* 76, 1–22.

North, B., Lehmann, A., and Dunbrack, R. J. (2011). A new clustering of antibody CDR loop conformations. *J. Mol. Biol.* 406, 228–256.

O'Brien, P. M., Aitken, R., O'Neil, B. W., and Campo, M. S. (1999). Generation of native bovine mAbs by phage display. *Proc. Natl. Acad. Sci. U.S.A.* 96, 640–645.

Ohara, R., Knappik, A., Shimada, K., Frisch, C., Ylera, F., and Koga, H. (2006). Antibodies for proteomic research: comparison of traditional immunization with recombinant antibody technology. *Proteomics* 6, 2638–2646.

Padlan, E. A. (1977). Structural basis for the specificity of antibody-antigen reactions and structural mechanisms for the diversification of antigen-binding specificities. *Q. Rev. Biophys.* 10, 35–65.

Padlan, E. A. (1994). Anatomy of the antibody molecule. *Mol. Immunol.* 31, 169–217.

Parvari, R., Avivi, A., Lentner, F., Ziv, E., Tel-Or, S., Burstein, Y., et al. (1988). Chicken immunoglobulin gamma-heavy chains: limited VH gene repertoire, combinatorial diversification by D gene segments and evolution of the heavy chain locus. *EMBO J.* 7, 739–744.

Parvari, R., Ziv, E., Lantner, F., Heller, D., and Schechter, I. (1990). Somatic diversification of chicken immunoglobulin light chains by point mutations. *Proc. Natl. Acad. Sci. U.S.A.* 87, 3072–3076.

Parvari, R., Ziv, E., Lantner, F., Tel-Or, S., Burstein, Y., and Schechter, I. (1987a). A few germline genes encode the variable regions of chicken immunoglobulin light and gamma-heavy chains. *Prog. Clin. Biol. Res.* 238, 15–26.

Parvari, R., Ziv, E., Lentner, F., Tel-Or, S., Burstein, Y., and Schechter, I. (1987b). Analyses of chicken immunoglobulin light chain cDNA clones indicate a few germline V lambda genes and allotypes of the C lambda locus. *EMBO J.* 6, 97–102.

Persson, H., Lantto, J., and Ohlin, M. (2006). A focused antibody library for improved hapten recognition. *J. Mol. Biol.* 357, 607–620.

Pini, A., Viti, F., Santucci, A., Carnemolla, B., Zardi, L., Neri, P., et al. (1998). Design and use of a phage display library. Human antibodies with subnanomolar affinity against a marker of angiogenesis eluted from a two-dimensional gel. *J. Biol. Chem.* 273, 21769–21776.

Prassler, J., Steidl, S., and Urlinger, S. (2009). *In vitro* affinity maturation of HuCAL antibodies: complementarity determining region exchange and RapMAT technology. *Immunotherapy* 1, 571–583.

Prassler, J., Thiel, S., Pracht, C., Polzer, A., Peters, S., Bauer, M., et al. (2011). HuCAL PLATINUM, a synthetic Fab library optimized for sequence diversity and superior performance in mammalian expression systems. *J. Mol. Biol.* 413, 261–278.

Raaphorst, F. M., Raman, C. S., Nall, B. T., and Teale, J. M. (1997). Molecular mechanisms governing reading frame choice of immunoglobulin diversity genes. *Immunol. Today* 18, 37–43.

Rada, C., Ehrenstein, M. R., Neuberger, M. S., and Milstein, C. (1998). Hot spot focusing of somatic hypermutation in MSH2-deficient mice suggests two stages of mutational targeting. *Immunity* 9, 135–141.

Rader, C., Ritter, G., Nathan, S., Elia, M., Gout, I., Jungbluth, A. A., et al. (2000). The rabbit antibody repertoire as a novel source for the generation of therapeutic human antibodies. *J. Biol. Chem.* 275, 13668–13676.

Ragunathan, G., Smart, J., Williams, J., and Almagro, J. (2012). Antigen-binding site anatomy and somatic mutations in antibodies that recognize different types of antigens. *J. Mol. Recognit.* 25, 103–113.

Rajewsky, K., Förster, I., and Cumano, A. (1987). Evolutionary and somatic selection of the antibody repertoire in the mouse. *Science* 238, 1088–1094.

Ramirez-Benitez, M. C., and Almagro, J. C. (2001). Analysis of antibodies of known structure suggests a lack of correspondence between the residues in contact with the antigen and those modified by somatic hypermutation. *Proteins* 45, 199–206.

Ratcliffe, M. J. (2006). Antibodies, immunoglobulin genes and the bursa of Fabricius in chicken B cell development. *Dev. Comp. Immunol.* 30, 101–118.

Reichert, J. (2012). Marketed therapeutic antibodies compendium. *MAbs* 4, 413–415.

Reynaud, C. A., Anquez, V., Dahan, A., and Weill, J. C. (1985). A single rearrangement event generates most of the chicken immunoglobulin light chain diversity. *Cell* 40, 283–291.

Reynaud, C. A., Anquez, V., Grimal, H., and Weill, J. C. (1987). A hyperconversion mechanism generates the chicken light chain preimmune repertoire. *Cell* 48, 379–388.

Reynaud, C. A., Anquez, V., and Weill, J. C. (1991). The chicken D locus and its contribution to the immunoglobulin heavy chain repertoire. *Eur. J. Immunol.* 21, 2661–2670.

Reynaud, C. A., Dahan, A., Anquez, V., and Weill, J. C. (1989). Somatic hyperconversion diversifies the single Vh gene of the chicken with a high incidence in the D region. *Cell* 59, 171–183.

Reynaud, C. A., Dahan, A., and Weill, J. C. (1983). Complete sequence of a chicken lambda light chain immunoglobulin derived from the nucleotide sequence of its mRNA. *Proc. Natl. Acad. Sci. U.S.A.* 80, 4099–4103.

Riechmann, L., and Muyldermans, S. (1999). Single domain antibodies: comparison of camel VH and camelised human VH domains. *J. Immunol. Methods* 231, 25–38.

Rothe, C., Urlinger, S., Lohning, C., Prassler, J., Stark, Y., Jager, U., et al. (2008). The human combinatorial antibody library HuCAL GOLD combines diversification of all six CDRs according to the natural immune system with a novel display method for efficient selection of high-affinity antibodies. *J. Mol. Biol.* 376, 1182–1200.

Sanz, I. (1991). Multiple mechanisms participate in the generation of diversity of human H chain CDR3 regions. *J. Immunol.* 147, 1720–1729.

Saphire, E., Parren, P., Pantophlet, R., Zwick, M., Morris, G., Rudd, P., et al. (2001). Crystal structure of a neutralizing human IGG against HIV-1: a template for vaccine design. *Science* 293, 1155–1159.

Schäble, K., Thiebe, R., Bensch, A., Brensing-Küppers, J., Heim, V., Kirschbaum, T., et al. (1999). Characteristics of the immunoglobulin Vkappa genes, pseudogenes, relics and orphons in the mouse genome. *Eur. J. Immunol.* 29, 2082–2086.

Schäble, K., Thiebe, R., Flügel, A., Meindl, A., and Zachau, H. (1994). The human immunoglobulin kappa locus: pseudogenes, unique and repetitive sequences. *Biol. Chem. Hoppe Seyler.* 375, 189–199.

Schroeder, H. W. Jr. (2006). Similarity and divergence in the development and expression of the mouse and human antibody repertoires. *Dev. Comp. Immunol.* 30, 119–135.

Schroeder, H. W. Jr., Hillson, J. L., and Perlmutter, R. M. (1987). Early restriction of the human antibody repertoire. *Science* 238, 791–793.

Schroeder, H. W. Jr., Hillson, J. L., and Perlmutter, R. M. (1990). Structure and evolution of mammalian VH families. *Int. Immunol.* 2, 41–50.

Schroeder, H. W. Jr., Ippolito, G. C., and Shiokawa, S. (1998). Regulation of the antibody repertoire through control of HCDR3 diversity. *Vaccine* 16, 1383–1390.

Schroeder, H. W. Jr., Mortari, F., Shiokawa, S., Kirkham, P. M., Elgavish, R. A., and Bertrand, F. E. 3rd. (1995). Developmental regulation of the human antibody repertoire. *Ann. N.Y. Acad. Sci.* 764, 242–260.

Shi, L., Wheeler, J. C., Sweet, R. W., Lu, J., Luo, J., Tornetta, M., et al. (2010). *De novo* selection of high-affinity antibodies from synthetic fab libraries displayed on phage as pIX fusion proteins. *J. Mol. Biol.* 397, 385–396.

Shirai, H., Kidera, A., and Nakamura, H. (1996). Structural classification of CDR-H3 in antibodies. *FEBS Lett.* 399, 1–8.

Sidhu, S. S., and Fellouse, F. A. (2006). Synthetic therapeutic antibodies. *Nat. Chem. Biol.* 2, 682–688.

Sidhu, S. S., Li, B., Chen, Y., Fellouse, F. A., Eigenbrot, C., and Fuh, G. (2004). Phage-displayed antibody libraries of synthetic heavy chain complementarity determining regions. *J. Mol. Biol.* 338, 299–310.

Silacci, M., Brack, S. S., Spath, N., Buck, A., Hillinger, S., Arni, S., et al. (2006). Human monoclonal antibodies to domain C of tenascin-C selectively target solid tumors *in vivo*. *Protein Eng. Des. Sel.* 19, 471–478.

Silacci, M., Brack, S., Schirru, G., Marlind, J., Ettorre, A., Merlo, A., et al. (2005). Design, construction, and characterization of a large synthetic human antibody phage display library. *Proteomics* 5, 2340–2350.

Sinclair, M. C., Gilchrist, J., and Aitken, R. (1997). Bovine IgG repertoire is dominated by a single diversified VH gene family. *J. Immunol.* 159, 3883–3889.

Smith, G. P. (1985). Filamentous fusion phage: novel expression vectors that display cloned antigens on the virion surface. *Science* 228, 1315–1317.

Stanfield, R. L., Dooley, H., Flajnik, M. F., and Wilson, I. A. (2004). Crystal structure of a shark single-domain antibody V region in complex with lysozyme. *Science* 305, 1770–1773.

Stanfield, R. L., Dooley, H., Verdino, P., Flajnik, M. F., and Wilson, I. A. (2007). Maturation of shark single-domain (IgNAR) antibodies: evidence for induced-fit binding. *J. Mol. Biol.* 367, 358–372.

Stanfield, R. L., and Wilson, I. A. (2010). "Antibody molecular structure," in *Therapeutic Monoclonal Antibodies: From Bench to Clinic,* ed Z. An (John Wiley and Sons, Inc.), 51–66.

Stephens, S., Emtage, S., Vetterlein, O., Chaplin, L., Bebbington, C., Nesbitt, A., et al. (1995). Comprehensive pharmacokinetics of a humanized antibody and analysis of residual anti-idiotypic responses. *Immunology* 85, 668–674.

Thiebe, R., Schäble, K., Bensch, A., Brensing-Küppers, J., Heim, V., Kirschbaum, T., et al. (1999). The variable genes and gene families of the mouse immunoglobulin kappa locus. *Eur. J. Immunol.* 29, 2072–2081.

Tomlinson, I. M., Cox, J. P., Herardi, G. E., Lesk, A. M., and Chothia, C. (1995). The structural repertoire of the human V kappa domain. *EMBO J.* 14, 4628–4638.

Tomlinson, I. M., Walter, G., Jones, P. T., Dear, P. H., Sonnhammer, E. L., Winter, G. (1996). The imprint of somatic hypermutation on the repertoire of human germline V genes. *J. Mol. Biol.* 256, 813–817.

Tomlinson, I. M., Walter, G., Marks, J. D., Llewelyn, M. B., and Winter, G. (1992). The repertoire of human germline VH sequences reveals about fifty groups of VH segments with different hypervariable loops. *J. Mol. Biol.* 227, 776–798.

Tonegawa, S. (1983). Somatic generation of antibody diversity. *Nature* 14, 575–581.

Tsurushita, N., Park, M., Pakabunto, K., Ong, K., Avdalovic, A., Fu, H., et al. (2004). Humanization of a chicken anti-IL-12 monoclonal antibody. *J. Immunol. Methods* 295, 9–19.

Vandenbroucke, K., de Haard, H., Beirnaert, E., Dreier, T., Lauwereys, M., Huyck, L., et al. (2010). Orally administered L. lactis secreting an anti-TNF Nanobody demonstrate efficacy in chronic colitis. *Mucosal Immunol.* 3, 49–56.

Vargas-Madrazo, E., Lara-Ochoa, F., and Almagro, J. C. (1995). Canonical structure repertoire of the antigen-binding site of immunoglobulins suggests strong geometrical restrictions associated to the mechanism of immune recognition. *J. Mol. Biol.* 254, 497–504.

Virnekas, B., Ge, L., Pluckthun, A., Schneider, K. C., Wellnhofer, G., and Moroney, S. E. (1994). Trinucleotide phosphoramidites: ideal reagents for the synthesis of mixed oligonucleotides for random mutagenesis. *Nucleic Acids Res.* 22, 5600–5607.

Viti, F., Nilsson, F., Demartis, S., Huber, A., and Neri, D. (2000). Design and use of phage display libraries for the selection of antibodies and enzymes. *Meth. Enzymol.* 326, 480–505.

Weill, J. C., and Reynaud, C. A. (1992). Early B-cell development in chickens, sheep and rabbits. *Curr. Opin. Immunol.* 4, 177–180.

Weinstein, J., Jiang, N., White, R. R., Fisher, D., and Quake, S. (2009). High-throughput sequencing of the zebrafish antibody repertoire. *Science* 324, 807–810.

Wesolowski, J., Alzogaray, V., Reyelt, J., Unger, M., Juarez, K., Urrutia, M., et al. (2009). Single domain antibodies: promising experimental and therapeutic tools in infection and immunity. *Med. Microbiol. Immunol.* 198, 157–174.

Williams, A., and Barclay, A. (1988). The immunoglobulin superfamily–domains for cell surface recognition. *Annu. Rev. Immunol.* 6, 381–405.

Wilson, I. A., and Stanfield, R. L. (1994). Antibody-antigen interactions: new structures and new conformational changes. *Curr. Opin. Struct. Biol.* 4, 857–867.

Wilson, P. C., Bouteiller, O. D., Liu, Y.-J., Potter, K., Banchereau, J., Capra, J. D., et al. (1998). Somatic hypermutation introduces insertions and deletions into immunoglobulin V genes. *J. Exp. Med.* 187, 59–70.

Wong, S. E., Sellers, B. D., and Jacobson, M. P. (2011). Effects of somatic mutations on CDR loop flexibility during affinity maturation. *Proteins* 79, 821–829.

Wu, L., Oficjalska, K., Lambert, M., Fennell, B. J., Darmanin-Sheehan, A., Ni Shuilleabhain, D., et al. (2011). Fundamental characteristics of the immunoglobulin VH repertoire of chickens in comparison with those of humans, mice, and camelids. *J. Immunol.* 188, 322–333.

Wu, T., Johnson, G., and Kabat, E. (1993). Length distribution of CDRH3 in antibodies. *Proteins* 16, 1–7.

Wu, T. T., and Kabat, E. A. (1970). An analysis of the sequences of the variable regions of Bence Jones proteins and myeloma light chains and their implications for antibody complementarity. *J. Exp. Med.* 132, 211–250.

Yamanaka, H. I., Inoue, T., and Ikeda-Tanaka, O. (1996). Chicken monoclonal antibody isolated by a phage display system. *J. Immunol.* 157, 1156–1162.

Zemlin, M., Klinger, M., Link, J., Zemlin, C., Bauer, K., Engler, J. A., et al. (2003). Expressed murine and human CDR-H3 intervals of equal length exhibit distinct repertoires that differ in their amino acid composition and predicted range of structures. *J. Mol. Biol.* 334, 733–749.

Zhai, W., Glanville, J., Fuhrmann, M., Mei, L., Ni, I., Sundar, P. D., et al. (2011). Synthetic antibodies designed on natural sequence landscapes. *J. Mol. Biol.* 412, 55–71.

Zhao, S., and Lu, J. (2010). A germline knowledge based computational approach for determining antibody complementarity determining regions. *Mol. Immunol.* 47, 694–700.

Zhu, D., Lossos, C., Chapman-Fredricks, J., Matthews, J., Ikpatt, O., Ruiz, P., et al. (2011). Biased use of the IGHV4 family and evidence for antigen selection in *Chlamydophila psittaci*-negative ocular adnexal extranodal marginal zone lymphomas. *PLoS ONE* 6:e29114. doi: 10.1371/journal.pone.0029114

17

Dynamical and mechanistic reconstructive approaches of T lymphocyte dynamics: using visual modeling languages to bridge the gap between immunologists, theoreticians, and programmers

Véronique Thomas-Vaslin[1,2]*, Adrien Six[1,2], Jean-Gabriel Ganascia[3,4] and Hugues Bersini[5]

[1] UPMC Univ Paris 06, UMR7211, Immunology, Immunopathology, Immunotherapy (I3), Integrative Immunology, Paris, France
[2] CNRS, UMR 7211, Immunology-Immunopathology-Immunotherapy (I3) Integrative Immunology, Paris, France
[3] UPMC Univ Paris 06, UMR 7606, ACASA-LIP6, Paris, France
[4] CNRS, UMR 7606, ACASA-LIP6, CNRS, Paris, France
[5] Université Libre de Bruxelles, IRIDIA-Code, Bruxelles, Belgium

Edited by:
Rob J. de Boer, Utrecht University, Netherlands

Reviewed by:
Christopher E. Rudd, University of Cambridge, UK
Yoram Louzoun, Bar-Ilan University, Israel
Hillel Kugler, Microsoft Research, UK

***Correspondence:**
Véronique Thomas-Vaslin, UMR 7211, Immunology, Immunopathology, Immunotherapy, Integrative Immunology, UPMC-CNRS, 83 Boulevard de l'Hôpital, Paris 75013, France
e-mail: veronique.thomas-vaslin@upmc.fr

Dynamic modeling of lymphocyte behavior has primarily been based on populations based differential equations or on cellular agents moving in space and interacting each other. The final steps of this modeling effort are expressed in a code written in a programing language. On account of the complete lack of standardization of the different steps to proceed, we have to deplore poor communication and sharing between experimentalists, theoreticians and programmers. The adoption of diagrammatic visual computer language should however greatly help the immunologists to better communicate, to more easily identify the models similarities and facilitate the reuse and extension of existing software models. Since immunologists often conceptualize the dynamical evolution of immune systems in terms of "state-transitions" of biological objects, we promote the use of unified modeling language (UML) state-transition diagram. To demonstrate the feasibility of this approach, we present a UML refactoring of two published models on thymocyte differentiation. Originally built with different modeling strategies, a mathematical ordinary differential equation-based model and a cellular automata model, the two models are now in the same visual formalism and can be compared.

Keywords: state-transition diagram, computer modeling, cell dynamics, agent-based model, complex system

The perspective is to encourage immunologists involved into mathematical modeling or software productions, to adopt a visual graphical language, here mainly the unified modeling language (UML) "state-transition" diagram to ease the communication, the reuse and the extension of their models.

COMPLEXITY OF THE IMMUNE SYSTEM

The immune system is a complex biological adaptive, highly diversified, robust and resilient system, characterized by complexity at different levels. Lymphocytes are the central actors of the immune system, in the middle of a multi-scale biological organization, "from molecule to organism". Multi-scale modeling remains a challenge, as for other biological systems (1). Despite recent systems biology initiatives to understand and model the immune system (2), we are still far from having the appropriate tools to understand its dynamics and to easily communicate among various researchers who observe this system at different levels of granularity and attempt through software modeling to answer different questions. Several complementary experimental methods and models have been used to explore lymphocyte dynamics and turnover (3, 4) and to model it in health, aging and diseases (5).

DRAWBACKS OF CURRENT DYNAMICS LYMPHOCYTE MODELING AND EVOLUTION

System dynamics models deal with time, formalized with two distinct concepts as "discrete time," by a succession of time points and intervals, or as "continuous time" (6). Models of lymphocyte population dynamics and turnover (3) have primarily been based on mechanistic reconstruction with continuous time models. The fluxes of cell populations are then described by differential equations. These mathematical models describe for example the thymocyte differentiation and selection (7), until the thymic export (8–10), the homeostasis of CD4/CD8 T cells (11, 12), the CD8 immune response (13, 14), or the Bromodeoxyuridine or deuterium labeling (15) to account for turnover. Up to now, simulations and validation of some of these models reveal interesting T cell dynamics properties: how the system grows, self-maintains as well as the effects of perturbations, i.e. how the system reacts to antigens, collapses and reorganizes. However, integrating the heterogeneity of cell populations, phenotypes, lineages, cell location and interactions, cell differentiation across generations (16) in the different biological, and time scales, is problematic in such a mathematical form, which make these models particularly difficult to handle.

The evolution of homogeneous mathematical model of cell populations (17) toward "spatialized," discrete, and heterogeneous software models (18) has allowed the reproduction and observation of more detailed and thus complex behaviors. For example, this made possible to model lymphocyte dynamics from thymic selection (19, 20) up to quantitative modeling of immune responses, as extensively reviewed (21) with development of agent-based and automata models (22). However, both population-based mathematical model (a top-down approach) and discrete cell-based model (a bottom-up approach) and the various platforms developed have limitations (23). Conversely, the Statecharts language (24) and the visual reactive tools (25) such as biocharts (26) and reactive animation applied to various systems (27) developed by Harel et al. are a powerful way to simulate complex dynamical biological behavior with more didactic representation than equations. Such models have revealed emergent properties during thymic differentiation (28) pancreatic islet organogenesis but also the immune response in lymph node (29).

LACK OF INTEROPERABILITY, UNDER-USE OF SOFTWARE MODELS

Although in Immunology there is more than 20-years tradition of software and mathematical modeling, very few of them have been the object of further exploitation once published and made available (30). Models are often under-used because experimentalists can be reluctant to entertain mathematical formalization and because published models are largely disposable: rapidly forgotten after being published, instead of providing a foundation to build upon. Moreover, the various expressions of these models with different mathematical descriptions, programing languages, software libraries and graphical packages, require much effort in understanding and running the software and prevent interoperability.

USING VISUAL LANGUAGE TO COMMUNICATE AND EXECUTE MODELS

Immunologists often conceptualize the dynamical evolution of their systems in terms of "state-transitions" of biological objects and do it by means of personalized and informal graphical illustrations. Thus, the adoption of a more formal and standard type of state-transition diagram could improve the current situation to not only help biologists to better understand each other but also to facilitate the production and the reading of software code executing these visual transitions, at level of populations or agents (31).

Thus, in this paper, we promote the development and usage of a visual, computational approach more comprehensible than mathematical equations and programing instructions. This should improve our understanding of lymphocyte dynamics, the exchange on this understanding and simplify the implementation of models by non-specialists delivered from the production of executable code or mathematical equations, to concentrate to *in silico* experiments.

LEVEL OF ABSTRACTION AND MULTI-SCALE MODELING

A model describes a complex system from the "real word" and thus requires abstraction. This abstraction is performed as the immunologist decides about an experimental protocol in order to observe selected objects at different scales and to follow them in time and space. For example, the capacities of the immune system to preserve the homeostasis and to provide rapid adaptation to an antigen and anamnestic responses can be observed at the organism level, through physiological or pathological clinical observations that relate to lower scale levels. At molecular level, the somatic generation of the diversity of an immuno-receptor, as the TCR, allows for a dynamic network of interactions with antigens. At the cell level, this leads to clonal selection, activation and division. At the organ level, the fluidity of the system insures constant tissue redistribution of cells and molecules, cell migration from thymus to spleen and lymph nodes.

Thus, models of lymphocyte population dynamics and turnover consist in reconstructing the components or "entities" of the system across various scales, from molecules to organisms, to determine the relations/interactions through space (varying from micrometer to meters) and "processes" through time (varying between microseconds to years) as explained below. However, the formalization and abstraction of the immune objects as entities undergoing processes, with the help of spatial and dynamic ontologies, respectively defined as SNAP and SPAN (32), as well as cell/molecule interactions (33), is rarely done, maintaining a language-barrier between biologists and theoreticians. In the following, some examples will be given to help the immunologists with the transition between current mathematical models to computer ones and with the terms currently used in modeling.

DEFINE ENTITIES, STATES, LOCATION, INTERACTIONS, GRANULARITY

The immune "entities" could be described according to the language used by the modeler. A cell exists in one "state": it could be quiescent or in a given phase of the cell cycle or dead. In addition the phenotype and/or a function of a cell define a given state, as CD4 helper T cells. Cells are "located" in various tissues and are in "relation" with other entities. Finally, cells can be considered at various level of "granularity." For example, T lymphocyte populations are "aggregation" of T cells according to criteria of phenotype, structure or function, although heterogeneity still prevails inside these populations at lower granularity. Accordingly, cells can be modeled at population level (with continuous model as ordinary equation) or at cell level according to space (with discrete model as automata or multi-agent system).

DEFINE PROCESSES

According to ontologies, cells participate to various processes, such as division, activation, differentiation, interaction, clonotype selection, apoptosis or migration. According to the states of the cells, their evolution can thus be modeled as "state-transition" that can be applied to various processes in parallel: for example, a thymocyte can differentiate while migrating in cortex and medulla. Note that processes at other levels like molecular or organ levels can similarly be described and modeled. Finally, all these process will determine the global cell dynamics and turnover.

THE UNIFIED MODELING LANGUAGE FOR HIGH-LEVEL MODELING

"High-level programing languages" are based on abstraction and use of natural language that is easier to understand as compared to "low level programing language," based on codes. Thus, visual modeling language considers biological-object as conceptual abstract-objects that endure processes. The level of abstraction allowed by these diagrams makes possible to distinguish more easily the "entities" as T cells and the "processes" that occur at different levels such as differentiation, migration and cell cycle. Moreover, such "state-transition diagrams" allow computing parallel pathways at various scales to avoid redundancy that is inherent in the formal description of multi-level, heterogeneous and concurrent systems and to model heterogeneity in a very simplified and economical form (as compared to mathematical equations) (31).We have thus used the well-established Unified Modelling Language (UML – a sofware standard) that still remains approachable to the lab-immunologist, convenient for the theoretician and that can be directly adopted for the high-level graphical depiction (31, 34). The adoption of UML state-transition diagrams that transcends any programing language or computer platform, will allow both experimentalists and theorists to work together at a higher level than writing software code or mathematical equations. This final step is progressively more and more automatized out of the diagrams. Example of basic transformations of mathematical equations into state-transition diagrams including elementary, parallel, independent, or coupled state transition have been given (31), to familiarize biologists with the general approach.

REFACTORING FROM LOW LEVEL (CODE, EQUATIONS) TO HIGH-LEVEL (DIAGRAM) MODELING LANGUAGES

To convince the immunologist of the feasibility of this approach as well as the benefit gained by adopting it, we sketch in the rest of the paper how existing "low level programed" immune models should gain in readability and accessibility by adopting a "high-level graphical" representation under the form of "state-transition diagrams." We present a "refactoring" of two published models of T cell biology in the thymus. Refactoring consists in restructuring the code or equations of a model to improve its expression, readability and extensibility, without changing its external behavior. One model consists in cell population differentiation modeling with differential equations (continuous model). The other one is a discrete model. Originally it was an automata model consisting of a discrete lattice, where each site (cell) in a given state, follows some rules in space and time that depends on local neighbors (18). It has been refactorized as an agent-based model (ABM), depicting individual cell behavior through thymus differentiation and migration. It would be much too long and redundant to describe in details the behavior of these two models. We do not pretend here to modify at all the results obtained by the running of these models (the readers interested in these results are invited to access the original papers). We have just reshape them into a state-transition diagrammatic form that allows execution of simulations reproducing the original results with similar parameter values.

POPULATION-BASED MODEL DESCRIBING THE CONVEYOR-BELT T CELL DIFFERENTIATION IN THYMUS

The original model (8) is a compartmentalized ordinary differential equation (ODE) model, rather complex to read and manage by immunologists. This model reflects the conceptual "conveyor belt" model of thymic T cell differentiation, schematically represented by immunologists by the continuous ordered transition of cells through the different stages with time (35–37). **Figure 1** represents a biological schema, originally published and the "state-transition" description of the model (in a UML state-transition diagram) as it is proposed now. Although the original model is composed of 30 differential equations, the whole mathematical description and the code that captures it, can easily be deduced and regenerated from the **Figure 1**. Conversely, the mathematical equations can be automatically generated from the state-transition diagram as previously described (38). In essence, the model is summarized by the input, transition and output from the thymus, by "parallel processes" that occur concomitantly, as differentiation, cell cycle, proliferation and death, and by exit from the thymus. Note that these parallel processes concern various biological levels and time scales. The "differentiation" process represents each stage of the conveyor belt, from double negative (DN) to single positive (SP) cells, with flows into and from a particular stage according to the general equation:

$$dx_i/dt = 2\gamma\, px_{i-1} - \left(p + d + u\,(i)\right)x_i$$

p, d, and u represent proliferation, death, and differentiation, respectively, and x_i represents the ith stage. The model mainly consists of constant hematopoietic progenitor influx in thymus (Sn); differentiation between thymocyte developmental phenotypes DN and double-positive (DP) cells differentiation into $CD4^+$ or $CD8^+$ cells, then egression of SP stage, either, to the periphery [Us4(i), Us8(i)]; proliferation [Pn(y), Pp(y), and Ps(y)]; positive and negative selection (a4, a8); and natural cell death (Dn, Dp, and Ds). In parallel, the "cell cycle" is represented: the cell switches between quiescence (G0) and cycle with division (S/M). The parameter γ set to 1 represents the cell division into two daughter cells. There is the possibility to induce a perturbation into the system through the specific depletion of T cells entering the S/M cycle phase (p), if γ is set to 0. This represents the presence or absence of a pharmacogenetic conditional treatment by ganciclovir that induces apoptosis related to the incorporation of a nucleotide analog during DNA elongation. This rule applies to all cell populations except in late DP quiescent cells as indicated in the schema. The "proliferation" depicts that the daughters of a proliferating cell transit into the next generational compartment, except during treatment ($\gamma = 0$) when dividing cells die by apoptosis and are lost from the model. The parameter u is an increasing function of generation (G1 to n), making cells more likely to differentiate between phenotypic compartments as they progress through the cell generations.

The parallelism in this graphical model largely simplifies the original formulation of ODEs while remaining faithful to it. Hierarchy and compound states are present again clearly reducing the diagram clutter. Other representation of the model depicting the differentiation with linear cell generations is also possible (31).

DISCRETE MODEL DESCRIBING THE DIFFERENTIATION ALONG THE MIGRATION OF T CELLS IN THE THYMUS IN A 2-D ENVIRONMENT

The original model (20) is a discrete-based "cellular automata" computer model. The model depicts the behavior of individual thymocytes that evolve in the 2-D epithelial cell network, guided by chemokines gradients. The current model (**Figure 2**) is now an Agent-Based Model (ABM). Again, the interested reader is referred to the original paper for a detailed understanding of the simulation. Although available for download, the 40 pages of FORTRAN source code are far from easy to understand. After refactoring, the transition rules of any agent (thymocytes) map onto a parallel

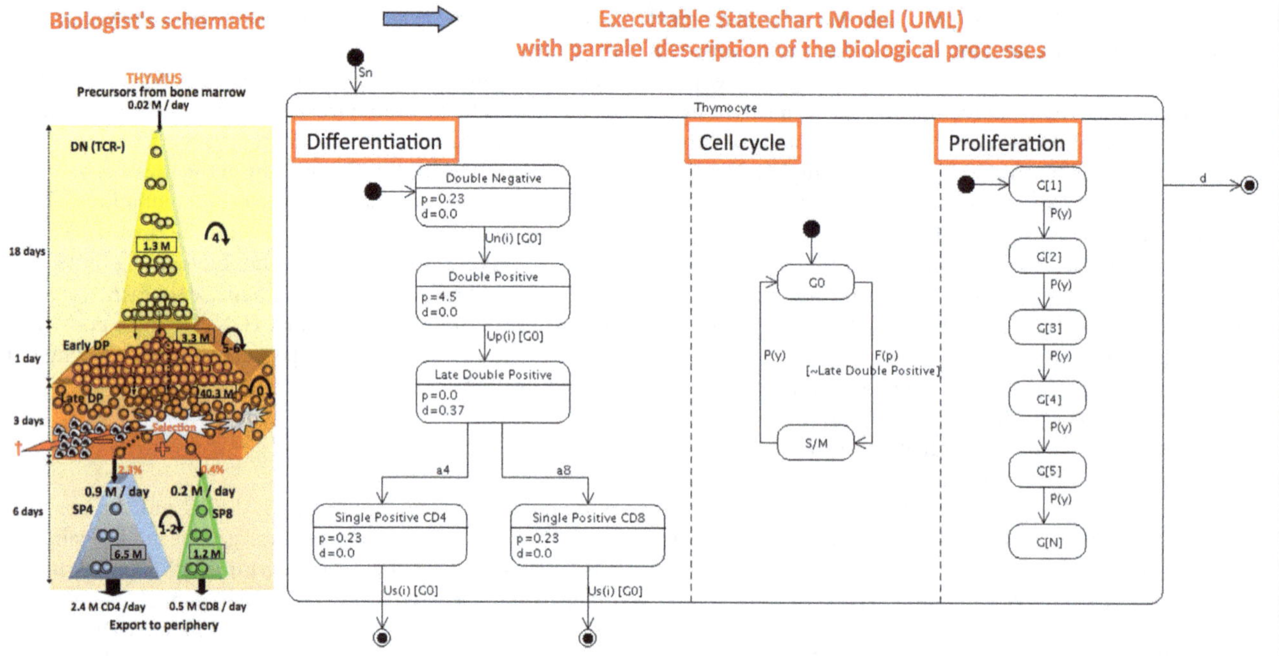

FIGURE 1 | Refactoring the continuous population (ODE) conveyor-belt model of thymocyte differentiation (8) into a computer executable visual language: The «biological schema »of thymocyte dynamics originally proposed is transformed into a UML state-transition diagram. This diagram represents the evolution of cell populations in the thymus, represented by their state from DN to SP, with UML figuration of the input (close circle arrow) and output representing death and thymus exit (open circle arrow) and transitions (oriented arrows). Parallel processes (underlined with red box) as differentiation, cell cycle and proliferation are depicted more explicitly in this representation than with the original 30 mathematical equations. Annotation with the proliferation and death rates values indicated in each state are values from the best scenario observed in the original paper.

state-transition diagram. The conception of the state-transition diagram, as done here, should considerably improve the understanding of the model (even for the original programmer) allowing the researchers to progress further with the existing simulator. A complete description of the model includes additional implementation details that are abstractions of the mechanisms behind cell decisions to differentiate. The parallel state-transition diagram represents the different simultaneous transitions taking place in the model and coded as various cellular automata rules: a cell in the model as it differentiates transits in successive states, it may be bound or not to thymic epithelial cells via TCR/MHC, it moves and may be located into one of several anatomical compartments of the thymus. As indicated in the boxes, the gradient of chemokines (k) orients the migration of cells for each specific stage of differentiation, and chemokines are localized in specific areas of the thymus. A T cell sums up the time and number of interactions with the same or different epithelial cells. This sum value determines whether the T cell is positively or negatively selected. DP and SP phenotypes have their own threshold parameters. They cannot differentiate until they cross a threshold number of interactions. If, after a given time, a DP cell has not reached this threshold, it enters apoptosis by neglect. If the time is too long, it is negatively selected. A threshold parameter simulates the phenotype decision. With this “signal-duration” hypothesis, long duration TCR-MHC interactions promote the CD4 phenotype and short duration promotes the CD8 phenotype.

It is important to notice that both refactored models, population-based and ABM can now be compared, are directly executable and can provide simulations of physiology, pathologies, and treatment, while not being the scope of this paper. Moreover, their parameters can be automatically tuned to fit experimental data. Any ABM model can also be run as a population version to save time in simulation (McEwan et al., manuscript in preparation). Moreover, the flexibility of these diagrams allows assembling the parts of the biological puzzle piece after piece and improving the models.

PERSPECTIVES

As shown here, state-transition diagrams can represent high-level semantics suitable to clarify immunological concepts and to aid communication among interdisciplinary researchers. It can also represent low levels quantitative information suitable for individual-based ABM and population-based ODE modeling. Organization of immune knowledge using a standardized, diagrammatic formal language should greatly improve knowledge integration at multi-scale levels and sharing between experimentalist and theoretician collaborators, rendering their software more readable, scalable, and usable. We are currently working on ways of automatically generating executable code out of these state-transition diagrams. State-transition diagrams supports the extension and interoperability of published models. This will help for dynamic computational modeling of lymphocyte behavior

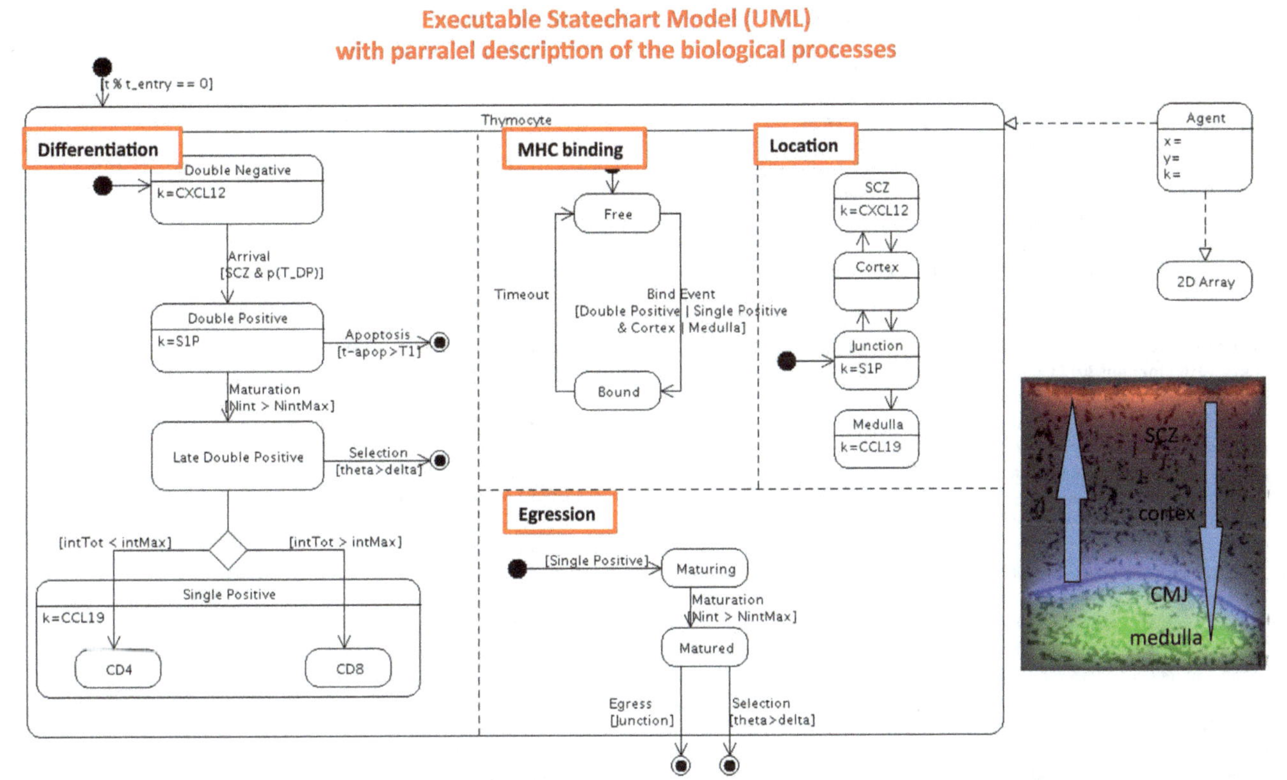

FIGURE 2 | Refactoring the automata single-cell model of thymocyte differentiation and migration (20) into a computer executable visual language. The 40 pages of Fortran code is transformed in computer UML state-transition diagram. This diagrams describes the experimentally observable heterogeneity, and the biologically relevant parallel processes (underlined in red box). As in **Figure 1**, input, output, and oriented transitions are described in the state-transition diagram. Parallel state-transitions represent the evolution of single cells in the thymus, represented by their differentiation from DN to SP stage, sequential binding event of TCR/MHC peptide on epithelial cells, thymic location, egression of cell when matured. Additional qualitative abstractions for computational model of individual cells in semi-realistic environment are represented by the 2-D array: cells are allowed migrating sequentially through the epithelial cell network (black network) across the various thymic areas, guided by chemokine gradients CXCL12 (red), CCL19/CCL21 (green), S1P (blue).

in health and diseases, and for "*in silico*" experiments to predict and explain the puzzling T cells dynamics and the effect of immunological perturbations.

AUTHOR CONTRIBUTIONS

Véronique Thomas-Vaslin and Hugues Bersini designed the project and wrote the article, Adrien Six and Jean-Gabriel Ganascia participated to discussions.

ACKNOWLEDGMENTS

The authors thank C. McEwan for computer modeling developments and discussions, B. Zerath, B. Horsmans for early refactoring of models, W. Chaara, and E. Mariotti-Ferrandiz from critical reading of the manuscript. Hugues Bersini is an invited Professor at UPMC. Financial supports: Emergence-UPMC program, PHC Tournesol EGIDE, CNRS PEPS BMI, Investissements d'Avenir program (ANR-11-IDEX-0004-02), LabEx Transimmunom.

REFERENCES

1. Lavelle C, Berry H, Beslon G, Ginelli F, Giavitto J, Kapoula Z, et al. From molecules to organisms: towards multiscale integrated models of biological systems. *Theor Biol Insights* (2008) **1**:13–22.
2. Germain RN, Meier-Schellersheim M, Nita-Lazar A, Fraser ID. Systems biology in immunology: a computational modeling perspective (*). *Annu Rev Immunol* (2011) **29**:527–85. doi:10.1146/annurev-immunol-030409-101317
3. Thomas-Vaslin V, Six A, Bellier B, Klatzmann D. Lymphocytes dynamics repertoires, modeling. In: Dubitzky W, Wolkenhauer O, Cho KH, Yokota H, editors. *Encyclopedia of Systems Biology*. New York: Springer (2013). p. 1149–62. doi:10.1007/978-1-4419-9863-7_96
4. Thomas-Vaslin V, Six A, Bellier B, Klatzmann D. Lymphocyte dynamics and repertoire, biological methods. In: Dubitzky W, Wolkenhauer O, Cho KH, Yokota H, editors. *Encyclopedia of Systems Biology*. New York: Springer (2013). p. 1145–49. doi:10.1007/978-1-4419-9863-7_95
5. Asquith B, Borghans JA, Ganusov VV, Macallan DC. Lymphocyte kinetics in health and disease. *Trends Immunol* (2009) **30**(4):182–9. doi:10.1016/j.it.2009.07.013
6. Ossimitz G, Mrotzek M. The basics of system dynamics: discrete vs. continuous modelling of time. *Proceedings of the 26th International Conference of the System Dynamics Society*. Wiley-Blackwell (July 2008) (2008). Available from: http://teoriasistemas.mex.tl/imagesnew/6/6/4/5/2/SimulaciondiscretavsContinua.pdf
7. Mehr R, Globerson A, Perelson AS. Modeling positive and negative selection and differentiation processes in the thymus. *J Theor Biol* (1995) **175**(1):103–26. doi:10.1006/jtbi.1995.0124
8. Thomas-Vaslin V, Altes HK, de Boer RJ, Klatzmann D. Comprehensive assessment and mathematical modeling of T cell population dynamics and homeostasis. *J Immunol* (2008) **180**(4):2240–50.

9. Bains I, Thiebaut R, Yates AJ, Callard R. Quantifying thymic export: combining models of naive T cell proliferation and TCR excision circle dynamics gives an explicit measure of thymic output. *J Immunol* (2009) **183**(7):4329–36. doi:10.4049/jimmunol.0900743
10. den Braber I, Mugwagwa T, Vrisekoop N, Westera L, Mögling R, de Boer AB, et al. Maintenance of peripheral naive T cells is sustained by thymus output in mice but not humans. *Immunity* (2012) **36**(2):288–97. doi:10.1016/j.immuni.2012.02.006
11. Mehr R, Perelson AS. Blind T-cell homeostasis and the CD4/CD8 ratio in the thymus and peripheral blood. *J Acquir Immune Defic Syndr Hum Retrovirol* (1997) **14**(5):387–98. doi:10.1097/00042560-199704150-00001
12. Almeida AR, Amado IF, Reynolds J, Berges J, Lythe G, Molina-París C, et al. Quorum-sensing in CD4+ T cell homeostasis: a hypothesis and a model. *Front Immunol* (2012) **3**:125. doi:10.3389/fimmu.2012.00125
13. Chao DL, Davenport MP, Forrest S, Perelson AS. A stochastic model of cytotoxic T cell responses. *J Theor Biol* (2004) **228**(2):227–40. doi:10.1016/j.jtbi.2003.12.011
14. Terry E, Marvel J, Arpin C, Gandrillon O, Crauste F. Mathematical model of the primary CD8 T cell immune response: stability analysis of a nonlinear age-structured system. *J Math Biol* (2012) **65**(2):263–91. doi:10.1007/s00285-011-0459-8
15. De Boer RJ, Perelson AS, Ribeiro RM. Modelling deuterium labelling of lymphocytes with temporal and/or kinetic heterogeneity. *J R Soc Interface* (2012) **9**(74):2191–200. doi:10.1098/rsif.2012.0149
16. Yamanaka YJ, Gierahn TM, Love JC. The dynamic lives of T cells: new approaches and themes. *Trends Immunol* (2013) **34**(2):59–66. doi:10.1016/j.it.2012.10.006
17. Louzoun Y. The evolution of mathematical immunology. *Immunol Rev* (2007) **216**:9–20.
18. Celada F, Seiden PE. A computer model of cellular interactions in the immune system. *Immunol Today* (1992) **13**:56. doi:10.1016/0167-5699(92)90135-T
19. Morpurgo D, Serentha R, Seiden PE, Celada F. Modelling thymic functions in a cellular automaton. *Int Immunol* (1995) **7**(4):505–16. doi:10.1093/intimm/7.4.505
20. Souza-e-Silva H, Savino W, Feijoo RA, Vasconcelos AT. A cellular automata-based mathematical model for thymocyte development. *PLoS One* (2009) **4**(12):e8233. doi:10.1371/journal.pone.0008233
21. Cohn M, Mata J. Quantitative modeling of immune responses. *Immunol Rev* (2007) **216**(1):5–8.
22. Chavali AK, Gianchandani EP, Tung KS, Lawrence MB, Peirce SM, Papin JA. Characterizing emergent properties of immunological systems with multi-cellular rule-based computational modeling. *Trends Immunol* (2008) **29**(12):589–99. doi:10.1016/j.it.2008.08.006
23. Bianca C, Pennisi M. Immune system modelling by top-down and bottom-up approaches. *Int Math Forum* (2012) **7**(3):109–28.
24. Harel D. Statecharts: a visual formalism for complex systems. *Sci Comput Program* (1987) **8**(3):231–74. doi:10.1016/0167-6423(87)90035-9
25. Efroni S, Harel D, Cohen IR. Toward rigorous comprehension of biological complexity: modeling, execution, and visualization of thymic T-cell maturation. *Genome Res* (2003) **13**(11):2485–97. doi:10.1101/gr.1215303
26. Kugler H, Larjo A, Harel D. Biocharts: a visual formalism for complex biological systems. *J R Soc Interface* (2010) **7**(48):1015–24. doi:10.1098/rsif.2009.0457
27. Vainas O, Harel D, Cohen IR, Efroni S. Reactive animation: from piecemeal experimentation to reactive biological systems. *Autoimmunity* (2011) **44**(4):271–81. doi:10.3109/08916934.2010.523260
28. Efroni S, Harel D, Cohen IR. Emergent dynamics of thymocyte development and lineage determination. *PLoS Comput Biol* (2007) **3**(1):e13. doi:10.1371/journal.pcbi.0030013
29. Swerdlin NI, Cohen IR, Harel D. The lymph node B cell immune response: dynamic analysis in-silico. *Proc IEEE* (2008) **96**(8):1421–43. doi:10.1109/JPROC.2008.925435
30. Bersini H, editor. Object-oriented refactoring of existing immune models. In: *Artificial Immune Systems. Lecture notes in Computer Science*. Berlin: Springer-Verlag (2009). p. 27–40.
31. Bersini H, Klatzmann D, Six A, Thomas-Vaslin V. State-transition diagrams for biologists. *PLoS One* (2012) **7**(7):e41165. doi:10.1371/journal.pone.0041165
32. Grenon P, Smith B. SNAP and SPAN: towards dynamic spatial ontology. *Spat Cogn Comput* (2004) **4**(1):69–104. doi:10.1207/s15427633scc0401_5
33. Pappalardo F, Lefranc MP, Lollini PL, Motta S. A novel paradigm for cell and molecule interaction ontology: from the CMM model to IMGT-ONTOLOGY. *Immunome Res* (2010) **6**(1):1. doi:10.1186/1745-7580-6-1
34. Bersini H. UML for ABM. *J Artif Soc Soc Simul* (2012) **15**(1):
35. Penit C, Vasseur F. Sequential events in thymocyte differentiation and thymus regeneration revealed by a combination of bromodeoxyuridine DNA labeling and antimitotic drug treatment. *J Immunol* (1988) **140**(10):3315–23.
36. Penit C, Lucas B, Vasseur F. Cell expansion and growth arrest phases during the transition from precursor (CD4-8-) to immature (CD4+8+) thymocytes in normal and genetically modified mice. *J Immunol* (1995) **154**(10):5103–13.
37. Scollay R, Godfrey D. Thymic emigration: conveyor belts or lucky dips? *Immunol Today* (1995) **16**:268–74. doi:10.1016/0167-5699(95)80179-0
38. McEwan CH, Bersini H, Klatzmann D, Thomas-Vaslin V, Six A. A computational technique to scale mathematical models towards complex heterogeneous systems. *COSMOS Workshop ECAL 2011 Conference*; Paris: Luniver Press (2011).

18

A new-age for biologic therapies: long-term drug-free therapy with BiP?

Adrian M. Shields, Gabriel S. Panayi and Valerie M. Corrigall*

Department of Academic Rheumatology, Centre for Molecular and Cellular Biology of Inflammation, King's College London, London, UK

Edited by:
Willem Van Eden, Utrecht University, Netherlands

Reviewed by:
Miriam Wittmann, University of Leeds, UK
Bernard R. Lauwerys, Université Catholique de Louvain, Belgium
Ruurd Van Der Zee, Universiteit Utrech, Netherlands

****Correspondence:***
Valerie M. Corrigall, Department of Academic Rheumatology, Centre for Molecular and Cellular Biology of Inflammation, 1st Floor New Hunts House, Guy's Campus, King's College London, SE1 1UL London, UK.
e-mail: valerie.corrigall@kcl.ac.uk

Heat shock proteins (HSPs) and other members of the much broader stress protein family have been shown to play important roles in coordinating multiple phases of immunological reactions; from facilitating immunological recognition, to promoting and regulating immunological responses and finally augmenting the resolution of inflammation and return to immunological homeostasis. In this review, we consider the challenges facing the stress protein field as we enter 2012; in particular we consider the role that HSPs and stress proteins may play in the initiation and termination of immunological responses. Special attention is afforded to the resolution-associated molecular pattern, binding immunoglobulin protein (BiP, also known as glucose regulated protein-78). We review the evidence that resolution-promoting proteins such as BiP may herald a new generation of biologics for inflammatory disease and reflect on the challenges of achieving clinical remission in rheumatoid arthritis with novel therapeutics and correlating clinical remission with immunological parameters of resolution of inflammation.

Keywords: binding immunoglobulin protein, resolution-associated molecular patterns, inflammation, resolution of inflammation, immunotherapy, rheumatoid arthritis, immune networks

INTRODUCTION

Heat shock proteins (HSP) and stress proteins are a collection of highly evolutionarily conserved proteins, grouped by molecular weight, with intracellular functions involving protein chaperoning and folding and protection of the cell during physiologically stressful conditions, including heat-shock, hypoxia, hypoglycemia, and intracellular electrolyte abnormalities. The term "stress protein" provides an umbrella for all those proteins upregulated in response to physiological stress, while HSP refers to the sub-family of proteins that have specific promoters allowing them to respond to heat shock. Stress proteins may be intracellular, cell surface expressed, and/or extracellular proteins and, therefore, have access to multiple subcellular and extracellular compartments. Consequently, there has been much discussion around potential roles that stress proteins may play in innate and adaptive immune responses.

Immunological responses may be grouped into four overlapping and interdependent phases: recognition, response, regulation, and resolution. Much data suggest that stress proteins play important roles in all of the phases of the immunological response. In this review, we briefly discuss how stress proteins can influence the resolution of inflammation, in particular, with respect to binding immunoglobulin protein (BiP, also known as glucose regulated protein-78). We also explore the concept of third generation biologic therapies for immunological diseases such as rheumatoid arthritis (RA). The third generation of biologics for immune-mediated diseases will be therapeutic agents that significantly modulate the dysregulated immune system, restoring immune homeostasis for prolonged periods without further biologic administration. We believe that BiP and other members of the recently defined resolution associated molecular pattern (RAMP) family (Shields et al., 2011) may herald a new generation of such novel biologics.

ELEPHANTS IN THE LABORATORY; A 2011 VIEW OF THE STRESS PROTEIN FIELD

Extensive research has now shown that stress proteins are involved in multiple stages of the immune response (**Figure 1**): stress proteins participate in the recognition of immunological danger, facilitate peptide carriage between cells and subsequent cross presentation of antigen, can modulate the immunological profile of myeloid lineage cells in both a pro- and anti-inflammatory direction and promote the regulation and resolution of inflammation. However, research in the stress protein field has been dogged by two controversies for many years. Firstly, there remains suspicion that stress protein family members possess no intrinsic immunological activity and all observed activity is the consequence of bacterial contaminants, particularly endotoxin, within the protein preparation (Wallin et al., 2002; Gao and Tsan, 2003a,b; Ye and Gan, 2007). Secondly, compounding this problem, is the ever-increasing variety of cell surface receptors identified for HSP. Using HSP70 as an example, the broad array of putative receptors include, TLR2, TLR4, CD14, CD40, CD91, CCR5, LOX-1, SREC-1 (Calderwood et al., 2007). However, there remain inconsistencies when trying to replicate HSP binding to null cells transfected with some of these specific molecules, such as CD14, TLR2, and TLR4, thus throwing doubt on whether they are true receptors (Theriault et al., 2005).

The major challenge facing the stress protein field is consolidating and refining the results of the extensive body of research conducted to date into a more comprehensive theory of how stress protein networks facilitate the initiation, progression, and resolution of an immunological event. To achieve this, careful

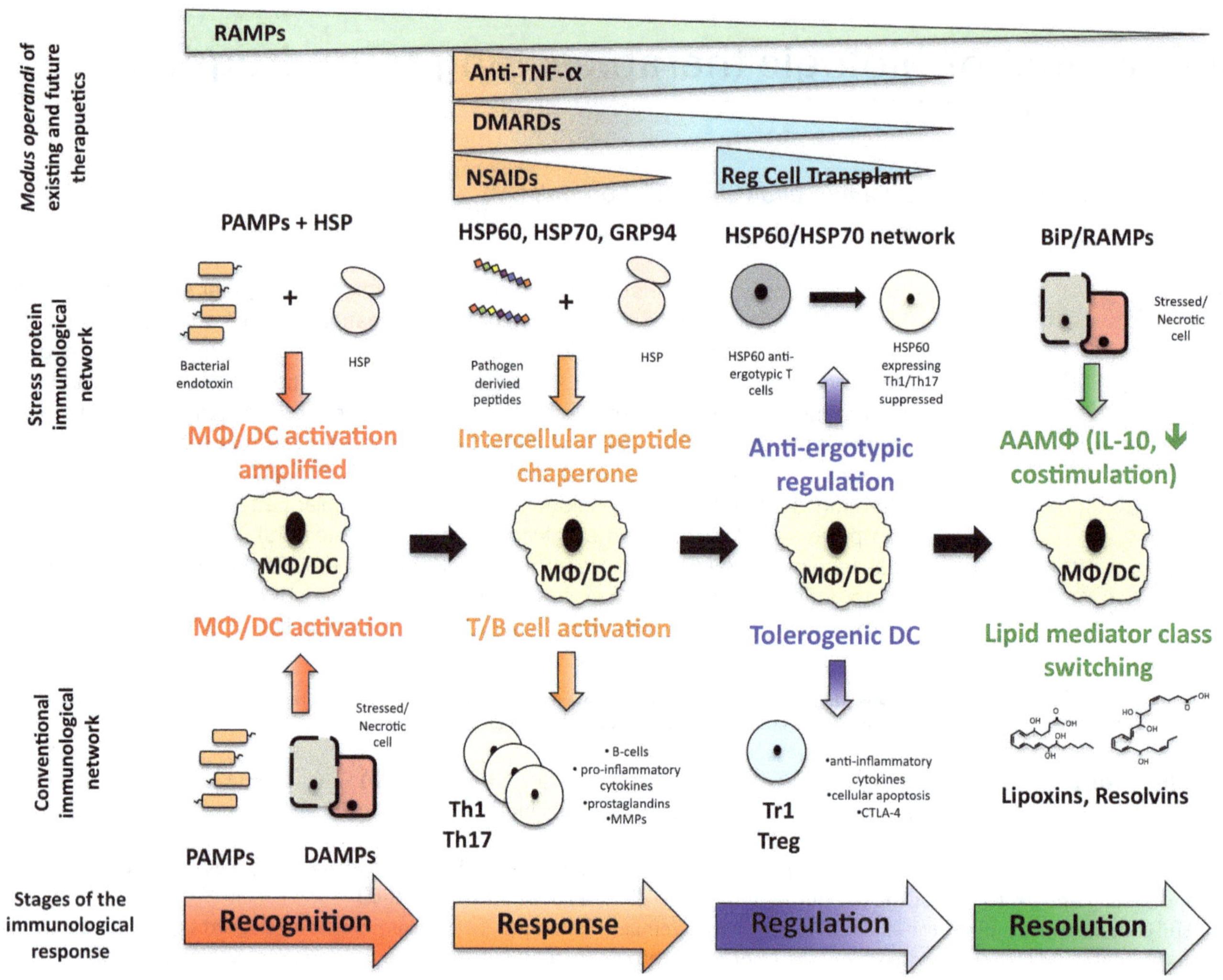

FIGURE 1 | How stress protein networks influences immunological reactions. Immunological events can be broken down into a series of interdependent phases: immunological recognition, an immunological response following by regulation of that response and resolution of inflammation leading to a return to homeostasis. The stress protein network influences each phase of the immunological event and ultimately, resolution-associated molecular patterns may help facilitate the return to immunological homeostasis. The different phases at which existing and future therapeutics act are also illustrated.

distinctions should be made between the immunological activity of mycobacterial HSP and mammalian HSP and, more pertinently, between the immunological effects derived from whole extracellular stress protein molecules and those effects caused by peptides derived from stress protein molecules coordinating the generation or expansion of self-reactive HSP T cells.

Moreover, stress protein researchers must address the elephants in their experimental data. It is increasingly clear that stress proteins bind bacterial products; however, the potential immunological implications of stress protein–bacterial product interactions have been over-shadowed by heated debate as to the immunological activity of ultra-pure stress protein preparations and their role as damage-associated molecular patterns (DAMP; Gao and Tsan, 2003a,b; Osterloh et al., 2004; Henderson et al., 2010). More recently, further discussion has arisen surrounding subtle differences between danger-associated and DAMP (van Eden et al., 2011), with van Eden et al. convincingly arguing that HSP should be excluded from the DAMP family given the paucity of evidence that they alone can activate an immunological response. Yet, the very fact that HSP are upregulated in response to cellular stress and can associate with pathogen associated molecular patterns (PAMP) is of great immunological significance in it's own right, particularly with respect to the danger hypothesis, for the following reasons:

(1) Cellular stress is synonymous with potential threats to tissue viability and is therefore synonymous with immunological danger, in accordance with the danger hypothesis (Matzinger, 2002). Cellular stress can arise from infectious and non-infectious sources (Macario and Conway de Macario, 2005; Rath and Haller, 2011) and results in the upregulation and redistribution of stress proteins, including members of the

HSP family, to the cell surface and beyond, into the extracellular fluid (Multhoff and Hightower, 1996; Delpino and Castelli, 2002; Mambula and Calderwood, 2006; Corrao et al., 2010; Merendino et al., 2010; Sreekumar et al., 2010).

(2) Cell surface HSP and other stress proteins (e.g., gp96) signal immunological danger by inducing and/or enhancing inflammatory cytokine production, dendritic cell (DC) maturation, and NK cell activity (Chen et al., 2002; Liu et al., 2003; Osterloh et al., 2004). While this does not qualify the molecules as DAMPs, as laid out in the criteria defined by Kono and Rock (2008), it emphasizes their importance in signaling immunological danger. Furthermore, while on the cell surface, it has been hypothesized that stress proteins associate with PAMPs and thus serve as a primitive antigen presentation system (Li et al., 2002).

(3) There is considerable evidence to suggest that extracellular HSP60, HSP70, HSP90, and gp96 bind to LPS and potentiate its immunostimulatory effects (Triantafilou et al., 2001; Warger et al., 2006; Osterloh et al., 2007). High-mobility group box protein-1 has shown similar properties (Pisetsky et al., 2008). This suggests that stress proteins may facilitate the recognition of a pathogenic infection, particularly if that infection has caused direct cellular insult. This may be of significance in maintaining immunological homeostasis at epithelial surfaces.

(4) Beyond the cell, stress protein family members appear to bind multiple extracellular protein and receptor targets (Calderwood et al., 2007). The immunological significance of these protein–protein interactions remain unclear. However, HSP do appear to be "sticky" proteins. Given their interaction with PAMPs, this promiscuity may facilitate the containment of shed bacterial products, preventing their dissemination, while providing a localized cache of PAMPs permitting a more anatomically targeted immunological response.

In summary, the specific properties of an extracellular stress protein are likely to depend both on the protein itself, the surrounding extracellular environment and the nature of the tissue from which the stress protein was released. Furthermore, the possibility that the extracellular environment modulates the activity of stress proteins during the course of an immunological response requires further attention; one could envisage a paradigm where extracellular stress proteins evolve from poachers, inciting inflammation, and tissue destruction, into gamekeepers, promoting regulation, and resolution during the course of an immunological event. Indeed a post-translational modification of high-mobility G protein-1 (HMGB1) caused by oxidation attenuates pro-inflammatory functions and makes the protein anti-inflammatory (Urbonaviciute et al., 2009). However, since stress proteins exhibit such radically different extracellular functions it should not be surprising that they show different affinities for a variety of receptors and may even bind different receptors depending on cell type. Such activity would enhance their flexibility and diversity of function (Calderwood et al., 2007). Hence, a greater understanding of how the stress protein network interacts with wider immunological networks would be extremely beneficial, however, a systems biology approach will likely be necessary to extend our knowledge further.

THE THIRD GENERATION OF BIOLOGICS: PROMOTING RESOLUTION

At present all therapies for immune-mediated diseases – autoimmune or allotransplant – require either continuous administration of immunosuppressive drugs or intermittent dosing at frequent intervals. For example, despite the effectiveness of anti-TNF-α therapy at suppressing inflammation in RA, cessation of therapy is associated with clinical relapse and radiological progression (Quinn et al., 2005) and although there is some *in vitro* evidence that anti-TNF-α therapy may modulate adaptive immune responses, particularly with respect to regulatory T cells (Ehrenstein et al., 2004), there is little evidence that long-term therapy alters the underlying immunological mechanisms that contribute to the chronic autoimmune state. Indeed, even after achieving low disease activity following long-term infliximab treatment, 45% of patients displayed further radiological disease progression within just a year of cessation of therapy (Tanaka et al., 2010).

Nevertheless, the transplantation field has offered hope that physicians can induce a state of tolerance to alloantigen in the absence of long-term immunosuppression. The best-characterized example of this phenomenon is liver transplantation: 20% of liver transplant recipients are capable of achieving a state of clinical operational tolerance (defined as a well functioning graft, without histological signs of rejection following the complete cessation of immunosuppression for over 1 year; Orlando et al., 2009). Tolerance is rarer with other solid-organ transplants, but has been reported in renal transplantation (Orlando et al., 2010); immunologists are beginning to describe biomarkers and molecular signatures that characterize and can be used to monitor clinical operational tolerance which include reduced co-stimulatory molecule expression, immune quiescence, apoptosis, and memory T cell responses are important in the maintenance of operational tolerance (Brouard et al., 2007; Hernandez-Fuentes and Lechler, 2010).

With respect to RA, the clinical goal is not a tolerogenic state *per se*, but the induction of drug-free remission. The ACR–EULAR agreed definition of disease remission in RA is a simplified disease activity index (SDAI) of ≤13.3 at any one time, or a total joint count of ≤1, and a swollen joint count ≤1, and a CRP ≤1 mg/dl and a patient global assessment score of ≤1 (Bykerk, 2011). Remission of RA, may indeed involve the re-establishment of immunological tolerance to cognate autoantigens. However, extensive cell–cell interactions between immune and stromal cells within the synovial architecture add a layer a complexity beyond the extracelluar cytokine and stress protein networks that drive the pathogenesis and maintain chronic inflammation within the rheumatoid joint (McInnes and Schett, 2011).

Currently, rheumatologists do not possess any immunological biomarkers to predict which patients will achieve or maintain a state of disease-free remission or indeed the mechanisms by which clinical remission is achieved (Isaacs, 2010). Thus, the attainment of drug-free remission in RA is the premier challenge facing rheumatologists and immunologist in the twenty-first century.

Early, aggressive intervention in the disease process is now the gold-standard for achieving maximum clinical response and potential remission in the RA patient (Quinn et al., 2005). B-cell depletion therapy has also offered a glimpse that more permanent changes to the immunological phenotype are possible. For example, rituximab, a B-cell depleting anti-CD20 monoclonal antibody, induces enduring clinical responses that do not correlate with peripheral blood levels of $CD20^+$ B cells after treatment (Breedveld et al., 2007). Multiple potential therapies and possible mechanisms for the re-establishment of immune tolerance and subsequent resolution of chronic inflammation have been discussed at length elsewhere (Albani et al., 2011). Needless to say that, like the conditions necessary for operational tolerance of renal grafts, tolerance in the rheumatoid patient involves modification of DC function such that T regulatory cells, of various phenotypes and mode of action are generated.

Since stress proteins have pleiotropic functions, and have been called "moonlighting" proteins (Huberts and van der Klei, 2010), it may be that the immune down regulating properties of some of them are due to an effect on DCs. Hence when used for the treatment of human disease they may be able to produce prolonged drug-free disease remissions or even tolerance. What is the evidence for this dramatic claim? Examination of the multiple extracellular functions of BiP may provide an answer.

BiP – A BRIEF HISTORY

Binding immunoglobulin protein is a member of the HSP70 family and an ubiquitously expressed, endogenous protein. BiP is constitutively expressed in the endoplasmic reticulum (ER), and essential for the correct folding of many nascent peptides (Gething, 1999). BiP is also the master regulator of the unfolded protein response (UPR), a transcriptional program designed to relieve ER stress by promoting the correct folding of ER luminal proteins (Hendershot, 2004). BiP, therefore, is regulated at two levels, constitutive and stress induced. Stress induced upregulation occurs in environments of high cellular activity in inadequately vascularized tissue, for example, during inflammation or neoplasia, pathologies characterized by relative hypoglycemia and hypoxia (Lee, 2007). Principally, during perturbation of the ER, BiP protects the cell from the accumulation of misfolded and denatured proteins and, thus, prevents apoptosis. Testament to the fundamental importance of BiP is the fact that BiP knock-out mice and mice where BiP is constitutively targeted to the incorrect subcellular compartment are not viable (Luo et al., 2006; Mimura et al., 2007). Many previous reviews have covered the intracellular chaperone function and protective role of BiP, during health and disease, so these aspects of BiP biology will not be reviewed here.

In contrast, our work for the last decade has focused exclusively on the extracellular properties of cell-free human BiP and its immunoregulatory role in inflammation. Like many other stress proteins, BiP is now known to be cell surface expressed and detectable at relatively high concentrations in serum, synovial fluid and oviductal fluid (Delpino and Castelli, 2002; Corrigall et al., 2004; Marin-Briggiler et al., 2010). As such, BiP has several physiological properties. Although BiP is a member of the HSP70 family we have previously hypothesized that, unlike HSP70 itself, BiP acts as a RAMP (Shields et al., 2011). RAMPs are protein molecules released alongside DAMPs from stressed or necrotic cells, which provide negative inputs into immunological networks, antagonizing pro-inflammatory mediators, and helping restore the immune system to homeostasis. Unlike the "DAMPing" or regulatory effect that HSPs exert on the immune system which appear to act via HSP derived peptides expanding sets of HSP-specific regulatory T cells (van Eden et al., 2005; Quintana and Cohen, 2011), the RAMP family members act predominantly on the myeloid lineage, setting the scene for the resolution of inflammation. Furthermore, what makes these molecules unique, is that unlike the increasing number of resolution inducing molecules being described (e.g., lipoxins and resolvins), the protein members of the RAMP family are constitutively expressed and thus able to affect the course of inflammation from the outset (Shields et al., 2011).

BiP: DRIVING RESOLUTION OF INFLAMMATION

What sets BiP apart from other potential biologic therapeutics appears to be its mode of action. Our research provides evidence that BiP offers long-lasting prophylactic, and therapeutic protection from disease in the murine model of collagen induced arthritis (CIA; Corrigall et al., 2001; Brownlie et al., 2006). Adoptive transfer studies confirm that the end-point of the mode of action involves immunological changes to cell function and suggests that regulatory T cells are induced rapidly by BiP either in naïve animals, following intravenous injection of BiP, or *in vitro*, when their splenocytes and lymph nodes are cultured in the presence of BiP (Corrigall et al., 2001; Brownlie et al., 2006). Importantly, the message from these studies is that BiP-treated cells, when adoptively transferred into arthritic mice are therapeutic and give long-term relief in the absence of repeated administration.

Another indicator that BiP is a potentially successful therapeutic in RA arises from our experimental pre-clinical investigation into a xenogeneic model where small pieces of inflamed synovium from RA patients were transplanted subcutaneously into severe combined immunodeficient (SCID) mice (Yoshida et al., 2011). Following successful vascular anastomosis of the graft, a single intravenous dose of BiP significantly reduced histological features of inflammation in the synovial explants. In addition, the histological expression of pro-inflammatory cytokines (TNF-α and IL-6) and the co-stimulatory molecules HLA-DR and CD86 was significantly down regulated in the grafts from the BiP-treated animals (Yoshida et al., 2011). The down-regulation of co-stimulatory molecules would significantly reduce the efficiency of antigen presentation. This SCID/RA synovial membrane chimera has been used to validate other biologic therapies, anti-TNF-α neutralizing antibody inhibitor and anti-soluble IL-6 receptor, that are now in the clinic.

Binding immunoglobulin protein treatment induces key changes in T cell and monocyte development. Firstly, T cell development is skewed to a Th2 profile with the production of IL-4, IL-5, and IL-10 (Bodman-Smith et al., 2003). Human BiP-specific T cell clones derived from healthy PBMC are predominantly $CD8^+$ and produce little or no interferon γ while splenocyte and lymph node cell suspensions from BiP-treated CIA mice also show a Th2 profile of cytokine release, IL-4, IL-5, and IL-10, on re-stimulation with BiP *in vitro* (Brownlie et al., 2006). Serum samples from these mice suggest that BiP suppresses the production of the pathogenic anti-collagen type II antibodies, which drive CIA, while stimulating the production of non-pathogenic IgG1 isotype antibodies indicative of a Th2 environment (Brownlie et al., 2006). Secondly, BiP is capable of binding to a receptor expressed by >95% human peripheral blood monocytes, up to 50% B cells and 10% T cells (Corrigall et al., 2003). Currently, the identity of this receptor(s) remains elusive. The immediate result of BiP stimulation, in human peripheral blood mononuclear cells, is the attenuation of TNF-α production after 7 h and increased IL-10 production to a plateau lasting over 96 h (Corrigall et al., 2004). On being stimulated by BiP, monocytes show phenotypic changes similar to deactivated macrophages. Macrophage deactivation is achieved via the stimulation of macrophages with IL-10, TGF-β, steroids, or interactions between CD200 and CD200R and CD47 and CD172a; the consequences of deactivation include increased production of IL-10, TGF-β, PGE-2, and reduced expression of MHC-II molecules (Gordon and Taylor, 2005). The various differentiation pathways and activation states of the monocyte–macrophage lineage remain under intense investigation, however, BiP induced changes are temporally different from those induced exclusively by IL-10. The major effect is the complete inhibition of TNF-α production with increased production of IL-10, soluble TNF receptors, and IL-1 receptor antagonist (Corrigall et al., 2004). Ultimately, the consequence of BiP stimulation is non-phlogistic activation of the monocyte–macrophage. Monocytes cultured in the presence of IL-4 and GM-CSF and BiP fail to differentiate into mature DC (Corrigall et al., 2009). Remarkably these BiP-treated cells were highly positive for indoleamine 2,3-dioxygenase (IDO), a characteristic of tolerogenic DC. When these DCs were co-cultured with autologous T cells they induced regulatory CTLA-4^{+} T cells. This process was attributable to IDO up regulation because CTLA-4 up regulation was reversible in the presence of 1 methyl tryptophan, the IDO inhibitor. On separation from the DC the CTLA-4^{+} T cells showed regulatory T cell function capable of suppressing T cell stimulation by anti-CD3. Although BiP was essential for the induction of the DCs, no additional BiP was required in the secondary cultures in which regulatory T cell function was assessed (Corrigall et al., 2009). The mechanism underlying the induction of regulatory T cells by BiP is under investigation by our laboratory. There are three possible scenarios: firstly, that there is direct action on the T cell via a receptor mediated process, but this is unlikely given the relative lack of extracellular BiP protein in the culture system during DC–T cell col-culture; secondly, that BiP drives the induction of DC of a tolerogenic phenotype, including increasing IDO expression, which we have shown directly leads to upregulated CTLA-4^{+} regulatory T cells, either in the presence or absence of peptide presentation. Finally BiP-specific peptide presentation may expand existing regulatory T cells in a peptide dependent process. Cross-reactivity with peptides from other HSP70 family members is a possibility in this case as 68% amino acid homology exists between HSP70 and BiP. If cross-reactivity between HSP70 and BiP occurs and is responsible for any of the T-cell dependent regulatory effects of either protein, it lends further weight to the hypothesis that an intricate network of extracellular stress proteins exists which facilitates the maintenance of immunological homeostasis (Panayi et al., 2004).

These studies are all in immunological models. In the TNF-α transgenic mouse a spontaneous arthritis develops that resembles RA in many of its features (Li and Schwarz, 2003) although the joint inflammation and destruction is independent on immune mechanisms. However, since BiP deactivates monocytes both at the transcriptional and the translational level a prediction would be that BiP would also have a therapeutic effect in this model. Indeed a single intraperitoneal dose of BiP was able to significantly suppress joint inflammation and systemic bone damage for several weeks (Corrigall et al., manuscript submitted).

The spontaneous arthritis observed in the transgenic mice is almost certainly induced by TNF-α activation of transcription factors including NF-κB, which is responsible for the induction of many of the major inflammatory cytokines. Intracellularly, BiP and NF-κB are counter regulated (Pahl and Baeuerle, 1995). A recent review by Kitamura (2011) has reported that although early UPR activity may drive NF-κB activation later UPR involvement tends to attenuate NF-κB function. As an extracellular protein we have shown that BiP acts to inhibit MAPK phosphorylation (Corrigall et al., manuscript submitted) and downregulates protein levels of these signaling molecules. As a stress protein, BiP is upregulated intracellularly in response to ER stress prior to its release into the extracellular environment. Thus, both the intracellular and extracellular actions of BiP may operate to diminish the pro-inflammatory effects of NF-κB thus helping the resolution of acute inflammation.

THE OTHER RESOLUTION-ASSOCIATED MOLECULAR PATTERNS

Binding immunoglobulin protein is just one member of a family of proteins we have recently defined as the RAMPs. We have extensively reviewed the properties of the RAMP family elsewhere (Shields et al., 2011). Needless to say, we believe this family of proteins, whose founder members include HSP10, HSP27, and α-B-crystallin may have great potential as resolution-promoting therapeutics. Resolution-promoting regulatory signals are subtly different from immunoregulatory immunological signals; resolution-promoting signals are those that specifically promote the non-phlogistic activation of macrophages, the phagocytosis of apoptotic neutrophils, the prevention of influx of inflammatory cells and the restoration of parenchymal cells to the non-inflammatory state (Serhan et al., 2007). The crux of resolution is, therefore, centered around myeloid lineage cells and the parenchyma. This is why we believe the RAMP family, which principally exert their immunological effects via the myeloid lineage (thus affecting antigen presentation, co-stimulatory molecule expression, myeloid cell differentiation, and anti-inflammatory cytokine secretion (De et al., 2000; Corrigall et al., 2004, 2009; Banerjee et al., 2011; Shields et al., 2011)), have the potential to exert resolution-promoting effects, rather than simply immunoregulatory effects.

Clinical trials of HSP10 have already yielded promising results (Vanags et al., 2006; Williams et al., 2008) and pre-clinical models have shown α-B-crystallin to be an extremely effective therapeutic in a variety of different inflammatory disease models including experimental autoimmune encephalomyelitis, ischemic optic neuropathy and stroke (Ousman et al., 2007; Arac et al., 2011; Pangratz-Fuehrer et al., 2011). Further investigations are necessary to fully understand how the RAMP family exert their immunological effects and under what circumstance they might be used in clinical practice.

CONCLUSION

To develop the third generation of biologics, a great deal of investment will need to be made in correlating the clinical parameters of remission from chronic inflammatory disease and the immunological parameters of resolution from inflammation. Experience from the rheumatological field has shown us that aggressive immunosuppressive and biological therapy can induce remission in early RA. However, the longer the disease progresses, the more unlikely this strategy is to succeed because the mechanisms controlling the regulation and resolution of inflammation fail in chronic inflammation. Therapy in chronic inflammation can reduce ongoing inflammation but does not resolve the underlying immunological defect.

Evidence from our laboratory suggests that a single administration of BiP in models of inflammatory arthritis is sufficient to regulate and resolve chronic inflammation. The planned Stage I/II clinical trial of BiP in RA patients will teach us more regarding the properties of BiP as a therapy in human disease. However, it may be that resolution-promoting biologic therapies will have to be administered in conjunction with other biologics, which can control ongoing inflammation and set-the-scene for immunological resolution and restoration of homeostasis to occur.

ACKNOWLEDGMENTS

Prof. Gabriel Panayi is a shareholder in Immune Regulation Ltd., which holds the patent rights for BiP for the treatment of rheumatoid arthritis. Dr. Valerie Corrigall is a shareholder in Immune Regulation Ltd. Funding Statement: As a review, this manuscript has not received direct funding although Dr. Adrian Shields received an Oliver Bird Rheumatism Foundation PhD studentship for the duration of his doctoral studies (completed July 2010) and the Corrigall laboratory receives funding from Arthritis Research UK.

REFERENCES

Albani, S., Koffeman, E. C., and Prakken, B. (2011). Induction of immune tolerance in the treatment of rheumatoid arthritis. *Nat. Rev. Rheumatol.* 7, 272–281.

Arac, A., Brownell, S. E., Rothebard, J. B., Chen, C., Ko, R. M., Pereira, M. P., Albers, G. W., Steinman, L., and Steinberg, G. K. (2011). Systemic augmentation of αB-crystallin provides therapeutic benefit twelve hours post-stroke onset via immune modulation. *Proc. Natl. Acad. Sci. U.S.A.* [Epub ahead of print].

Banerjee, S., Lin, C. F., Skinner, K. A., Schiffhauer, L. M., Peacock, J., Hicks, D. G., Redmond, E. M., Morrow, D., Huston, A., Shayne, M., Langstein, H. N., Miller-Graziano, C. L., Strickland, J., O'Donoghue, L., and De, A. K. (2011). Heat shock protein 27 differentiates tolerogenic macrophages that may support human breast cancer progression. *Cancer Res.* 71, 318–327.

Bodman-Smith, M. D., Corrigall, V. M., Kemeny, D. M., and Panayi, G. S. (2003). BiP, a putative autoantigen in rheumatoid arthritis, stimulates IL-10-producing CD8-positive T cells from normal individuals. *Rheumatology (Oxford)* 42, 637–644.

Breedveld, F., Agarwal, S., Yin, M., Ren, S., Li, N. F., Shaw, T. M., and Davies, B. E. (2007). Rituximab pharmacokinetics in patients with rheumatoid arthritis: B-cell levels do not correlate with clinical response. *J. Clin. Pharmacol.* 47, 1119–1128.

Brouard, S., Mansfield, E., Braud, C., Li, L., Giral, M., Hsieh, S. C., Baeten, D., Zhang, M., Ashton-Chess, J., Braudeau, C., Hsieh, F., Dupont, A., Pallier, A., Moreau, A., Louis, S., Ruiz, C., Salvatierra, O., Soulillou, J. P., and Sarwal, M. (2007). Identification of a peripheral blood transcriptional biomarker panel associated with operational renal allograft tolerance. *Proc. Natl. Acad. Sci. U.S.A.* 104, 15448–15453.

Brownlie, R. J., Myers, L. K., Wooley, P. H., Corrigall, V. M., Bodman-Smith, M. D., Panayi, G. S., and Thompson, S. J. (2006). Treatment of murine collagen-induced arthritis by the stress protein BiP via interleukin-4-producing regulatory T cells: a novel function for an ancient protein. *Arthritis Rheum.* 54, 854–863.

Bykerk, V. P. (2011). Rheumatoid arthritis: 2011 remission criteria are a new benchmark for RA therapy. *Nat. Rev. Rheumatol.* 7, 317–318.

Calderwood, S. K., Theriault, J., Gray, P. J., and Gong, J. (2007). Cell surface receptors for molecular chaperones. *Methods* 43, 199–206.

Chen, X., Tao, Q., Yu, H., Zhang, L., and Cao, X. (2002). Tumor cell membrane-bound heat shock protein 70 elicits antitumor immunity. *Immunol. Lett.* 84, 81–87.

Corrao, S., Campanella, C., Anzalone, R., Farina, F., Zummo, G., Conway De Macario, E., Macario, A. J., Cappello, F., and La Rocca, G. (2010). Human Hsp10 and Early Pregnancy Factor (EPF) and their relationship and involvement in cancer and immunity: current knowledge and perspectives. *Life Sci.* 86, 145–152.

Corrigall, V. M., Bodman-Smith, M. D., Brunst, M., Cornell, H., and Panayi, G. S. (2004). Inhibition of antigen-presenting cell function and stimulation of human peripheral blood mononuclear cells to express an anti-inflammatory cytokine profile by the stress protein BiP: relevance to the treatment of inflammatory arthritis. *Arthritis Rheum.* 50, 1164–1171.

Corrigall, V. M., Bodman-Smith, M. D., Fife, M. S., Canas, B., Myers, L. K., Wooley, P., Soh, C., Staines, N. A., Pappin, D. J., Berlo, S. E., Van Eden, W., Van Der Zee, R., Lanchbury, J. S., and Panayi, G. S. (2001). The human endoplasmic reticulum molecular chaperone BiP is an autoantigen for rheumatoid arthritis and prevents the induction of experimental arthritis. *J. Immunol.* 166, 1492–1498.

Corrigall, V. M., Bodman-Smith, M. D., and Panayi, G. S. (2003). The stress protein, immunoglobulin binding protein (BiP), has a specific receptor (abstract). *Rheumatology (Oxford)* 42, 43.

Corrigall, V. M., Vittecoq, O., and Panayi, G. S. (2009). Binding immunoglobulin protein-treated peripheral blood monocyte-derived dendritic cells are refractory to maturation and induce regulatory T-cell development. *Immunology* 128, 218–226.

De, A. K., Kodys, K. M., Yeh, B. S., and Miller-Graziano, C. (2000). Exaggerated human monocyte IL-10 concomitant to minimal TNF-alpha induction by heat-shock protein 27 (Hsp27) suggests Hsp27 is primarily an antiinflammatory stimulus. *J. Immunol.* 165, 3951–3958.

Delpino, A., and Castelli, M. (2002). The 78 kDa glucose-regulated protein (GRP78/BIP) is expressed on the cell membrane, is released into cell culture medium and is also present in human peripheral circulation. *Biosci. Rep.* 22, 407–420.

Ehrenstein, M. R., Evans, J. G., Singh, A., Moore, S., Warnes, G., Isenberg, D. A., and Mauri, C. (2004). Compromised function of regulatory T cells in rheumatoid arthritis and reversal by anti-TNFalpha therapy. *J. Exp. Med.* 200, 277–285.

Gao, B., and Tsan, M. F. (2003a). Endotoxin contamination in recombinant human heat shock protein 70 (Hsp70) preparation is responsible for the induction of tumor necrosis factor alpha release by murine macrophages. *J. Biol. Chem.* 278, 174–179.

Gao, B., and Tsan, M. F. (2003b). Recombinant human heat shock protein 60 does not induce the release of tumor necrosis factor alpha from murine macrophages. *J. Biol. Chem.* 278, 22523–22529.

Gething, M. J. (1999). Role and regulation of the ER chaperone BiP. *Semin. Cell Dev. Biol.* 10, 465–472.

Gordon, S., and Taylor, P. R. (2005). Monocyte and macrophage heterogeneity. *Nat. Rev. Immunol.* 5, 953–964.

Hendershot, L. M. (2004). The ER function BiP is a master regulator of ER function. *Mt. Sinai J. Med.* 71, 289–297.

Henderson, B., Calderwood, S. K., Coates, A. R., Cohen, I., Van Eden, W., Lehner, T., and Pockley, A. G. (2010). Caught with their PAMPs down? The extracellular signalling actions of molecular chaperones are not due to microbial contaminants. *Cell Stress Chaperones* 15, 123–141.

Hernandez-Fuentes, M. P., and Lechler, R. I. (2010). A "biomarker signature" for tolerance in transplantation. *Nat. Rev. Nephrol.* 6, 606–613.

Huberts, D. H., and van der Klei, I. J. (2010). Moonlighting proteins: an intriguing mode of multitasking. *Biochim. Biophys. Acta* 1803, 520–525.

Isaacs, J. D. (2010). The changing face of rheumatoid arthritis: sustained remission for all? *Nat. Rev. Immunol.* 10, 605–611.

Kitamura, M. (2011). Control of NF-kappaB and inflammation by the unfolded protein response. *Int. Rev. Immunol.* 30, 4–15.

Kono, H., and Rock, K. L. (2008). How dying cells alert the immune system to danger. *Nat. Rev. Immunol.* 8, 279–289.

Lee, A. S. (2007). GRP78 induction in cancer: therapeutic and prognostic implications. *Cancer Res.* 67, 3496–3499.

Li, P., and Schwarz, E. M. (2003). The TNF-alpha transgenic mouse model of inflammatory arthritis. *Springer Semin. Immunopathol.* 25, 19–33.

Li, Z., Menoret, A., and Srivastava, P. (2002). Roles of heat-shock proteins in antigen presentation and cross-presentation. *Curr. Opin. Immunol.* 14, 45–51.

Liu, B., Dai, J., Zheng, H., Stoilova, D., Sun, S., and Li, Z. (2003). Cell surface expression of an endoplasmic reticulum resident heat shock protein gp96 triggers MyD88-dependent systemic autoimmune diseases. *Proc. Natl. Acad. Sci. U.S.A.* 100, 15824–15829.

Luo, S., Mao, C., Lee, B., and Lee, A. S. (2006). GRP78/BiP is required for cell proliferation and protecting the inner cell mass from apoptosis during early mouse embryonic development. *Mol. Cell. Biol.* 26, 5688–5697.

Macario, A. J., and Conway de Macario, E. (2005). Sick chaperones, cellular stress, and disease. *N. Engl. J. Med.* 353, 1489–1501.

Mambula, S. S., and Calderwood, S. K. (2006). Heat shock protein 70 is secreted from tumor cells by a nonclassical pathway involving lysosomal endosomes. *J. Immunol.* 177, 7849–7857.

Marin-Briggiler, C. I., Gonzalez-Echeverria, M. F., Munuce, M. J., Ghersevich, S., Caille, A. M., Hellman, U., Corrigall, V. M., and Vazquez-Levin, M. H. (2010). Glucose-regulated protein 78 (Grp78/BiP) is secreted by human oviduct epithelial cells and the recombinant protein modulates sperm-zona pellucida binding. *Fertil. Steril.* 93, 1574–1578.

Matzinger, P. (2002). The danger model: a renewed sense of self. *Science* 296, 301–305.

McInnes, I. B., and Schett, G. (2011). The pathogenesis of rheumatoid arthritis. *N. Engl. J. Med.* 365, 2205–2219.

Merendino, A. M., Bucchieri, F., Campanella, C., Marciano, V., Ribbene, A., David, S., Zummo, G., Burgio, G., Corona, D. F., Conway De Macario, E., Macario, A. J., and Cappello, F. (2010). Hsp60 is actively secreted by human tumor cells. *PLoS ONE* 5, e9247. doi:10.1371/journal.pone.0009247

Mimura, N., Hamada, H., Kashio, M., Jin, H., Toyama, Y., Kimura, K., Iida, M., Goto, S., Saisho, H., Toshimori, K., Koseki, H., and Aoe, T. (2007). Aberrant quality control in the endoplasmic reticulum impairs the biosynthesis of pulmonary surfactant in mice expressing mutant BiP. *Cell Death Differ.* 14, 1475–1485.

Multhoff, G., and Hightower, L. E. (1996). Cell surface expression of heat shock proteins and the immune response. *Cell Stress Chaperones* 1, 167–176.

Orlando, G., Hematti, P., Stratta, R. J., Burke, G. W. III, Di Cocco, P., Pisani, F., Soker, S., and Wood, K. (2010). Clinical operational tolerance after renal transplantation: current status and future challenges. *Ann. Surg.* 252, 915–928.

Orlando, G., Soker, S., and Wood, K. (2009). Operational tolerance after liver transplantation. *J. Hepatol.* 50, 1247–1257.

Osterloh, A., Kalinke, U., Weiss, S., Fleischer, B., and Breloer, M. (2007). Synergistic and differential modulation of immune responses by Hsp60 and lipopolysaccharide. *J. Biol. Chem.* 282, 4669–4680.

Osterloh, A., Meier-Stiegen, F., Veit, A., Fleischer, B., Von Bonin, A., and Breloer, M. (2004). Lipopolysaccharide-free heat shock protein 60 activates T cells. *J. Biol. Chem.* 279, 47906–47911.

Ousman, S. S., Tomooka, B. H., Van Noort, J. M., Wawrousek, E. F., O'Connor, K. C., Hafler, D. A., Sobel, R. A., Robinson, W. H., and Steinman, L. (2007). Protective and therapeutic role for alphaB-crystallin in autoimmune demyelination. *Nature* 448, 474–479.

Pahl, H. L., and Baeuerle, P. A. (1995). A novel signal transduction pathway from the endoplasmic reticulum to the nucleus is mediated by transcription factor NF-kappa B. *EMBO J.* 14, 2580–2588.

Panayi, G. S., Corrigall, V. M., and Henderson, B. (2004). Stress cytokines: pivotal proteins in immune regulatory networks; opinion. *Curr. Opin. Immunol.* 16, 531–534.

Pangratz-Fuehrer, S., Kaur, K., Ousman, S. S., Steinman, L., and Liao, Y. J. (2011). Functional rescue of experimental ischemic optic neuropathy with alphaB-crystallin. *Eye (Lond.)* 25, 809–817.

Pisetsky, D. S., Erlandsson-Harris, H., and Andersson, U. (2008). High-mobility group box protein 1 (HMGB1): an alarmin mediating the pathogenesis of rheumatic disease. *Arthritis Res. Ther.* 10, 209.

Quinn, M. A., Conaghan, P. G., O'Connor, P. J., Karim, Z., Greenstein, A., Brown, A., Brown, C., Fraser, A., Jarret, S., and Emery, P. (2005). Very early treatment with infliximab in addition to methotrexate in early, poor-prognosis rheumatoid arthritis reduces magnetic resonance imaging evidence of synovitis and damage, with sustained benefit after infliximab withdrawal: results from a twelve-month randomized, double-blind, placebo-controlled trial. *Arthritis Rheum.* 52, 27–35.

Quintana, F. J., and Cohen, I. R. (2011). The HSP60 immune system network. *Trends Immunol.* 32, 89–95.

Rath, E., and Haller, D. (2011). Inflammation and cellular stress: a mechanistic link between immune-mediated and metabolically driven pathologies. *Eur. J. Nutr.* 50, 219–233.

Serhan, C. N., Brain, S. D., Buckley, C. D., Gilroy, D. W., Haslett, C., O'Neill, L. A., Perretti, M., Rossi, A. G., and Wallace, J. L. (2007). Resolution of inflammation: state of the art, definitions and terms. *FASEB J.* 21, 325–332.

Shields, A. M., Panayi, G. S., and Corrigall, V. M. (2011). Resolution-associated molecular patterns (RAMP): RAMParts defending immunological homeostasis? *Clin. Exp. Immunol.* 165, 292–300.

Sreekumar, P. G., Kannan, R., Kitamura, M., Spee, C., Barron, E., Ryan, S. J., and Hinton, D. R. (2010). AlphaB crystallin is apically secreted within exosomes by polarized human retinal pigment epithelium and provides neuroprotection to adjacent cells. *PLoS ONE* 5, e12578. doi:10.1371/journal.pone.0012578

Tanaka, Y., Takeuchi, T., Mimori, T., Saito, K., Nawata, M., Kameda, H., Nojima, T., Miyasaka, N., and Koike, T. (2010). Discontinuation of infliximab after attaining low disease activity in patients with rheumatoid arthritis: RRR (remission induction by Remicade in RA) study. *Ann. Rheum. Dis.* 69, 1286–1291.

Theriault, J. R., Mambula, S. S., Sawamura, T., Stevenson, M. A., and Calderwood, S. K. (2005). Extracellular HSP70 binding to surface receptors present on antigen presenting cells and endothelial/epithelial cells. *FEBS Lett.* 579, 1951–1960.

Triantafilou, K., Triantafilou, M., and Dedrick, R. L. (2001). A CD14-independent LPS receptor cluster. *Nat. Immunol.* 2, 338–345.

Urbonaviciute, V., Meister, S., Furnrohr, B. G., Frey, B., Guckel, E., Schett, G., Herrmann, M., and Voll, R. E. (2009). Oxidation of the alarmin high-mobility group box 1 protein (HMGB1) during apoptosis. *Autoimmunity* 42, 305–307.

van Eden, W., Spiering, R., Broere, F., and Van Der Zee, R. (2011). A case of mistaken identity: HSP are no DAMPs but DAMPERs. *Cell Stress Chaperones.* [Epub ahead of print].

van Eden, W., van Der Zee, R., and Prakken, B. (2005). Heat-shock proteins induce T-cell regulation of chronic inflammation. *Nat. Rev. Immunol.* 5, 318–330.

Vanags, D., Williams, B., Johnson, B., Hall, S., Nash, P., Taylor, A., Weiss, J., and Feeney, D. (2006). Therapeutic efficacy and safety of chaperonin 10 in patients with rheumatoid arthritis: a double-blind randomised trial. *Lancet* 368, 855–863.

Wallin, R. P., Lundqvist, A., More, S. H., Von Bonin, A., Kiessling, R., and Ljunggren, H. G. (2002). Heat-shock proteins as activators of the innate immune system. *Trends Immunol.* 23, 130–135.

Warger, T., Hilf, N., Rechtsteiner, G., Haselmayer, P., Carrick, D. M., Jonuleit, H., Von Landenberg, P., Rammensee, H. G., Nicchitta, C. V., Radsak, M. P., and Schild, H. (2006). Interaction of TLR2 and TLR4 ligands with the N-terminal domain of Gp96 amplifies innate and adaptive immune responses. *J. Biol. Chem.* 281, 22545–22553.

Williams, B., Vanags, D., Hall, S., McCormack, C., Foley, P., Weiss, J., Johnson, B., Latz, E., and Feeney, D. (2008). Efficacy and safety of chaperonin 10 in patients with moderate to severe plaque psoriasis: evidence of utility beyond a single indication. *Arch. Dermatol.* 144, 683–685.

Ye, Z., and Gan, Y. H. (2007). Flagellin contamination of recombinant heat shock protein 70 is responsible for its activity on T cells. *J. Biol. Chem.* 282, 4479–4484.

19

Automated cleaning and pre-processing of immunoglobulin gene sequences from high-throughput sequencing

Miri Michaeli[1], Hila Noga[1], Hilla Tabibian-Keissar[1,2], Iris Barshack[2] and Ramit Mehr[1]*

[1] *The Mina and Everard Goodman Faculty of Life Sciences, Bar-Ilan University, Ramat Gan, Israel*
[2] *Department of Pathology, Sheba Medical Center and Sackler School of Medicine, Tel Aviv University, Tel Aviv, Israel*

Edited by:
Harry W. Schroeder, University of Alabama at Birmingham, USA

Reviewed by:
Harry W. Schroeder, University of Alabama at Birmingham, USA
Michael Zemlin, Philipps University Marburg, Germany

****Correspondence:***
Ramit Mehr, The Mina and Everard Goodman Faculty of Life Sciences, Bar-Ilan University, Ramat-Gan 52900, Israel.
e-mail: ramit.mehr@biu.ac.il

High-throughput sequencing (HTS) yields tens of thousands to millions of sequences that require a large amount of pre-processing work to clean various artifacts. Such cleaning cannot be performed manually. Existing programs are not suitable for immunoglobulin (Ig) genes, which are variable and often highly mutated. This paper describes Ig High-Throughput Sequencing Cleaner (Ig-HTS-Cleaner), a program containing a simple cleaning procedure that successfully deals with pre-processing of Ig sequences derived from HTS, and Ig Insertion—Deletion Identifier (Ig-Indel-Identifier), a program for identifying legitimate and artifact insertions and/or deletions (indels). Our programs were designed for analyzing Ig gene sequences obtained by 454 sequencing, but they are applicable to all types of sequences and sequencing platforms. Ig-HTS-Cleaner and Ig-Indel-Identifier have been implemented in Java and saved as executable JAR files, supported on Linux and MS Windows. No special requirements are needed in order to run the programs, except for correctly constructing the input files as explained in the text. The programs' performance has been tested and validated on real and simulated data sets.

Keywords: B cell receptor, computer programs, high-throughput sequencing, immunoglobulin (Ig) genes, insertions and deletions (indels)

INTRODUCTION

Studying the generation, development and selection of lymphocyte repertoires, and their functions during immune responses, is essential for understanding the function of the immune system in healthy individuals, and in monitoring and intervening with the immune system in immune deficient, autoimmune disease or cancer patients. The recent development of high-throughput sequencing (HTS) enables researchers to obtain large numbers of sequences from several samples simultaneously (Galan et al., 2010). HTS has a great advantage over classical sequencing methods in the field of immunoglobulin (Ig) gene research, as it enables us to extract more sequences per sample and it is sensitive enough so we can identify different unique sequences. Ig genes encode the B cell receptors (BCR) and tend to accumulate point mutations in their sequences in order to improve the BCRs affinity to antigens. Mutation analysis, which is one aspect of Ig gene research, enables the tracking of mutation accumulation in the BCRs and hence analysis of the diversification of Ig gene sequences that originate from the same ancestor. Thus, HTS presents us now, for the first time, with the ability to analyze and compare large samples of mutated Ig gene repertoires in health, aging and disease (Campbell et al., 2008; Boyd et al., 2009; Gibson et al., 2009; Scheid et al., 2009; Ademokun et al., 2010; Dunn-Walters and Ademokun, 2010). However, the huge numbers of sequences obtained require a large amount of pre-processing work to clean out artifacts, sort sequences according to sample according to their molecular identification (MID) tags, identify primers, and discard sequences that do not contain enough information, such as sequences much shorter or longer than the expected length of an Ig variable region gene, or sequences with average quality scores below a defined threshold. Several programs are already used by the scientific community to study the B cell mutational patterns, such as SoDA (Volpe et al., 2006), SoDA2 (Munshaw and Kepler, 2010), and iHMMune-Align (Gaëta et al., 2007) which perform V(D)J segment identification; identification of clonally-related Ig gene sequences using clustering methods (Chen et al., 2010); ClustalW2 (Larkin et al., 2007), for alignment of clonally-related sequences; and IgTree (Barak et al., 2008), for creating lineage trees from the sets of aligned clonally-related sequences. However, in order to use these programs and receive reliable results that are not affected by sequencing artifacts, one must first make sure that all such artifacts are cleaned out of the input data.

Although HTS has already been available for several years, there are very few such cleaning programs available for users, and none that can deal with the cleaning of Ig genes. For example, the program CANGS (Pandey et al., 2010) has a very good pipeline of cleaning sequences, but it discards unique sequences and searches for primers and MID tags with perfect matches only, while it is known that tags and primers are often incomplete or sequenced incorrectly. Another program that could be used for Ig gene data cleaning is SeqTrim (Falgueras et al., 2010). This program does all the desired cleaning processes, but has two main disadvantages: one is that it runs on sequences that were inserted in vectors, so the program identifies the inserts only according to vector sequences found in databases such as NCBI's UniVec, EMBL's emvec, or BLAST. The user does not have the option to insert the ends of the genes, e.g., primers, as an input. Therefore, this program is suitable only for researchers that use sequencing with vectors. A second disadvantage is that SeqTrim requires other external programs. Ngs_backbone (Blanca et al., 2011) is another program that can be used for cleaning Ig gene sequences, but it requires external softwares. Additionally, there are several programs that trim the adapters (primers used in HTS) and the template-specific primers (MID tags or barcodes). One of them is TagCleaner (Schmieder et al., 2010), but this program takes all the input sequences, aligns them in order to identify the most frequent sequences at both ends that are supposed to be the adapters/tags and trims them. TagCleaner and similar programs are therefore ineffective when sequences come from several samples and hence contain several tag combinations; tags are composed of different sequences, so no consensus sequence can be deduced correctly using this method. In addition, highly homologous or, in contrast, highly variable sequences may yield erroneous alignments and therefore false identification of adapters. We have tested TagCleaner on our Ig genes data but this program could not correctly identify the tags. Another program is TagDust (Lassmann et al., 2009), but this program identifies artifact reads by comparing all reads to a library of sequences and checking for significant match. It is not possible to create such library for Ig gene sequences, as they undergo somatic hypermutation (SHM) in a high rate, and thus can diverge (Cook and Tomlinson, 1995; Rajewsky, 1996). EA-utils (Aronesty, 2011), Scythe (Buffalo, n.d.), SeqPrep (John, n.d.), FASTX (Gordon, n.d.), and Trim Galore! (Krueger, n.d.) are additional programs that are used to trim adapters among other functions; however, it is not possible to identify adapters in the 5′ end of the reads and to search for multiple different adapters using these programs. Using trimLRPatterns [one tool of ShortRead, (Morgan et al., 2009)] lacks the option to search for multiple different adapters. Trimmomatic (Bolger and Giorgi, n.d.) does not allow identifying adapters in the 5′ end of the reads, and anyway is compatible to Illumina sequencing only. FAR [The Flexible Adapter Remover, (Unknown, n.d.)] is capable of searching for multiple adapters using a simple global alignment algorithm, but it does not record the combination of adapters (or barcodes or MIDs) if found and cut. This is important when sequencing several different samples in the same sequencing run. Cutadapt (Martin, 2011) offers an easy-to-use command-line program that searches for multiple adapters and trim them, and is specialized for small RNA sequences. However, cutadapt currently does not support using a configuration file in which, for example, a list of adapters can be specified; hence, inputting several adapter sequences is via the command-line, which makes it slightly cumbersome. AdapterRemoval (Lindgreen, 2012) can search for multiple adapters in both 5′ and 3′ ends of the reads and discards reads that do not exceed a minimum length given by the user. However, none of the above mentioned programs assign the reads to their original samples according to their MIDs (barcodes), although the search of adapters should be similar to the identification of MIDs. Btrim (Kong, 2011) presents the closest cleaning options to our desired ones. In addition to trimming adapters and low quality regions as some of the above programs do, it can also identify barcodes and assign the reads to their original samples. However, Btrim has several shortcomings. First, it is limited to Linux. Second, similar to some of the above-mentioned programs, it requires some knowledge regarding the use with the command-line. A program with a user interface or even a double-click program is preferable, as its use can be included in an automated pipeline easy to operate even by users with little experience with computers. Moreover, it can search for multiple adapters or barcodes, and it can work with a configuration file containing all the adapters or barcodes to search, but it requires this file to contain pairs of 5′ and 3′ adapters or barcodes. This way, if barcodes were used in several combinations for samples, as we do, this file should contain all possible combinations of barcodes.

Thus, we needed—and created—a program that can clean the sequences of artifacts, and would be suitable for use with Ig genes in spite of their unique characteristics. We present here the Ig-HTS-Cleaner program, which enables the user to give the ends of the genes (primers and MID tags) as input no matter what their origin is, can handle multiple tags, and does not require any additional programs in order to run. Our Ig-HTS-Cleaner program does not require any knowledge in programming nor complicated installation, only a simple input file which contains the parameters for run. Moreover, the FASTA output files enable easy downstream analyses of the sequences.

Sequencing of complete Ig genes can currently be carried out only by the 454 pyrosequencing sequencing platform or the illumina platform. The reason is the maximum sequencing length required in order to get the full Ig gene. Only 454 or illumina currently reach a maximum read length of 500 nucleotides. Other platforms can reach such lengths only by using the paired-ends method, when only the ends of the gene are sequenced and the middle is inferred by comparing to a reference gene. This, of course, is not valid with Ig genes, due to their huge variability and the lack of a reference gene. Other platforms require assembly of complete sequences from shorter reads, which is also a problem due to the high mutation load and large numbers of similar but not identical sequences in Ig genes. When other sequencing platforms reach the same read length, our programs may be used on the data generated by them as well.

One of the shortcomings of pyrosequencing is that during the sequencing of homopolymer tracts (HPTs, repeats of the same nucleotide), the polymerase can add or delete one or more nucleotides from these repeats, or alternatively, the signal of poly-nucleotide incorporation can be misread (Huse et al., 2007). These errors may result in insertions/deletions (indels) that are a result of the sequencing and therefore are considered as artifacts (Margulies et al., 2005). In Ig gene research, it is very important to distinguish between artifact indels and legitimate indels that are a result of normal SHM and affinity maturation of B cells, although naturally occurring indels are very rare. Legitimate indels should be taken into account when analyzing mutations of the B cell Ig genes, and artifact indels should be discarded from the analysis. There are several common approaches for dealing with indels. Campbell et al. used an algorithm that discards sequences with insertions, deletions or substitutions that occurred near or in HPTs, unless the indel or the substitution was seen in both the forward and reverse reads (Campbell et al., 2008). In other studies, all sequences with any type of indel are excluded from analysis (Boyd et al., 2010; Wu et al., 2010) or included without accounting for indels (Wu et al., 2010). CANGS (Pandey et al., 2010) identifies indels that appear only in HPTs near the primers and discards them. The program does not identify indels occurring far from the primers. VarScan (Koboldt et al., 2009) and VARiD (Dalca et al., 2010) can identify indels, but these programs deal with variability and single nucleotide polymorphism (SNP) identification, and do not distinguish between legitimate and artifact indels, and are hence less suitable for identifying and discarding artifact indels from Ig genes. Recently, two methods for distinguishing true indels from sequencing artifacts have been developed. Dindel (Albers et al., 2011) utilizes a probabilistic method that accounts for the increased indel rates near HPTs. However, Dindel detects indels from short reads generated by Illumina sequencing and aligns the reads to a specific region in the genome. Hence, Dindel is not suitable for Ig genes because they are longer than Illumina reads and they cannot be aligned to a specific region in the genome due to the enormous variability and randomness of Ig gene rearrangements. PiCALL (Bansal and Libiger, 2011) also detects indels using a probabilistic method, but it works on a population of diploid individuals. Therefore, piCALL is not suitable for Ig gene sequences, in which different cells have different Ig genes.

Sometimes, discarding all the indels causes loss of information. For example, if an indel appears in a unique sequence, most of the algorithms would discard this sequence because no other sequence contains this indel. Nevertheless, there is a chance that this indel is legitimate, and we refer to such cases as uncertain indels. Because in several of our studies we perform sequencing on DNA from preserved tissue samples which do not yield large enough amounts of DNA (Tabibian-Keissar et al., 2008), we do not want to simply discard all unique sequences. Since there is no absolute way to identify all sequencing errors, and because we have limited sequencing data, we intend to save as many sequences as possible, and still avoid as many artificial indels and point mutations as possible. To address this issue, we developed Ig-Indel-Identifier, a program that identifies legitimate and artifact indels and does not discard sequences that contain uncertain indels. Hence, we may decide to keep these uncertain sequences for maximal information utilization.

This paper describes both Ig-HTS-Cleaner and Ig-Indel-Identifier. Our programs were designed to process Ig genes, but they are easily applicable to all types of sequences.

MATERIALS AND METHODS

Ig-HTS-Cleaner and Ig-Indel-Identifier have been programmed in Java on the Windows operating system and is saved as an executable JAR file. The JAR files support Linux and Microsoft Windows. An executable file for each of our programs is available at http://immsilico2.lnx.biu.ac.il/Software.html. To execute the program, the user should double-click on the program symbol after saving it in the same directory where the input files are saved. No special requirements are needed in order to run them, except for correctly constructing the input files as explained below.

Ig-HTS-Cleaner INPUT AND OUTPUT

The program receives as an input the following files, which should be saved in the same directory as the program. (1) A group of *.fna files (*denotes any desirable name) containing the FASTA sequence reads—see **Figure 1** for the structure of a typical read. (2) Quality (*.qual) files containing the scores for the sequences (both file types are received from the sequencing platform). (3) An input.txt file created and updated by the user, containing the parameters for the cleaning, such as the MID tags and the primer sequences, the length range within which the sequence is considered legitimate, the samples (in case more than one sample was sequenced), etc. A detailed explanation on how to fill the input.txt file can be found in **Figure 2**. The input file should be created precisely according to these instructions.

As output, the program generates the following files:

1. FailedInFindMIDs.txt—a FASTA file containing all the sequences in which the program could not find one or both MID tags, or the MID combination did not match the table in the input file.
2. FailedInFindPrimers.txt—a FASTA file containing all the sequences in which the program could not find one or both primers, such that only sequences with identifiable MIDs and primers are included in further analysis.
3. FailedInCheckLength.txt—a FASTA file containing all the sequences for which L2 (sequence length between the primers) was not within the allowed range.
4. FailedInQuality.txt—contains all sequences that had identifiable primers at both ends and were within the allowed length range, but the average quality score of the sequence was lower than the input threshold.
5. Log.txt—a tab-delimited text file that assembles details of the run in two parts. The first part (**Figure 3A**) contains a table of the samples that were sequenced and the following numbers per each sample: total number of sequences found, number of failed sequences in finding primers, percent of the last value out of the total, number of failed sequences in length, percent of the last value out of total, and out of the total after the previous stage, number of sequences with lower quality than threshold, percent of the last value out of total and out of the total after the previous stage, total remaining number of sequences, average quality score. The second part (**Figure 3B**) contains information regarding the total numbers of the run, such as (partial list): how many sequences failed in the MID tags finding step, how many failed in the primers finding step, how many failed in the length check, how many failed in the quality check, how many are in the sense or antisense orientation, and a short review of the parameters of the run.
6. A text file for each sample, containing the sequences that passed all the checks and were identified as belonging to that

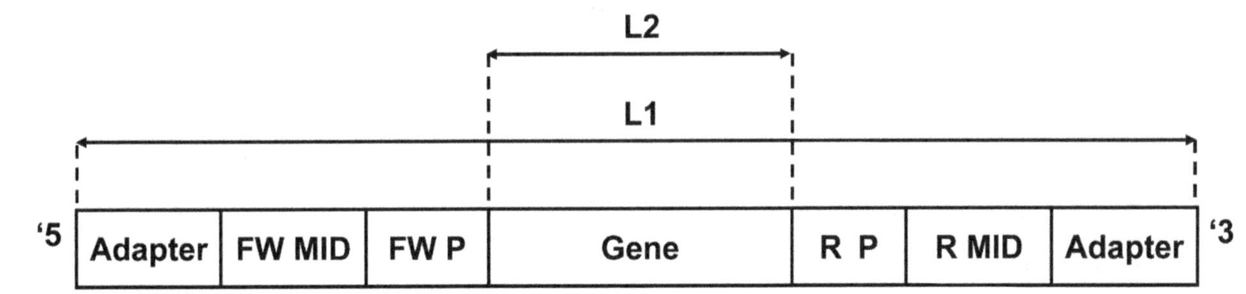

FIGURE 1 | A typical sequencer output (e.g., 454) read consists of the following segments (ordered from the 5′ end to the 3′ end): adapter: sequencer adapters. FW MID denotes the forward molecular identifier (tag). FW P denotes the forward polymerase chain reaction (PCR) primer. Gene is the target sequence. R P denotes the reverse PCR primer. R MID denotes the reverse molecular identifier (tag). L1: Sequence length before first filtering—should be in the allowed range defined by the first minimum and maximum values (minL1 < L1 < maxL1, for example, 200 and 400 in **Figure 2**). L2: Sequence length after primers were cut—should be in the allowed range defined by the second minimum and maximum values (minL2 < L2 < maxL2, for example, 150 and 360 in **Figure 2**). These ranges can be changed in the input file according to the data set and the specific requirements of each study.

sample according to their MID tag combination (given as input, **Figure 2**).

7. A text file for each sample, containing the quality score sequence of each sequence belonging to the sample, with the scores referring to the gene sequence only (without scores for the MID tags, primers, etc.).

Ig-HTS-Cleaner ALGORITHM

The program works according to the following outline (**Figure 4**):

1. Read input file and initiate parameters for the run.
2. Read .fna and .qual files and parse them for the run.
3. For each sequence, if it is longer or shorter than the allowed range given in the input file, discard it from analysis.
4. For each sequence that passed the previous step, do the following:
    - 4.1. Find tags (MIDs) at both ends of the sequence. If found, go to 4.2, else go to 4.5.
    - 4.2. Find Primers at both ends of the sequence. If found, go to 4.3, else go to 4.5.
    - 4.3. Check whether the length of the sequence between the primers is within the input range. If so, go to 4.4, else go to 4.5.
    - 4.4. Check the average quality score of the sequence. If the average quality score is below the input threshold, go to 4.5, else go to 4.6.
    - 4.5. A sequence that failed in one of the above stages will be written to a discard file according to the reason of failure.
    - 4.6. A sequence that succeeded in all the above stages will be written to an output file according to its MID combination.

MID tag finding

The goal of the first step is to find the MID tags for each sequence. Each 454 run enables the sequencing of several, pooled samples, as long as we mark each sequence according to its sample using known combinations of MID tags at both ends of the sequence (because sequencing may start at each end of the sequence). To use this feature, the genes must undergo preliminary PCR with primers that are connected to specific 10-base oligonucleotides, representing the MID tags. These tags were composed by the sequencing company to provide different oligosequences that are distinguishable. In addition, the reads also contain adapter sequences at their ends that are required for starting the sequencing (**Figure 1**). Since the number of tags that are sufficiently distinguishable from each other (see below) is limited, one can use primers with a known combination of forward and reverse MID tags for each sample. This way, one can obtain different sequences from many different samples at one run, and later correctly attribute the sequences to the original samples by identifying the MID tag combination in each sequence. If either MID tag cannot be identified, the program would not be able to attribute the sequence to a sample and thus will reject it as a failed sequence. The program searches each sequence for a perfect match to each MID tag (taken from the input file) at both ends of the sequence, which are the regions where we expect the MID tags to be found (and not in the middle of the read, for example). The search is executed on a limited range of nucleotides, given in the input file. If a perfect match is achieved, the number of the tag is noted. If not, the program searches for a perfect match of the minimal MID length that the user has inserted in the input file. This minimal MID length represents the number of consecutive nucleotides of the tag on the side closer to the primers (the inner side of the sequence) that enables unambiguous identification of the tag. This is done because the sequencer more often inserts errors close to the sequence boundaries, so the tags might have been trimmed or contain errors at their outer edges. We found that five consecutive nucleotides are the lowest number of nucleotides that can still distinguish between the different MID tags we used (basic set—Hamming distance: 6, **Table 1**). However, the minimal MID length is dependent on the Hamming distance of the MID set used, and should be assigned correctly by the user. The program prioritizes a perfect match, thus in case of a perfect match to the minimal MID length of one MID tag, the program will continue the search

```
organism
human
chain
h
quality threshold
20
maximum mismatches allowed
2
fraction of primer to search
0.75
range to search primers in
50
minimal mid length
5
mids
ACGAGTGCGT
ACGCTCGACA
AGACGCACTC
#
forward
TGCGMCAGGCCCCYGGACAAR
ARGRAAGGCCCTGGAGTGG
CCGCCAGGCTCCAGGSAAG
MGGGAAGGGRCTGGAGTGG
GAAAGGCCTGGAGTGGATGGG
TTGAGTGGCTGGGRAGGAC
#
reverse
TGACCRKGGTHCCYTGGCCC
#
minimum length
200
150
maximum length
400
360
table
1	1	sample1
2	2	sample2
3	3	sample3
1	2	sample4
2	3	sample5
1	3	sample6
3	2	sample7
2	1	sample8
3	1	sample9
#
```

FIGURE 2 | An example of the input.txt file content. In bold- words/characters that should always appear. **Organism**—represents the organism to which the sequences belong, "**Human**" in this example. **Chain**—represents the chain of the Ig (h, heavy as in this example; l, lambda; k, kappa). **Quality threshold**—the minimal average score for a sequence allowed. **Maximum mismatches allowed**—the number of mismatches the user allows when primers are being searched. "2" means that when primers are being searched, the sequence can contain 2 insertions/deletions or substitutions in the primer's sequence. **Fraction of primer to search**—in case the full primer was not found, the program searches only the given fraction of the primer from the side closer to the gene. **Range to search primers in**—the search is executed on a limited range of bases at the ends of the read. **Minimal MID length**—in case the full MID was not found, the program searches for a perfect match of the minimal length of the MID from the side closer to the gene. **Mids**—a list of the MID tags that have been used in the current sequencing. The program automatically numbers the MID tags according to the insertion order. At the end of each list, a "**#**" should appear, see example. In case no MIDs

(Continued)

FIGURE 2 | Continued

were used, leave only the title and the "#". **Forward**—a list of the forward primers that have been used in the current sequencing, used for identification of the primers. At the end of each list, a "#" should appear, see example. **Reverse**—a list of the reverse primers that have been used in the current sequencing, used for identification of the primers. At the end of each list, a "#" should appear, see example. **Minimum length**—two values, the first is the minimal length for the first filtering of the data (minL1). The second value represents the minimal length that is legitimate for the genes in between the primers (minL2). **Maximum length**—two values, the first is the maximal length for the first filtering of the data (maxL1). The second value represents the maximal length that is allowed for the genes in between the primers (maxL2). **Table**—contains the MID tag combination per each sample that was sequenced. MID tag numbers should coordinate with their serial number in the above list. This enables the program to attribute each sequence to its corresponding sample. Each line should contain: number of the forward MID tag/tab/number of the reverse MID tag/tab/sample id (see example). At the end of each list, a "#" should appear, see example. In case no MIDs were used, put 0 as the number of forward and reverse MIDs.

for a perfect match of the rest of the MID tags. Although rare, in case a perfect match of one MID tag and a perfect match of the minimal MID length of other MID tags are found in the same read-end, the program prefers the perfect match of the full MID tag.

A legitimate sequence contains a legitimate combination of tags (according to the input file) with the tag at the 5′ end found in the sense orientation and at the one 3′ end found in the anti-sense orientation. Each search for tags is performed using both the tags and their complementary sequences, in order to identify tags at both ends. If a match of two tags, one at each edge of the sequence, is found, the tag numbers are noted and the sequence in between the MID tags is passed on to the next stage of cleaning. Otherwise, the sequence is discarded from further analysis, and written to a file containing all the sequences that failed in this stage. It is important to note that Ig-HTS-Cleaner can also work in case no MIDs are listed (for example, when the sequencing was carried out on a single sample). The program will then search directly for primers, but it is important that the input file is written properly as detailed in **Figure 2**.

Primer identification

In this stage, the sequence between the MID tags (after MID tags have been removed) is searched for primers at both ends. Again, the search is executed on a limited range of nucleotides, given in the input file. The program runs using the primer lists given in the input file and searches for a perfect match of both forward and reverse primers in the current sequence. The program searches both the primer and its complementary sequence. If one or both primers were not found with a perfect match, the program searches for a partial match between the sequence and the primers, after the latter are trimmed (from the side furthest from the gene) leaving a fraction of the original primers' length, given in the input file (e.g., 75% of the original length). Sometimes PCR and/or sequencing trim the primer ends. Searching only the primer fraction closer to the gene enables the program to identify even primers which contain errors or were trimmed at the ends distal to the gene. This is useful when

A

Sample	Total	Failed in primers	% out of total	Failed in length	% out of total	% out of remaining	Failed in quality	% out of total	% out of remaining	Total remaining	Average score
Sample1	2097	22	1.05	0	0	0	1	0.048	0.048	2074	21
Sample2	1579	760	48.13	0	0	0	1	0.063	0.122	818	21
Sample3	2461	73	2.97	0	0	0	0	0.000	0.000	2388	21
Sample4	664	240	36.14	0	0	0	0	0.000	0.000	424	23
Sample5	749	30	4.01	0	0	0	0	0	0	719	22

B

Total number of reads: 641574
How many reads were not within the first length boundaries and were discarded from further analysis: 253030
How many did not have MIDs at both ends of the sequence: 3970
How many did not have primers at both ends of the sequence (either forward or reverse primer, or both): 4380
How many were not within the second length range: 258
How many were shorter than the range: 258
How many were longer than the range: 0
How many sequences had average quality scores below the threshold: 7
How many sequences are in a sense orientation out of the ok sequences: 67234
How many sequences are in a antisense orientation out of the ok sequences: 59665
How many succeeded in partial match of forward primer: 17519
How many succeeded in partial match of reverse primer: 18098
How many failed in finding a forward primer: 1280
How many failed in finding a reverse primer: 1856
How many had primers, but both were sense or antisense, which probably means these are chimeric sequences: 1549
How many have different MID combinations than those given in the input, out of those that have MIDs: 1572
How many out of the total sequences could not be identified by their MIDs (percent): 4
MIDs were searched 5 nts from the side closer to the primers in order to address cases of deletion of the edges.
The partial match was based on the following criteria:
taking 0.75 of primer length from the side closer to the gene,
searching for it in the 50 nts at the edges of the gene- depending on the orientation of the primer,
allowing a maximum of 2 mismatches (insertions/ deletions/ substitutions).
The threshold for the average quality score per sequence was: 20

FIGURE 3 | A sample of an Ig-HTS-Cleaner log.txt output file. (A) The first part of the file (after importing the .txt file into a table). "Sample" is the sample name, inserted in the input file. "Total" represents the total number of sequences received from the sequencer before cleaning (as counted after MID identification). "Failed in primers" represents the number of sequences without primers at both ends. "% out of total" means the % of the "Failed in primers" column out of the total column. "Failed in length" represents the number of sequences with length not in between the input range. "% out of total" means the % of the "Failed in length"column out of the total column. "% of the remaining" for the "Failed in length" column represents the % after we subtract the number of sequences failed in primers from the total and calculate the % from that. "Failed in quality" represents the number of sequences with an average quality score below the threshold. "% out of total" means the % of the "Failed in quality" column out of the total column. "% of the remaining" for the "Failed in quality" column represents the % after we subtract the number of sequences failed in primers and in length from the total and calculate the % from that. "Total remaining" represents the number of sequences that have passed all cleaning steps successfully. "Average score" is the average score for the sample. First, the average score for each sequence is calculated by an average of the scores per base, given in the .qual files in the 454 output. Then, the average score of the sample is calculated as the average of the scores of all sequences belonging to the sample. **(B)** The second part of the file, containing information and statistics regarding the run.

the reads are from one sample and thus there was no use in MID tags. The partial match allows the number of mismatches per primer defined by the user input. The larger the number of allowed mismatches, the more erroneous primer identifications would occur. Therefore, one should decide on the maximal number of mismatches allowed for the data, according to this trade-off. We examined this parameter on data sets from human and mouse tissues (data not shown). We ran each data set in Ig-HTS-Cleaner with different values between 1 and 10 for the number of allowed mismatches. For our human data set, we found that a value of two allowed mismatches is the best cut-off which minimizes both the loss of sequences and the gain of erroneous sequences with falsely identified primers. For our mouse data set, we found that a value of four allowed mismatches is the best cut-off. This type of analysis may be performed on other data sets with Ig-HTS-Cleaner, to decide on the best value for each data set.

The partial match uses dynamic programming of local alignment of the sequence with each forward or reverse primer, based on the Smith–Waterman algorithm. If both forward and reverse primers are found, the gene orientation is known, hence the MID tag order is known as well, so the sample identity is known.

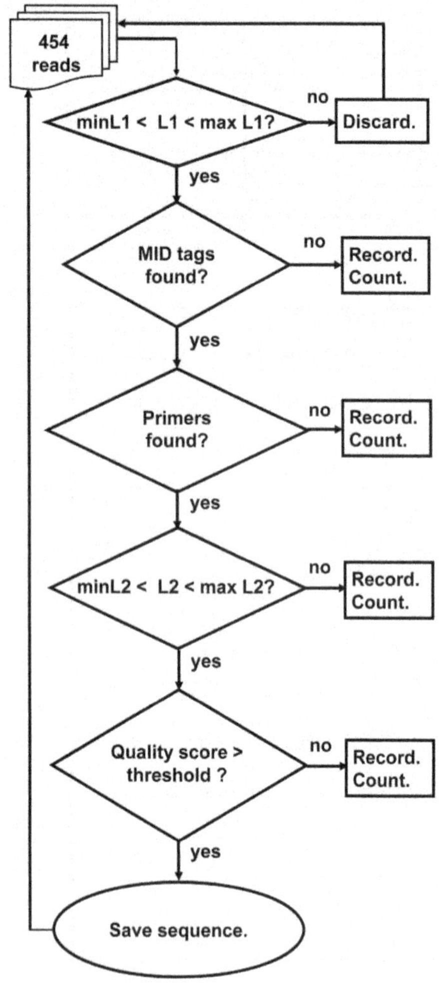

FIGURE 4 | A schematic outline of the Ig-HTS-Cleaner program algorithm. "Discard" means: discard the read because it is not likely to be an immunoglobulin gene sequence. "Record" means: write the sequence to a file containing all sequences that failed in this stage. "Count" means: count the number of failed sequences. In case the failure is in the last two stages, the counts are done per sample. "MID tags found?" means: "Is there an identifiable MID tag at each end of the sequence?", "Primers found?" means: "Is there an identifiable primer at each end of the sequence?" Checks of L1 and L2 are as described in **Figures 1** and **2**. "Quality score > threshold?" means: "Is the average quality score of the sequence larger than the threshold score given in the input file?" "Save sequence" means: "Write the sequence to the corresponding sample file. Advance the counter of sequences per sample."

Table 1 | List of MID tags, forward and reverse primers used for Ig-HTS-Cleaner validation[a].

	MID tags (5′ to 3′)[b]	ACGAGTGCGT ACGCTCGACA AGACGCACTC AGCACTGTAG ATCAGACACG ATATCGCGAG CGTGTCTCTA CTCGCGTGTC TAGTATCAGC
Human	Forward primers (5′ to 3′)	TGCGMCAGGCCCCYGGACAAR ARGRAAGGCCCTGGAGTGG CCGCCAGGCTCCAGGSAAG MGGGAAGGGRCTGGAGTGG GAAAGGCCTGGAGTGGATGGG TTGAGTGGCTGGGRAGGAC
	Reverse primer (5′ to 3′)	TGACCRKGGTHCCYTGGCCC
Mouse—heavy chain	Forward primers (5′ to 3′)	AGRTYCARCTGCARCAGYC TGCAGCTKMAGSAGTCAG GARGTGAAGCTKSTSGAGTC GAGGAGTCTGGAGGAGGCTT CTGGGATATTGCAGCCCTCC AGGTGTGCATTGTGAGGTGC GTSAGGTGCAGCTKGTRGA CAATCCCAGGTTCACCTACAA
	Reverse primer (5′ to 3′)	GTGGTBCCTTSGCCCCAG
Mouse—light chain	Forward primers (5′ to 3′)	MTGATGACCCARTCTCCA SRGATATTGTGATGACGCAGG AWTGTDCTSACCCARTCTCC CCTGTGGRGACATTGTGAT AYCCVGATGACYCAGTCT CCAGATGTGAYRTYCARATG BCAGTGTGACATCCRVAT ACACAGGCTCCAGCTTCTCT TCCCAGGCTGTTGTGACTC CAACTTGTGCTCACTCAGTC CTCTAGGAAGCACAGTCAAAC
	Reverse primer (5′ to 3′)	GTGGTBCCTTSGCCCCAG

[a]*Key to degenerate nucleotides:* $R = A + G$; $M = A + C$; $W = A + T$; $K = G + T$; $S = G + C$; $Y = C + T$; $H = A + T + C$; $B = G + T + C$; $D = G + A + T$; $N = A + C + G + T$; $V = G + A + C$.

[b]*We used the basic set, with Hamming distance = 6.*

The sequence then proceeds to the next stage. If one or both primers were not found, the sequence is discarded from further analysis, and written to a file containing all the sequences that failed in this stage.

Length check

This is the last check before the sequence is accepted as legitimate. If the sequence length between the primers is within the allowed range, the sequence is written to the file of the sample corresponding to its MID tag combination; each file represents one sample. Otherwise, the sequence is discarded, and written to a file containing all the sequences that failed in this stage.

Quality check

For each sequence, a file containing the sequencing quality scores per each base is generated during the sequencing run. When using the 454 platform, each nucleotide in each sequence gets a score between 0 and 40 that represents the confidence level of the sequencer that a specific nucleotide is the correct one. In other words, the higher the score per base (or average score per sequence), the better the quality of the sequencing. For each read, a sequence of numbers between 0 and 40 in the original length of the read is generated. The file with all the score sequences is the .qual file.

In addition to cleaning the sequence of tags and primers, a calculation of the quality score per sequence is performed in Ig-HTS-Cleaner using the .qual files. One can either look at each position to investigate its quality (for example, when examining point mutations), or can look at the average quality score per sequence or even per sample to evaluate the quality of sample sequencing (for example, when dealing with preserved tissue samples where DNA is often denaturated). For each sequence, the quality score is calculated as the average score for all bases of the sequence, after tags and primers were removed. Then, the quality score of each sample is calculated, as the average score of the sample's sequences.

The calculation of minimal and average quality scores of one sample or a group of samples is also important for downstream analyses. For example, in Ig-Indel-Identifier (see below for more details), point mutations are checked for their quality score, and if the latter is lower than the threshold given by the user, the sequence can be discarded. In **Figure 5**, we show as an example the quality score analyses of four samples from human lymph nodes (LN).

In this example, many (42.81%) of the sequences in the LN samples had an average quality score of 37–38, which is considered a very high score (**Figure 5A**). On the other hand, many of the sequences also contained nucleotides with low quality scores (11–12, **Figure 5B**). These analyses led us to conclude that in our LN data, we could use the average quality score threshold of 30 without losing to many sequences. However, as most of the sequences appear to have a low minimal quality score (mostly lower than 20, with a peak in 11–12), we could not use a minimal threshold larger than 10.

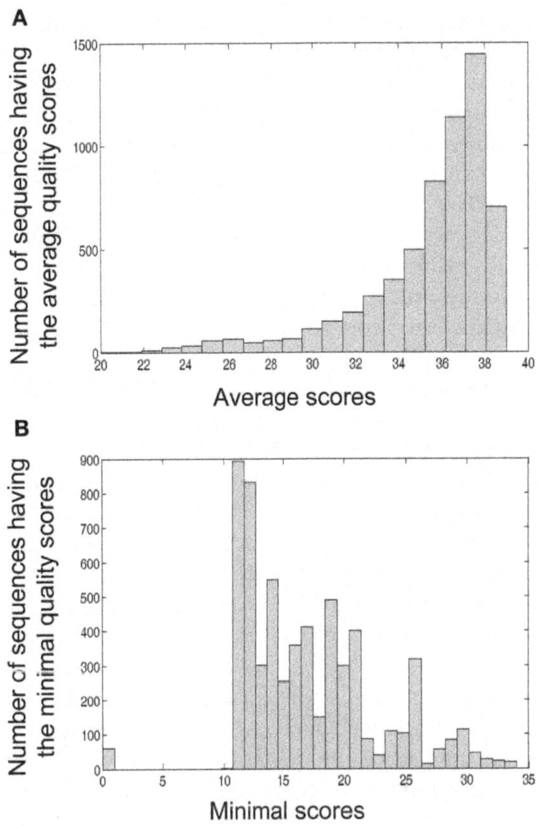

FIGURE 5 | Four formalin-fixed paraffin-embedded (FFPE) reactive lymph node tissues, archived about 10 years ago, from adult patients, were used as part of a study that dealt with Ig repertoire analysis of gastric lymphomas. In the current paper we used these samples in order to demonstrate quality scores obtained by the 454 platform using FFPE tissues. **(A)** Average quality score distribution of sequences obtained from four LN samples. For each sequence, the average quality score was calculated as the sum of all base scores divided by the length of the sequence. **(B)** Minimal quality score distribution of sequences obtained from four LN samples. For each sequence, the minimal quality score was calculated as the minimal base score value of all base scores in the sequence.

Ig-Indel-Identifier INPUT AND OUTPUT

To identify indels created by the sequencer, the sequences are usually compared to some reference gene. In the case of Ig genes, where no reference gene can be used, the sequences should be organized by clones, according to their germline (GL) segment identifications. Then, a consensus sequence can be created for each clone based on all sequences in the clone, and serve as the reference gene. In our analysis pipeline, we first identify the GL segments for every sequence using SoDA (Volpe et al., 2006). Then we group the sequences (from the same sample) that use the same GL segments into one clone, and find the consensus sequence for the N-regions of this clone. In each position of the N-regions, the consensus GL contained the most frequent nucleotide in all the aligned sequences that belonged to the same clone. In the data presented below, we identified clones only based on their V(D)J GL segments for the purpose of demonstration of the action of Ig-Indel-Identifier. However, for proper data analysis, these groups of sequences are aligned and examined, as more than one clone may have the same V(D)J combination. For this purpose, one may use the clustering-based program created by Gaeta et al. (Chen et al., 2010), which deals with groups of sequences that share the same V(D)J segments, and checks whether they belong to one or more clones. After the clonally-related groups of sequences are identified, the sequences from each clone are aligned, along with the "root" sequence composed of the GL segments and N-region consensus, using ClustalW2 (Larkin et al., 2007). The output files from ClustalW2 (*.txts files in the PIR format, which is an alignment format) serve as the input files for Ig-Indel-Identifier.

In addition to cleaning artifact indels, Ig-Indel-Identifier identifies point mutations (mismatches) by comparing to the reference gene or GL, and decides whether they are sequencing artifacts or may be derived from natural mutation processes. For each point mutation, Ig-Indel-Identifier checks the quality score of the base, given in the *.qual files. One of the parameters that are given by the user is the minimal quality score. This parameter is used when Ig-Indel-Identifier compares the quality score of the point mutation to the given minimal quality score. If the quality score of the point mutation is lower than the user's threshold, and if this point mutation appears in fewer sequences in the clone than the number given in the input.txt file, the sequence is discarded. Moreover, Ig-Indel-Identifier identifies whether a point mutation occurred inside activation-induced cytidine deaminase (AID) motifs that contain HPT [AACA or the complementary TGTT (MacCarthy et al., 2009)]. If so, the sequence shall not be discarded even if its quality score is lower than the threshold. If the user is not interested in identifying such mismatches, the value of the minimal quality score given in the input.txt file should be set to −1.

Ig-Indel-Identifier receives as input *.txts files, each containing an alignment of a group of clonally-related sequences with their consensus GL sequence; an *.input file, containing all the sequences from the current sample in the FASTA format; and a *.qual file, corresponding to the *.input file, which contains the quality score sequences of the sequences in *.input file. Ig-HTS-Cleaner generates these files automatically. In addition, the user should prepare a file called "input.txt," with integer values for three parameters, as follows:

1. The minimum number of sequences in a clone that must share the same indel or a low quality score point mutation for this indel or mutation to be considered legitimate. Before discarding a sequence, the user may decide that in case more sequences contain the same indel or low quality score point mutation, the suspected sequence shall not be discarded. The user can choose how many sequences in a clone must share that particular indel or mutation in order to save this sequence. The higher this threshold number, the fewer suspected sequences would be saved.
2. HPT length: the user can decide on the minimum length of same-nucleotide stretch that will be considered a HPT. The longer the HPT length, the more sequences would be saved, since fewer indels would be identified as near-HPT indels.
3. The minimal quality score for a point mutation to be considered legitimate. The higher the minimal quality score, the more sequences would be discarded. If the user is not interested in identifying such mismatches, the value of the minimal quality score given in the input.txt file should be set to −1.

To use Ig-Indel-Identifier on non-Ig gene sequences, one should create a consensus sequence of all sequences that should be checked. This can be done using several programs, such as ClustalW2 (Larkin et al., 2007). A consensus sequence is composed of the most frequent base in each position of the aligned sequences. Then, the consensus and the sequences should be run in ClustalW2 to create the *.txts file that contains the alignment. Ig-Indel-Identifier will work on this file together with the *.input file that should contain the sequences. When using ClustalW2 in order to align each of the sequences with its reference gene, each gap (of one or more nucleotides), in either the GL or the tested sequence, anywhere in the sequence, is designated as an indel that would be checked by Ig-Indel-Identifier.

As output, the program generates the following files for each input file:

1. "(Name-of-input-file)-WithoutIndels.txt"—a FASTA file that contains a list of all sequences from the current input file which contain neither artifact nor uncertain indels.
2. "(Name-of-input-file)-CloneOfSize1WithIndels.txt"—a FASTA file that contains a list of sequences that contain suspected indels, but do not belong to a larger clone, so we cannot decide whether each indel is an artifact or not. We call these "uncertain indels," and keep these sequences separately, so one can perform the analysis either with or without them, as desired.
3. "(Name-of-input-file)-IllegitimateIndels.txt"—a FASTA file that contains a list of the sequences with artifact indels, which are part of a large clone, hence these indels are certainly artifact and not uncertain indels (this list has no overlap with output file number 2).
4. "(Name-of-input-file)-SeqsWithLowQualPointMuts.txt"—a FASTA file that contains a list of sequences that contain point mutations with quality scores lower than the minimal quality score given by the user, and which appeared in fewer sequences in the clone than set by the user.
5. "(Name-of-input-file)-Ig-Indel-Identifier.log"—a file containing the report of the run.

Ig-Indel-Identifier ALGORITHM

The program works according to the following outline (**Figure 6**):

1. For each sequence in each clone, do:

    1.1. Search for indels or point mutations by comparing the sequence to the corresponding GL (or consensus) sequence position by position, from the last indel or point mutation checked (or, in a new sequence—from the first position of the alignment) until the alignment ends. If an indel is found, go to 1.2. If a point mutation is found, go to 1.9, else go to 1.7.

    1.2. If this indel appears near a HPT (see below), go to 1.3, else go to 1.6.

    1.3. This indel is suspected to be an illegitimate (artifact) indel. If this indel is unique, i.e., no other sequence in its clone shares the same indel, go to 1.4, else go to 1.6.

    1.4. If the sequence is the single one in its clone go to 1.8, else go to 1.5.

    1.5. The sequence has an artifact indel and hence is discarded from further analyses. Write it to the appropriate file and go to the next sequence (step 1).

    1.6. This indel is considered as a legitimate indel. Go to 1.1.

    1.7. Sequence is OK. Write it to the appropriate file and go to the next sequence (step 1).

    1.8. Sequence has an uncertain indel. Mark as uncertain. Go to 1.1.

    1.9. Check if the quality score of the point mutation base is lower than the threshold given by the user as input. If so, go to 1.10, else go to 1.1.

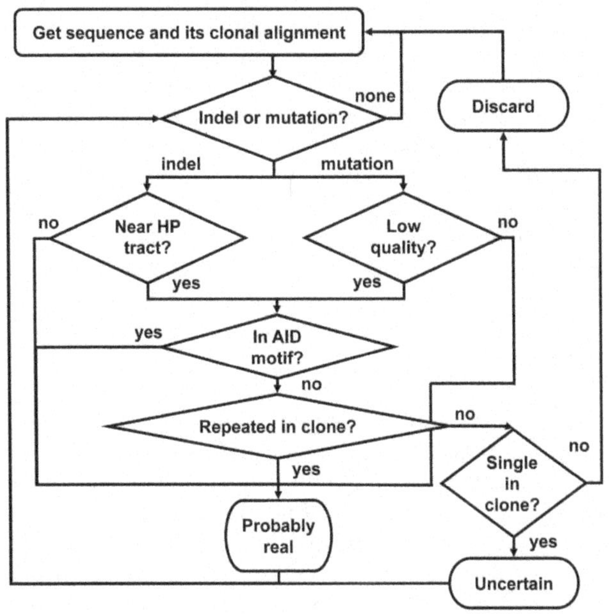

FIGURE 6 | A schematic outline of the Ig-Indel-Identifier program. "Indel or mutation?" means: "Are there (more) indels or mutations in the sequence?" "Low quality?" means: "Did the point mutation have a quality score lower than the input threshold?" "Near HP tract?" means: "Is the indel near a HPT?" "In AID motif?" means: "Is the indel or point mutation detected inside the known AID motif (AACA or the complementary TGTT)?" "Repeated in clone?" means: "Are there more sequences in the clone with the same indel?" "Single in clone?" means: "Is this the only sequence in the clone?" "Discard" means: "Discard the sequence because it has an artifact indel." "Uncertain" means: save the sequence separately as it is suspected to have artifact indel(s), but there are no other sequences in this clone, hence we cannot be sure. "Probably real" means: save the sequence as it has a legitimate indel according to our definitions.

1.10. Check if the point mutation is inside the AID motif (AACA or the complementary TGTT). If so, go to 1.1, else go to 1.11.
1.11. Check the number of sequences in the clone that share the same point mutation. If there are more sequences in the clone but no other sequence shares the same point mutation, go to 1.12. Else, go to 1.1.
1.12. The sequence has an artifact point mutation and hence is discarded from further analyses. Write it to the appropriate file and go to the next sequence (step 1).

2. Write the sequences to the output files.

In order to decide whether an indel is near or inside a HPT of a length that equals or exceeds the minimum length given by the user, we test the GL sequence to find whether one or more of the following conditions are fulfilled:

- The indel is inside a HPT.
- The indel is 5′ to a HPT.
- The indel is 3′ to a HPT.

We chose to first define HPTs by at least two identical nucleotides. Although this definition is very broad, as pairs of identical nucleotides are very common in all sequences, we preferred to check more indels than to leave sequences with illegitimate ones in the dataset. However, the user can choose the minimal length defining a HPT. If any of the above three conditions is fulfilled, this indel is suspected to be a sequencing artifact. A suspected indel is denoted as an artifact if fewer than the threshold number of sequences that share this indel exist in the clone.

Creating a simulated dataset for testing Ig-Indel-Identifier

In order to check the Ig-Indel-Identifier program, we collected 504 real sequences without indels from previous 454 HTS studies. This dataset contained either groups of clonally-related sequences or single sequences, all already aligned to their GL. We simulated the artificial induction of deletions (see below) on this dataset, creating a new and larger dataset of sequences, each with one deletion at most, near or inside HPTs of different lengths. The simulation was not created in order to reflect the "natural" generation of indels by the sequencer, but simply in order to have sequences with no more than one deletion, near or inside HPTs of different lengths, in order to test the Ig-Indel-Identifier program and analyze the results more easily. The simulation works as follows. For each sequence, the simulation decides whether to introduce a deletion or not. In case a deletion should be introduced, the simulation draws a value (2–10) for the length of HPT that the deletion should occur in. If the sequence does not contain any HPTs with that length, the simulation keeps drawing a value until at least one HPT with the drawn length is found in the sequence. From the list of positions contained in the chosen HPT, the simulation draws one position in one HPT to introduce the deletion in. A deletion (and indels in general) can occur 5′ to the HPT, 3′ to the HPT, or in its middle. Hence, the simulation draws the exact position for the deletion, according to the length of HPT drawn in the first step. Deletions were not allowed at the beginning or at the end of a sequence. Deletions were introduced by replacing the character (A/C/G/T) in the desired position of the aligned sequence by "–". Ig-Indel-Identifier identifies insertions and deletions according to the alignment of the clonally-related sequences and their GL, and hence a "–" sign in the GL is considered as an insertion, and in the sequence, it is considered as a deletion). Introducing only deletions during the simulation should not affect identification of indels by Ig-Indel-Identifier, and we used only deletions for convenience. After introducing a deletion to the sequence, the simulation draws a value (0–10) for the number of duplicate sequences carrying the same deletion that will be generated. One of our assumptions for correctly identifying artifact indels is that indels that appear in more than one sequence in the same clone are probably real and thus are not designated as suspect. The exact number of sequences carrying the same indel, which are needed for accurately identifying an indel, can change between datasets and observations. It is important to note that all the deletions introduced into the sequences during the simulation were artifact indels, and hence were all expected to be identified by Ig-Indel-Identifier and evaluated based on their frequency within the clone.

The simulation algorithm is as follows:

1. For each sequence (not GL) in a clone do:
   1.1. Decide whether the sequence will undergo a deletion. If so, go to 1.2. Else go to the next sequence (step 1).
   1.2. Draw a value (2–10) for the length of HPTs to search for in the sequence. If no HPT in the drawn value is found, repeat step 1.2. Else, go to 1.3.
   1.3. Draw one HPT from the sequence (there can be several, but only one is chosen).
   1.4. Draw the specific position near or inside the HPT (this depends on the HPT's length).
   1.5. Replace the character in the chosen position (A/C/G/T) with a "–".
   1.6. Draw the number of duplicate sequences carrying the same indel (0–10).
   1.7. Generate the new sequence(s) and write them into a new file.

RESULTS

Ig-HTS-Cleaner—PERFORMANCE AND VALIDATION

We tested the performance of Ig-HTS-Cleaner on real data from 454 HTS. Twenty-nine DNA samples (from a study that will be published elsewhere) were subject to Ig gene amplification by PCR and the products were sequenced on the Roche 454 FLX Titanium platform to yield a total of 44,617 reads. We ran Ig-HTS-Cleaner on this data set with the following parameters: average quality score threshold of 20, 2 allowed mismatches in the primer search, 75% of the primer's length to search, and a range of 50 bases at the ends of the read for the MIDs and primers search (denoted as "combination 1," see **Table 2**). Out of the 44,617 reads, 35,453 reads contained MID tags at both ends of the read. In the next step, Ig-HTS-Cleaner discarded 2504 sequences that did not contain identifiable primers at both ends, because in such sequences we cannot identify sequence orientation. It is important to identify primers at both ends, not only in order to identify where the gene is positioned inside the read, but also to identify the orientation of both primers, in order to discard those chimeric sequences—created during the PCR or the sequencing—that contain both primers in the same orientation rather than opposite orientations. These artifact sequences can be identified by primers with the same orientation. Only one read did not have a length within the requested range and was discarded. The reason the latter number was so low is that all Ig genes are of similar lengths, such that if the whole gene between the primers was sequenced, it is highly likely to have the correct length. Much shorter or longer reads could be chimeric sequences (discussed below). Only seven sequences did not pass the average quality threshold, which we set to be 20. This is not surprising, as most of the nucleotides were sequenced with a quality score of 20–40 (see **Figure 5**). The user may decide whether to assign this threshold a higher value, and thus to discard more sequences. Finally, when Ig-HTS-Cleaner had finished running, we were left with 32,941 remaining sequences (**Table 2**, parameter combination 1). The list of MID tags and primers used in this specific run can be found in **Table 1**.

We ran Ig-HTS-Cleaner on the same data set with four different combinations of parameters (numbered 2–5 in **Table 2**), in order to demonstrate the influence of each parameter on the cleaning process. Parameter combination number 2 had the same parameter values as the original run (number 1) except for allowing up to 4 mismatches. It is not surprising that fewer reads were discarded in the stage of primer search (because more mismatches were allowed), thus there were more sequences attributed to MID tag combinations. In addition, six reads were included due to the lenient primer search, but two were discarded due to insufficient length, and 4 were discarded due to a low average quality score. Parameter combination number 3 had the same parameter values as the original run (number 1) except for the fraction of primer to search, which was set to 100%—that is, the program would search only for the full primer. It was obvious that in this case, more reads would be discarded, as we searched for the full primer sequence and allowed only 2 mismatches. There were fewer reads with low average quality scores, because some were already discarded in the primer search step. Parameter combination number 4 had the same parameter values as the original run (number 1) except for the range of 25 bases at the ends of the read for the MID and primers search. In this case, which took longer than previous runs (see below regarding run times), more reads were subjected to partial match, which allows mismatches, and thus fewer reads were discarded. Parameter combination number 5 had the same parameter values as the combination number 4 except for the fraction of primer to search, which was set to 100%. In this case, more reads were discarded than in the previous run, because the program searched only for the full primer. However, fewer reads were discarded than in runs 1 and 3, because more reads were subjected to partial match.

Table 2 | A summary of the Ig-HTS-Cleaner results in each parameter combination: human data set of 44K sequences.

Parameter combination	Number of sequences received	Number of sequences with tags	Number of sequences without primers	Number of sequences that failed due to length	Number of sequences that failed in quality check	Number of remaining sequences
1	44,617	35,453	2504	1	7	32,941
2	44,617	35,891	1662	3	11	34,215
3	44,617	35,114	3528	1	3	31,582
4	44,617	36,246	439	0	8	35,799
5	44,617	35,911	1684	0	4	34,223

See text for parameter combinations.

Validation of Ig-HTS-Cleaner results was done manually. Each cleaning step was examined individually. We checked for false negatives by looking at 50 reads that were discarded due to lack of MID tags and manually checked whether they do contain MID tags. None of the sequences was found to be false negative in this step. False positives were also not found when we performed manual checks on about 10 sequences from each sample (a total of ~200 sequences), which had successfully passed this step. The same validation steps were performed on ~150 sequences lacking primers and on ~100 sequences at both ends of which primers were found. This step was more complicated due to the use of dynamic programming for identifying primers with less than 100% match. About 50 sequences that did not contain 100% match of a primer were also checked to validate the dynamic programming algorithm's accuracy. All of the sequences that proceeded to the next cleaning step contained primers at both ends. Discarded sequences in this step indeed lacked one or more primers at their edges. Length checks were done automatically: a simple script validated that the lengths of all sequences that had passed the length check are truly within the allowed range, and that the sequences that had failed this step really were outside the allowed length range. We also validated that the sequences that were discarded due to lower quality score had indeed an average quality scores below the threshold. We collected these sequences and automatically calculated their average quality scores.

Applying Ig-HTS-Cleaner on the first data set of 44,617 reads, with a range of 50 nucleotides at each end to search primers in, took approximately 3–4 min to run on an Intel® core™2 CPU 6700, 2 GB RAM 2.67 GHz. When the primer search range was decreased to 25, Ig-HTS-Cleaner run took almost 1 h on the same computer. The longer run time is because when the primer search range decreases, primers that were located not in the first 25 bases but closer to the inner side of the sequence would not be found. Hence, the program would search for partial match of the primer(s), and that would take much longer. We then proceeded to test Ig-HTS-Cleaner on larger data sets, obtained from human and mouse DNA samples and together representing ~527,000 reads that were assigned into samples. However, for this number of reads we could not use the above-described computer due to memory shortage, and needed to run Ig-HTS-Cleaner on our UNIX server, which is equipped with larger RAM (16 GB). An Ig-HTS-Cleaner run on the ~527,000 reads took approximately 5 min on our UNIX server. Hence, we recommend using Ig-HTS-Cleaner on UNIX machines or on PCs with large internal memory. Regarding memory complexity, the program saves the reads for the whole running time in a special data structure, representing $O(n \times k)$ memory, where n represents the length of a sequence, k represents the number of sequences, and $n \ll k$, hence $O(k)$ memory is required. For each instance of dynamic programming used in finding a partial primer match, we have $O(n \times m)$, where n represents the sequence length and $m \ll n$ represents the primer length. Actually, when the program searches for the primer, it searches it in a window shorter from the full sequence length at each side of the sequence, and not in the whole sequence, as we expect the primers to be on the sides of the sequence and not in the middle. Thus, $O(n \times m)$ is limited to a finite number. Moreover, a partial match search was carried out in less than 10% of the reads, reducing the complexity in one order of magnitude. To summarize, a run of ~500,000 sequences performed on a computer equipped with large internal memory (16 GB) would yield results within a short time (5 min). **Table 3** presents the cleaning results of both human and mouse data sets with an average quality score threshold of 20, and 2 and 4 allowed mismatches of primers for the human and mouse data sets, respectively. The two data sets were sequenced in the same run, but in different lanes. We present here the numbers of sequences attributed to each dataset and the cleaning results using Ig-HTS-Cleaner. The list of MID tags and primers used in this specific run can be found in **Table 1**.

Ig-Indel-Identifier—PERFORMANCE AND VALIDATION

We tested the performance of Ig-Indel-Identifier on the first dataset described above. The original study included 29 samples, but after cleaning with Ig-HTS-Cleaner, five samples out of the 29 yielded fewer than 30 sequences each, and these sequences were discarded from further analyses due to lack of interest. Data from 24 samples, which originally contained 36,944 sequences, were taken from the output of Ig-HTS-Cleaner. Out of these sequences, 33,767 sequences did not contain indels at all; this is reasonable, since SHM inserts mostly single base substitutions (Liu and Schatz, 2009; Steele, 2009). On the other hand, 3177 sequences contained indels (both uncertain and artifact), representing 8.6% of all sequences. Of the latter, 93 sequences with uncertain indels and 3084 with artifact indels were found (**Table 4**).

Applying Ig-Indel-Identifier on the data set of 44,617 reads took approximately 5 min to run on an Intel® core™2 CPU 6700, 2 GB RAM 2.67 GHz. Regarding memory complexity, the program saves the reads for the whole running time in a special data structure, representing $O(n \times k)$ memory, where n represents the length of a sequence and k represents the number of sequences. For each sequence, both the sequence and its GL (consensus) sequence are being compared, representing additional $O(n)$ memory space.

Table 3 | A summary of the Ig-HTS-Cleaner results: human and mouse data sets of 500 K sequences together.

Organism	Number of sequences with tags	Number of sequences without primers	Number of sequences that failed in due to length	Number of sequences that failed in quality check	Number of remaining sequences
Human	116,546	3248	4	10	113,284
Mouse	410,352	143,729	271	4	266,348

Table 4 | Numbers of sequences after Ig-Indel-Identifier cleaning.

Total	Number of sequences w/o indels	Total number of sequences with indels	% of sequences with indels	Number of uncertain indels[a]	Number of sequences with artifact indels[b]
36,944	33,767	3177	8.6	93	3084

[a]*An uncertain indel is an indel in a single sequence that does not belong to a multi-sequence clone.*

[b]*An artifact indel is an indel near a HPT, where no other sequences in the same clone contain the same indel (and is not in a single sequence).*

TESTING Ig-Indel-Identifier ON SIMULATED DATA

We collected 504 sequences without indels, from 85 clones with sizes ranging from a single sequence to 73 sequences. These sequences were taken from seven different samples from the dataset described above. The simulation ran on each clone 10 independent times, each time with different random variables as described above, in order to extend the dataset. These simulations yielded a total of 10,475 sequences, out of which 10,308 sequences had artifact deletions.

We then ran Ig-Indel-Identifier on each clone from the simulated dataset, using all possible combinations of the following program parameters: the minimum HPT length (with values ranging between 2 and 5) and the required number of sequences sharing the same indel for an indel to be considered a legitimate indel (with values ranging between 1 and 12). The former value range was based on our finding that there were no HPTs of length higher than five in our dataset.

For each parameter combination, we recorded how many artifact deletions were identified and calculated the percentage of accuracy (the number of identified deletions divided by the total number of artifact deletions and multiplied by 100).

As expected, the higher the value for HPT length, the lower the number of identified artifact deletions. This is reasonable since the probability of a HPT to be found in a sequence decreases with its length (HPTs of length two are much more frequent than HPTs of length five).

On the contrary, but also as expected, the higher the required number of sequences sharing the same deletion, the more artifact deletions were identified, designated as suspect and finally discarded. This is also reasonable, since the higher the required number of sequences sharing the same indel, the more stringent the requirements, and hence more indels (and sequences) do not fulfill these requirements.

Table 5 presents the average required number of sequences sharing the same deletion in each HPT length that was needed to identify 50% of the artifact deletions, or to identify all the artifact deletions—or as many as the program managed to identify. Due to the fact that Ig-Indel-Identifier was run individually on different samples (in our case we used seven different samples to collect the initial dataset of clones and sequences without indels from), and since each Ig-Indel-Identifier run included all combinations as explained above, the results in **Table 5** represent the average numbers out of 336 ($7 \times 4 \times 12$) runs.

When the minimal HPT length was 2, 50% of the artifact deletions were identified only when we required more than five sequences sharing the same deletion (on average) for a deletion to be considered legitimate. The maximal number of the artifact deletions identified out of the total deletions in the dataset was

Table 5 | The numbers of sequences sharing an indel within a clone that are required in order for it to be considered legitimate, that allow the indicated level of artifact indel identification.

HPT length	50% identification	Maximal identification
2	5	10
3	7	10
4	–	9*
5	–	7*

**Numbers marked with a "*" indicate that for the indicated HPT length, the program achieved less than 50% identification even with the indicated number of required sequences. Higher values gave the same results, so the minimal values of the required number of sequences in a clone that share the same indel were chosen.*

obtained only when we required more than 10 sequences sharing the same deletion (on average). Similarly, when the HPT length was 3 (or 4), 50% of the artifact deletions were identified when we required more than 7 (or 9) sequences sharing the same deletion (on average). For HPT = 3, the maximal number of the artifact deletions identified out of the total deletions in the dataset was when we required more than 10 sequences sharing the same deletion (on average). With HPTs of length 4–5, no required number of sequences sharing the same indel could help identify more than 50% of the artifact indels. If the HPT length is set to 4 in Ig-Indel-Identifier, the program does not consider HPTs of length less than 4 and hence "misses" those indels, which brings the % identification down no matter now many sequences we require. When the HPT length was 5, the maximal number of the artifact deletions identified out of the total deletions in the dataset was when we required more than seven sequences sharing the same deletion (on average). Again, most of the deletions occurred near or inside HPTs of length less than 5, thus, no matter what the number of sequences sharing the same indel was, most of the indels were missed. Based on these results, our conclusion is that one should consider using either 2 or 3 as the values for HPT length in Ig-Indel-Identifier; otherwise the program would miss many artifact indels. Of course, it would be more efficient for each user to investigate their data for appearances of indels near or inside HPTs and lengths of the latter, in order to decide on the appropriate parameter values. We also recommend demanding as many sequences to share the same indel as possible (each user should optimize this number for their specific dataset).

In addition, we tested Ig-Indel-Identifier performance on 2355 Ig Sanger sequences from data published on B cells from autoimmune diseases (AI) (Zuckerman et al., 2010a,b) and lymphomas (Zuckerman et al., 2010c). The Sanger sequences barely contained

Table 6 | Numbers of Sanger and 454 sequences after Ig-Indel-Identifier cleaning.

Sequencing method	Sample (number of sequences in the sample)	Number of indels found in the sample	Number of sequences with artifact indels[a]	Number of uncertain indels[a]	Number of sequences w/o indels or with legitimate indels	Total number of point mutations in the sample	Number of point mutations in AID targeting motifs
Sanger	MG (33)	24	2	0	31	459	11
	MS (78)	4	0	0	78	2709	25
	Myositis-Bradshaw (33)	25	4	0	29	781	0
	RA-Gause (28)	7	1	2	25	356	6
	RA-Miura (123)	125	10	73	41	2495	29
	SS-Gellrich (70)	2	0	0	70	1269	13
	SS-Jacobi (190)	94	14	58	118	1226	22
	BL-Chapman (22)	0	0	0	22	465	1
	MZL-Zhu (72)	0	0	0	72	587	8
	DLBCL (708)	98	17	0	692	19,416	209
	FL (772)	87	31	0	741	19,249	226
	PCNSL (226)	4	2	0	224	7204	127
454	LN-1 (507)	2276	24	1	482	4631	2
	LN-2 (913)	8164	82	1	837	5682	0
	LN-3 (585)	5803	30	0	557	3019	0
	LN-4 (1137)	17,831	280	2	887	5744	0

[a]*Same as in* ***Table 4****.*

MG, Myasthenia Gravis; MS, Multiple Sclerosis; RA, Rheumatoid Arthritis; SS, Sjögren's Syndrome; BL, Burkitt's Lymphoma; MZL, Marginal Zone Lymphoma; DLBCL, Diffuse Large B Cell Lymphoma; FL, Follicular Lymphoma; PCNSL, Primary Central Nervous System Lymphoma; LN, Lymph Node.

For the original studies from which the sequences were taken, see Zuckerman et al. (2010a,b,c).

indels (**Table 6**). However, when they did, most of the indels were uncertain, due to the small numbers of sequences sampled using the Sanger method. Only a small proportion of the sequences contained artifact indels. Therefore, the many indels observed in the 454 sequences and identified by Ig-Indel-Identifier are probably sequencing errors.

DISCUSSION

HTS is increasingly popular in various research fields such as immunology, cancer research, and evolutionary biology. The enormous amounts of data generated by HTS require the development of new and efficient data processing algorithms. There are already several tools for cleaning and analysis of HTS data, but no dedicated program for Ig genes has been made publicly available up to this work. In this paper, we present Ig-HTS-Cleaner, a program that successfully performs the pre-processing of Ig sequences derived from HTS, and Ig-Indel-Identifier, a program that precisely distinguishes between legitimate and artifact indels which are typical of 454 HTS (and discards the latter), and also discards sequences containing point mutations with low quality score that appear only once in a clone. The two programs are independent of each other or any other tools, and are applicable to other sequences, in addition to Ig genes, and other sequencing platforms in addition to 454.

While the rules defined in Ig-Indel-Identifier do not guarantee that we identify all sequencing artifacts, it is known that HTS using the 454 platform mostly introduces indels near HPTs (Huse et al., 2007), while SHM of Ig genes mostly introduces point mutations rather than indels (Liu and Schatz, 2009; Steele, 2009). Moreover, most features of the SHM process are studied through analysis of point mutations (Zuckerman et al., 2010a,b,c). Thus, on one hand, the elimination of a large fraction of the artifact indels helps us retain the legitimate sequences that—having fewer indels—are easier to align and analyze further. On the other hand, the remaining artifact indels that may have not been eliminated do not affect the measurements of mutation characteristics.

The next step in analyzing Ig genes is to identify the GL V(D)J segments used in the unmutated (ancestor) sequences, and then assign the sequences into clonally-related groups. For gene segment identification, we use either SoDA (Volpe et al., 2006) or iHMMune-align (Gaëta et al., 2007). Our automated pipeline, which follows the above-described processes of cleaning the data, removing indels and identifying GL segments, contains our program "Ig_Clone_Finder©," which groups the sequences into clones based only on their V, D, and J segments. The weakness of this method is that two different rearrangements using the same V(D)J segments may be grouped together into the same clone; this necessitates manual checking of groups that clearly segregate into two or more different clones. A more sophisticated method, based on sequence clustering and the use of an empirical cut-off, was recently published by Chen et al. (2010); however, it has yet to be tested on large data sets.

Another weak point of HTS analysis is identifying chimeric (hybrid) sequences generated during PCR or HTS. It is essential to discard such sequences before performing repertoire and hypermutation analyses. Although there are a few existing tools that identify and discard chimeric sequences from HTS data (Huber et al., 2004), these programs are not suitable for use with Ig gene sequences. These programs depend on reference sequences that do not exist for Ig gene sequences, due to the complexity of Ig gene rearrangements and mutations, which make almost each sequence unique. There are several reasons why such a tool has not been fully developed yet for Ig genes, although HTS is already available and is extensively used. One major reason is the large homology between V segments. In order to find a chimeric sequence, one must recognize the two most probable V segments [obtained by e.g., SoDA2 (Munshaw and Kepler, 2010) or iHMMune-Align (Gaëta et al., 2007)] that are likely to have been merged to create the suspected sequence. The problem is that GL genes from the same family can only diverge by up to 25% (by definition) and are usually much more similar, while mutated Ig genes can diverge by several tens of mutations (Cook and Tomlinson, 1995; Rajewsky, 1996). Thus, it is often impossible to identify whether the mismatches in the alignment are due to SHM of the suspected sequence, or due to SNPs that distinguish between the two almost identical V segments. Due to these reasons, we still search for chimeric sequences manually. However, discarding sequences that are too short or too long to be legitimate Ig gene sequences, as we do, probably gets rid of some obvious chimeras.

Technologies for HTS and the amounts of sequences generated using them continue to evolve. For this reason, we developed Ig-HTS-Cleaner and Ig-Indel-Identifier, two independent programs for cleaning high-throughput sequences. We hope these programs would be useful to the research community.

ACKNOWLEDGMENTS

The authors are indebted to Dr. Deborah Dunn-Walters for critical reading of the manuscript. This work was supported in parts by an Israel Science Foundation [grant number 270/09, to Ramit Mehr and Iris Barshack]; and a Human Frontiers Science Program Research Grant [to Ramit Mehr]. The work was part of Miri Michaeli's studies toward the MSc degree in Bar-Ilan University, and she was supported by a Combined Technologies Scholarship from the Israeli Council for Higher Education.

REFERENCES

Ademokun, A., Wu, Y.-C., and Dunn-Walters, D. K. (2010). The ageing B cell population: composition and function. *Biogerontology* 11, 125–137.

Albers, C. A., Lunter, G., Macarthur, D. G., McVean, G., Ouwehand, W. H., and Durbin, R. (2011). Dindel: accurate indel calls from short-read data. *Genome Res.* 21, 961–973.

Aronesty, E. (2011). *ea-utils: Command-line Tools for Processing Biological Sequencing Data.* Available online at: http://code.google.com/p/ea-utils

Bansal, V., and Libiger, O. (2011). A probabilistic method for the detection and genotyping of small indels from population-scale sequence data. *Bioinformatics* 27, 2047–2053.

Barak, M., Zuckerman, N. S., Edelman, H., Unger, R., and Mehr, R. (2008). IgTree: creating Immunoglobulin variable region gene lineage trees. *J. Immunol. Methods* 338, 67–74.

Blanca, J. M., Pascual, L., Ziarsolo, P., Nuez, F., and Cañizares, J. (2011). ngs _ backbone: a pipeline for read cleaning, mapping and SNP calling using next generation sequence. *BMC Genomics* 12:285. doi: 10.1186/1471-2164-12-285

Bolger, A., and Giorgi, F. *Trimmomatic: A Flexible Read Trimming Tool for Illumina NGS Data.* Available online at: http://www.usadellab.org/cms/index.php?page=trimmomatic

Boyd, S. D., Gaëta, B. A., Jackson, K. J. L., Fire, A. Z., Marshall, E. L., Merker, J. D., et al. (2010). Individual variation in the germline Ig gene repertoire inferred from variable region gene rearrangements. *J. Immunol.* 184, 6986–6992.

Boyd, S. D., Marshall, E. L., Merker, J. D., Maniar, J. M., Zhang, L. N., Sahaf, B., et al. (2009). Measurement and clinical monitoring of human lymphocyte clonality by massively parallel V-D-J pyrosequencing. *Sci. Transl. Med.* 1, 12ra23.

Buffalo, V. *Scythe.* Available online at: https://github.com/vsbuffalo/scythe

Campbell, P. J., Pleasance, E. D., Stephens, P. J., Dicks, E., Rance, R., Goodhead, I., et al. (2008). Subclonal phylogenetic structures in cancer revealed by ultra-deep sequencing. *Proc. Natl. Acad. Sci. U.S.A.* 105, 13081–13086.

Chen, Z., Collins, A. M., Wang, Y., and Gaëta, B. A. (2010). Clustering-based identification of clonally-related immunoglobulin gene sequence sets. *Immunome Res.* 6(Suppl. 1), S4.

Cook, G. P., and Tomlinson, I. M. (1995). The human immunoglobulin VH repertoire. *Immunol. Today* 16, 237–242.

Dalca, A. V., Rumble, S. M., Levy, S., and Brudno, M. (2010). VARiD: a variation detection framework for color-space and letter-space platforms. *Bioinformatics* 26, i343–i349.

Dunn-Walters, D. K., and Ademokun, A. (2010). B cell repertoire and ageing. *Curr. Opin. Immunol.* 22, 514–520.

Falgueras, J., Lara, A. J., Fernández-Pozo, N., Cantón, F. R., Pérez-Trabado, G., and Claros, M. G. (2010). SeqTrim: a high-throughput pipeline for pre-processing any type of sequence read. *BMC Bioinformatics* 11:38. doi: 10.1186/1471-2105-11-38

Gaëta, B. A., Malming, H. R., Jackson, K. J. L., Bain, M. E., Wilson, P., and Collins, A. M. (2007). iHMMune-align: hidden Markov model-based alignment and identification of germline genes in rearranged immunoglobulin gene sequences. *Bioinformatics* 23, 1580–1587.

Galan, M., Guivier, E., Caraux, G., Charbonnel, N., and Cosson, J.-F. (2010). A 454 multiplex sequencing method for rapid and reliable genotyping of highly polymorphic genes in large-scale studies. *BMC Genomics* 11:296. doi: 10.1186/1471-2164-11-296

Gibson, K. L., Wu, Y.-C., Barnett, Y., Duggan, O., Vaughan, R., Kondeatis, E., et al. (2009). B-cell diversity decreases in old age and is correlated with poor health status. *Aging cell* 8, 18–25.

Gordon, A. *FASTX-Toolkit.* Available online at: http://hannonlab.cshl.edu/fastxtoolkit/

Huber, T., Faulkner, G., and Hugenholtz, P. (2004). Bellerophon: a program to detect chimeric sequences in multiple sequence alignments. *Bioinformatics* 20, 2317–2319.

Huse, S. M., Huber, J. A., Morrison, H. G., Sogin, M. L., and Welch, D. M. (2007). Accuracy and quality of massively parallel DNA pyrosequencing. *Genome Biol.* 8, R143–R151.

John, J. S. *SeqPrep*. Available online at: https://github.com/jstjohn/SeqPrep

Koboldt, D. C., Chen, K., Wylie, T., Larson, D. E., McLellan, M. D., Mardis, E. R., et al. (2009). VarScan: variant detection in massively parallel sequencing of individual and pooled samples. *Bioinformatics* 25, 2283–2285.

Kong, Y. (2011). Btrim: a fast, lightweight adapter and quality trimming program for next-generation sequencing technologies. *Genomics* 98, 152–153.

Krueger, F. *Trim Galore!* Available online at: http://www.bioinformatics.babraham.ac.uk/projects/trimgalore/

Larkin, M. A., Blackshields, G., Brown, N. P., Chenna, R., McGettigan, P. A., McWilliam, H., et al. (2007). Clustal W and Clustal X version 2.0. *Bioinformatics* 23, 2947–2948.

Lassmann, T., Hayashizaki, Y., and Daub, C. O. (2009). TagDust—a program to eliminate artifacts from next generation sequencing data. *Bioinformatics* 25, 2839–2840.

Lindgreen, S. (2012). *AdapterRemoval: Easy Cleaning of Next Generation Sequencing Reads.* Available online at: http://code.google.com/p/adapterremoval/

Liu, M., and Schatz, D. G. (2009). Balancing AID and DNA repair during somatic hypermutation. *Trends Immunol.* 30, 173–181.

MacCarthy, T., Kalis, S. L., Roa, S., Pham, P., Goodman, M. F., Scharff, M. D., et al. (2009). V-region mutation *in vitro, in vivo,* and in silico reveal the importance of the enzymatic properties of AID and the sequence environment. *Proc. Natl. Acad. Sci. U.S.A.* 106, 8629–8634.

Margulies, M., Egholm, M., Altman, W. E., Attiya, S., Bader, J. S., Bemben, L. A., et al. (2005). Genome sequencing in microfabricated high-density picolitre reactors. *Nature* 437, 376–380.

Martin, M. (2011). Cutadapt removes adapter sequences from high-throughput sequencing reads. *EMBnet J.* 17, 10–12.

Morgan, M., Anders, S., Lawrence, M., Aboyoun, P., Pagès, H., and Gentleman, R. (2009). ShortRead: a bioconductor package for input, quality assessment and exploration of high-throughput sequence data. *Bioinformatics* 25, 2607–2608.

Munshaw, S., and Kepler, T. B. (2010). SoDA2: a Hidden Markov Model approach for identification of immunoglobulin rearrangements. *Bioinformatics* 26, 867–872.

Pandey, R. V., Nolte, V., and Schlötterer, C. (2010). CANGS: a user-friendly utility for processing and analyzing 454 GS-FLX data in biodiversity studies. *BMC Res. Notes* 3:3. doi: 10.1186/1756-0500-3-3

Rajewsky, K. (1996). Clonal selection and learning in the antibody system. *Nature* 381, 751–758.

Scheid, J. F., Mouquet, H., Feldhahn, N., Seaman, M. S., Velinzon, K., Pietzsch, J., et al. (2009). Broad diversity of neutralizing antibodies isolated from memory B cells in HIV-infected individuals. *Nature* 458, 636–640.

Schmieder, R., Lim, Y. W., Rohwer, F., and Edwards, R. (2010). TagCleaner: identification and removal of tag sequences from genomic and metagenomic datasets. *BMC Bioinformatics* 11:341. doi: 10.1186/1471-2105-11-341

Steele, E. J. (2009). Mechanism of somatic hypermutation: critical analysis of strand biased mutation signatures at A:T and G:C base pairs. *Mol. Immunol.* 46, 305–320.

Tabibian-Keissar, H., Zuckerman, N. S., Barak, M., Dunn-Walters, D. K., Steiman-Shimony, A., Chowers, Y., et al. (2008). B-cell clonal diversification and gut-lymph node trafficking in ulcerative colitis revealed using lineage tree analysis. *Eur. J. Immunol.* 38, 2600–2609.

Unknown. *FAR – The Flexible Adapter Remover.* Available online at: http://sourceforge.net/apps/mediawiki/theflexibleadap/

Volpe, J. M., Cowell, L. G., and Kepler, T. B. (2006). SoDA: implementation of a 3D alignment algorithm for inference of antigen receptor recombinations. *Bioinformatics* 22, 438–444.

Wu, Y.-C., Kipling, D., Leong, H. S., Martin, V., Ademokun, A., and Dunn-Walters, D. K. (2010). High-throughput immunoglobulin repertoire analysis distinguishes between human IgM memory and switched memory B-cell populations. *Blood* 116, 1070–1078.

Zuckerman, N. S., Hazanov, H., Barak, M., Edelman, H., Hess, S., Shcolnik, H., et al. (2010a). Somatic hypermutation and antigen-driven selection of B cells are altered in autoimmune diseases. *J. Autoimmun.* 35, 325–335.

Zuckerman, N. S., Howard, W. A., Bismuth, J., Gibson, K. L., Edelman, H., Berrih-Aknin, S., et al. (2010b). Ectopic GC in the thymus of myasthenia gravis patients show characteristics of normal GC. *Eur. J. Immunol.* 40, 1150–1161.

Zuckerman, N. S., McCann, K. J., Ottensmeier, C. H., Barak, M., Shahaf, G., Edelman, H., et al. (2010c). Immunoglobulin gene diversification and selection in follicular lymphoma, diffuse large B cell lymphoma and primary central nervous system lymphoma revealed by lineage tree and mutation analyses. *Int. Immunol.* 22, 875–887.

20

HSP: bystander antigen in atopic diseases

Joost A. Aalberse[1]*, Berent J. Prakken[1]* and Berber Kapitein[2]

[1] Department of Pediatric Immunology, Center for Molecular and Cellular Intervention, Wilhelmina Children's Hospital, University Medical Center, Utrecht, Netherlands
[2] Pediatric Intensive Care Unit, Sophia Children's Hospital, Rotterdam, Netherlands

Edited by:
Willem Van Eden, Utrecht University, Netherlands

Reviewed by:
Miriam Wittmann, University of Leeds, UK
Cristina Bonorino, Pontificia Universidade Catolica do Rio Grande do Sul, Brazil

***Correspondence:**
Joost A. Aalberse and Berent J. Prakken, Wilhelmina Children's Hospital, University Medical Centre, Department of Pediatric Immunology, Center for Molecular and Cellular Intervention, Eureka Institute for Translational Medicine, KC.03.063.0, PO Box 85090, Utrecht, The Netherlands.
e-mail: jaalber2@umcutrecht.nl; bprakken@umcutrecht.nl

Over the last years insight in the complex interactions between innate and adaptive immunity in the regulation of an inflammatory response has increased enormously. This has revived the interest in stress proteins; proteins that are expressed during cell stress. As these proteins can attract and trigger an immunological response they can act as important mediators in this interaction. In this respect, of special interest are proteins that may act as modulators of both innate and adaptive immunity. Heat shock proteins (HSPs) are stress proteins that have these, and more, characteristics. More than two decades of studies on HSPs has revealed that they are part of intrinsic, "natural" mechanisms that steer inflammation. This has provoked comprehensive explorations of the role of HSPs in various human inflammatory diseases. Most studies have focused on classical autoimmune diseases. This has led to the development of clinical studies with HSPs that have shown promise in Phase II/III clinical trials. Remarkably, only very little is yet known of the role of HSPs in atopic diseases. In allergic disease a number of studies have investigated the possibility that allergen-specific regulatory T cell (Treg) function is defective in individuals with allergic diseases. This raises the question whether methods can be identified to improve the Treg repertoire. Studies from other inflammatory diseases have suggested HSPs may have such a beneficial effect on the T cell repertoire. Based on the immune mechanisms of atopic diseases, in this review we will argue that, as in other human inflammatory conditions, understanding immunity to HSPs is likely also relevant for atopic diseases. Specifically, we will discuss why certain HSPs such as HSP60 connect the immune response to environmental antigens with regulation of the inflammatory response. Thus they provide a molecular link that may eventually even help to better understand the immune pathological basis of the hygiene hypothesis.

Keywords: allergic disease, atopic disease, stress proteins, heat shock protein, HSP60, regulatory T cells, hygiene hypothesis, inflammation

INTRODUCTION

Over the last years insight in the complex interactions between innate and adaptive immunity in the regulation of an inflammatory response has increased enormously. This has revived the interest in stress proteins; proteins that are expressed during cell stress. As these proteins can attract and trigger an immunological response they can act as important mediators in this interaction. In this respect, of special interest are proteins that may act as modulators of both innate and adaptive immunity. Heat shock proteins (HSPs) are stress proteins that have these, and more, characteristics. More than two decades of studies on HSPs has revealed that they are part of intrinsic, "natural" mechanisms that steer an inflammatory response (Pockley, 2003; van Eden et al., 2005). This has provoked comprehensive explorations of the role of HSPs in various human inflammatory diseases. Most of these studies have focused on classical autoimmune diseases such as type I diabetes (IDDM), rheumatoid arthritis (RA), and juvenile idiopathic arthritis (JIA; Abulafia-Lapid et al., 1999; de Kleer et al., 2003, 2004). This has led to the development of clinical studies with HSPs that have shown promise in Phase II/III clinical trials in both IDDM and RA (Albani et al., 1995a; Raz et al., 2001; Prakken et al., 2004).

Remarkably, only very little is yet known of the role of HSPs in atopic diseases. Based on the immune mechanisms of atopic diseases, in this review we will argue that, as in other human inflammatory conditions, understanding immunity to HSPs is likely also relevant for atopic diseases. Specifically, we will discuss why certain HSPs such as HSP60 connect the immune response to environmental antigens with regulation of the inflammatory response. Thus, they provide a molecular link that may eventually even help to better understand the immune pathological basis of the hygiene hypothesis: an important concept relating the increase in the prevalence of atopic disease with exposure to microbes or microbial products early in life.

ALLERGY

Atopy is the predisposition to develop allergic diseases like atopic dermatitis, food allergy, asthma, and allergic rhinitis. It is characterized by a predominant typical T helper 2 (Th2)-like immune response (Umetsu et al., 2003). Firstly, an environmental allergen, like an inhalant or food allergen interacts with the innate immune system. After uptake by antigen-presenting cells, subsequent T cell priming leads to the stimulation of type 2 cytokines such as interleukin (IL)-4, IL-5, and IL-13. These cytokines interact with their receptors to induce a class switch toward IgE production and to increase the number of eosinophils and mast cells. In immediate hypersensitivity reactions IgE binds to its receptors and causes mast cells to degranulate. Apart from IgE, increased levels of IgG4 are often measured in allergic individuals. IgG4 is considered as an antibody with anti-inflammatory activity (van der Neut et al., 2007). The levels of IgG4 are usually elevated in serum from people that are repeatedly exposed to the same antigen, like beekeepers, or subjects receiving increased doses of antigen during specific immune therapy (SIT). In addition to this humoral immune response, allergy is characterized by a cellular response, mostly mediated by Th2 cells (Del Prete, 1992; Ozdemir et al., 2010), but also by Th1 cells (like in atopic dermatitis) and regulatory T cells.

The combination of these humoral and cellular responses, both innate and adaptive, leads to an allergic inflammatory reaction (Yazdanbakhsh et al., 2002). Here we will discuss various aspects of the allergic immune responses in the context of the possible role of environmental antigens such as HSPs in steering this immune response.

ALLERGY AND THE HYGIENE HYPOTHESIS

The prevalence of atopic disease has increased tremendously in the second half of the twentieth century (Peat et al., 1994). Although the cause of this increase is not known though, a genetic cause is unlikely due to the time span in which the increase took place. Therefore environmental changes are more likely causes of this observed increase. Strachan (1989) first proposed the concept of the hygiene hypothesis. This hypothesis states that the increase in the prevalence of atopic disease is due to a decreased exposure to microbes or microbial products early in life, especially in western societies. The concept was supported by the observation of an inverse association between both atopic dermatitis and hay fever and the number of children in a household. Although the hygiene hypothesis and its proposed immune mechanism are still under debate, in the 1990s numerous of studies have been published supporting this hypothesis. For example, these observations relate the number of siblings, the number of infections and exposure to endotoxins on the farm, with the incidence of atopic diseases (Jarvis et al., 1997; Bodner et al., 1998; von Mutius et al., 1999; Wickens et al., 1999; Braun-Fahrlander et al., 2002).

IMMUNE MECHANISMS OF THE HYGIENE HYPOTHESIS

What could be the immunological cause of this inverse relation between exposure to environmental antigens and the incidence of allergic disease? The explanation takes us back to the original observations in the eighties of Mosmann and Coffman who defined two main subtypes of helper T lymphocytes: Th1 and Th2 cells. Th2 cells are characterized by their production of cytokines like IL-4, IL-5, IL-9, and IL-13 and chemokines like TARC and MDC. They are involved in mediating allergic responses and host defense against parasitic infection (Mosmann and Coffman, 1989).

During fetal life and shortly after birth a predominant Th2 response is present (Wegmann et al., 1993). During life, a shift to a predominant Th1 response occurs in non-allergic subjects, but this shift may be incomplete in allergic individuals. As a consequence, an allergic individual will develop a Th2 response to an allergen leading to IgE production and typical type 2 cytokine production (IL-4, IL-5, and IL-13) and ultimately to a clinical allergic reaction, whereas non-allergic subjects develop a Th1 response leading to a protective IgG response and production of IFN-γ (Larche, 2007). This is the basis for the immunological explanation of the hygiene hypothesis, as exposure to microbes and microbial products would stimulate a Th1 response. Those individuals that were not enough exposed to these stress factors would be more prone to develop predominant Th2 responses, and thus an allergic response. Obviously this is still a simplification of the immune pathogenesis that does not explain all observations. For example, a Th1 response in allergic individuals would implicate the development of late hypersensitivity responses, whereas healthy individuals do not respond to allergens with a clinically noticeable response (Chen et al., 2004).

The hygiene hypothesis also does not explain why not only the incidence of allergic diseases is increasing but also that of auto immune diseases like RA and IDDM (Sheikh et al., 2003). These diseases are obviously known as typical Th1-like diseases.

TRIGGERING AN ALLERGIC IMMUNE RESPONSE

In order to fully assess and better appreciate the value of the hygiene hypothesis it is important to understand which cells are responsible for the initial trigger leading to the characteristic allergic immune response. First, naive T cells have to be activated, in a way that promotes the classical Th2 like response. There is recent evidence that basophils may play a crucial role in antigen recognition and processing. When recruited to lymph nodes they are able to induce Th2 cell differentiation through the release of IL-4 (Sokol et al., 2009; Falcone et al., 2011). Other cells also have the capacity to process and present allergens, including mast cells, macrophages, eosinophils, and natural helper cells. Natural helper cells are innate cell populations that include innate Th2 cells and are activated by IL-25 and IL-33 to secrete Th2 cytokines (Saenz et al., 2010).

There is an increasing realization that Th2 cells are not the only cells involved in the pathophysiology of allergic disease, as particularly in severe disease other cells than Th2 play a role in aggravating and perpetuating the immune response (**Table 1**; Lloyd and Hessel, 2010).

First of all, whereas Th2 cytokines have a clear role in initiating an allergic response, especially Th1 cells have been implicated in more chronic severe allergic disease, both in atopic dermatitis and allergic asthma (Krug et al., 1996; Ong and Leung, 2006; Yamanaka and Mizutani, 2011).

Secondly, in addition to the Th2 cytokines IL-4, IL-5, and IL-13, recently also IL-9 was shown to play an important role in asthma. At first IL-9 was discussed as a new Th2 cytokine. It was shown that Th9 cells are dependent on both IL-4 and transforming growth factor-beta (TGF-β) for their development. Interestingly, like Th2 cells, also Th9 cells are regulated by IL-25, predominantly seen in lung inflammation (Devos et al., 2006; Hauber et al., 2007; Soroosh and Doherty, 2009; Angkasekwinai et al., 2010). IL-25 (like IL-33 and thymic stromal lymphopoietin) is a type II initiating cytokine (Oliphant et al., 2011). In addition to the role of

Table 1 | Different subtypes described to play a role in the pathogenesis of allergic diseases.

Cell	Main transcription factor	Activating cytokines	Effector cytokines	Role in allergic diseases
Th1	T-Bet	IL-12	IFNγ	Possible role in chronic asthma or atopic dermatitis
Th2	GATA-3	IL-4, IL-25, IL-33, TSLP	IL-4, IL-5, IL-13, IL-25	Eosinophil production; IgE induction
Th9	PU-1	IL-4, TGFβ, IL-10, IL-25	IL-9, IL-10	Mucus production, lung inflammation, dermatitis
Th17	Batf	TGFβ, IL-1β IL-6, IL-21	IL-6, IL-8, IL-17, IL-22	Possibly related to steroid resistant asthma; related to neutrophil production
Th22	RORγT(?)	?	IL-22	Limiting airway inflammation in mice. Negative association with Th2 cytokines
Tr1	FOXP3	TGFβ	IL-5, IL-10, IL-13, TGFβ	Regulatory function on B cells by suppression of allergen-specific IgE and induction of IgG4 and IgA
Tregs	FOXP3	TGFβ	IL-10	Diminished function and number in allergic individuals

IL-25 in lung inflammation, it is also of importance in atopic dermatitis and food allergy (Aalberse et al. unpublished data; Hvid et al., 2011). Although IL-25 (also known as IL-17E) is a cytokine from the IL-17 family it has opposite effects of IL17A (IL-17).

Thirdly, Th17 cells (named after their main effector cytokine; IL-17) like Th1 cells may be associated with more severe asthma and mediate a more neutrophilic pattern of inflammation.

Fourthly, it was recently shown that IL-22 (also produced by Th17 cells), is produced by a distinct set of CD4+ cells, named Th22-cells. These cells have been implicated as being protective in a mouse model of allergic lung inflammation (Souwer et al., 2010) and may play a role in the severity of atopic dermatitis in humans (Nograles et al., 2009).

Finally, a lot of attention has recently focused on a subset of T cells with the capacity to suppress other T cells, namely regulatory T cells (Treg). Two types of regulatory T cells will be discussed below, namely IL-10 producing regulatory cells and FOXP3 expressing regulatory cells.

REGULATORY T CELLS

Here we will discuss two types of regulatory T cells; FOXP3 expressing Tregs and IL-10 producing regulatory T cells. However, it has to be emphasized that the distinction between these two types is not absolute, as for example FOXP3 expressing Tregs are also capable of producing IL-10. Moreover, many different regulatory T cells, may even act in concert in a single immune response.

IL-10 PRODUCING REGULATORY T CELLS

As discussed above, exposure to an allergen leads to the development of sensitization in a susceptible individual. Upon a next encounter, a typical Th2 reaction will follow, including a humoral (IgE and IgG4) response. In contrast, when healthy (non-allergic) individuals are exposed to an allergen it was long thought that (in line with the Th1/Th2 dichotomy) instead of a Th2 response a Th1 response would develop. However it has become clear that, in fact, this is not the only difference between a normal and an allergic response to an allergen. Though indeed some IFN-γ responses to allergens are present in healthy individuals, a study by Akdis et al. (2004) showed that this is a simplification of the reality. They isolated CD4 T cells specific to several food- and aeroallergens from healthy and allergic individuals according to their IL-4, IFN-γ, and IL-10 secretion profile. Interestingly, allergen-specific T cells that belong to all three secretion profiles were detectable in both healthy and allergic individuals, with allergen-specific IL-10-secreting T cells being the predominant subset in healthy individuals. They regarded these IL-10 producing CD4+ T cells as T regulatory cell type 1 (Tr1 cells). Seemingly, low Tr1 numbers and high Th2 cell numbers resulted in an allergic response, whereas in healthy individuals a mixed Th1/Th2 response is associated with a strong IL-10 response (Larche, 2007). The crucial role for IL-10 in allergy is also suggested by other studies on food and inhalant allergies. In cow's milk allergy, T-cell clones derived from children that are persistently allergic produced Th2 cytokines (IL-4, IL-13), whereas allergic control subjects that are cow milk tolerant produced a mixed Th1/Th2 response associated with markedly elevated IL-10 levels (Tiemessen et al., 2004).

Similar observations of elevated IL-10 levels associated with less allergy symptoms were made in inhalation allergies. Children raised in a house with a cat are less likely to become allergic to cat allergen than those who only get indirect exposure. Many of these highly exposed children had an IgG and IgG4 response to the major cat allergen Fel d 1 without production of specific IgE. This induction of high levels of allergen-specific IgG4 in the relative absence of IgE has been referred to as a modified Th2 response (Platts-Mills et al., 2004). Interestingly also in the peripheral blood of these non-allergic children, T cell response to the allergens are characterized by an elevated level of IL-10. Comparable indications for a role for IL-10-producing Tr1 cells in the maintenance of tolerance to allergens can be found in individuals exposed to relatively high doses of allergen like bee keepers and allergic patients undergoing immunotherapy. Bee keepers with a repeated exposure to bee venom during the bee-keeping season demonstrate a marked increase in allergen-specific IL-10 secretion from peripheral blood T cells as the season progresses, while allergen-specific IgE is seen especially in the beginning of the season. Interestingly, reactions to stings disappear during the season, simultaneously with the increased IL-10 production by T-cells (Akdis and Blaser, 1999). Apart from IL-10, also TGF-β, another cytokine that can be produced by Tr1 cells, is reported to be induced by SIT, while both IL-10 and TGF-β are associated respectively with the blocking antibodies IgG4 and IgA (Larche et al., 2006; Taylor et al., 2006).

FOXP3 REGULATORY T CELLS

Not only IL-10 producing T cells but also FOXP3+ Tregare associated with an allergic response. The important role of the transcription factor FOXP3 for maintaining immune tolerance stems for multiple basic studies, mainly in experimental models. This importance of FOXP3+ Treg in human disease was underscored by the IPEX syndrome (immunodysregulation, polyendocrinopathy, and enteropathy, X-linked). In IPEX patients a genetic mutation causes the FOXP3 transcription factor to be defective. Patients with IPEX have symptoms that fit both generalized autoimmunity and allergy (Bennett et al., 2001; Patel, 2001). The relevance of FOX P3 Treg has been extensively demonstrated in mice models, showing an inverse correlation to Treg and diseases like RA, inflammatory bowel disease, MS, and IDDM (Shevach, 2000; Fontenot et al., 2003; Sakaguchi, 2005). Not only in autoimmune diseases but also in allergic disease various studies have suggested a possible defective suppressive function of Tregs (Viglietta et al., 2004; Sakaguchi et al., 2006). In addition to the bee keeper model also the season-dependent antigen exposure during the pollen season offers a model to study responses in the same individuals with and without exposure. Whereas in several studies it was shown that both non-allergic as allergic individuals have CD4+CD25+ Treg, in the allergic subjects, these cells still produced IL-5 and IL-13 cytokines (Grindebacke et al., 2004; Ling et al., 2004). Further related experiments demonstrated that both dose and type of allergen appear to have effects on the ability of CD4+CD25+ T cells to suppress responses. At the time of these studies $CD25^b$ expression on CD4 T cells was used as a surrogate marker of FOXP3+ Treg. Later studies using FOXP3 as a direct marker seemed to confirm these data. During venom immunotherapy the increased allergen-specific IgG4 and reduced IgE correlated with circulating FOXP3 positive Treg (Pereira-Santos et al., 2008). A recent study even suggested that Treg function may be impaired in patients with allergic diseases and that this function can be enhanced by specific immunotherapy (Palomares et al., 2010).

Thus, altogether, there are ample suggestions that the presence of allergen-specific T cells with a regulatory phenotype (either expressing FOXP3, and/or capable of producing IL-10 and TGF-β) may have a beneficial effect on allergic diseases. However in some atopic diseases, like atopic dermatitis and asthma, the specific trigger is often not known. This raises the question whether methods can be identified to improve the Treg repertoire, when the triggering allergen is unknown. Studies from other inflammatory diseases, like JIA and RA, have suggested that a certain group of antigens, called HSPs, are present at the site of inflammation and may have such a beneficial effect on the T cell repertoire.

HEAT SHOCK PROTEINS

The Treg repertoire is both formed in the thymus (so-called *natural Treg*) and generated in the periphery upon encounter with an antigen (induced or *adaptive Treg*). Both self and non-self antigens can induce Treg in the periphery, although the repertoire of Treg might be biased toward self antigens (Romagnoli et al., 2002).

In 1991, Cohen and Young (1991) proposed that a select group of self antigens is especially important for the maintenance of peripheral tolerance). He described the presence of auto reactive immune responses in a healthy individual to a limited set of self molecules, formed by auto reactive T cells and antibodies, which he called the immunological homunculus. The self antigens of this "homunculus" are all evolutionary highly conserved between the self and the non-self homolog of these proteins. According to Cohen, the immune system utilizes these self antigens to form an immunological picture of self which is crucial for the balance of the immune system. One of these homunculus' self proteins is human HSP60 (van Eden et al., 2005). HSPs are indeed evolutionarily highly conserved proteins and either present constitutively, functioning as chaperones, or induced upon cell stress caused by, for instance, heat, oxidative stress, and hypoxia (Craig et al., 1993). Several HSPs have been identified and, according to their size, organized into six families: HSP100, HSP90, HSP70, HSP60, HSP40, and HSP10. In this review we focus on the immune responses of HSP60 in atopic disease. It has to be stressed that as only very little data are available right now on HSPs and allergic disease, and thus we need to deduce the role of HSP in atopic disorders mostly on what is known about HSP reactivity on other diseases.

IMMUNITY TO HSPs AND INFLAMMATION

Humoral and cellular immune responses to HSP60 have been detected both in patients with an inflammatory disease, such as autoimmune and allergic diseases, as well as in healthy subjects. After these initial discoveries the perception was that HSP's may be involved in the development of autoimmunity through antigenis mimicry: an immune response toward a microbial HSP could lead to a cross-reactive response to a self-HSP and thus cause autoimmunity. However, after further studies it quickly became clear that the immune responses toward self HSP60 were more involved in the regulation and not in the induction of autoimmunity. Indeed, a wealth of data obtained in the last decade both in experimental models and from observations in human diseases point to a regulatory role of immunity to self HSP60 (van Eden et al., 2005).

The presence of self-HSP-reactive cells was first shown in animal studies by immunization of rats with mammalian HSP60 (Lopez-Guerrero et al., 1993). Though immunization could induce self-HSP-specific antibodies and T cells, a self-HSP-reactive immune repertoire was also shown to be present in the absence of immunization. The cause for this could be previous contact with homologous bacterial HSPs, for example in the mucosa of the gastro intestinal tract. The first report that immune responses to self HSP60 may have a regulatory role in inflammatory diseases was in mycobacteria-induced adjuvant arthritis. In this model the induction of a self HSP60, cross-reactive T cells response was responsible for the observed protection of HSP60 peptide immune therapy. After these initial findings, protective effects of various (conserved) microbial HSPs were seen in many other experimental disease models, including arthritis, atherosclerosis, allergic encephalomyelitis, and allergic asthma (Anderton et al., 1995; Birnbaum et al., 1998; Harats et al., 2002; Rha et al., 2002).

In vitro experiments show that immune responses modulated by HSPs can result in the induction of various cytokines like IFNγ and TNFα, as well as IL-10. HSPs are strong immune modulators and are able to influence the impact and direction of immune responses (Kaufmann et al., 1987). Moreover, HSP60 has the capacity to steer both innate and humoral immunity.

In human diseases, antibody responses to HSP60 were previously described in skin lesions of patients with Behçets disease, whereas HSP60 has been described as a target for T-cells in autoimmune diseases such as IDDM and JIA (Albani et al., 1995b; Ergun et al., 2001; Raz et al., 2001). Data in the experimental models have pointed out that the protective effect of HSP60 was independent of an antigenic relationship (antigen mimicry) between HSP60 and the disease-inducing antigen. Instead it seemed that HSP60 could confer protection through so-called bystander suppression (Horner et al., 2001; Larche et al., 2006). Inflammation causes local damage and cell stress leading to upregulation of stress proteins such as HSP60. Next, these bystander (self) antigens can become the target of subsequent, possibly suppressive immune responses. So, it is possible that immune responses to HSPs could be involved in the control of human chronic inflammatory diseases that have distinct, although as-yet-unknown, initiating auto-antigens, or even allergens.

HSP RESPONSES IN EARLY LIFE

Apparently, responses to HSP60 are important for maintaining peripheral tolerance in the adult immune system. It is unknown when during live these specific T cells arise. It would seem reasonable to expect that they are primed after birth upon encounter with homologous microbial HSP in the gut. However, there are indications that self HSP60 reactivity is present at birth. In a study by Ramage et al. (1999) it was shown that cord blood cells proliferate in response to an *in vitro* challenge with the self HSP60. This supported the hypothesis that this reactivity is part of the normal naive immune repertoire. A more recent study by Merbl et al. (2007) put these findings also in a different perspective. They found that normal cord blood contains IgM and IgA auto-antibodies directed against a relatively uniform set of auto-antigens, such as auto-antigens related to immune regulation such as HSP60. This obviously benign autoimmune self reactivity, present at birth, may have a dual function. On the one hand it may provide the basis for autoimmunity in later life, while on the other hand the "inborn" autoimmunity to regulatory self antigens such as HSP60 may actually serve to protect against autoimmune disease. Intrigued by these studies, we questioned whether CD4+ T cells specific for HSP60 are already detectable at birth before exposure to the microbial flora, and if so, to what type of immune response these "inborn" autoreactive CD4+ T cells have upon exposure to the self antigen HSP60. We found that HSP60 specific T cells are indeed present at birth. Moreover, stimulation of CBMC with HSP60 leads to CD4+ T cell proliferation and cytokine production, and induces T cells with an *in vitro* regulatory phenotype that are functionally suppressive (Aalberse et al., 2011).

HSP60 AND ALLERGY

Thus, HSP60 is a self-protein, recognized already at birth in healthy subjects, but also in individuals with chronic inflammatory diseases. Thereby a correlation between self-HSP reactivity and diminished disease activity is seen both in experimental as in human autoimmunity. This has already led to the successful exploration of HSP60 immune therapy in human disease, firstly in IDDM. It is not known yet if the levels and responses to HSP60 are different in individuals developing chronic inflammatory disease later in life.

For once, priming of HSP60 T cell responsiveness takes places primarily in the gut through contact with microbial HSP60 (van Eden et al., 2005). Thus, priming of HSP60 immunity early in life through contact with microbiota leads to more self HSP60 mediated immune regulation. This could be one of possibly multiple mechanisms that explain why individuals exposed to more microbial triggers early in life, could be less prone to develop immune mediated diseases. Thus it may very well fit the concept of the hygiene hypothesis.

For that reason we set out to study the role of HSP60 immunity in human atopic diseases. Obviously the first pre-requisite for a potential role of self HSP60 in dermatitis is the (preferably increased) expression of HSP60 at the site of inflammation. Indeed we were able to show that self HSP60 is increased expressed in the skin of patients with atopic dermatitis (Kapitein and Aalberse submitted for publication). Moreover, *in vitro* stimulation with self HSP60 induced FOXP3 positive T cells, as well as T cells producing IL-10 and IFN-γ.

It has to be emphasized that this increased expression by no means is very specific for atopic diseases (Seung et al., 2007). Still it could be highly relevant for atopic disease as the characterization of an antigen present at the site of inflammation, without being the disease-causing antigen has therapeutic possibilities through, as previously mentioned, "antigen driven bystander suppression." Bystander suppression as a mechanism is especially important in human autoimmune diseases, because often the immunizing trigger is unknown.

Theoretically, in allergic diseases this could also be an interesting option for intervention. Although often at least one of the allergens triggering the disease is known, mono-sensitization is rare which would imply multi-antigen immune therapy. Immune therapy with a single bystander antigen might undermine this issue.

NOVEL IMMUNE THERAPEUTIC POSSIBILITIES IN ALLERGIC DISEASE

Various novel immune therapeutic approaches to diminish allergic symptoms have been or are being studied. Of these new interventions, blocking of effector cytokines (such as IL-4 and IL-5) and IgEis the most important. As IL-5 is important for the priming and survival of eosinophils and these cells play an important role in the pathophysiology of allergic disease, blocking IL-5 seemed logical. However only a highly selected patient group with severe asthma, shown as sputum eosinophilia, had profit from this therapy (Busse et al., 2010). Also blocking IL-4 and IL-13 has not yet been shown to be of clinical benefit in asthma (Oh et al., 2010). Thus, so far, the experiences with blocking antibodies to effector cytokines suggest that either the cytokines cannot be fully blocked or that not one of these cytokines is solely responsible for the allergic response. As mentioned above in recent years Th2 induction cytokines have been described among which IL-25. IL-25 is strongly elevated in a subgroup of peanut allergic subjects (Aalberse et al., submitted for publication). Moreover, in mouse models blocking IL-25 has a positive effect on bronchial hyperreactivity (Ballantyne et al., 2007). Apart from blocking cytokines that are important in the pathophysiology of allergic disease, in the last decade various studies in asthmatic patients have been performed in which an IgE-blocker was used (Rodrigo et al., 2011). Although the first results look promising, the effect is not present in all patients, underlining again the complexity of chronic allergic diseases.

Antigen SIT, in which an allergic individual is exposed to increasing doses of the allergen triggering disease, has been used for over a century. It is one of the earliest and most effective forms of human immune therapy. Although for long the mechanisms behind this clearly effective immune intervention was not fully understood, we now know that IgG4, IL-10, and Treg probably play an important role. A disadvantage of this approach in which the eliciting protein is used, is the chance of a severe anaphylactic reaction, as has been described following immune therapy in peanut allergic subjects (Reid et al., 1993).

To tackle this issue, recent work has focused on allergy peptide therapy, showing good results. Mice studies showed that after immunization with Der p 2, the house dust mite allergen, down-regulation of T cell and antibody responses was seen to Der p 2. Similar results were seen using Fel d 1 (cat allergen) and Bet v 1 (birch allergen) peptide therapy. As most patients are not sensitized to just one allergen, it is now studied if combination immune therapy is also effective. Another approach is the use of a peptide of an antigen present at the site of inflammation, without being the triggering antigen. This is the concept of the previous mentioned antigen bystander suppression model (Horner et al., 2001; Larche et al., 2006).

Based on the development of immune therapies usingHSP60 for other human inflammatory diseases and encouraged by recent data showing that HSP60 expression is increased in the skin in patients with atopic dermatitis, it is tempting to suggest that HSP60 may also be a potential candidate for bystander therapy in allergic diseases.

REFERENCES

Aalberse, J. A., Kapitein, B., de Roock, S., Klein, M. R., de Jager, W., van der Zee, R., Hoekstra, M. O., van Wijk, F., and Prakken, B. J. (2011). Cord blood CD4+ T cells respond to self heat shock protein 60 (HSP60). *PLoS ONE* 6, e24119. doi:10.1371/journal.pone.0024119

Abulafia-Lapid, R., Elias, D., Raz, I., Keren-Zur, Y., Atlan, H., and Cohen, I. R. (1999). T cell proliferative responses of type I diabetes patients and healthy individuals to human hsp60 and its peptides. *J. Autoimmun.* 12, 121–129.

Akdis, C. A., and Blaser, K. (1999). IL-10-induced anergy in peripheral T cell and reactivation by microenvironmental cytokines: two key steps in specific immunotherapy. *FASEB J.* 13, 603–609.

Akdis, M., Verhagen, J., Taylor, A., Karamloo, F., Karagiannidis, C., Crameri, R., Thunberg, S., Deniz, G., Valenta, R., Fiebig, H., Kegel, C., Disch, R., Schmidt-Weber, C. B., Blaser, K., and Akdis, C. A. (2004). Immune responses in healthy and allergic individuals are characterized by a fine balance between allergen-specific T regulatory 1 and T helper 2 cells. *J. Exp. Med.* 199, 1567–1575.

Albani, S., Keystone, E. C., Nelson, J. L., Ollier, W. E., La Cava, A., Montemayor, A. C., Weber, D. A., Montecucco, C., Martini, A., and Carson, D. A. (1995a). Positive selection in autoimmunity: abnormal immune responses to a bacterial dnaJ antigenic determinant in patients with early rheumatoid arthritis. *Nat. Med.* 1, 448–452.

Albani, S., Keystone, E. C., Nelson, J. L., Ollier, W. E., La, C. A., Montemayor, A. C., Weber, D. A., Montecucco, C., Martini, A., and Carson, D. A. (1995b). Positive selection in autoimmunity: abnormal immune responses to a bacterial dnaJ antigenic determinant in patients with early rheumatoid arthritis. *Nat. Med.* 1, 448–452.

Anderton, S. M., van der Zee, R., Prakken, B., Noordzij, A., and van Eden, W. (1995). Activation of T cells recognizing self 60-kD heat shock protein can protect against experimental arthritis. *J. Exp. Med.* 181, 943–952.

Angkasekwinai, P., Chang, S. H., Thapa, M., Watarai, H., and Dong, C. (2010). Regulation of IL-9 expression by IL-25 signaling. *Nat. Immunol.* 11, 250–256.

Ballantyne, S. J., Barlow, J. L., Jolin, H. E., Nath, P., Williams, A. S., Chung, K. F., Sturton, G., Wong, S. H., and McKenzie, A. N. (2007). Blocking IL-25 prevents airway hyperresponsiveness in allergic asthma. *J. Allergy Clin. Immunol.* 120, 1324–1331.

Bennett, C. L., Christie, J., Ramsdell, F., Brunkow, M. E., Ferguson, P. J., Whitesell, L., Kelly, T. E., Saulsbury, F. T., Chance, P. F., and Ochs, H. D. (2001). The immune dysregulation, polyendocrinopathy, enteropathy, X-linked syndrome (IPEX) is caused by mutations of FOXP3. *Nat. Genet.* 27, 20–21.

Birnbaum, G., Kotilinek, L., Miller, S. D., Raine, C. S., Gao, Y. L., Lehmann, P. V., and Gupta, R. S. (1998). Heat shock proteins and experimental autoimmune encephalomyelitis. II: environmental infection and extra-neuraxial inflammation alter the course of chronic relapsing encephalomyelitis. *J. Neuroimmunol.* 90, 149–161.

Bodner, C., Godden, D., and Seaton, A. (1998). Family size, childhood infections and atopic diseases. The Aberdeen WHEASE Group. *Thorax* 53, 28–32.

Braun-Fahrlander, C., Riedler, J., Herz, U., Eder, W., Waser, M., Grize, L., Maisch, S., Carr, D., Gerlach, F., Bufe, A., Lauener, R. P., Schierl, R., Renz, H., Nowak, D., and von Mutius, E. (2002). Environmental exposure to endotoxin and its relation to asthma in school-age children. *N. Engl. J. Med.* 347, 869–877.

Busse, W. W., Ring, J., Huss-Marp, J., and Kahn, J. E. (2010). A review of treatment with mepolizumab, an anti-IL-5 mAb, in hypereosinophilic syndromes and asthma. *J. Allergy Clin. Immunol.* 125, 803–813.

Chen, L., Martinez, O., Overbergh, L., Mathieu, C., Prabhakar, B. S., and Chan, L. S. (2004). Early up-regulation of Th2 cytokines and late surge of Th1 cytokines in an atopic dermatitis model. *Clin. Exp. Immunol.* 138, 375–387.

Cohen, I. R., and Young, D. B. (1991). Autoimmunity, microbial immunity and the immunological homunculus. *Immunol. Today* 12, 105–110.

Craig, E. A., Gambill, B. D., and Nelson, R. J. (1993). Heat shock proteins: molecular chaperones of protein biogenesis. *Microbiol. Rev.* 57, 402–414.

de Kleer, I. M., Kamphuis, S. M., Rijkers, G. T., Scholtens, L., Gordon, G., de Jager, W., Hafner, R., van de Zee, R., van Eden, W., Kuis, W., and Prakken, B. J. (2003). The spontaneous remission of juvenile idiopathic arthritis is characterized by CD30+ T cells directed to human heat-shock protein 60 capable of producing the regulatory cytokine interleukin-10. *Arthritis Rheum.* 48, 2001–2010.

de Kleer, I. M., Wedderburn, L. R., Taams, L. S., Patel, A., Varsani, H., Klein, M., de Jager, W., Pugayung, G., Giannoni, F., Rijkers, G., Albani, S., Kuis, W., and Prakken, B. (2004). CD4+CD25bright regulatory T cells actively regulate inflammation in the joints of patients with the remitting form of juvenile idiopathic arthritis. *J. Immunol.* 172, 6435–6443.

Del Prete, G. (1992). Human Th1 and Th2 lymphocytes: their role in the pathophysiology of atopy. *Allergy* 47, 450–455.

Devos, S., Cormont, F., Vrtala, S., Hooghe-Peters, E., Pirson, F., and Snick, J. (2006). Allergen-induced interleukin-9 production in vitro: correlation with atopy in human adults and comparison with interleukin-5 and interleukin-13. *Clin. Exp. Allergy* 36, 174–182.

Ergun, T., Ince, U., Eksioglu-Demiralp, E., Direskeneli, H., Gurbuz, O., Gurses, L., Aker, F., and Akoglu, T. (2001). HSP 60 expression in mucocutaneous lesions of Behcet's disease. *J. Am. Acad. Dermatol.* 45, 904–909.

Falcone, F. H., Knol, E. F., and Gibbs, B. F. (2011). The role of basophils in the pathogenesis of allergic disease. *Clin. Exp. Allergy* 41, 939–947.

Fontenot, J. D., Gavin, M. A., and Rudensky, A. Y. (2003). Foxp3 programs the development and function of CD4+CD25+ regulatory T cells. *Nat. Immunol.* 4, 330–336.

Grindebacke, H., Wing, K., Andersson, A. C., Suri-Payer, E., Rak, S., and Rudin, A. (2004). Defective suppression of Th2 cytokines by CD4CD25 regulatory T cells in birch allergics during birch pollen season. *Clin. Exp. Allergy* 34, 1364–1372.

Harats, D., Yacov, N., Gilburd, B., Shoenfeld, Y., and George, J. (2002). Oral tolerance with heat shock protein 65 attenuates *Mycobacterium tuberculosis*-induced and high-fat-diet-driven atherosclerotic lesions. *J. Am. Coll. Cardiol.* 40, 1333–1338.

Hauber, H. P., Bergeron, C., Toda, M., Kontolemos, M., Holroyd, K. J., Levitt, R. C., and Hamid, Q. (2007). Up-regulation of interleukin-9 and the interleukin-9-associated calcium-activated chloride channel hCLCA1 in nasal mucosa following in vivo allergen challenge. *Allergy Asthma Clin.Immunol.* 3, 19–23.

Horner, A. A., Datta, S. K., Takabayashi, K., Belyakov, I. M., Hayashi, T., Cinman, N., Nguyen, M. D., Van Uden, J. H., Berzofsky, J. A., Richman, D. D., and Raz, E. (2001). Immunostimulatory DNA-based vaccines elicit multifaceted immune responses against HIV at systemic and mucosal sites. *J. Immunol.* 167, 1584–1591.

Hvid, M., Vestergaard, C., Kemp, K., Christensen, G. B., Deleuran, B., and Deleuran, M. (2011). IL-25 in atopic dermatitis: a possible link between inflammation and skin barrier dysfunction? *J. Invest. Dermatol.* 131, 150–157.

Jarvis, D., Chinn, S., Luczynska, C., and Burney, P. (1997). The association of family size with atopy and atopic disease. *Clin. Exp. Allergy* 27, 240–245.

Kaufmann, S. H., Vath, U., Thole, J. E., Van Embden, J. D., and Emmrich, F. (1987). Enumeration of T cells reactive with *Mycobacterium tuberculosis* organisms and specific for the recombinant mycobacterial 64-kDa protein. *Eur. J. Immunol.* 17, 351–357.

Krug, N., Madden, J., Redington, A. E., Lackie, P., Djukanovic, R., Schauer, U., Holgate, S. T., Frew, A. J., and Howarth, P. H. (1996). T-cell cytokine profile evaluated at the single cell level in BAL and blood in allergic asthma. *Am. J. Respir. Cell Mol. Biol.* 14, 319–326.

Larche, M. (2007). Regulatory T cells in allergy and asthma. *Chest* 132, 1007–1014.

Larche, M., Akdis, C. A., and Valenta, R. (2006). Immunological mechanisms of allergen-specific immunotherapy. *Nat. Rev. Immunol.* 6, 761–771.

Ling, E. M., Smith, T., Nguyen, X. D., Pridgeon, C., Dallman, M., Arbery, J., Carr, V. A., and Robinson, D. S. (2004). Relation of CD4+CD25+ regulatory T-cell suppression of allergen-driven T-cell activation to atopic status and expression of allergic disease. *Lancet* 363, 608–615.

Lloyd, C. M., and Hessel, E. M. (2010). Functions of T cells in asthma: more than just T(H)2 cells. *Nat. Rev. Immunol.* 10, 838–848.

Lopez-Guerrero, J. A., Lopez-Bote, J. P., Ortiz, M. A., Gupta, R. S., Paez, E., and Bernabeu, C. (1993). Modulation of adjuvant arthritis in Lewis rats by recombinant vaccinia virus expressing the human 60-kilodalton heat shock protein. *Infect. Immun.* 61, 4225–4231.

Merbl, Y., Zucker-Toledano, M., Quintana, F. J., and Cohen, I. R. (2007). Newborn humans manifest autoantibodies to defined self molecules detected by antigen microarray informatics. *J. Clin. Invest.* 117, 712–718.

Mosmann, T. R., and Coffman, R. L. (1989). TH1 and TH2 cells: different patterns of lymphokine secretion lead to different functional properties. *Annu. Rev. Immunol.* 7, 145–173.

Nograles, K. E., Zaba, L. C., Shemer, A., Fuentes-Duculan, J., Cardinale, I., Kikuchi, T., Ramon, M., Bergman, R., Krueger, J. G., and Guttman-Yassky, E. (2009). IL-22-producing T22 T cells account for upregulated IL-22 in atopic dermatitis despite reduced IL-17-producing TH17 T cells. *J. Allergy Clin. Immunol.* 123, 1244–1252.

Oh, C. K., Geba, G. P., and Molfino, N. (2010). Investigational therapeutics targeting the IL-4/IL-13/STAT-6 pathway for the treatment of asthma. *Eur. Respir. Rev.* 19, 46–54.

Oliphant, C. J., Barlow, J. L., and McKenzie, A. N. (2011). Insights into the initiation of type 2 immune responses. *Immunology* 134, 378–385.

Ong, P. Y., and Leung, D. Y. (2006). Immune dysregulation in atopic dermatitis. *Curr. Allergy Asthma Rep.* 6, 384–389.

Ozdemir, C., Akdis, M., and Akdis, C. A. (2010). T-cell response to allergens. *Chem. Immunol. Allergy* 95, 22–44.

Palomares, O., Yaman, G., Azkur, A. K., Akkoc, T., Akdis, M., and Akdis, C. A. (2010). Role of Treg in immune regulation of allergic diseases. *Eur. J. Immunol.* 40, 1232–1240.

Patel, D. D. (2001). Escape from tolerance in the human X-linked autoimmunity-allergic disregulation syndrome and the Scurfy mouse. *J. Clin. Invest.* 107, 155–157.

Peat, J. K., van den Berg, R. H., Green, W. F., Mellis, C. M., Leeder, S. R., and Woolcock, A. J. (1994). Changing prevalence of asthma in Australian children. *BMJ* 308, 1591–1596.

Pereira-Santos, M. C., Baptista, A. P., Melo, A., Alves, R. R., Soares, R. S., Pedro, E., Pereira-Barbosa, M., Victorino, R. M., and Sousa, A. E. (2008). Expansion of circulating Foxp3+D25bright CD4+ T cells during specific venom immunotherapy. *Clin. Exp. Allergy* 38, 291–297.

Platts-Mills, T. A., Woodfolk, J. A., Erwin, E. A., and Aalberse, R. (2004). Mechanisms of tolerance to inhalant allergens: the relevance of a modified Th2 response to allergens from domestic animals. *Springer Semin. Immunopathol.* 25, 271–279.

Pockley, A. G. (2003). Heat shock proteins as regulators of the immune response. *Lancet* 362, 469–476.

Prakken, B. J., Samodal, R., Le, T. D., Giannoni, F., Yung, G. P., Scavulli, J., Amox, D., Roord, S., de Kleer, I., Bonnin, D., Lanza, P., Berry, C., Massa, M., Billetta, R., and Albani, S. (2004). Epitope-specific immunotherapy induces immune deviation of proinflammatory T cells in rheumatoid arthritis. *Proc. Natl. Acad. Sci. U.S.A.* 101, 4228–4233.

Ramage, J. M., Young, J. L., Goodall, J. C., and Gaston, J. S. (1999). T cell responses to heat-shock protein 60: differential responses by CD4+ T cell subsets according to their expression of CD45 isotypes. *J. Immunol.* 162, 704–710.

Raz, I., Elias, D., Avron, A., Tamir, M., Metzger, M., and Cohen, I. R. (2001). Beta-cell function in new-onset type 1 diabetes and immunomodulation with a heat-shock protein peptide (DiaPep277): a randomised, double-blind, phase II trial. *Lancet* 358, 1749–1753.

Reid, M. J., Lockey, R. F., Turkeltaub, P. C., and Platts-Mills, T. A. (1993). Survey of fatalities from skin testing and immunotherapy 1985–1989. *J. Allergy Clin. Immunol.* 92(Pt 1), 6–15.

Rha, Y. H., Taube, C., Haczku, A., Joetham, A., Takeda, K., Duez, C., Siegel, M., Aydintug, M. K., Born, W. K., Dakhama, A., and Gelfand, E. W. (2002). Effect of microbial heat shock proteins on airway inflammation and hyperresponsiveness. *J. Immunol.* 169, 5300–5307.

Rodrigo, G. J., Neffen, H., and Castro-Rodriguez, J. A. (2011). Efficacy and safety of subcutaneous omalizumab vs placebo as add-on therapy to corticosteroids for children and adults with asthma: a systematic review. *Chest* 139, 28–35.

Romagnoli, P., Hudrisier, D., and van Meerwijk, J. P. (2002). Preferential recognition of self antigens despite normal thymic deletion of CD4(+)CD25(+) regulatory T cells. *J. Immunol.* 168, 1644–1648.

Saenz, S. A., Noti, M., and Artis, D. (2010). Innate immune cell populations function as initiators and effectors in Th2 cytokine responses. *Trends Immunol.* 31, 407–413.

Sakaguchi, S. (2005). Naturally arising Foxp3-expressing CD25+CD4+ regulatory T cells in immunological tolerance to self and non-self. *Nat. Immunol.* 6, 345–352.

Sakaguchi, S., Setoguchi, R., Yagi, H., and Nomura, T. (2006). Naturally arising Foxp3-expressing CD25+CD4+ regulatory T cells in self-tolerance and autoimmune disease. *Curr. Top. Microbiol. Immunol.* 305, 51–66.

Seung, N. R., Park, E. J., Kim, C. W., Kim, K. H., Kim, K. J., Cho, H. J., and Park, H. R. (2007). Comparison of expression of heat-shock protein 60, Toll-like receptors 2 and 4, and T-cell receptor gammadelta in plaque and guttate psoriasis. *J. Cutan. Pathol.* 34, 903–911.

Sheikh, A., Smeeth, L., and Hubbard, R. (2003). There is no evidence of an inverse relationship between Th2 mediated atopy and Th1 mediated autoimmune disorders: Lack of support for the hygiene hypothesis. *J. Allergy Clin. Immunol.* 111, 131–135.

Shevach, E. M. (2000). Regulatory T cells in autoimmmunity*. *Annu. Rev. Immunol.* 18, 423–449.

Sokol, C. L., Chu, N. Q., Yu, S., Nish, S. A., Laufer, T. M., and Medzhitov, R. (2009). Basophils function as antigen-presenting cells for an allergen-induced T helper type 2 response. *Nat. Immunol.* 10, 713–720.

Soroosh, P., and Doherty, T. A. (2009). Th9 and allergic disease. *Immunology* 127, 450–458.

Souwer, Y., Szegedi, K., Kapsenberg, M. L., and de Jong, E. C. (2010). IL-17 and IL-22 in atopic allergic disease. *Curr. Opin. Immunol.* 22, 821–826.

Strachan, D. P. (1989). Hay fever, hygiene, and household size. *BMJ* 299, 1259–1260.

Taylor, A., Verhagen, J., Blaser, K., Akdis, M., and Akdis, C. A. (2006). Mechanisms of immune suppression by interleukin-10 and transforming growth factor-beta: the role of T regulatory cells. *Immunology* 117, 433–442.

Tiemessen, M. M., Van Ieperen-Van Dijk, A. G., Bruijnzeel-Koomen, C. A., Garssen, J., Knol, E. F., and Van Hoffen, E. (2004). Cow's milk-specific T-cell reactivity of children with and without persistent cow's milk allergy: key role for IL-10. *J. Allergy Clin. Immunol.* 113, 932–939.

Umetsu, D. T., Akbari, O., and Dekruyff, R. H. (2003). Regulatory T cells control the development of allergic disease and asthma. *J. Allergy Clin. Immunol.* 112, 480–487.

van der Neut, K. M., Schuurman, J., Losen, M., Bleeker, W. K., Martinez-Martinez, P., Vermeulen, E., den Bleker, T. H., Wiegman, L., Vink, T., Aarden, L. A., De Baets, M. H., van de Winkel, J. G., Aalberse, R. C., and Parren, P. W. (2007). Anti-inflammatory activity of human IgG4 antibodies by dynamic Fab arm exchange. *Science* 317, 1554–1557.

van Eden, W., van der Zee, R., and Prakken, B. (2005). Heat-shock proteins induce T-cell regulation of chronic inflammation. *Nat. Rev. Immunol.* 5, 318–330.

Viglietta, V., Baecher-Allan, C., Weiner, H. L., and Hafler, D. A. (2004). Loss of functional suppression by CD4+CD25+ regulatory T cells in patients with multiple sclerosis. *J. Exp. Med.* 199, 971–979.

von Mutius, E., Illi, S., Hirsch, T., Leupold, W., Keil, U., and Weiland, S. K. (1999). Frequency of infections and risk of asthma, atopy and airway hyperresponsiveness in children. *Eur. Respir. J.* 14, 4–11.

Wegmann, T. G., Lin, H., Guilbert, L., and Mosmann, T. R. (1993). Bidirectional cytokine interactions in the maternal-fetal relationship: is successful pregnancy a TH2 phenomenon? *Immunol. Today* 14, 353–356.

Wickens, K., Crane, J., Pearce, N., and Beasley, R. (1999). The magnitude of the effect of smaller family sizes on the increase in the prevalence of asthma and hay fever in the United Kingdom and New Zealand. *J. Allergy Clin. Immunol.* 104(Pt 1), 554–558.

Yamanaka, K., and Mizutani, H. (2011). The role of cytokines/chemokines in the pathogenesis of atopic dermatitis. *Curr. Probl. Dermatol.* 41, 80–92.

Yazdanbakhsh, M., Kremsner, P. G., and van Ree, R. (2002). Allergy, parasites, and the hygiene hypothesis. *Science* 296, 490–494.

21

Immunoglobulin Analysis Tool: a novel tool for the analysis of human and mouse heavy and light chain transcripts

Tobias Rogosch[1], Sebastian Kerzel[1], Kam Hon Hoi[2], Zhixin Zhang[3], Rolf F. Maier[1], Gregory C. Ippolito[4] and Michael Zemlin[1]*

[1] *Department of Pediatrics, Philipps-University Marburg, Marburg, Germany*
[2] *Department of Biomedical Engineering, University of Texas at Austin, Austin, TX, USA*
[3] *Department of Pathology and Microbiology, Eppley Institute for Research in Cancer, University of Nebraska Medical Center, Omaha, NE, USA*
[4] *Section of Molecular Genetics and Microbiology, University of Texas at Austin, Austin, TX, USA*

Edited by:
Harry W. Schroeder, University of Alabama at Birmingham, USA

Reviewed by:
John D. Colgan, University of Iowa, USA
Deborah K. Dunn-Walters, King's College London School of Medicine, UK

****Correspondence:***
Michael Zemlin, University Children's Hospital, Baldingerstrasse, D-35033 Marburg, Germany.
e-mail: zemlin@med.uni-marburg.de

Sequence analysis of immunoglobulin (Ig) heavy and light chain transcripts can refine categorization of B cell subpopulations and can shed light on the selective forces that act during immune responses or immune dysregulation, such as autoimmunity, allergy, and B cell malignancy. High-throughput sequencing yields Ig transcript collections of unprecedented size. The authoritative web-based IMGT/HighV-QUEST program is capable of analyzing large collections of transcripts and provides annotated output files to describe many key properties of Ig transcripts. However, additional processing of these flat files is required to create figures, or to facilitate analysis of additional features and comparisons between sequence sets. We present an easy-to-use Microsoft® Excel® based software, named Immunoglobulin Analysis Tool (IgAT), for the summary, interrogation, and further processing of IMGT/HighV-QUEST output files. IgAT generates descriptive statistics and high-quality figures for collections of murine or human Ig heavy or light chain transcripts ranging from 1 to 150,000 sequences. In addition to traditionally studied properties of Ig transcripts – such as the usage of germline gene segments, or the length and composition of the CDR-3 region – IgAT also uses published algorithms to calculate the probability of antigen selection based on somatic mutational patterns, the average hydrophobicity of the antigen-binding sites, and predictable structural properties of the CDR-H3 loop according to Shirai's *H3-rules*. These refined analyses provide in-depth information about the selective forces acting upon Ig repertoires and allow the statistical and graphical comparison of two or more sequence sets. IgAT is easy to use on any computer running Excel® 2003 or higher. Thus, IgAT is a useful tool to gain insights into the selective forces and functional properties of small to extremely large collections of Ig transcripts, thereby assisting a researcher to mine a data set to its fullest.

Keywords: immunoglobulin heavy chain gene, immunoglobulin light chain gene, rearrangement, somatic mutation, sequence analysis software, antibody repertoire, high-throughput analysis, deep sequencing

INTRODUCTION

The fate of a B cell largely depends on the B cell receptor, or immunoglobulin (Ig), which it expresses on its surface (Rajewsky, 1996; Kurosaki et al., 2010). Thus, the analysis of Ig gene transcripts can give important insights into the selective forces that act upon B cells during cellular maturation or during physiological or pathological immune reactions (Schroeder and Cavacini, 2010). For example, repertoire studies of Ig transcripts have revealed that the length and composition of the Ig heavy chain third complementarity determining region (CDR-H3) is strictly regulated during ontogeny, and somatic mutations are rare during the perinatal period even in secondary antibody repertoires (Schroeder et al., 1987, 2001; Cuisinier et al., 1993; Brezinschek et al., 1997; Zemlin et al., 2001, 2007; Kolar et al., 2004; Souto-Carneiro et al., 2005; Schelonka et al., 2007; Richl et al., 2008; Prabakaran et al., 2012). It has also been shown that the composition of the antigen-binding site plays a key role during B cell maturation and during the recruitment into various B cell subsets (Schelonka et al., 2007; Arnaout et al., 2011) and during protective immune responses (Rajewsky, 1996; Frolich et al., 2010). Moreover, studies of Ig repertoires can give valuable insights into the immune dysregulation that underlies the development of autoimmunity (Dorner and Lipsky, 2005; Vrolix et al., 2010; Zuckerman et al., 2010; Kalinina et al., 2011) and allergies (Snow et al., 1998; Takhar et al., 2007; Kerzel et al., 2010).

The antigen-binding site of the antibody is endowed with an almost unlimited theoretical diversity due to the imprecise junction of Variable, Joining, and (in the case of the Ig heavy chain) Diversity gene segments (Tonegawa, 1983). The random exonucleolytic truncation of the rearranged gene segments and the insertion of non-encoded N-nucleotides and P-nucleotides, the shuffling of light and heavy chains, and the insertion of somatic mutations during the germinal center reaction further expands the potential diversity exponentially. Theoretically, these mechanisms

Table 1 | Estimate of the maximum size of sequence collections that can be processed.

Excel version	Operation system	Max. memory	No. of sequences
Excel 2003	Windows XP Windows 7 (32/64-bit)	1 Gigabyte	~40,000
Excel 2007 Excel 2010 (32-bit)	Windows XP Windows 7 (32/64-bit)	2 Gigabyte	~60,000
Excel 2010 (64-bit)	Windows 7 (64-bit)	8 Terabyte	150,000 (max. no. of IMGT/HighV-QUEST)

The restrictions are caused by limited addressable memory by Excel. Excel versions prior 2007 can not address more than 1 GB of memory. 32-bit versions of Excel 2007/2010 can use 2 GB of memory, while the 64-bit versions are virtually unrestricted.

allow the production of more than 10^{15} different antigen-binding sites (Schroeder and Cavacini, 2010). Although seemingly limitless in theoretical potential, the human antibody response probably does not exploit more than 1% of its potential diversity (Boyd et al., 2009; Glanville et al., 2009; Arnaout et al., 2011). Thus, it seems unlikely that the expressed antibody repertoire would represent merely a random selection of the theoretical diversity.

In order to discover potential biases within repertoires that may have been coined by selective forces, it is desirable to study large numbers of Ig gene transcripts. With the advent of next generation sequencing (NGS) technologies, such as Roche 454 pyrosequencing, the direct large-scale sampling of sequence collections of 10^4, 10^5, and even greater numbers, is now obtainable within the span of a few days (Boyd et al., 2009; Reddy et al., 2010; Wu et al., 2010; Zuckerman et al., 2010; Jiang et al., 2011; Ippolito et al., 2012). Previously published semi-automated instruments cannot be used for such large collections or state-of-the-art characterizations due to significant quantitative and qualitative advances in Ig gene analysis (Shannon, 1997; Johnson and Wu, 2000; Zemlin et al., 2003). Thus, novel analysis tools are required which can handle extremely large sequence batches.

The online repository "International ImMunoGeneTics Information System®" (IMGT®[1], founder and director: Marie-Paule Lefranc, Montpellier, France (Brochet et al., 2008; Lefranc et al., 2009) offers IMGT/HighV-QUEST, a free online tool to assign Variable, Diversity, and Joining gene segments to each individual full-length Ig transcript in batches up to 150,000 sequences. In addition, IMGT/HighV-QUEST provides numerous descriptors for each individual sequence, such as assignment of N- and P-nucleotides, amino acid translation, position of somatic mutations, isoelectric point, and many others (Giudicelli et al., 2011; Alamyar et al., 2012). The output files of these analyses contain descriptions of each individual sequence and can be downloaded as text files in comma separated values (CSV) format for documentation and further analysis.

[1]http://www.imgt.org

Our aim was to create an easy-to-use software tool for the generation of informative statistics and publication-ready figures derived from the HighV-QUEST text-only output files. Moreover, we sought to include new and important analyses of higher order antibody features. For instance, although Shirai's *H3-rules* have been formulated for the sequence-based prediction of CDR-H3 structural properties (Shirai et al., 1999), and whereas complex algorithms have been published to determine the probability by which a somatic mutation profile might arise non-randomly from antigen-driven selection (Chang and Casali, 1994; Lossos et al., 2000), there are at present no software tools available to the research community for high-throughput application of these rules and algorithms.

Here we present Immunoglobulin Analysis Tool (IgAT), a novel and user-friendly software tool for the extensive analysis and graphical presentation of very large collections of Ig transcripts which have been pre-analyzed by IMGT/HighV-QUEST. IgAT additionally calculates the probability of antigen-driven selection within Ig repertoires and predicts structural properties of the antigen-binding site. IgAT can be used to analyze up to 150,000 human or murine heavy or light chain transcripts in a single run of the application and automatically generates 25 Microsoft® PowerPoint® graphics files illustrating key characteristics of the Ig repertoire, such as VDJ gene utilization, amino acid use, CDR-H3 junctional diversity, and average hydrophobicity, as well as the quantitation of somatic mutation among Ig heavy chain transcripts, to name but a few. IgAT is available free of charge.

When applied to two or more sequence collections (e.g., samples from multiple individuals, different cell subsets, or identical cell subsets but under differing immunological conditions), IgAT readily yields the necessary data to allow statistical and graphical comparisons between various repertoires.

METHODS

IgAT is a Microsoft® Excel® workbook containing the analysis functions as Visual Basic® for Applications (VBA) code. Each sheet is described in the results section. The workbook was created in Excel 2010 on Microsoft Windows® XP but should be compatible with Excel versions down to Excel 2003 with some limitations (**Table 1**). IgAT is not compatible with Excel for Mac®. The file can be found at: www.uni-marburg.de/neonat/igat

RESULTS

In the following, we present the features offered by IgAT, using exemplarily a previously published collection of 78,569 murine Ig heavy chain sequences that contained 18,403 functional sequences (Reddy et al., 2010). These sequences were obtained from $CD138^+$ plasma-cell-enriched bone marrow mRNA of two BALB/c mice immunized with human complement serine protease (C1S; NCBI Entrez Gene ID: 716).

Begin with a text file of FASTA-formatted Ig DNA sequences as can be obtained from a Roche 454 experimental run or other techniques. When submitting the sequence batch to IMGT/HighV-QUEST, under the advanced parameters setting, "Nb of accepted D-GENE in JUNCTION" must be set to the default (1) as IgAT will only process IMGT output files that assign a maximum of one single D-gene to each V-D_H-J junction. IMGT individual result files are not necessary for the analysis with IgAT.

INPUT

As input, IgAT takes the 11 CSV text output files standardly generated by IMGT/HighV-QUEST derived from its analysis of raw 454 sequence data uploaded by the researcher. IgAT imports the folder containing the IMGT/HighV-QUEST CSV text output files through the cell "C6" of the "input" worksheet. (Alternatively, the IgAT program may be copied and pasted into the folder, which already contains the IMGT files.) Optionally, sequences marked as "unproductive" by IMGT/HighV-QUEST can be deleted. Deleting unproductive sequences will improve performance but might discard functional transcripts as Roche 454 sequencing is prone to homopolymer errors due to technical reasons.

The species (human or mouse), the Ig chain (heavy, lambda, or kappa), the minimum number of non-mutated nucleotides that are required to identify a diversity (D) gene, and the option to calculate the Taq-error must be chosen before starting the analysis. The Ig isotype is needed to calculate the Taq-error (**Figure 1**).

To start the analysis simply press the button "analyze data." If "convert formulas to text" is checked, most formulas will be replaced by their values, resulting in reduced file size and recalculation time. In this case, however, additional changes will not have any effect on the analysis output. Once the sequence analysis is complete, the graphs can be exported as Microsoft PowerPoint® files (.ppt) by pressing "save graphs as ppt."

The workbook was created in Excel 2010 and tested in Excel 2003 and 2010. To determine if your Microsoft Office® software meets this requirement, press "check office version." It might be compatible with other versions (not tested).

SUMMARY

The number of total, non-functional, functional, and unique sequences, as well as the number of clonotypes is listed in the "summary" worksheet (**Figure 2**). Deep sequencing technologies usually yield a significant proportion of incomplete or otherwise defective sequences. IgAT counts the sequences which were labeled "unproductive," "no result," or "unknown" by IMGT/HighV-QUEST.

Sequences are considered clonally related if they (i) use the same V and J genes, (ii) have an identical CDR-3 length, and (iii) a highly homologous CDR-3 region. The default definition of "highly homologous CDR-3 region" is ≤10% difference in nucleotide sequence. IgAT gives the user the flexibility to choose another percentage difference in nucleotide sequence, or a total number of nucleotide matches, or a percentage or total number difference in amino acid sequence when defining clonotypic parameters.

DATA

The "Data" worksheet contains the imported data of the IMGT/HighV-QUEST output files. IgAT uses the taxonomy and numbering of the IMGT repository (Lefranc et al., 2009).

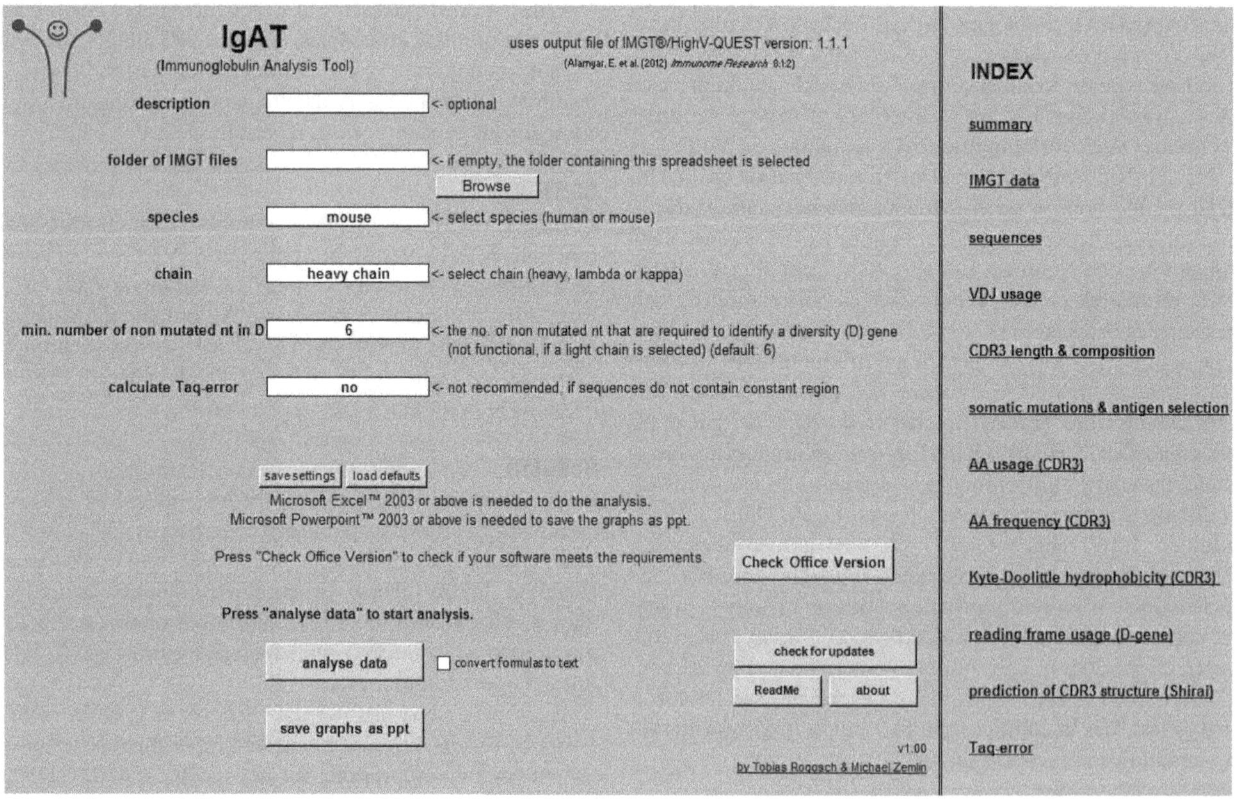

FIGURE 1 | Screenshot of the "input" worksheet.

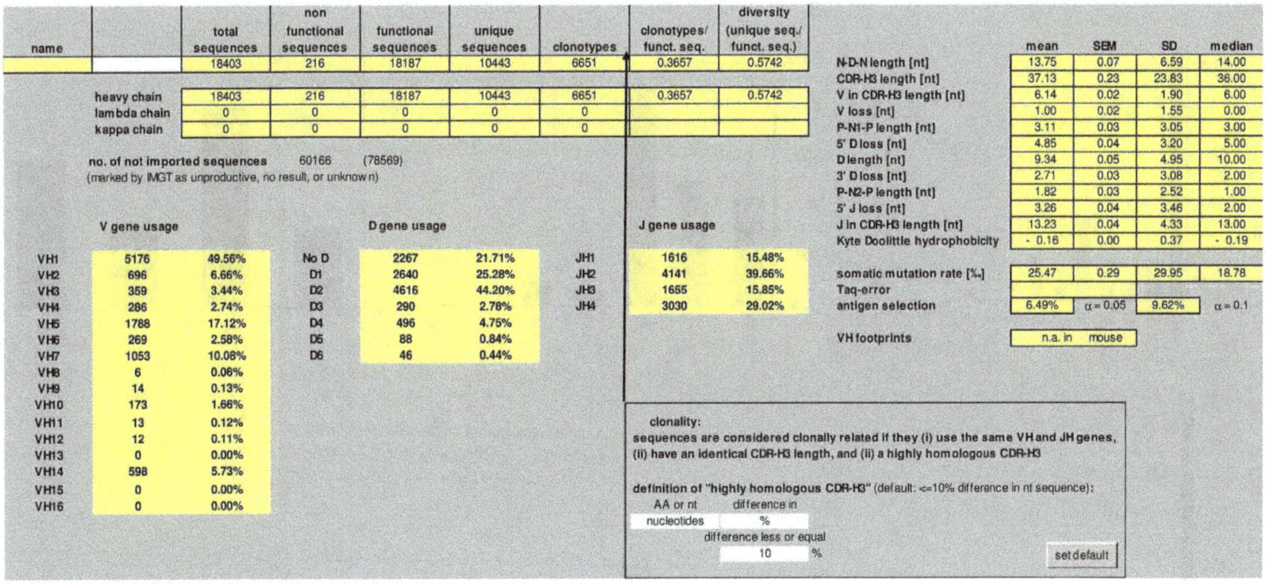

FIGURE 2 | Screenshot of the "summary" worksheet of IgAT.

SEQUENCE

In this worksheet, each nucleotide sequence occurs in an individual row and is split into framework regions (FR) 1–4 and complementarity determining regions 1–3. The sequences are ordered by functionality, which is defined by the existence of an open reading frame throughout the sequence, and by V gene segment utilization. Furthermore, the "Sequence" worksheet provides the length and amino acid translation for CDR-3, number of clonotypes, and identifies sequences with potential "V_H-replacement footprints" (only human sequences) that can originate from V_H replacement during receptor editing according to Zhang et al. (2003). In addition, sequences can be tagged with the sample ID. Based on sample IDs, the analysis can be confined to one or several samples or the transcripts can be divided into two groups for comparison.

VDJ

The "VDJ" worksheet contains absolute numbers, percentages, and graphs of the V-, D_H-, and J-gene families and individual genes in the order of their localization in the germline (**Figure 3**).

CDR-3_LENGTH

The "CDR-3_length" worksheet displays the nucleotide length distribution of CDR-3, N1-, and N2-nucleotides within the analyzed sequence collection (**Figure 4**). In addition, the average lengths of the components of CDR-3, namely V length, P-nucleotides 3′ of V, N1-nucleotides, P-nucleotides 5′ of D, D length, P-nucleotides 3′ of D, N2-nucleotides, P-nucleotides 3′ of J, and J length are displayed in a deconstruction graph. A separate graph displays the deconstruction of those sequences without an identifiable D-gene. As a default for the IgH chain, CDR-H3 is defined as amino acids 105–117, according to the IMGT unique numbering system. The descriptive statistics given in the "CDR_length" worksheet can be used for comparative statistics with other sequence collections.

SOMAT_MUT

This worksheet displays the somatic mutation rate of each transcript (mutations per 1,000 nt), as well as the average mutational frequency (**Figure 5A**). In addition, the probability of antigen selection is analyzed by assessing the distribution of replacement and silent mutations between FRs and CDRs (only available for heavy chains). Using the method of Lossos et al. (2000), we determined the replacement frequency and the relative length of FR and CDR of each germline V_H gene. The average probability that a random mutation would allocate in CDR was calculated to be 0.23 ± 0.012, and the sequence-inherent probability that a mutation in the CDR would be a replacement mutation was estimated to be 0.79 ± 0.01. Therefore, the chance for a random mutation to introduce a replacement mutation into the CDR was 0.18. The binomial distribution method of Chang and Casali (1994) was used to calculate the 90 and 95% confidence limits for the ratio of replacement mutations in the CDR (R_{CDR}) to the number of total mutations in the V region (M_V) as described by Dahlke et al. (2006). These confidence intervals are shown as dark (90%) and light gray (95%) shaded area in **Figure 5B**. A data point falling outside these confidence limits represents a sequence that has a high proportion of replacement mutations in the CDR. Therefore, an allocation above the upper or below the lower confidence limit is considered indicative of Ag-driven selection. It should be mentioned that refined methods for calculation of antigen selection have been published and are available to the public (Hershberg et al., 2008; Uduman et al., 2011). However, at the present IgAT is not suitable to include this type of analyses, because sequence alignments in large sequence collections would require a different software environment.

AA

This worksheet shows the amino acid distribution and frequency of the CDR-3 loop for sequences with the same CDR-3 length as

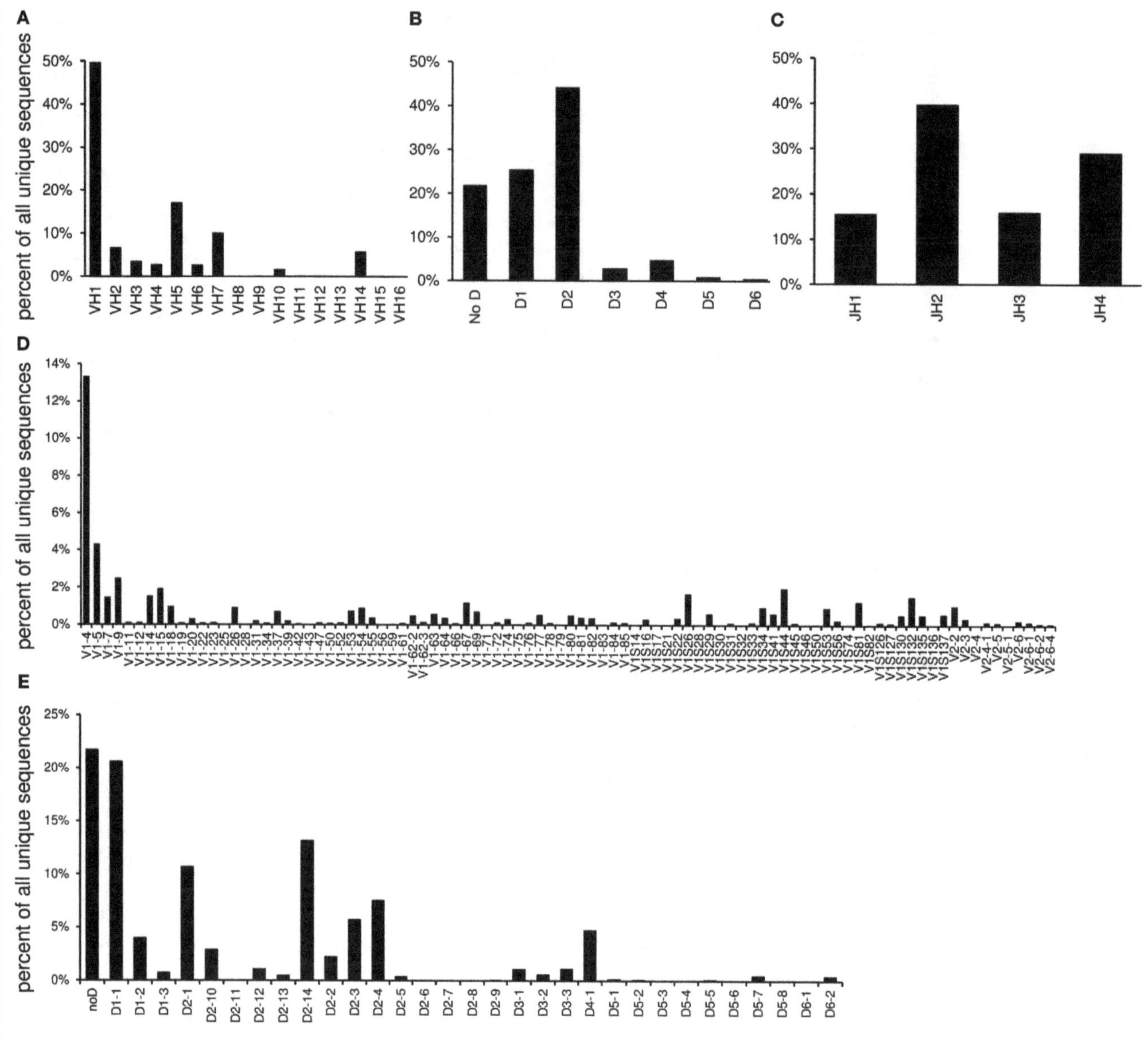

FIGURE 3 | The "VDJ" worksheet contains graphs displaying the relative utilization of V_H families (A), D_H families (B), and J_H gene segments (C) as well as individual V gene segments (D) and D_H gene segments (E).

entered in cell "G3" and different resulting amino acid variability plot (Shannon entropy, a measure of amino acid variability at a given position of aligned protein sequences, and Kabat–Wu plot, the number of different amino acids observed at a position divided by the frequency of the most common amino acid; Shannon, 1997; Johnson and Wu, 2000; Zemlin et al., 2003; **Figure 6**).

AA_FREQUENCY

This diagram shows the amino acid frequencies of the CDR-3 loop for all sequences (**Figure 7**). The frequency is given as percent of all amino acids encoded by CDR-3 from all unique sequences studied. As a default for the IgH chain, the CDR-H3 loop is defined as the amino acids 107–114, according to the IMGT unique numbering system, but the definition of the loop can be modified by the user by entering the limits into the worksheet "AA," cells N5 and N6.

KYTE–DOOLITTLE

The normalized Kyte–Doolittle scale assigns one value to each amino acid. Negative numbers represent polar/hydrophilic amino acids and positive values represent hydrophobic amino acids (Kyte and Doolittle, 1982; Eisenberg, 1984). **Figure 8** displays the distribution of average CDR-3 hydrophobicities according to the normalized Kyte–Doolittle scale.

IGHD

This worksheet displays the D_H gene reading frame usage (**Figure 9**). For each D_H segment there is one reading frame

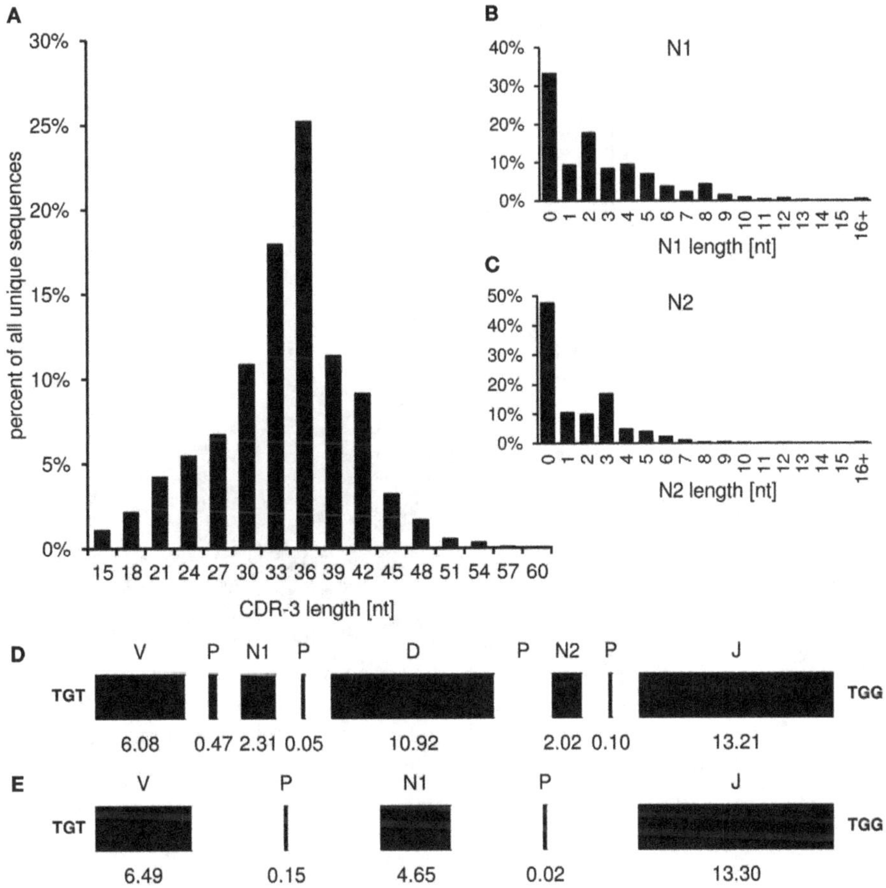

FIGURE 4 | The graphs in the "CDR-3_length" (positions 105–117) worksheet display the length distribution of CDR-H3 (A), N1 (B), N2 (C), and deconstruction graphs for CDR-H3 with (D) or without (E) identifiable D_H gene segment. Lengths are given in nucleotides.

encoding predominantly hydrophilic residues (especially tyrosine and serine; RF1), followed by a hydrophobic reading frame (RF2), and lastly a third reading frame that often encodes a stop codon (RF3). Thus, the third reading frame can be used only if either somatic mutations or else nucleotide losses during VDJ recombination delete the germline stop codon.

SHIRAI

In this worksheet the predicted structural features of the CDR-H3 are displayed (**Figure 10**). The "H3-rules" by Shirai (Shirai et al., 1999; Kuroda et al., 2008) are used to predict the structure of the CDR-H3 loop and base classified upon amino acid sequence, localization, and characteristics like hydrophobicity and size of the amino acid side chain. The structure of the base can be either extended, kinked, or extra kinked. In case of the latter two, the H3-rules may predict whether an intact hydrogen bond ladder or a deformed hairpin is formed within the loop.

TAQ-ERROR

This worksheet calculates the Taq-error rate. To exclude a relevant biasing of the somatic mutation frequency by Taq polymerase errors, IgAT calculates the Taq-error rate within the stretches of the Ig constant region when it is included in the PCR amplificates.

DISCUSSION

Since the discovery of the Ig genes, as well as the fundamental mechanisms describing their combinatorial somatic rearrangement, numerous studies have been published with the goal of understanding the selective forces which might govern B cell and T cell development and the diversification of their lymphocyte receptor repertoires. Whereas B and T cells share a common mode of initial diversification (VDJ recombination), it is only B cells which include additional postrecombination diversification mechanisms such as V_H replacement and somatic hypermutation. Furthermore, whereas the selective forces shaping the receptor repertoire of developing T cells have been well established (Morris and Allen, 2012), the same cannot be said for the antibody receptor repertoire of B cells. For instance, mechanisms of positive selection are not clearly defined for B cell antibody repertoires; however, on the contrary, there are clear examples of negative selective mechanisms (deletion, anergy, and follicular exclusion) as well as additional mechanisms (average amino acid hydrophobicity of CDR-H3, preferential V gene utilization, V_H gene replacement) which act to constrain the diversity of the antibody repertoire.

Early pioneering efforts involved laborious cloning and classic Sanger DNA/cDNA sequencing which yielded sequence collections of modest size on the order of tens to a few hundreds.

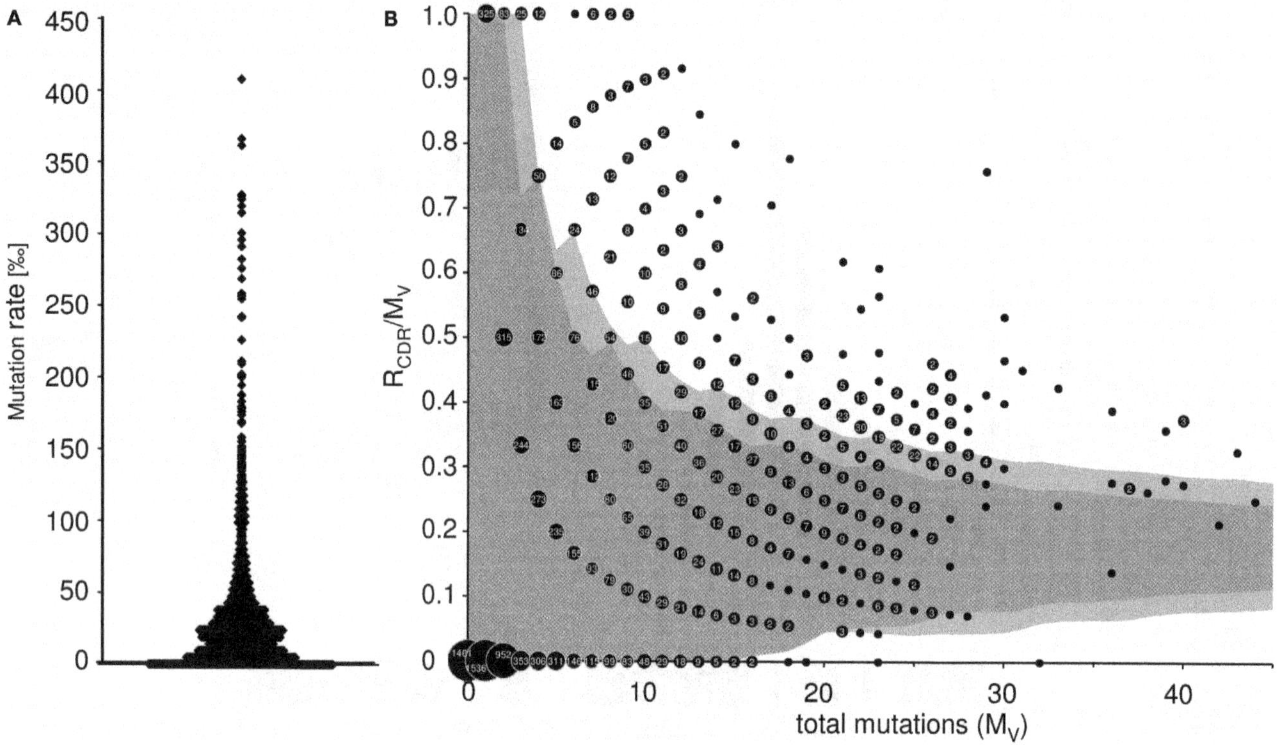

FIGURE 5 | (A) Somatic mutation frequency of Ig transcripts (mutations per 1000 nt). Each data point represents the somatic mutation frequency of one sequence. **(B)** Inference of Ag selection in Ig transcripts. Shown is the ratio of replacement mutations in CDR-H1 and CDR-H2 (R_{CDR}) to the total number of mutations in the V region (M_V) plotted against M_V. The dark shaded area represents the 90% confidence limits and the light gray shaded area the 95% confidence limits for the probability of random mutations. A data point falling outside these confidence limits represents a sequence that has a high proportion of replacement mutations in the CDR. The probability that such a sequence has accumulated as many replacement mutations in the CDR by mere random mutation is $p = 0.1$ and $p = 0.05$, respectively. An allocation above the upper confidence limit was considered indicative of Ag selection. Data points are accompanied by their observed frequency. 6.5% ($\alpha = 0.05$) of the sequences were Ag selected ($\alpha = 0.1$: 9.6%).

Novel antibody repertoire studies employ high-throughput deep sequencing technologies which can yield collections of unprecedented sizes on the order of thousands to millions of raw sequence reads (reviewed in Benichou et al., 2011). To facilitate such studies, the web-based IMGT/HighV-QUEST™program is capable of analyzing large collections of transcripts (up to 150,000 per analysis) by comparison with the known V, D_H, and J germline gene segments. Here we present IgAT, a novel easy-to-use Microsoft Excel based Visual Basic code for the summary, interrogation, and further processing of IMGT/HighV-QUEST output files. IgAT presents the data as organized spreadsheets, yields ready-to-publish statistics and figures, and allows the standardized comparison of multiple sequence batches.

Conventional and Roche 454 deep sequencing of Ig heavy chain transcripts has been used to better understand the maturation of B cells, their selection into various maturational subsets (Wu et al., 2010), to determine the degree to which the repertoire might be genetically predetermined (Glanville et al., 2009; Ippolito et al., 2012), to characterize protective antibody responses (e.g., tetanus-toxoid neutralizing antibodies (Frolich et al., 2010) or HIV neutralizing antibodies (Wu et al., 2011), autoimmunity (Dorner and Lipsky, 2005; Vrolix et al., 2010; Zuckerman et al., 2010; Kalinina et al., 2011), allergies (Kerzel et al., 2010), and especially a push to monitor minimal residual disease in B cell neoplasias (Boyd et al., 2009; Logan et al., 2011). In such studies, IgAT could help indicate to what extent the repertoire has been influenced by antigen-driven selection. The detailed analyses provided by IgAT can be used to speculate about the nature of the antigen epitope(s) that evoked a biasing of the repertoire during an antibody response.

In this report we have used as an example a previously published collection of >18,000 Ig heavy chain (IgH) sequences from mice immunized with the human complement serine protease C1S (Reddy et al., 2010). Although we have focused exclusively upon an analysis of heavy chain sequences in this example, IgAT is also capable of analyzing human and murine Ig kappa and lambda light chain (IgL) repertoires.

CLONOTYPIC DIVERSITY AS A MEASURE OF RESTRICTION OF THE EXPRESSED REPERTOIRE VERSUS A RANDOM REPERTOIRE

In theory, a diversity of more than 1×10^{15} antibodies can be established from the human and murine Ig germline loci, respectively (Schroeder, 2006). However, several antigen-independent and antigen-dependent mechanisms restrict the expressed antibody repertoires to probably less than 1% of the theoretically available diversity. Current theory holds that during B cell development in

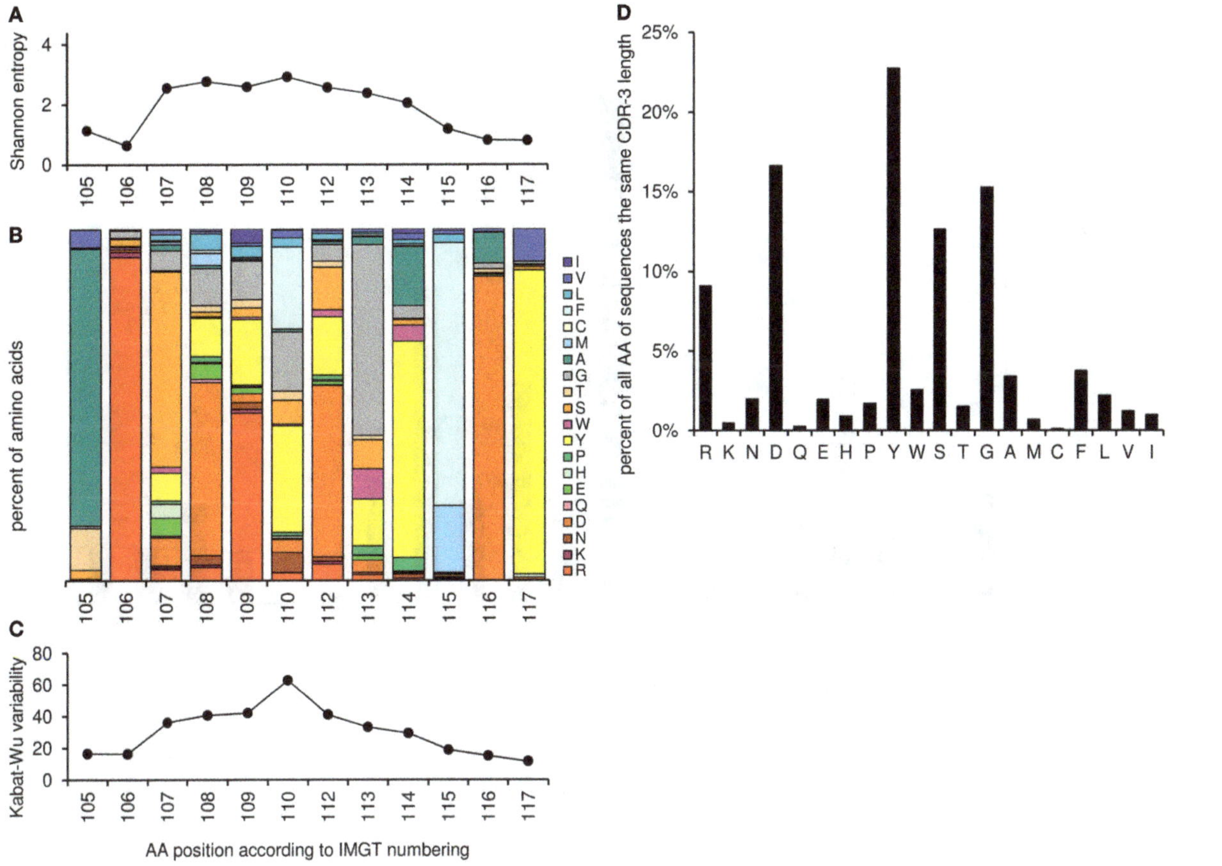

FIGURE 6 | Graphic output of the analysis of amino acid frequencies and variability, using as an example the CDR-H3 sequences with the length of 12 amino acids (positions 105–117, $n = 2572$). (A) The Shannon entropy for each position in the CDR-H3 region (the higher the score the more variable the position in terms of amino acids). **(B)** Relative amino acid frequencies at the positions 105–117 for CDR-H3 region. Each bar represents 100% of the amino acid residues found at this specific position. The amino acid residues are stacked in the order of their hydrophobicity according to a normalized Kyte–Doolittle Index (Eisenberg, 1984). Charged amino acid residues are at the bottom, and hydrophobic amino acid residues at the top of each bar as presented previously (Zemlin et al., 2003). **(C)** The Kabat–Wu variability for each position in the CDR-3 region (the higher the score the more variable the position). **(D)** Overall amino acid frequencies within the CDR-3 loop (positions 107–114).

the bone marrow, restrictions are required to avoid the production of harmful or unnecessary antibodies while focusing on potentially protective antibodies. Current data obtained from the deep sequencing of human and mouse IgH repertoires suggests that primary antibody repertoires, while highly diverse, are nonetheless constrained by genetic mechanisms imposed during antigen-independent B cell development (Arnaout et al., 2011; Glanville et al., 2011; Ippolito et al., 2012). A second shift imposed upon the antibody repertoire occurs during the response to antigen. As an indirect measure of divergence from a totally random repertoire, IgAT calculates the clonotypic diversity (clonotypes per functional sequences) and also the sequence diversity (unique sequences per functional sequences). In the example given here, the clonotypic diversity of the IgH chain repertoire after immunization against C1S amounts to 36.6%. In previous studies, we found clonotypic diversities ranging from 27% in extremely immature IgG repertoires from preterm neonates or 30% in IgE transcripts from allergic children up to 81% in peripheral blood IgM repertoires (Zemlin et al., 2007; Kerzel et al., 2010). Although the clonotypic diversity and sequence diversity are essential descriptors of a given sequence collection, the absolute values should only be compared between sequence collections that were obtained with the same method, because (a) increasing rounds of PCR increase the risk of overamplification of a non-representative set of sequences and (b) degenerate V primers may not recognize all V genes with equivalent affinity, leading to a possible underestimation of the true repertoire diversity. Thus, a low clonal diversity might reflect a focusing of the repertoire during oligoclonal or even monoclonal B cell proliferations, but could also be caused by a low number of PCR targets or by suboptimal PCR conditions. Ademokun et al. (2011) have suggested that the reduced clonal diversity observed in peripheral blood IgM, IgG, and IgA repertoires in the elderly might reflect a weaker response to vaccines when compared to young individuals (Ademokun et al., 2011). Moreover, changes of the clonal diversity of the antibody response can be studied longitudinally to characterize the maturation of the antibody repertoire during ontogeny (Zemlin et al., 2007; Kerzel et al., 2010).

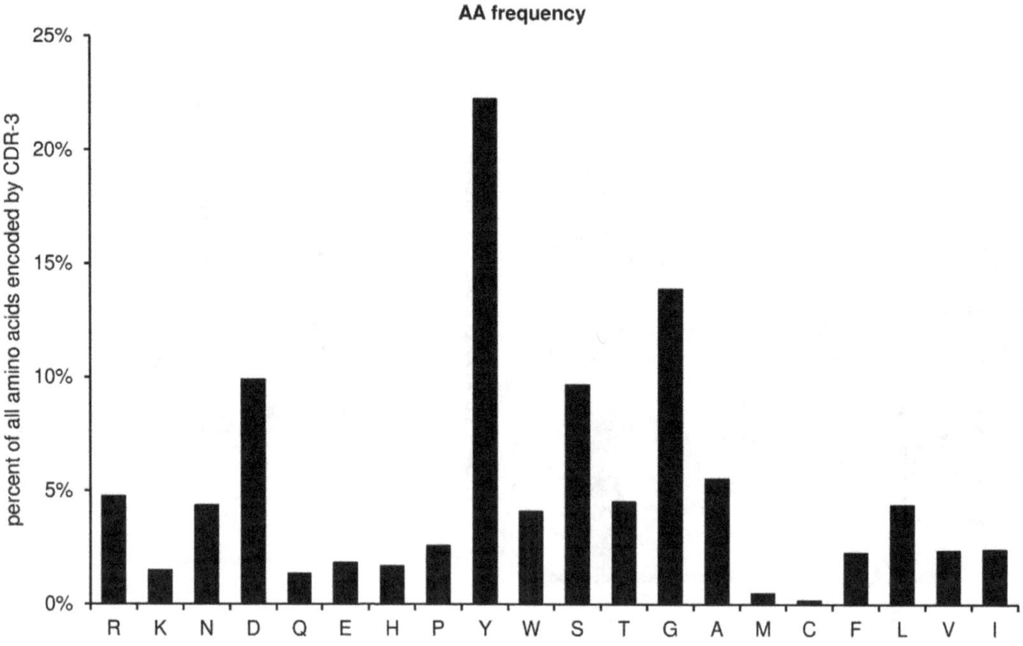

FIGURE 7 | Amino acid frequencies of the CDR-H3 loop for all unique sequences (positions 107–114).

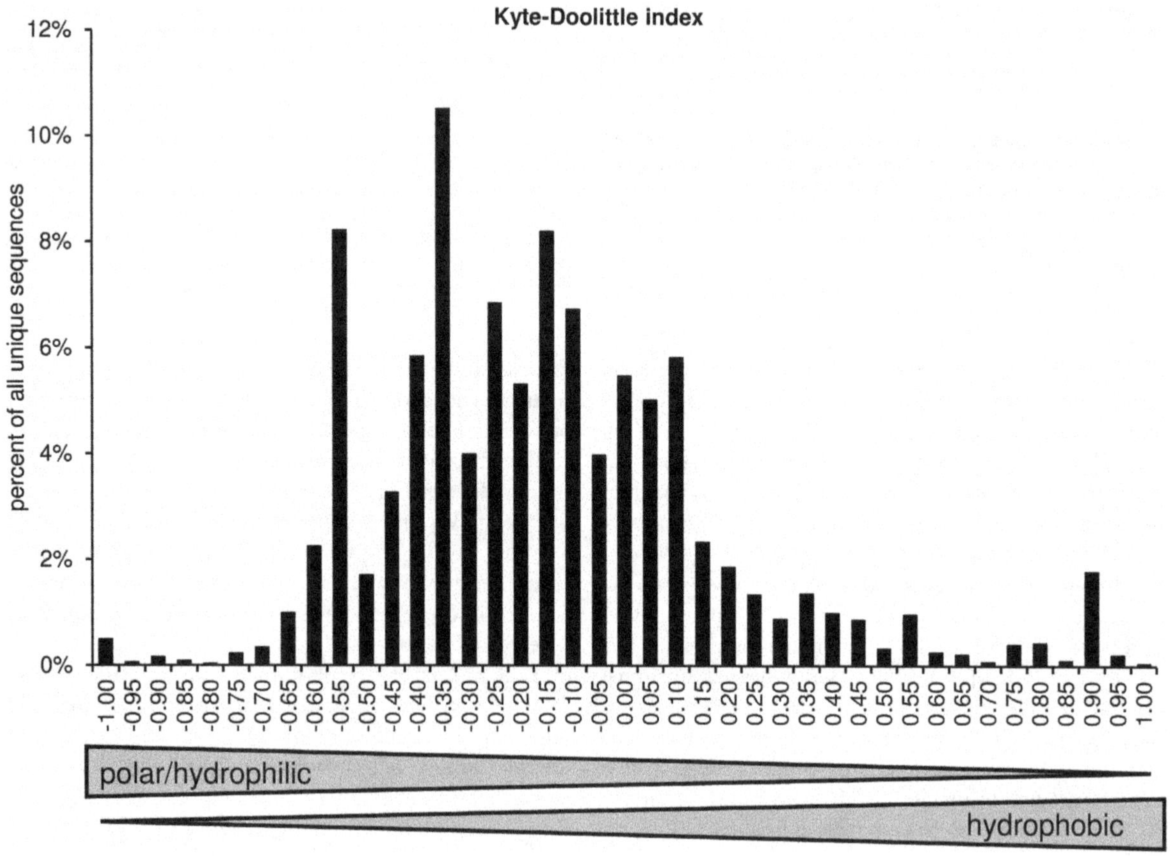

FIGURE 8 | Distribution of average CDR-H3 loop hydrophobicities according to a normalized Kyte–Doolittle scale (positions 107–114; Eisenberg, 1984).

IgAT HELPS IDENTIFYING BIASES IN V, D_H, AND J GENE UTILIZATION THAT CAN INDICATE SUPERANTIGEN-DRIVEN SELECTION OR FREQUENT V_H GENE REPLACEMENT

IgAT summarizes the frequency of V and D_H gene families and individual V, D_H, and J genes. The V_H and V_L gene segments encode for four of the six complementarity determining regions and can thus have great influence on the recognition of classical antigens or superantigens. One reason for contradictory results regarding V gene utilization is the observation that southern blot probes or oligonucleotide primers may not have equal affinity to all V_H gene segments, in particular when somatic mutations affect the primer binding site. To overcome this limitation, Vale et al. (2012) have suggested a novel technique for a less biased analysis of V_H gene usage. A true predominance of one V gene family or V gene segment can arise from the positive selection of the repertoire for a particular classical antigen or by a superantigen (Zouali, 1995) and has also been described in Ig transcripts of B cell neoplasias (Sasso et al., 1989; Coker et al., 2005; Steininger et al., 2012). The use of individual V_H genes can depend on the position of the V_H gene segments in the germline as well as on epigenetic influences and the multidimensional genomic architecture of the locus (Feeney, 2011). The Ig transcripts studied here as an example were highly polarized toward utilization of the VH1-4 gene segment. Previous analyses demonstrated that this bias reflected the preferred expansion of plasma cells that produced antibodies directed against the antigen used for immunization, C1S (Reddy et al., 2010). Studying V gene expression can also indicate "gaps" in the V gene repertoire that can be a putative cause for increased susceptibility to particular infections such as *Haemophilus influenzae* type B (Feeney et al., 1996). Interestingly, V gene utilization of the Ig heavy and light chains can shift during V gene replacement because only an upstream V gene can replace a downstream V gene (Radic and Zouali, 1996; Zhang et al., 2003). To give a visual impression of a potential 5′ shift of V gene usage, IgAT displays V gene segment usage according to each segment's unique position in the germline.

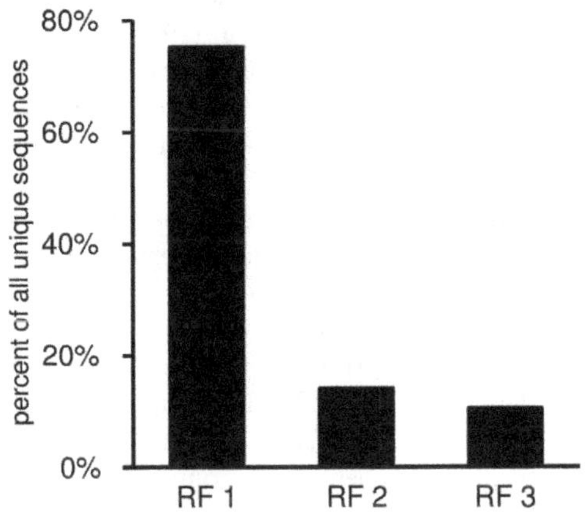

FIGURE 9 | Reading frame utilization given as percent of all unique sequences with identifiable D_H gene segment. The D_H reading frames are defined according to the nomenclature of Ichihara et al. (1989).

BIASES IN AMINO ACID FREQUENCIES AND AVERAGE HYDROPHOBICITY OF CDR-H3 CALCULATED BY IgAT REVEAL RESTRICTIONS WITH POTENTIAL RELEVANCE FOR ANTIGEN RECOGNITION

In the example presented here, IgAT calculated a slightly hydrophilic average hydrophobicity according to a normalized Kyte–Doolittle Hydrophobicity scale for the CDR-H3 region, which is representative for a typical murine primary antibody

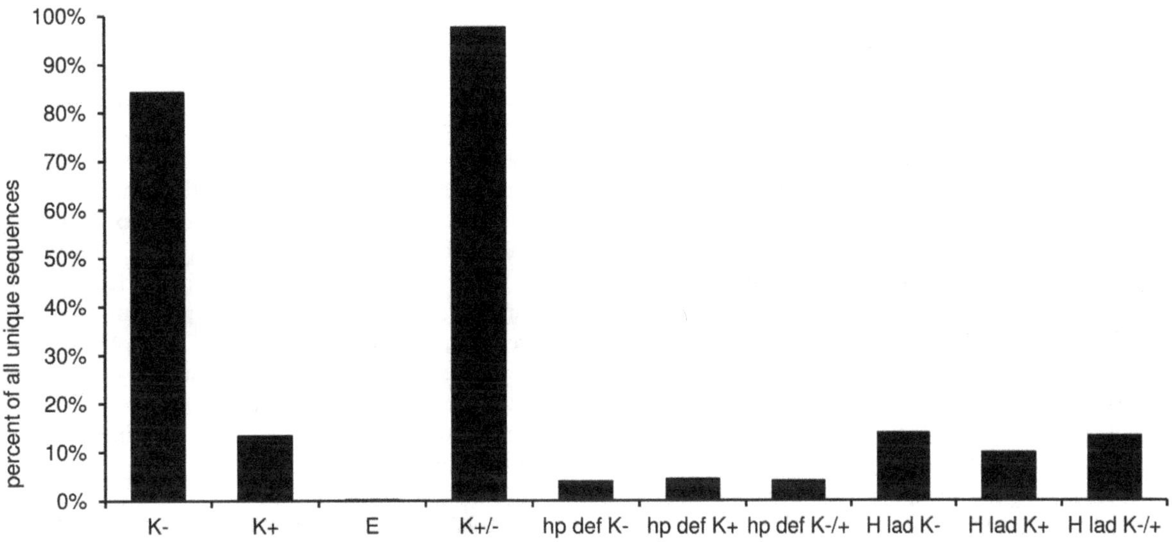

FIGURE 10 | Predicted structural features of the CDR-3 according to the "H3-rules" by Shirai et al. (1999). (K–, kinked base; K+, extra kinked base; K–/+, kinked or extra kinked base; E, extended base; hp def K–, deformed hairpin in sequences with kinked base; hp def K+, deformed hairpin in sequences with extra kinked base; hp def K–/+, deformed hairpin in sequences with kinked and extra kinked base; H lad K–, intact hydrogen bond ladder in sequences with kinked base; H lad K+, intact hydrogen bond ladder in sequences with extra kinked base; H lad K–/+, intact hydrogen bond ladder in sequences with kinked and extra kinked base).

repertoire (Zemlin et al., 2003). The hydrophobicity profile of the CDR-H3 region in mice has been shown to be crucial for conservation of global features of a normal antibody repertoire, for generation of normal B cell differentiation, and for the maintenance of normal adaptive immunity to model antigens and pathogens (Ippolito et al., 2006). For example, the position of positively charged amino acids correlates with the specificity against (negatively charged) double strand-DNA in pathogenic autoantibodies (Krishnan et al., 1996) and triplets of hydrophobic amino acids within the CDR-H3 have been implicated with disturbed B cell repertoire formation during a porcine viral infection (Butler et al., 2008). CDR-H3 hydrophobicity is mainly regulated by D_H gene reading frame utilization (reviewed in: Schroeder et al., 2010). The D_H gene segments frequently encode for the core of the CDR-H3, which prototypically lies at the center of the classical antigen-binding site and which therefore can make direct contact with antigen and principally determines Ig specificity (Kabat and Wu, 1991; Padlan, 1994; Xu and Davis, 2000; Collis et al., 2003). Unlike the V and J genes of IgH and IgL loci, the D_H genes are unique in their potential to be used in three forward and three reverse reading frames. The D_H reading frames are characterized by differing hydrophobicity signatures: the first forward reading frame predominantly encodes for hydrophilic amino acids, such as tyrosine, glycine, and serine, and is the most frequent across evolution among jawed vertebrate species, while the hydrophobic second and the often non-functional third reading frame are significantly under-represented (Gu et al., 1991).

Shifts in reading frame usage can be identified by IgAT and may indicate a selective bias regarding the hydrophobicity profile of the antigen-binding site. Moreover, the overall amino acid frequencies of CDR-H3 regions and the frequency of each amino acid per position in CDR-H3 sequences of identical length are presented in bar diagrams by IgAT to characterize a given collection of Ig transcripts and to compare collections that were generated under differing selective pressure.

IgAT ANALYZES THE LENGTH OF CDR-H3 AND ITS COMPONENTS AND CALCULATES PREDICTIONS FOR STRUCTURAL PROPERTIES OF CDR-H3

The CDR-H3 loop can assume an almost unlimited diversity of differing three dimensional shapes which are grouped into canonical structures (Morea et al., 1998). In general, a CDR-H3 region of more than 14 amino acids protrudes into the solvent, while shorter CDR-H3 regions form an antigen-binding groove together with the other CDRs (Ramsland et al., 2001). The three dimensional structure of the antigen-binding site is of great significance for antigen recognition. For example, antibodies directed against virus antigens contain longer CDR-H3 regions on average than antibodies directed against haptens (Collis et al., 2003). Crystallization of antibodies has allowed identifying rules for the prediction of several important structural properties of the H3 loop and of the H3-hairpin based on the deduced amino acid sequence (Shirai et al., 1996, 1999; Kuroda et al., 2008). IgAT applies Shirai's "H3-rules" to predict a kinked, extra kinked or extended shape for the H3 base. The category of the H3 base is mainly determined by the 5′ nt of CDR-H3 which are often encoded by the J_H gene. Moreover, for a subset of sequences, the Shirai rules allow the prediction whether the H3 loop can establish an intact hydrogen bond ladder or a deformed hairpin. In previous studies, we found that intact hydrogen bond ladders were significantly more frequent in IgG heavy chains from preterm neonates than from adults (Zemlin et al., 2007). In both mouse and man, one reason for reduced CDR-H3 length during fetal development is a reduction in the average number of non-templated N-nucleotide additions (Schroeder et al., 1987). Thus, the structural diversity of the H3 loop is heavily restricted during early ontogeny, potentially contributing to the low affinity and poly-reactivity that characterizes the cord blood antibody repertoire.

Besides elucidating the ontogeny of antibody repertoires, the deconstruction of CDR-H3 components provided by IgAT can also give insights into the selective mechanisms during antigen responses. For example, Dorner et al. (1998a) have found that CDR-H3s are generally shorter in non-functional than in functional Ig transcripts and Rosner et al. (2001) observed that mutated Ig transcripts contain shorter CDR-H3s than non-mutated Ig transcripts.

Moreover, IgH receptor editing by the mechanism of V_H replacement result in increased CDR-H3 length due to retention of a portion of the 3′ end of the original V_H segment (Zhang et al., 2003). IgAT identifies these "V_H footprints" which tend to accumulate within the V_H-D_H junction during V_H replacement and which typically encode for highly charged amino acids (R, E, and D) at the 5′ end of CDR-H3 (Zhang et al., 2003). V_H replacement seems to occur more frequently in autoimmunity (Dorner et al., 1998b).

THE NATURE AND DISTRIBUTION OF SOMATIC MUTATIONS INDICATES ANTIGEN-DRIVEN SELECTION

An enrichment of replacement mutations within the CDRs compared to the FRs is indicative of antigen selection (Berek et al., 1985; Chang and Casali, 1994; Rajewsky, 1996; Lossos et al., 2000). IgAT uses the algorithms created by Chang and Casali (1994), and by Lossos et al. (2000), to identify sequences reflective of antigen-driven selection. In the example given here, 6.5% of the sequences were antigen-selected. This relatively low percentage is plausible since in this experiment, the bone marrow plasma cells were harvested 1 week after immunization, thus before it could be expected that the cells would have undergone excessive class switch recombination and affinity-driven maturation. In previous studies we found that the percentage of antigen-selected transcripts in humans ranged from 9% (IgM) to 29% (IgE) in peripheral blood (Kerzel et al., 2010) and in mice from 0.6% (IgM) to 15% (IgE) in splenic B cells (Rogosch et al., 2010). With this analysis, IgAT quantitatively visualizes the extent to which antigen-mediated selection has impinged upon the B cell repertoire during the course of an immune response.

IN CONJUNCTION WITH IMGT/HIGHV-QUEST, IgAT SIGNIFICANTLY ACCELERATES THE CHARACTERIZATION OF LARGE COLLECTIONS OF Ig TRANSCRIPTS

Fifteen years ago, a researcher needed ~1 h to assign V_H-, D_H-, and J_H-gene segments, N- and P-nucleotides, and somatic mutations to one single Ig heavy chain gene transcript (personal observation). Today, using the freely available IMGT/HighV-QUEST software and the immunoglobulin gene analysis tool, IgAT, which we present here, it is possible to perform much more detailed analyses on $>10^5$ sequences within hours and $>10^6$ sequences within one day. This comprises only a few minutes of work for the researcher while the remaining time is spent by automated data transfer and analyses. The sequence set used in this report consists of ~18,000 functional sequences. Results from IMGT/HighV-QUEST were received after ~2 h. The calculation time of IgAT depends on the hardware and software configuration of the computer. For example, the analysis takes merely 20 min on an Intel® Pentium® 4 (3 GHz) and 4 GB memory machine running Windows XP (32-bit) and Excel 2010 (32-bit) and 15 min on a AMD® Athlon® 4850e (2.5 GHz) and 4 GB memory machine running Windows 7 (64-bit) and Excel 2010 (32-bit).

In conclusion, IgAT can be used to summarize and further analyze large sequence collections that have been pre-analyzed with IMGT/HighV-QUEST. IgAT delivers publication-ready figures and descriptive statistics that can be used to compare multiple sequence collections. Thus, IgAT can be used to characterize selective forces that act upon Ig repertoires during B cell maturation, protective immune responses, and dysregulated immune responses, such as autoimmunity, allergies, and B cell neoplasias.

ACKNOWLEDGMENTS

We thank Jason M. Link for helpful discussions. This work was funded by the German Research Foundation, SFB/TR22, TPA17 (to Michael Zemlin).

REFERENCES

Ademokun, A., Wu, Y. C., Martin, V., Mitra, R., Sack, U., Baxendale, H., Kipling, D., and Dunn-Walters, D. K. (2011). Vaccination-induced changes in human B-cell repertoire and pneumococcal IgM and IgA antibody at different ages. *Aging Cell* 10, 922–930.

Alamyar, E., Giudicelli, V., Li, S., Duroux, P., and Lefranc, M. P. (2012). IMGT/HighV-QUEST: the IMGT® web portal for immunoglobulin (IG) or antibody and T cell receptor (TR) analysis from NGS high throughput and deep sequencing. *Immunome Res.* 8, 26.

Arnaout, R., Lee, W., Cahill, P., Honan, T., Sparrow, T., Weiand, M., Nusbaum, C., Rajewsky, K., and Koralov, S. B. (2011). High-resolution description of antibody heavy-chain repertoires in humans. *PLoS ONE* 6, e22365. doi:10.1371/journal.pone.0022365

Benichou, G., Yamada, Y., Yun, S. H., Lin, C., Fray, M., and Tocco, G. (2011). Immune recognition and rejection of allogeneic skin grafts. *Immunotherapy* 3, 757–770.

Berek, C., Griffiths, G. M., and Milstein, C. (1985). Molecular events during maturation of the immune response to oxazolone. *Nature* 316, 412–418.

Boyd, S. D., Marshall, E. L., Merker, J. D., Maniar, J. M., Zhang, L. N., Sahaf, B., Jones, C. D., Simen, B. B., Hanczaruk, B., Nguyen, K. D., Nadeau, K. C., Egholm, M., Miklos, D. B., Zehnder, J. L., and Fire, A. Z. (2009). Measurement and clinical monitoring of human lymphocyte clonality by massively parallel VDJ pyrosequencing. *Sci. Transl. Med.* 1, 12ra23.

Brezinschek, H. P., Foster, S. J., Brezinschek, R. I., Dorner, T., Domiati-Saad, R., and Lipsky, P. E. (1997). Analysis of the human VH gene repertoire. Differential effects of selection and somatic hypermutation on human peripheral CD5(+)/IgM+ and CD5(-)/IgM+ B cells. *J. Clin. Invest.* 99, 2488–2501.

Brochet, X., Lefranc, M. P., and Giudicelli, V. (2008). IMGT/V-QUEST: the highly customized and integrated system for IG and TR standardized V-J and V-D-J sequence analysis. *Nucleic Acids Res.* 36, W503–W508.

Butler, J. E., Wertz, N., Weber, P., and Lager, K. M. (2008). Porcine reproductive and respiratory syndrome virus subverts repertoire development by proliferation of germline-encoded B cells of all isotypes bearing hydrophobic heavy chain CDR3. *J. Immunol.* 180, 2347–2356.

Chang, B., and Casali, P. (1994). The CDR1 sequences of a major proportion of human germline Ig VH genes are inherently susceptible to amino acid replacement. *Immunol. Today* 15, 367–373.

Coker, H. A., Harries, H. E., Banfield, G. K., Carr, V. A., Durham, S. R., Chevretton, E., Hobby, P., Sutton, B. J., and Gould, H. J. (2005). Biased use of VH5 IgE-positive B cells in the nasal mucosa in allergic rhinitis. *J. Allergy Clin. Immunol.* 116, 445–452.

Collis, A. V., Brouwer, A. P., and Martin, A. C. (2003). Analysis of the antigen combining site: correlations between length and sequence composition of the hypervariable loops and the nature of the antigen. *J. Mol. Biol.* 325, 337–354.

Cuisinier, A. M., Gauthier, L., Boubli, L., Fougereau, M., and Tonnelle, C. (1993). Mechanisms that generate human immunoglobulin diversity operate from the 8th week of gestation in fetal liver. *Eur. J. Immunol.* 23, 110–118.

Dahlke, I., Nott, D. J., Ruhno, J., Sewell, W. A., and Collins, A. M. (2006). Antigen selection in the IgE response of allergic and nonallergic individuals. *J. Allergy Clin. Immunol.* 117, 1477–1483.

Dorner, T., Brezinschek, H. P., Foster, S. J., Brezinschek, R. I., Farner, N. L., and Lipsky, P. E. (1998a). Delineation of selective influences shaping the mutated expressed human Ig heavy chain repertoire. *J. Immunol.* 160, 2831–2841.

Dorner, T., Foster, S. J., Farner, N. L., and Lipsky, P. E. (1998b). Immunoglobulin kappa chain receptor editing in systemic lupus erythematosus. *J. Clin. Invest.* 102, 688–694.

Dorner, T., and Lipsky, P. E. (2005). Molecular basis of immunoglobulin variable region gene usage in systemic autoimmunity. *Clin. Exp. Med.* 4, 159–169.

Eisenberg, D. (1984). Three-dimensional structure of membrane and surface proteins. *Annu. Rev. Biochem.* 53, 595–623.

Feeney, A. J. (2011). Epigenetic regulation of antigen receptor gene rearrangement. *Curr. Opin. Immunol.* 23, 171–177.

Feeney, A. J., Atkinson, M. J., Cowan, M. J., Escuro, G., and Lugo, G. (1996). A defective Vkappa A2 allele in Navajos which may play a role in increased susceptibility to *Haemophilus influenzae* type b disease. *J. Clin. Invest.* 97, 2277–2282.

Frolich, D., Giesecke, C., Mei, H. E., Reiter, K., Daridon, C., Lipsky, P. E., and Dorner, T. (2010). Secondary immunization generates clonally related antigen-specific plasma cells and memory B cells. *J. Immunol.* 185, 3103–3110.

Giudicelli, V., Brochet, X., and Lefranc, M. P. (2011). IMGT/V-QUEST: IMGT standardized analysis of the immunoglobulin (IG) and T cell receptor (TR) nucleotide sequences. *Cold Spring Harb. Protoc.* 2011, 695–715.

Glanville, J., Kuo, T. C., Von Budingen, H. C., Guey, L., Berka, J., Sundar, P. D., Huerta, G., Mehta, G. R., Oksenberg, J. R., Hauser, S. L., Cox, D. R., Rajpal, A., and Pons, J. (2011). Naive antibody gene-segment frequencies are heritable and unaltered by chronic lymphocyte ablation. *Proc. Natl. Acad. Sci. U.S.A.* 108, 20066–20071.

Glanville, J., Zhai, W., Berka, J., Telman, D., Huerta, G., Mehta, G. R., Ni, I., Mei, L., Sundar, P. D., Day, G. M., Cox, D., Rajpal, A., and Pons, J. (2009). Precise determination of the diversity of a combinatorial antibody library gives insight into the human immunoglobulin repertoire. *Proc. Natl. Acad. Sci. U.S.A.* 106, 20216–20221.

Gu, H., Kitamura, D., and Rajewsky, K. (1991). B cell development regulated by gene rearrangement: arrest of maturation by membrane-bound D mu protein and selection of DH element reading frames. *Cell* 65, 47–54.

Hershberg, U., Uduman, M., Shlomchik, M. J., and Kleinstein, S. H. (2008). Improved methods for detecting selection by mutation analysis of Ig V region sequences. *Int. Immunol.* 20, 683–694.

Ichihara, Y., Hayashida, H., Miyazawa, S., and Kurosawa, Y. (1989). Only DFL16, DSP2, and DQ52 gene families exist in mouse immunoglobulin heavy chain diversity gene loci, of which DFL16 and DSP2 originate from the same primordial DH gene. *Eur. J. Immunol.* 19, 1849–1854.

Ippolito, G. C., Hon Hoi, K., Reddy, S. T., Carroll, S. M., Ge, X., Rogosch, T., Zemlin, M., Shultz, L. D., Ellington, A. D., Vandenberg, C. L., and Georgiou, G. (2012). Antibody repertoires in humanized NOD-scid-IL2Rg-null mice and human B cells reveals human-like diversification and tolerance checkpoints in the mouse. *PLoS ONE.* 7, e35497. doi: 10.1371/journal.pone.0035497

Ippolito, G. C., Schelonka, R. L., Zemlin, M., Ivanov, Ii, Kobayashi, R., Zemlin, C., Gartland, G. L., Nitschke, L., Pelkonen, J., Fujihashi, K., Rajewsky, K., and Schroeder, H. W. Jr. (2006). Forced usage of positively charged amino acids in immunoglobulin CDR-H3 impairs B cell development and antibody production. *J. Exp. Med.* 203, 1567–1578.

Jiang, N., Weinstein, J. A., Penland, L., White, R. A. III, Fisher, D. S., and Quake, S. R. (2011). Determinism and stochasticity during maturation of the zebrafish antibody repertoire. *Proc. Natl. Acad. Sci. U.S.A.* 108, 5348–5353.

Johnson, G., and Wu, T. T. (2000). Kabat database and its applications: 30 years after the first variability plot. *Nucleic Acids Res.* 28, 214–218.

Kabat, E. A., and Wu, T. T. (1991). Identical V region amino acid sequences and segments of sequences in antibodies of different specificities. Relative contributions of VH and VL genes, minigenes, and complementarity-determining regions to binding of antibody-combining sites. *J. Immunol.* 147, 1709–1719.

Kalinina, O., Doyle-Cooper, C. M., Miksanek, J., Meng, W., Prak, E. L., and Weigert, M. G. (2011). Alternative mechanisms of receptor editing in autoreactive B cells. *Proc. Natl. Acad. Sci. U.S.A.* 108, 7125–7130.

Kerzel, S., Rogosch, T., Struecker, B., Maier, R. F., and Zemlin, M. (2010). IgE transcripts in the circulation of allergic children reflect a classical antigen-driven B cell response and not a superantigen-like activation. *J. Immunol.* 185, 2253–2260.

Kolar, G. R., Yokota, T., Rossi, M. I., Nath, S. K., and Capra, J. D. (2004). Human fetal, cord blood, and adult lymphocyte progenitors have similar potential for generating B cells with a diverse immunoglobulin repertoire. *Blood* 104, 2981–2987.

Krishnan, M. R., Jou, N. T., and Marion, T. N. (1996). Correlation between the amino acid position of arginine in VH-CDR3 and specificity for native DNA among autoimmune antibodies. *J. Immunol.* 157, 2430–2439.

Kuroda, D., Shirai, H., Kobori, M., and Nakamura, H. (2008). Structural classification of CDR-H3 revisited: a lesson in antibody modeling. *Proteins* 73, 608–620.

Kurosaki, T., Shinohara, H., and Baba, Y. (2010). B cell signaling and fate decision. *Annu. Rev. Immunol.* 28, 21–55.

Kyte, J., and Doolittle, R. F. (1982). A simple method for displaying the hydropathic character of a protein. *J. Mol. Biol.* 157, 105–132.

Lefranc, M. P., Giudicelli, V., Ginestoux, C., Jabado-Michaloud, J., Folch, G., Bellahcene, F., Wu, Y., Gemrot, E., Brochet, X., Lane, J., Regnier, L., Ehrenmann, F., Lefranc, G., and Duroux, P. (2009). IMGT, the international ImMunoGeneTics information system. *Nucleic Acids Res.* 37, D1006–D1012.

Logan, A. C., Gao, H., Wang, C., Sahaf, B., Jones, C. D., Marshall, E. L., Buno, I., Armstrong, R., Fire, A. Z., Weinberg, K. I., Mindrinos, M., Zehnder, J. L., Boyd, S. D., Xiao, W., Davis, R. W., and Miklos, D. B. (2011). High-throughput VDJ sequencing for quantification of minimal residual disease in chronic lymphocytic leukemia and immune reconstitution assessment. *Proc. Natl. Acad. Sci. U.S.A.* 108, 21194–21199.

Lossos, I. S., Tibshirani, R., Narasimhan, B., and Levy, R. (2000). The inference of antigen selection on Ig genes. *J. Immunol.* 165, 5122–5126.

Morea, V., Tramontano, A., Rustici, M., Chothia, C., and Lesk, A. M. (1998). Conformations of the third hypervariable region in the VH domain of immunoglobulins. *J. Mol. Biol.* 275, 269–294.

Morris, G. P., and Allen, P. M. (2012). How the TCR balances sensitivity and specificity for the recognition of self and pathogens. *Nat. Immunol.* 13, 121–128.

Padlan, E. A. (1994). Anatomy of the antibody molecule. *Mol. Immunol.* 31, 169–217.

Prabakaran, P., Chen, W., Singarayan, M. G., Stewart, C. C., Streaker, E., Feng, Y., and Dimitrov, D. S. (2012). Expressed antibody repertoires in human cord blood cells: 454 sequencing and IMGT/HighV-QUEST analysis of germline gene usage, junctional diversity, and somatic mutations. *Immunogenetics* 64, 337–350.

Radic, M. Z., and Zouali, M. (1996). Receptor editing, immune diversification, and self-tolerance. *Immunity* 5, 505–511.

Rajewsky, K. (1996). Clonal selection and learning in the antibody system. *Nature* 381, 751–758.

Ramsland, P. A., Kaushik, A., Marchalonis, J. J., and Edmundson, A. B. (2001). Incorporation of long CDR3s into V domains: implications for the structural evolution of the antibody-combining site. *Exp. Clin. Immunogenet.* 18, 176–198.

Reddy, S. T., Ge, X., Miklos, A. E., Hughes, R. A., Kang, S. H., Hoi, K. H., Chrysostomou, C., Hunicke-Smith, S. P., Iverson, B. L., Tucker, P. W., Ellington, A. D., and Georgiou, G. (2010). Monoclonal antibodies isolated without screening by analyzing the variable-gene repertoire of plasma cells. *Nat. Biotechnol.* 28, 965–969.

Richl, P., Stern, U., Lipsky, P. E., and Girschick, H. J. (2008). The lambda gene immunoglobulin repertoire of human neonatal B cells. *Mol. Immunol.* 45, 320–327.

Rogosch, T., Kerzel, S., Sikula, L., Gentil, K., Liebetruth, M., Schlingmann, K. P., Maier, R. F., and Zemlin, M. (2010). Plasma cells and nonplasma B cells express differing IgE repertoires in allergic sensitization. *J. Immunol.* 184, 4947–4954.

Rosner, K., Winter, D. B., Tarone, R. E., Skovgaard, G. L., Bohr, V. A., and Gearhart, P. J. (2001). Third complementarity-determining region of mutated VH immunoglobulin genes contains shorter V, D, J, P, and N components than non-mutated genes. *Immunology* 103, 179–187.

Sasso, E. H., Silverman, G. J., and Mannik, M. (1989). Human IgM molecules that bind staphylococcal protein A contain VHIII H chains. *J. Immunol.* 142, 2778–2783.

Schelonka, R. L., Tanner, J., Zhuang, Y., Gartland, G. L., Zemlin, M., and Schroeder, H. W. Jr. (2007). Categorical selection of the antibody repertoire in splenic B cells. *Eur. J. Immunol.* 37, 1010–1021.

Schroeder, H. W. Jr. (2006). Similarity and divergence in the development and expression of the mouse and human antibody repertoires. *Dev. Comp. Immunol.* 30, 119–135.

Schroeder, H. W. Jr., and Cavacini, L. (2010). Structure and function of immunoglobulins. *J. Allergy Clin. Immunol.* 125, S41–S52.

Schroeder, H. W. Jr., Hillson, J. L., and Perlmutter, R. M. (1987). Early restriction of the human antibody repertoire. *Science* 238, 791–793.

Schroeder, H. W. Jr., Zemlin, M., Khass, M., Nguyen, H. H., and Schelonka, R. L. (2010). Genetic control of DH reading frame and its effect on B-cell development and antigen-specific antibody production. *Crit. Rev. Immunol.* 30, 327–344.

Schroeder, H. W. Jr., Zhang, L., and Philips, J. B. III. (2001). Slow, programmed maturation of the immunoglobulin HCDR3 repertoire during the third trimester of fetal life. *Blood* 98, 2745–2751.

Shannon, C. E. (1997). The mathematical theory of communication, 1963. *MD Comput.* 14, 306–317.

Shirai, H., Kidera, A., and Nakamura, H. (1996). Structural classification of CDR-H3 in antibodies. *FEBS Lett.* 399, 1–8.

Shirai, H., Kidera, A., and Nakamura, H. (1999). H3-rules: identification of CDR-H3 structures in antibodies. *FEBS Lett.* 455, 188–197.

Snow, R. E., Chapman, C. J., Holgate, S. T., and Stevenson, F. K. (1998). Clonally related IgE and IgG4 transcripts in blood lymphocytes of patients with asthma reveal differing patterns of somatic mutation. *Eur. J. Immunol.* 28, 3354–3361.

Souto-Carneiro, M. M., Sims, G. P., Girschik, H., Lee, J., and Lipsky, P. E. (2005). Developmental changes in the human heavy chain CDR3. *J. Immunol.* 175, 7425–7436.

Steininger, C., Widhopf, G. F. II, Ghia, E. M., Morello, C. S., Vanura, K., Sanders, R., Spector, D., Guiney, D., Jager, U., and Kipps, T. J. (2012). Recombinant antibodies encoded by IGHV1-69 react with pUL32, a phosphoprotein of cytomegalovirus and B-cell superantigen. *Blood* 119, 2293–2301.

Takhar, P., Corrigan, C. J., Smurthwaite, L., O'Connor, B. J., Durham, S. R., Lee, T. H., and Gould, H. J. (2007). Class switch recombination to IgE in the bronchial mucosa of atopic and nonatopic patients with asthma. *J. Allergy Clin. Immunol.* 119, 213–218.

Tonegawa, S. (1983). Somatic generation of antibody diversity. *Nature* 302, 575–581.

Uduman, M., Yaari, G., Hershberg, U., Stern, J. A., Shlomchik, M. J., and Kleinstein, S. H. (2011). Detecting selection in immunoglobulin sequences. *Nucleic Acids Res.* 39, W499–W504.

Vale, A. M., Foote, J. B., Granato, A., Zhuang, Y., Pereira, R. M., Lopes, U. G., Bellio, M., Burrows, P. D., Schroeder, H. W. Jr., and Nobrega, A. (2012). A rapid and quantitative method for the evaluation of V gene usage, specificities and the clonal size of B cell repertoires. *J. Immunol. Methods* 376, 143–149.

Vrolix, K., Fraussen, J., Molenaar, P. C., Losen, M., Somers, V., Stinissen, P., De Baets, M. H., and Martinez-Martinez, P. (2010). The auto-antigen repertoire in myasthenia gravis. *Autoimmunity* 43, 380–400.

Wu, X., Zhou, T., Zhu, J., Zhang, B., Georgiev, I., Wang, C., Chen, X., Longo, N. S., Louder, M., Mckee, K., O'Dell, S., Perfetto, S., Schmidt, S. D., Shi, W., Wu, L., Yang, Y., Yang, Z. Y., Yang, Z., Zhang, Z., Bonsignori, M., Crump, J. A., Kapiga, S. H., Sam, N. E., Haynes, B. F., Simek, M., Burton, D. R., Koff, W. C., Doria-Rose, N. A., Connors, M., Mullikin, J. C., Nabel, G. J., Roederer, M., Shapiro, L., Kwong, P. D., and Mascola, J. R. (2011). Focused evolution of HIV-1 neutralizing antibodies revealed by structures and deep sequencing. *Science* 333, 1593–1602.

Wu, Y. C., Kipling, D., Leong, H. S., Martin, V., Ademokun, A. A., and Dunn-Walters, D. K. (2010). High-throughput immunoglobulin repertoire analysis distinguishes between human IgM memory and switched memory B-cell populations. *Blood* 116, 1070–1078.

Xu, J. L., and Davis, M. M. (2000). Diversity in the CDR3 region of V(H) is sufficient for most antibody specificities. *Immunity* 13, 37–45.

Zemlin, M., Bauer, K., Hummel, M., Pfeiffer, S., Devers, S., Zemlin, C., Stein, H., and Versmold, H. T. (2001). The diversity of rearranged immunoglobulin heavy chain variable region genes in peripheral blood B cells of preterm infants is restricted by short third complementarity-determining regions but not by limited gene segment usage. *Blood* 97, 1511–1513.

Zemlin, M., Hoersch, G., Zemlin, C., Pohl-Schickinger, A., Hummel, M., Berek, C., Maier, R. F., and Bauer, K. (2007). The postnatal maturation of the immunoglobulin heavy chain IgG repertoire in human preterm neonates is slower than in term neonates. *J. Immunol.* 178, 1180–1188.

Zemlin, M., Klinger, M., Link, J., Zemlin, C., Bauer, K., Engler, J. A., Schroeder, H. W. Jr., and Kirkham, P. M. (2003). Expressed murine and human CDR-H3 intervals of equal length exhibit distinct repertoires that differ in their amino acid composition and predicted range of structures. *J. Mol. Biol.* 334, 733–749.

Zhang, Z., Zemlin, M., Wang, Y. H., Munfus, D., Huye, L. E., Findley, H. W., Bridges, S. L., Roth, D. B., Burrows, P. D., and Cooper, M. D. (2003). Contribution of VH gene replacement to the primary B cell repertoire. *Immunity* 19, 21–31.

Zouali, M. (1995). B-cell superantigens: implications for selection of the human antibody repertoire. *Immunol. Today* 16, 399–405.

Zuckerman, N. S., Hazanov, H., Barak, M., Edelman, H., Hess, S., Shcolnik, H., Dunn-Walters, D., and Mehr, R. (2010). Somatic hypermutation and antigen-driven selection of B cells are altered in autoimmune diseases. *J. Autoimmun.* 35, 325–335.

Permissions

All chapters in this book were first published in TEDAR, by Frontiers; hereby published with permission under the Creative Commons Attribution License or equivalent. Every chapter published in this book has been scrutinized by our experts. Their significance has been extensively debated. The topics covered herein carry significant findings which will fuel the growth of the discipline. They may even be implemented as practical applications or may be referred to as a beginning point for another development.

The contributors of this book come from diverse backgrounds, making this book a truly international effort. This book will bring forth new frontiers with its revolutionizing research information and detailed analysis of the nascent developments around the world.

We would like to thank all the contributing authors for lending their expertise to make the book truly unique. They have played a crucial role in the development of this book. Without their invaluable contributions this book wouldn't have been possible. They have made vital efforts to compile up to date information on the varied aspects of this subject to make this book a valuable addition to the collection of many professionals and students.

This book was conceptualized with the vision of imparting up-to-date information and advanced data in this field. To ensure the same, a matchless editorial board was set up. Every individual on the board went through rigorous rounds of assessment to prove their worth. After which they invested a large part of their time researching and compiling the most relevant data for our readers.

The editorial board has been involved in producing this book since its inception. They have spent rigorous hours researching and exploring the diverse topics which have resulted in the successful publishing of this book. They have passed on their knowledge of decades through this book. To expedite this challenging task, the publisher supported the team at every step. A small team of assistant editors was also appointed to further simplify the editing procedure and attain best results for the readers.

Apart from the editorial board, the designing team has also invested a significant amount of their time in understanding the subject and creating the most relevant covers. They scrutinized every image to scout for the most suitable representation of the subject and create an appropriate cover for the book.

The publishing team has been an ardent support to the editorial, designing and production team. Their endless efforts to recruit the best for this project, has resulted in the accomplishment of this book. They are a veteran in the field of academics and their pool of knowledge is as vast as their experience in printing. Their expertise and guidance has proved useful at every step. Their uncompromising quality standards have made this book an exceptional effort. Their encouragement from time to time has been an inspiration for everyone.

The publisher and the editorial board hope that this book will prove to be a valuable piece of knowledge for researchers, students, practitioners and scholars across the globe.

List of Contributors

Gennady Bocharov
Institute of Numerical Mathematics, Russian Academy of Sciences, Moscow, Russia

Tatyana Luzyanina
Institute of Mathematical Problems in Biology, Russian Academy of Sciences, Pushchino, Russia

Jovana Cupovic and Burkhard Ludewig
Institute of Immunobiology, Kantonal Hospital St. Gallen, St. Gallen, Switzerland

Sara E. Brownell
Department of Neurology and Neurological Sciences, Stanford University, Stanford, CA, USA
Department of Biology, Stanford University, Stanford, CA, USA

Rachel A. Becker and Lawrence Steinman
Department of Neurology and Neurological Sciences, Stanford University, Stanford, CA, USA

Taylor A. Kessinger and Richard A. Neher
Evolutionary Dynamics and Biophysics, Max Planck Institute for Developmental Biology, Tübingen, Germany

Alan S. Perelson
Theoretical Biology and Biophysics, Los Alamos National Laboratory, Los Alamos, NM, USA

Gabriele Multhoff
Department of Radiation Oncology, Klinikum rechts der Isar, Technische Universität München, Munich, Germany
Clinical Cooperation Group Innate Immunity in Tumor Biology, Helmholtz Zentrum München, Munich, Germany

Michael Molls
Department of Radiation Oncology, Klinikum rechts der Isar, Technische Universität München, Munich, Germany

Jürgen Radons
multimmune GmbH, Munich, Germany

Katherine J. L. Jackson, Marie J. Kidd, Yan Wang and Andrew M. Collins
School of Biotechnology and Biomolecular Sciences, University of New South Wales, Sydney, NSW, Australia

John E. Butler and Nancy Wertz
Department of Microbiology, Carver College of Medicine, University of Iowa, Iowa City, IA, USA

Gilad Liberman
Gonda Multidisciplinary Brain Research Center, Bar-Ilan University, Ramat Gan, Israel

Jennifer Benichou and Lea Tsaban
Department of Mathematics, Bar-Ilan University, Ramat Gan, Israel

Jacob Glanville
Protein Engineering and Applied Quantitative Genotherapeutics, Rinat-Pfizer Inc., South San Francisco, CA, USA

Yoram Louzoun
Gonda Multidisciplinary Brain Research Center, Bar-Ilan University, Ramat Gan, Israel
Department of Mathematics, Bar-Ilan University, Ramat Gan, Israel

Simon Fillatreau
Deutsches Rheuma-Forschungszentrum, Leibniz Institute, Berlin, Germany

Adrien Six
UPMC Univ Paris 06, UMR 7211, "Immunology, Immunopathology, Immunotherapy", F-75013 Paris, France
UMR 7211, "Immunology, Immunopathology, Immunotherapy," CNRS, Paris, France

Susanna Magadan, Rosario Castro and Pierre Boudinot
Virologie et Immunologie Moléculaires, Institut National de la Recherche Agronomique, Jouy-en-Josas, France

J. Oriol Sunyer
Department of Pathobiology, School of Veterinary Medicine, University of Pennsylvania, Philadelphia, PA, USA

Inbal Sela-Culang, Vered Kunik and Yanay Ofran
The Goodman Faculty of Life Sciences, Bar Ilan University, Ramat Gan, Israel

Jaya Vas and Caroline Grönwall
Laboratory of B Cell Immunobiology, Department of Medicine, New York University School of Medicine, New York, NY, USA

Gregg J. Silverman
Laboratory of B Cell Immunobiology, Department of Medicine, New York University School of Medicine, New York, NY, USA

Andrew M. Collins and Katherine J. L. Jackson
School of Biotechnology and Biomolecular Sciences, University of New South Wales, Sydney, NSW, Australia

Bryan S. Briney
Department of Pathology, Microbiology and Immunology, Vanderbilt University Medical Center, Nashville, TN, USA

James E. Crowe Jr.
Department of Pathology, Microbiology and Immunology, Vanderbilt University Medical Center, Nashville, TN, USA
Department of Pediatrics, Vanderbilt University Medical Center, Nashville, TN, USA
The Vanderbilt Vaccine Center, Vanderbilt University Medical Center, Nashville, TN, USA

Verônica Coelho
Laboratório de Imunologia, Instituto do Coração, Universidade de São Paulo, São Paulo, Brazil
Instituto de Investigação em Imunologia, Instituto Nacional de Ciência e Tecnologia, São Paulo, Brazil

Ana M. C. Faria
Instituto de Investigação em Imunologia, Instituto Nacional de Ciência e Tecnologia, São Paulo, Brazil
Departamento de Bioquímica e Imunologia, Instituto de Ciências Biológicas, Universidade Federal de Minas Gerais, Belo Horizonte, Brasil

Yu-Chang Bryan Wu and Deborah K. Dunn-Walters
Department of Immunobiology, King's College London School of Medicine, London, UK

David Kipling
Institute of Cancer and Genetics, School of Medicine, Cardiff University, Cardiff, UK

Daisuke Morito and Kazuhiro Nagata
Faculty of Life Sciences, Kyoto Sangyo University, Kyoto, Japan

William J. J. Finlay
Global Biotherapeutics Technologies, Pfizer, Dublin, Ireland

Juan C. Almagro
Centers for Therapeutic Innovation, Pfizer, Boston, MA, USA

Véronique Thomas-Vaslin and Adrien Six
UPMC Univ Paris 06, UMR7211, Immunology, Immunopathology, Immunotherapy (I3), Integrative Immunology, Paris, France
CNRS, UMR 7211, Immunology-Immunopathology-Immunotherapy (I3) Integrative Immunology, Paris, France

Jean-Gabriel Ganascia
UPMC Univ Paris 06, UMR 7606, ACASA-LIP6, Paris, France
CNRS, UMR 7606, ACASA-LIP6, CNRS, Paris, France

Hugues Bersini
Université Libre de Bruxelles, IRIDIA-Code, Bruxelles, Belgium

Adrian M. Shields, Gabriel S. Panayi and Valerie M. Corrigall
Department of Academic Rheumatology, Centre for Molecular and Cellular Biology of Inflammation, King's College London, London, UK

Miri Michaeli, Hila Noga and Ramit Mehr
The Mina and Everard Goodman Faculty of Life Sciences, Bar-Ilan University, Ramat Gan, Israel

Hilla Tabibian-Keissar
The Mina and Everard Goodman Faculty of Life Sciences, Bar-Ilan University, Ramat Gan, Israel
Department of Pathology, Sheba Medical Center and Sackler School of Medicine, Tel Aviv University, Tel Aviv, Israel

Iris Barshack
Department of Pathology, Sheba Medical Center and Sackler School of Medicine, Tel Aviv University, Tel Aviv, Israel

Joost A. Aalberse and Berent J. Prakken
Department of Pediatric Immunology, Center for Molecular and Cellular Intervention, Wilhelmina Children's Hospital, University Medical Center, Utrecht, Netherlands

Berber Kapitein
Pediatric Intensive Care Unit, Sophia Children's Hospital, Rotterdam, Netherlands

Tobias Rogosch, Sebastian Kerzel, Rolf F. Maier and Michael Zemlin
Department of Pediatrics, Philipps-University Marburg, Marburg, Germany

Kam Hon Hoi
Department of Biomedical Engineering, University of Texas at Austin, Austin, TX, USA

Zhixin Zhang
Department of Pathology and Microbiology, Eppley Institute for Research in Cancer, University of Nebraska Medical Center, Omaha, NE, USA

Gregory C. Ippolito
Section of Molecular Genetics and Microbiology, University of Texas at Austin, Austin, TX, USA

Index

P

R

S

T

V

www.ingramcontent.com/pod-product-compliance
Lightning Source LLC
LaVergne TN
LVHW060543210926
848485LV00005B/1246
9781639893751